A HISTORY OF TRANSGENDER MEDICINE IN THE UNITED STATES

From Margins to Mainstream

Edited by

Carolyn Wolf-Gould, Dallas Denny, Jamison Green, and Kyan Lynch

SUNY PRESS

Published by State University of New York Press, Albany

© 2025 State University of New York

All rights reserved

Printed in the United States of America

No part of this book may be used or reproduced in any manner whatsoever without written permission. No part of this book may be stored in a retrieval system or transmitted in any form or by any means including electronic, electrostatic, magnetic tape, mechanical, photocopying, recording, or otherwise without the prior permission in writing of the publisher.

Links to third-party websites are provided as a convenience and for informational purposes only. They do not constitute an endorsement or an approval of any of the products, services, or opinions of the organization, companies, or individuals. SUNY Press bears no responsibility for the accuracy, legality, or content of a URL, the external website, or for that of subsequent websites.

For information, contact State University of New York Press, Albany, NY
www.sunypress.edu

Library of Congress Cataloging-in-Publication Data

Names: Wolf-Gould, Carolyn, 1961– editor. | Denny, Dallas, 1949– editor. | Green, Jamison, 1948– editor. | Lynch, Kyan, 1989– editor.
Title: A history of transgender medicine in the United States : from margins to mainstream / edited by Carolyn Wolf-Gould, Dallas Denny, Jamison Green, and Kyan Lynch.
Description: Albany : State University of New York Press, [2025] | Includes bibliographical references and index.
Identifiers: LCCN 2024034012 | ISBN 9798855801224 (hardcover : alk. paper) | ISBN 9798855801231 (ebook) | ISBN 9798855801217 (pbk : alk. paper)
Subjects: LCSH: Gender-affirming care—United States—History. | Transgender people—United States—History. | Transgender people—United States—Social conditions.
Classification: LCC HQ77.95.U6 F76 2024 | DDC 306.76/80973—dc23/eng/20240816
LC record available at https://lccn.loc.gov/2024034012

For the trans pioneers who courageously spoke their truth, the healthcare pioneers who listened when others would not, and the partnerships they forged to expand the bounds of both gender and medicine.

CONTENTS

Acknowledgments   x

Introduction: Writing Trans History   1
    *Carolyn Wolf-Gould, Dallas Denny, Jamison Green,
    and Kyan Lynch*

Section I. The International Roots of Transgender Medicine

1. Precolonial Gender Identities and the International Roots of Transitional Practices   16
    Serena Nanda

2. The Rise of Sexology in Europe   41
    Clayton J. Whisnant

    2.1 PROFILE: The Chevalière d'Eon (1728–1810)   62
        Clayton J. Whisnant

3. Pioneering Scientists: Hirschfeld, Benjamin, and Kinsey   65
    Annette F. Timm and Jamison Green

    3.1 PROFILE: Lili Elbe (1882–1931)   91
        Carolyn Wolf-Gould

    3.2 PROFILE: Otto Spengler (1873–unknown)   93
        Christopher Wolf-Gould

    3.3 Establishing North American Cultural Norms: Early Transgender Colonists and Americans (1600–1930s)   98
        Carolyn Wolf-Gould

4. International Pioneers of Trans-Specific Care   105
   Alexander Boscia and Cecile A. Ferrando

      4.1 PROFILES: Michael Dillon (1915–1962) and
   Roberta Cowell (1918–2011)   123
   Alexander Boscia and Cecile A. Ferrando

      4.2 PROFILES: Coccinelle (1931–2006), April Ashley
   (1935–2021), and Jan Morris (1926–2020)   125
   Alexander Boscia and Cecile A. Ferrando

5. Two Spirit Health in North America   128
   Trudie Jackson

      5.1 PROFILE: Ashliana Hawelu (1969–)   161
   Ashliana Hawelu

Section II. From the Margins

6. The Beginnings of Trans-Affirming Care in the United States   169
   Tj Gundling

      6.1 Construction of the "Good" Transsexual and Those
   Who Did Not Fit the Bill   202
   Carolyn Wolf-Gould

7. Trans Circles of Knowledge and Intimacy   209
   Annette F. Timm and Jamison Green

      7.1 PROFILE: Louise Lawrence (1912–1976): Unsung
   Mother of the Trans Community   241
   Ms. Bob Davis and Jules Gill-Peterson

      7.2 PROFILE: Virginia Prince (1912–2009)   244
   Dallas Denny

      7.3 PROFILE: A Curbside Encounter with Harry Benjamin
   (1985–1986)   249
   Sharon Stuart (a.k.a. Thomas Heitz)

7.4 PROFILE: Louis G. Sullivan (1951–1991): Changing the Paradigm about Sex and Gender *Jamison Green*	251
8. Trans-Focused Psychology and Psychiatry in the United States: 1910–1990 *Dallas Denny, Jamison Green, and Hansel Arroyo*	255
8.1 PROFILE: Joseph Israel Lobdell (1829–1912) *Bambi Lobdell*	286
8.2 PROFILE: David O. Cauldwell (1897–1959) *Carolyn Wolf-Gould*	292
8.3 The Religious Response to Medical Interventions *Carolyn Wolf-Gould*	295
9. The Costs of Medicalization *Kyan Lynch, Carolyn Wolf-Gould, Dallas Denny, and Jennifer Lee*	299

Section III. Encounters with the Mainstream

10. Legitimizing Trans: Reed Erickson (1917–1992) and the Erickson Educational Foundation *Aaron Devor*	331
11. Blinded by the Binary: A Critique of the Mid-Twentieth Century Gender Clinics *Dallas Denny*	361
12. Trans Rights as Civil Rights *Carolyn Wolf-Gould*	397
12.1 PROFILE: Marsha P. Johnson (1945–1992) *Amanda Yijun Wang*	417
12.2 PROFILE: Silvia Rivera (1951–2002): "The Rosa Parks of the Modern Transgender Movement" *Teri Wilhelm and Carolyn Wolf-Gould*	420

    12.3 PROFILE: Dallas Denny (1949–)   425
      Kenneth Hubbell

    12.4 PROFILE: Jamison Green (1948–)   428
      Teri Wilhelm

13. The Evolution of Professional Organizations and Standards of Care: An Inside-Outsider's Perspective   435
    Jamison Green

14. The Biological Underpinnings of Gender Identity   474
    Carolyn Wolf-Gould and Joshua D. Safer

    14.1 PROFILE: Eugen Steinach (1861–1944) and His Clinical Trials   504
      Carolyn Wolf-Gould

    14.2 "Born This Way" Data: Biological Validation or Cultural Oppression?   508
      Carolyn Wolf-Gould

15. Developing Meaningful Transgender Health Research: A Journey toward Social Justice   517
    George R. Brown and Carolyn Wolf-Gould

    15.1 By Us and for Us: Bringing Ethics into Transgender Health Research   544
      Noah Adams, Ruth Pearce, Jaimie F. Veale, Asa Radix, Amrita Sarkar, and Dani Castro

    15.2 Transgender Veterans and the Veterans Health Administration   549
      Jillian Shipherd

Section IV. Establishing the Interdisciplinary Field of Transgender Health within the Medical Mainstream

16. The Evolution of Hormonal Care in the United States   555
    Asa Radix, Zil Goldstein, and Alexander B. Harris

 16.1 PROFILE: Jeanne Hoff (1938–2023)   571
 Noah Adams

 16.2 PROFILE: JoAnne Keatley (1951–)   574
 Teri Wilhelm

 16.3 PROFILE: Admiral Rachel Leland Levine (1957–)   577
 Dallas Denny

17. Changing the Body to Match the Mind: The Development of Gender-Affirming Surgery in the United States   583
Carolyn Wolf-Gould

 17.1 PROFILE: Alan Hart (1890–1962)   620
 Carolyn Wolf-Gould

 17.2 PROFILE: Elmer Belt (1893–1980)   623
 Amy Block

 17.3 PROFILE: Christine McGinn (1969–)   627
 Yongha Kim

18. The Treatment of Transgender and Gender-Diverse Children and Adolescents   630
Diane Ehrensaft

 18.1 The Pediatric Gender Management Service and Gender Surgery Center at Boston Children's Hospital   649
 David A. Diamond

 18.2 Adolescent Medical Care   653
 Tresne Hernandez and Katherine Blumoff Greenberg

19. A History of Gender-Affirming Voice and Communication Interventions   660
Jack Pickering and Terren Lansdaal

 19.1 PROFILE: Musings from a Trans Speech and Language Pathologist   683
 Terren Lansdaal

20. Hair Troubles: A History of Hair Removal and Replacement 685
    Dallas Denny and Yuki Arai

Section V. Our Future

21. The Future of Transgender Medicine 717
    Kyan Lynch

List of Contributors 731

Index 735

ACKNOWLEDGMENTS

While we would like to call attention to a few noteworthy individuals, we recognize that we could not possibly mention everyone who helped along the way. If you believe that you played a part in bringing this work into the world, you are probably right, and we are deeply grateful.

Renate Reeves Ellington, thank you for supporting this project financially. Your support played a vital role in realizing one of our key goals—including voices typically left out of the narrative.

Leah Squires, thank you for your brilliance and compassionate advice. Your editorial instincts and attention to detail helped us carve a book out of our block of marble.

Thank you to each of our forty-three contributing authors. We admire your work, your advocacy, your passion, and your dedication to building an ever more inclusive world. We would like to make particular mention of Dr. Serena Nanda, whose death preceded the book's publication. We are honored that this book will be listed among her final publications.

We are indebted to Matt Roslund, reference librarian extraordinaire, whose expertise was instrumental in creating a thoroughly researched volume.

An earlier version of chapters 3 and 7 was published by Annette Timm in *Others of My Kind: Transatlantic Transgender Histories*, 2020, Calgary Press. The seven lines of the poem Dark Testament by Pauli Murray (chapter 9) was originally published in *Dark Testament and other Poems*, used here by permission of the Liveright Publishing Corporation.

On October 5, 2020, the world lost an icon. Monica Roberts was a transgender activist, historian, and journalist. We are proud to include her among the pioneers featured in this book and deeply saddened that she did not live to see her name on its pages.

Finally, we are unendingly grateful to our spouses, family, friends, and pets, who rode by our side through the ups, downs, monotonous flat stretches, roundabouts, and hairpin turns on our road to publication.

INTRODUCTION
Writing Trans History

Carolyn Wolf-Gould, Dallas Denny, Jamison Green, and Kyan Lynch

The histories of transgender and gender-diverse[1] (TGD) people have been long repressed, often neglected, and rarely curated. From its inception, the field of transgender medical care in the United States rose as a lightning rod in the battlefield of American culture wars, and yet this compelling story of struggle and gain remains largely untold. Although transgender people have been described throughout the world since early recorded times, the history of modern medical interventions dates only to the start of the twentieth century. Researchers, clinicians, and transgender people themselves have spent the last one hundred years developing an understanding of trans experiences and the language used to guide medical treatment. The history of transgender medicine in the United States is tied to the history of medical research and technology, the law, the popular press, academic thought, and various human rights movements. It is peppered with accounts of extraordinary individuals whose voices have shaped social change, often at great personal risk. Despite evidence that TGD people have existed across time, cultures, and socioeconomic/ethnic groups, a constant theme has been the struggle to legitimize even basic and emergency medical care, let alone transition-related care. Patients face stigma and disrespect and have been viewed as mentally ill, and the providers who serve them often considered opportunists or quacks. No story is that simple. In this volume, we present a history of the relationship between transgender people and medical professionals and the contexts in which these interactions took place.

Long before recorded history, TGD people lived on the land currently referred to as the United States. As colonists and immigrants moved across the continent, some of them also TGD, they imposed or submitted to what became the dominant American culture, a specific set of norms shaped by European Judeo-Christian doctrine that included rigid expectations about gender roles and expression. People living in and moving about this vast region encountered various subgroups—Indigenous people, enslaved people, religious groups, populations from different parts of the world—and began to form an array of subcultures influenced by their geographic location, race, education, and the work of staying alive in diverse and distinctive regional environments. Members of these subcultures, in turn, heard stories of or encountered people who transgressed gender and sexual norms. Faced with those who differ from expected norms (including TGD individuals), people asked themselves the following questions:

1. What is this phenomenon?

2. What do we call it?

3. Why are people like this?

4. What is the appropriate response?[2]

These questions have been asked repeatedly over the last century by colonists, religious leaders, politicians, transgender people, researchers, clinicians, and others. In all cases, the answers were shaped by the gender, gender identity, and other intersecting identities of the people asking or answering the questions; the sociopolitical cultural climate; and the era and geographical place in which said queries were entertained. Responses included a range of judgments, from confusion, shock, revulsion, and outrage to acceptance, affirmation, and celebration.

It was within this multifaceted cultural context that, in the early 1900s, stories about the medical care for TGD people began to seep into the American consciousness. Before this, Americans heard, largely through the popular press, only occasional accounts about individuals whose existence challenged the prevalent concept of gender immutability. But after the turn of the twentieth century, European reports about surgical experiments crossed the Atlantic, enabling some Americans to consider descriptive language, theories on the etiology of transgenderism, and the possibility that doctors could surgically (and, later, medically) effect a gender change or a change of sex characteristics to support one's experienced gender. Clinicians within the dominant white, European-derived, cisnormative culture wrote the initial (largely pathologizing) medical literature, but over time TGD people began to influence and then control their own medical narratives—first women like Christine Jorgensen, who told their own stories, but largely conformed to white, feminine cultural expectations, and later people like Lou Sullivan, JoAnne Keatley, Monica Roberts, and Trudie Jackson who challenged dominant social mores to unveil the needs of marginalized TGD subgroups. More recently, over the last thirty-five years or so, TGD people and their allies have begun to drive the cultural change necessary to expand social acceptance, legal recognition, and the delivery of gender-affirming healthcare services.

Compared to the evolution of other medical disciplines, the development of transgender healthcare in the United States advanced rather more like that of a liberation movement. Typically, liberation movements generate powerful interactions between groups within the larger cultural whole; the struggle to develop appropriate care for TGD people is no exception. Throughout this history, the reactions of American cultural subgroups impacted the evolution of transgender healthcare, while information about evolving medical treatments for TGD people evoked impassioned cultural battles across the nation. In most medical fields, the development of knowledge and skills to diagnose and treat specific conditions grows within the confines of that field, expanding through the efforts of its researchers and clinicians. In the field of transgender medicine, the absence of much clinical research and guidance created a vacuum, a void that filled instead with zealous public judgments. The absence and/or denial of affirming healthcare until the late twentieth century serves as an indicator of the cultural disrespect and denial of humanity TGD people have faced in America. While access to care has improved in some regions of the United States, many TGD people continue to suffer from this legacy, finding it difficult or impossible to access competent care.

HOW THIS BOOK CAME ABOUT

Carolyn Wolf-Gould identified the need for this book in 2015, after she was asked to write a short synopsis on the history of transgender medicine in the United States (a topic she knew little about) for the *SAGE LGBTQ Encyclopedia*.[3] While researching this piece, she recognized significant gaps in this medical story. As she sought the historical perspective of transgender people, she discovered a slide presentation about the history of gender-affirming surgery presented by Dallas Denny at the 2015 Transgender Lives Conference in Farmington, Connecticut. Carolyn and Dallas, who knew one another from the annual transgender event Fantasia Fair,[4] discussed their various projects, decided to coedit a book, and then drafted an outline. Carolyn remembered attending a talk by endocrinologist Wylie Hembree in 2013 at the conference Transgender Health and Wellness: Providing Primary Care and Mental Health Services for Transgender People and Their Families, held in Albany, New York, on how transgender health had moved from the margins toward the mainstream during his career. She suggested incorporating this theme in the book title and included it in the mission and vision for her emerging gender practice. In 2018, Carolyn heard Kyan Lynch speak on the history of transgender medicine at the SPECTRUM conference in Albany, New York. She and Dallas asked Kyan to join their team. Later that day, Carolyn and Kyan connected with Rebecca Colesworthy from SUNY Press and formed a collaborative plan to create and publish this volume. Soon afterward, the three editors asked longtime trans activist and author Jamison Green to join them. Like Dallas, Jamison has not only described, but also shaped, the history of transgender medicine in the United States. The four then set out to research, find additional contributors, and edit this volume.

Carolyn is a family physician. She founded the Gender Wellness Center of Oneonta, New York, a rural-based interdisciplinary center that provides medical care, surgical care, mental healthcare, and advocacy for TGD youth and adults, conducts community-based research and trains healthcare students and clinicians. Dallas holds a master's degree in psychology[5] and possesses decades of experience as an activist, organizer, writer, and speaker on a range of trans-issues. Kyan is a physician and educator based at the University of Rochester Medical Center. There, he serves as assistant professor in the Department of Obstetrics and Gynecology. Kyan is the youngest member of the editorial team and considers himself honored and humbled to work alongside such distinguished trans activists. Jamison is a writer, legal scholar, policy consultant, educator, a past president of the World Professional Association for Transgender Health, and an accomplished, internationally acknowledged activist for transgender people; he holds an MFA in creative writing and a PhD in equalities law. Jamison and Kyan identify as trans men; Dallas, as both transgender and as a woman of transsexual experience; and Carolyn, as a cisgender woman. Their pronouns are she/her (Dallas and Carolyn) and he/him (Kyan and Jamison).

As a team, they met weekly for a period of several years, first outlining the history as they envisioned it early in the project, then soliciting authors, writing, and editing. As their knowledge grew, they addressed the need for additional material. Eventually, they began to work the various chapters and sidebars to fit into a narrative arc until it became the book you hold today.

EDITORIAL CONUNDRUMS

While writing and editing, we repeatedly faced questions about how best to describe transgender people and the field of transgender health throughout history. We asked ourselves: Given that these stories must be told, how can we, as an editorial team, write and edit with respect for the struggles of present-day transgender people, as well as for those in the past? Can we tell this story without worsening stigma or triggering pain? How do we address the anger a clumsy phrase or concept, even if it's historically accurate, might provoke in our readers or contributors?

To explore these questions, we held two discussion groups with members of the trans community and their allies: one hosted online by our publisher, SUNY Press in June 2021[6] and one in October 2021 at Fantasia Fair.[7] We sought to solicit guidance from the community on how best to present this history with its dynamic, evolving language and ethical dilemmas. Ultimately, we found some peace when those who attended these groups expressed certainty that our book will offend, no matter what language we employ or how we record stories. They told us to carry on, recognize that it takes courage to plow ahead, and take refuge in the knowledge that our missteps and the outrage that it will doubtless provoke will help inform the next generation of historians and storytellers. They encouraged us: "Just do it!"

The feedback we received from these groups to specific questions informed our approach to editing this volume, as presented below.

WHO SPEAKS FOR TRANS PEOPLE?

To ensure *From Margins to Mainstream* would be more than a reflection of our understandings and competencies, we enlisted authors for the various chapters with a mind toward expertise and diversity. We also wished to center the work of TGD people themselves. We recognize that despite differences in age, gender, and occupation, our editorial team is all white. We lack the lived experience of trans people of color and those with other intersectional identities. We tried and failed to recruit another editor with different perspectives to our team. We worked hard to include diverse voices in this volume but are aware our efforts fell short of our expressed hope to center the unheard voices of those who have been the most marginalized by colonialism, institutionalized racism, stigma, and minority stress and are generally left out of medical historiographies. We are inspired by Monica Roberts, who spent her life addressing the historical gaps in written history by documenting the stories of transgender people of color.

Should cisgender people speak for TGD people? As the sole cisgender member of the editorial team, Carolyn struggled with this question, as did several other cisgender authors of works in this text. Ultimately, our team recognized that the historical gains of this medical movement accrued from the collaborative work of TGD people and their allies. This history reflects this convergence of effort by including the voices and accounts of current and historical professional allies.

WHAT DO WE DO ABOUT THE PATHOLOGIZING OR EVOLVING TERMS USED TO DESCRIBE TGD PEOPLE THROUGHOUT HISTORY?

In this field of transgender medical history, new terms crop up and old terms are discarded as inaccurate, obsolete, or offensive. Some terms add to our increasingly nuanced understanding of gender diversity, while others denigrate trans experiences. We understand and regret that the pathologizing language often employed by early researchers and clinicians contributes to the current, pervasive cultural stigma that impedes efforts by TGD people to thrive and hampers clinicians struggling to establish affirming services. We recognize that members of the TGD community may also participate as enablers, perpetuating harmful language themselves.

We ask our readers to remember that the words to describe diverse gender identities—such as *transvestite, transsexual, transgender, Two Spirit, cisgender, nonbinary*—are all relatively new to this world and possess dynamic connotations, dependent on the speaker and the audience and on the particular time or place in which a word is uttered. Our team struggled to create a glossary of historical and contemporary terms, but these short definitions felt flat and lifeless. Our list failed to capture the subtle overtones the terms possessed in different settings over time. Some of our readers may be new to the field, and we encourage you to search online for definitions of unfamiliar terms. We invite all readers to consider how the development of increasingly nuanced language reflected and transformed medical practices.

Ultimately, we chose to use the antiquated terms people used during specific historical periods, keeping in mind that like us, the thinking of historical figures was shaped and constrained by the language available to them. When referring to studies or individuals from the past, you will find us using terms—for instance, *transsexual, transvestite, gender identity disorder*—that have become or are becoming obsolete. To do otherwise would be to create a revisionist history. We invite the reader to reflect on how language has contributed to the oppression of TGD people and how, as it changed, it began to transform medical practices and reveal increasingly nuanced understandings of trans experiences.

HOW DID WE DECIDE WHAT PRONOUNS TO USE WHEN REFERRING TO TRANS PIONEERS?

We struggled with pronoun use and identity labels when referring to TGD people from the past. Some historical figures clearly stated their preferred pronouns and identities, and in those cases, we honored that preference. Some left no record of the word(s) they used to describe themselves or their identities, or they kept their preferences private. Some spoke languages without gendered pronouns. Sometimes there was just not enough written about them or by them to allow us to make an educated guess.

Is it ethical to out someone after their death? And if yes, how should we refer to that person?[8] After speaking with authors, editing chapters, talking within our discussion groups, and reviewing current best practices, we elected (except where otherwise noted) to employ individuals' expressed pronouns throughout their lifespan when those individuals explicitly stated a preference. When individuals did not specify pronoun choice (for whatever reason), we elected not to assign them pronouns without their consent and employed the ones they publicly used at the time. In some cases, such as when gendered pronouns were not part of a language or cultural tradition, we deferred to our contributors to decide pronoun choice, with a footnote to explain their decision.

SHOULD PEOPLES' DEAD NAMES BE INCLUDED IN WRITTEN HISTORY?

When we met with the group at Fantasia Fair, we asked for advice on including a trans person's dead name in this history.[9] Is the dead name ever important or relevant? Should we avoid the use of dead names completely? We were surprised to learn that many attendees at our workshop at Fantasia Fair felt the use of dead names might sometimes be important; some felt that failure to acknowledge this part of an individual's history was a form of erasure. As one participant expressed, "I want all of me to be seen as important to my story." We followed their advice to let individual chapter authors decide on this usage, understanding that this decision might be offensive to some.

THE FRUITS OF OUR LABOR

The result is this volume, a collection of writings from more than forty authors who present a uniquely trans-focused interpretation of the history of transgender healthcare. Our authors are members of the TGD community themselves and/or committed allies in healthcare. They come from all walks of life; some are well-known clinicians, researchers, and academics; others are lesser-known allies or TGD community members with a commitment to healthcare activism. Our editorial team was purposeful in allowing each contributor's voice to shine through, an approach that results in a reading experience that allows for greater richness in perspective. We extend special gratitude to the TGD authors who shared their personal experiences with healthcare in their contributions.

We offer this book to members of the transgender community and their families, allies, students, scholars, historians, healthcare professionals, and anyone interested in how the field of transgender healthcare emerged in the United States and exists within today's medical mainstream. We especially devote this text to those of you who value and celebrate the richness of the trans experience and appreciate how the TGD community has enriched your worldview.

The book is comprised of five sections. The first, "The International Roots of Transgender Medicine," features chapters about our Indigenous and international ancestry and the cultural practices that continue to impact present-day medical care. Long before TGD medical care arrived in the United States, Indigenous North Americans developed their own understanding about the TGD people who lived in their tribes. We move from precolonial times to eighteenth-century Europe, where individuals contending with nonprocreative sexual activities gave rise to the field of sexology. In the 1920s and 1930s clinicians in Magnus Hirschfeld's Berlin Institute for Sexual Science developed new surgical techniques to change the body to match the mind. Hirschfeld's intimate connection to Harry Benjamin and Benjamin's connection to Alfred Kinsey brought ideas about the mutability of gender to the United States. Pioneering surgeons across the globe learned and refined their techniques as increasing numbers of patients sought care.

In section II, "From the Margins," we explore the emergence of gender-affirming care in the United States. Christine Jorgensen's arrival home to the United States after medically transitioning in Denmark brought the possibility of gender transitions to the American consciousness. Dr. Harry Benjamin offered to care for Jorgensen and for the hundreds of other TGD people who, transfixed by her story, sought similar care for themselves. As options for medical care increased, TGD people formed communities and worked to educate themselves and US clinicians about their lives and their struggles. Psychiatrists weighed into this evolving field, introducing many of the pathologizing tropes, some of which impede access to care to this day. Many TGD people, especially those who didn't conform to the white, middle-class, heterosexual expectations that the publicity around Jorgensen's transition created in the public eye, found it impossible to access the care that they needed.

In section III of this volume, "Encounters with the Mainstream," our authors document efforts to drive the field of transgender health from the margins into mainstream medical practice. This includes efforts by people like Reed Erickson, a wealthy transgender man who sought to legitimize care in the eyes of the public and the medical community. The first official gender clinic opened at Johns Hopkins University in 1966, prompting the rise (and later the closure) of dozens of such centers across the country. Clinicians from the fields of medicine, psychiatry, and surgery began to form interdisciplinary groups and professional guidelines that shaped this emerging field. Researchers grappled with the etiology of gender diversity, exploring psychological and biological underpinnings, and researchers began to describe their interactions with the TGD population.

Section IV, "Establishing the Interdisciplinary Field of Transgender Health Within the Medical Mainstream," describes the establishment of TGD healthcare within American mainstream medical care. This work required (and continues to require) efforts to dispel the legacy of entrenched pathologizing beliefs about TGD people and the care they require. Clinicians, acknowledging the biopsychosocial complexity of medical transitions, continued to build an interdisciplinary model of care, one that required collaboration with colleagues in surgery, medicine, psychiatry, and ancillary fields, such as voice modification and hair removal.

Section V, "The Future," written by the youngest member of our team, contemplates the future of transgender healthcare in the United States from the perspective of December 2022, when we completed this volume. Our book ends at that juncture; yet history continues to unfold before our eyes.

Throughout the book, we feature a series of short biographical profiles devoted to those individuals who purposefully or unknowingly shaped the arc of this evolving medical field. We included these accounts at the conclusion of chapters in which their work is most relevant. We embrace these pioneers, all heroes, and thank them for the ways their lives and/or work ensured that care became more accessible to those who followed. We similarly embrace the pioneers unmentioned in this volume—we know many of you, respect your hard work, and regret the page limits of our publisher. We also extend thanks and encouragement to those new to the field and those yet unborn, knowing full well you are the ones who will continue to shape the historical events of our future. We also include several short pieces at the end of some chapters that complement chapter information or provide additional information about the cultural response to the rise of transgender healthcare.

The field of transgender medicine arose in the United States because TGD people insisted that medical professionals acknowledge their authenticity and address their medically necessary embodiment needs. The field developed as TGD people collaborated with those (cisgender and trans) who devoted their lives and/or work to the understanding and alleviation of what we now call *Gender Dysphoria*—a term that may soon be referred to as *Gender Incongruence* (and eventually something else). This journey has twisted and turned; one step forward often resulted in several steps back before progress could occur again. Today, affirmative models of care replace many of the pathologizing paradigms of the past. Nonetheless, most transgender people across the United States still face enormous barriers while attempting to access affirming healthcare. As we prepared this manuscript for submission in December 2022, news media regularly reported advances in human rights for transgender people, that is, repeal of the military ban on transgender recruits and legislation to protect against workplace discrimination, as well as vicious attacks on basic rights such as healthcare (especially for youth), access to bathrooms, the ability to participate in sports, and the right to live and work without fear or discrimination. Transgender people continue to be murdered for simply being themselves.[10] Medical professionals face harassment and death threats for offering medical care for youth,[11] and some have been forced to close the doors of their gender clinics.[12] In 2024, as we prepare this manuscript for publication, we bear witness to an even more polarized political climate, one that centers rage and fear about TGD healthcare in political debate. Twenty-six states have legislated bans on best practices medical care for transgender youth (treatment that is evidence-based and endorsed by all major medical societies), effectively placing judges and politicians—not clinicians, youth, and their families—in charge of medical care for this vulnerable population.[13] Rage and fear sometimes also divide the trans community and its allies as we work to negotiate a difficult path forward.

We are aware that some readers may find this book overly supportive of the medical establishment, whereas others will find it too critical and particularly hard on the cisgender clinicians of previous times. We recognize that many of the early US clinicians, especially those who ran the gender clinics in the 1960s and 1970s, chose to work in this field with good intentions, big hearts, and a desire to help suffering people. And yet, the truth that many TGD people experienced trauma from their interactions with these clinicians and institutions cannot be ignored. We have tried to be careful of faulting doctors and scientists for using language typical of their time, place, and audience, knowing that past and present medical literature favors objectification and detachment. Language one finds disrespectful today may have been politically correct years ago. We attempt to judge the past with the same deference we hope to receive from those reading this book in the future.

We regret any unintended harm reading this book might cause those who have suffered from the particularly damaging historical trauma that has created the field of transgender health. We hope that readers will discover new knowledge and surprising insights in this remarkable history. We trust that our words will give voice to this painful, yet inspiring, legacy and instill a commitment to better healthcare in the future.

The scope of any book is limited; gaps remain, and we hope at a minimum to provide a foundation on which other TGD people, scholars, activists, medical providers, and researchers can enrich this history.

This work looks not only to the past but also toward the future and the hard work that lies ahead.

We have moved forward but have not yet arrived.

It is from a humble place that we offer our collected narratives.

—The Editors

NOTES

1. The term *transgender and gender-diverse* is presently accepted terminology in trans-affirming medical publications and is used throughout this volume. Given the rapid evolution of language, we understand this term may be outdated by the time of publication. When we use the descriptor *trans* or *transgender*, we generally meant it in a way that includes all TGD people.
2. Given this volume's particular focus on medical transgender history, we specifically interrogate this question from the clinical perspective, that is, "As a clinician, what is the appropriate response?"
3. Goldberg, *SAGE Encyclopedia*; Wolf-Gould, "History of Transgender Medicine," 508–12.
4. Established in 1975 and held annually in Provincetown, Massachusetts, Fantasia Fair (now Trans Week) is the longest-running transgender event in the United States.
5. Dallas' participation in her doctoral program was derailed by prejudice after her transition.
6. Denny et al., "*Who Speaks for Trans People?*" 2021.
7. Wolf-Gould and Denny, "Writing about Transgender History."
8. For example, civil rights icon Pauli Murray struggled privately with gender identity while publicly using the name and pronouns linked to her assigned sex at birth.
9. *Dead name* is a term that some have used to describe the birth names (or original names) of TGD people who have renamed themselves and established legal and/or cultural names with which they identify. The use of prior names is generally considered disrespectful and offensive, dishonoring the person.
10. HRC Foundation, "Fatal Violence."
11. Carlisle, "Pediatricians who Serve Trans Youth."
12. Yeomans, "Doctor That Specializes in Transgender Care."
13. Movement Advancement Project, "New Democracy Maps: Bans on Best Practice Medical Care for Transgender Youth."; GLAAD, "Medical Association Statements in Support of Health Care for Transgender People and Youth."

WORKS CITED

Carlisle, Madeleine. "Pediatricians Who Serve Trans Youth Face Increasing Harassment. Lifesaving Care Could Be on the Line." *Time*, February 16, 2022. Accessed on May 5, 2022. https://time.com/6146269/doctors-trans-youth-gender-affirming-care-harassment/.

Denny, Dallas, Jamison Green, Kyan Lynch, and Carolyn Wolf-Gould. "Writing Trans History: Who Speaks for Trans People?" Annual SPECTRUM Conference, Albany, NY, June 30, 2021.

GLAAD. "Medical Association Statements in Support of Health Care for Transgender People and Youth." June 26, 2024. Accessed August 22, 2024. https://glaad.org/medical-association-statements-supporting-trans-youth-healthcare-and-against-discriminatory/.

Goldberg, Abbie E., ed. *The SAGE Encyclopedia of LGBTQ Studies*. Thousand Oaks, CA: SAGE Publications, 2016.

HRC Foundation. "Fatal Violence against the Transgender and Gender Non-Conforming Community in 2021—Human Rights Campaign." *Human Rights Campaign: Resources*, 2021. Accessed on May 5, 2022. https://www.hrc.org/resources/fatal-violence-against-the-transgender-and-gender-non-conforming-community-in-2021.

Movement Advancement Project. "New Democracy Maps: Bans on Best Practice Medical Care for Transgender Youth." 2024. Accessed August 22, 2024. https://www.lgbtmap.org/equality-maps/healthcare_youth_medical_care_bans

Wolf-Gould, Carolyn. "History of Transgender Medicine in the United States." In *The SAGE Encyclopedia of LGBTQ Studies*, edited by Abbie E. Goldberg, 508–12. Thousand Oaks, CA: SAGE Publications, 2016.

Wolf-Gould, Carolyn, and Dallas Denny. "Some Issues When Writing about Transgender History: A Lively Discussion." Workshop conducted at Fantasia Fair/Transgender Week, Provincetown, MA, October 21, 2021.

Yeomans, Meredith. "Doctor that Specializes in Transgender Care Takes Employer to Court." *NBC 5 Dallas-Fort Worth*, March 16, 2022. Accessed on May 5, 2022. https://www.nbcdfw.com/news/local/doctor-that-specializes-in-transgender-care-takes-employer-to-court/2917139/.

Section I

THE INTERNATIONAL ROOTS OF TRANSGENDER MEDICINE

The stories of transgender and gender-diverse (TGD) people existed long before the United States formed as a nation, and the history of transgender medicine begins in ancient times within numerous world cultures. In section I of this volume, we trace what we now consider gender-affirming care through time and across the globe to discover its indigenous and international roots. Prior to the availability of modern Western medical practices, TGD people responded to their internal longings, explored their identities, formed communities, interfaced with their dominant cultures, and developed practices to soften gender-related discomfort and survive, often in a hostile world. Western medical practices originated in the psycho-medical-social explorations of researchers and theorists in Europe and spread to the United States through the personal connections between clinicians and TGD people.

In chapter 1, anthropologist Serena Nanda explores precolonial TGD communities across the world (many of which still exist today) and the impact of Western colonialism on these subcultures. Influences from these diverse global communities continue to influence contemporary medical practices. In chapter 2, historian Clayton Whisnant uncovers stories about Europeans from the late Renaissance period to the early 1900s who reckoned with the nonprocreative sexual activities that transgressed social norms, giving rise to the field of sexology. He describes the scholars, clinicians, and activists who developed terms and theories on same sex attraction and gender nonconformity and published etiologic hypotheses and moral judgments that inflamed cultural mores. In chapter 3, historians Annette Timm and Jamison Green describe the intimate connections that developed in the early twentieth century between clinician/

sexologists Magnus Hirschfeld (Berlin) and Harry Benjamin (US) and between Harry Benjamin and Alfred Kinsey (US). This chapter is followed by a short piece on the establishment of early American cultural norms about TGD people who lived in North America during colonial times and those who were exposed in the American popular press in the late 1800s and early 1900s.

In chapter 4, clinicians/scholars Alexander Boscia and Cecile Ferrando present accounts of Harold Gilles, Georges Burou, and Christian Hamburger, three physicians who pioneered contemporary medical and surgical practices. In chapter 5, American Indian scholar Trudie Jackson records historical beliefs and practices around sexual and gender diversity within Indigenous North American communities, the impact of colonization on Two Spirit people, and contemporary efforts to decolonize the resulting destructive medical and cultural systems.

Profiles highlighted in section I include the story of the Chevalière d'Eon, a diplomat and a spy for Louis XVI in the late 1700s; Lili Elbe, whose surgical transition in the 1930s—one of the first (after Dorchen Richter) at Magnus Hirschfeld's Institute of Sexual Science in Berlin—exposed an astonished world to new possibilities for gender transformation; Otto Spengler, who served as an early networking link between the trans community and LGBT activists in Berlin and in the US around the turn of the century; Michael Dillon, who underwent his own surgical transition with renowned surgeon Sir Harold Gilles from 1946 to 1949, and, in 1951, while a medical student, met and fell in love with Roberta Cowell and performed her orchiectomy; celebrities Coccinelle (France), April Ashley, and Jan Morris (both from the United Kingdom) underwent vaginoplasty with Georges Burou in Casablanca in the 1950s to 1970s; and Ashliana Hawelu describes the historical forces that shaped her present life as an Indigenous TGD Hawaiian.

1

PRECOLONIAL GENDER IDENTITIES AND THE INTERNATIONAL ROOTS OF TRANSITIONAL PRACTICES

Serena Nanda

> And God said unto Noah . . . [W]ith thee will I establish my covenant; And of every living thing of all flesh, two of every sort shalt thou bring into the ark to keep them alive with thee; they shall be *male and female*.
>
> —Genesis 6:13–19

A dominant theme in Euro-American culture, embedded in the Judeo-Christian religion, is that human beings are divided without remainder into two biological sexes: male and female.[1] This presumably permanent delineation takes place at birth, with sex ascribed based on the genitals. For more than 150 years, this concept of sex, recognized as a system of ascribed and invariant biological binary oppositions, has been largely taken for granted by Western people and their scientific and medical communities.[2] With few exceptions (notably in the work of cultural anthropologists Franz Boas, Ruth Benedict, and Margaret Mead[3]), Westerners also assumed *gender* (the psychological, social, and behavioral aspects of being male or female, referred to as masculine or feminine) and *sexuality* (sexual desire and practices) to be dichotomous, permanent, and biologically inherent.[4]

With the rise of feminist anthropology in the 1970s, the concepts of gender, sex, and sexuality were increasingly extricated from biological determinism.[5] Ethnographies about a wide range of non-Western cultures revealed a tremendous diversity of definitions, roles, patterns, and identities associated with male and female, masculinity and femininity, and hetero- and homosexuality around the world that went beyond the Western binary.[6] For example, the acceptance of sex and gender diversity was part of the cultures of ancient Greece and Rome, as well as medieval Europe.[7] Individuals in such cultures interacted with prevalent societal norms to define social systems and develop body modification practices that allowed them to exist and survive more comfortably.

While some of these diverse practices continue into the present, they have been impacted in complex ways by contact with Western cultures, both through colonialism and postcolonial global connections.[8] In this chapter, I describe the history of non-Western transfeminine communities from a personal and societal context and ask the reader to consider how these cutlural beliefs and practices might have also contributed to current Western social/medical practices.

The recognition of this global diversity led academics to rethink sex, gender, and sexuality, emphasizing them as sociocultural constructs rather than natural, permanent, biological aspects of humanity. This rethinking opened up the subject of sex/gender systems to psychological, sociological, historical, and ethnographic reexamination. It also impacted medical and psychological practices relating to treatment for individuals with diverse gender expression and identities.[9] As a result, by the early twentieth century, public, scientific, legal, and medical responses to gender-diverse individuals in the West changed from a largely negative view to one that was more accepting of sex/gender diversity. This shift enabled persons with nonbinary sex, gender, and sexual identities to accept themselves more positively, individually, and flexibly, which allowed previously marginalized communities to move closer to the cultural mainstream. Several societal transformations illustrate these changes: the increasing public recognition and affirmation of transgender identities, the establishment of the "medical necessity" of gender transitions,[10] a transformed approach to the medical treatment of intersexed individuals,[11] and the rise of global trans activism. Despite these trends, the view that sex, gender, and sexuality are dichotomous and unchanging over an individual's lifetime maintains significant influence over the biological and social sciences, as well as in psychological and medical treatment in the United States.

The many terms available to describe nonnormative roles relating to sex, gender, and sexuality reflect the tremendous complexity when defining these roles, indigenously and in the West, in academic discussions and as personal subjectivities.[12] Historically, English terms used to describe nonbinary genders and individuals include but are not limited to hermaphrodite, eunuch, intersex, nonbinary, gender-bending, male-bodied persons socially considered women, trans-queer, transsexual, transgender, AC/DC, gender-crossing, tomboi, alternative gender, unfixed, fluid, LBGTQ, LBGTQI, third (or more) gender, gay or lesbian, bi-sexual, non-heteronormative, homosexual, invert, liminal, betwixt and between, men who have sex with men, nonmainstream, transvestite, androgynous, androphilic, gynephilic, and Two Spirit. In my ethnographic descriptions, I use local terms (with English translations) as much as possible, and I also note the linguistic changes that result from the impact of Western colonialism, contemporary Western culture, and expanding global connections.

HIJRA

One widely known alternative gender role is that of the *hijra* of South Asia, including India, Bangladesh, Pakistan, and Nepal.[13] In India, hijras are defined outside the dominant Hindu sex/gender system, which is binary, hierarchical, and patriarchal and based on the biological differences between men and women, as described in classical Hindu medical and ritual texts.[14] However, Hinduism also acknowledges diverse sex/gender variants and transformations, "celebrating the idea that the universe is boundlessly various, and . . . that all possibilities may exist without excluding each other."[15] As early as the eighth century BCE, Hinduism recognized alternatively gendered persons; these people were primarily understood as sexually impotent males who were unable to procreate.[16] This historically deep Hindu acceptance of androgyny allows for the interchange of male and female qualities, transformations of sex and gender, the incorporation of male and female within one person, and alternative sex and gender roles among deities and humans. These positive themes from Hindu mythology, ritual, and art, which are expressed in sculptures in the ancient kingdoms of Harappa and Mohenjadaro,[17] still exist to this day.

A diversity of views and personal subjectivities exist to understand hijras, some contradictory. For example, hijras are neither man nor woman, yet also both man and woman. This diversity embraces biological sex, gender identity, and sexuality, all of which have changed historically and continue to change in contemporary South Asia.[18] Hijras are widely believed to be sexually impotent males who undergo removal of their male genitals to achieve the spiritual and ritual power that Hinduism attributes to sexual renunciation. Once cut, the severed genitals are kept in a pot. Later in the night, the pot is buried underneath some earth near a tree. Burying the genitals is an important sign of respect; otherwise, the severed genitals will turn into a snake and bite the emasculated hijra on doomsday. There is no evidence that all or most hijras are born impotent, and many hijras engage in sexual relations with non-hijra men and even marry them.[19] Although hijras often define themselves as men who have no (sexual) desire for women, they are distinguished from gender-conforming, cisgender men who identify by their same-sex sexual orientation.[20]

Traditionally, hijras are employed as singers and dancers at marriages and at the birth of a male child, where they bless the bridal couple and child for fertility and prosperity. This ritual is carried out in the name of their goddess Bahuchara Mata, who is associated with male transvestism and transgenderism. In return, the hijras receive payments of money, sweets, and cloth. Hijra are widely known, both in the past and present, for also engaging in sex work, a lucrative source of income but also a basis of disrespect, criminal charges, and sometimes police violence.

Even as hijras are understood as man minus man, they are also man plus woman: they wear women's clothing and accessories; keep their hair long; imitate women's walk, gestures, voice, and language; take women's names; and experience themselves as the objects of men's sexual desires. But if hijras are "like women," they are also "not-women."[21] Their feminine dress and mannerisms are often exaggerations, and their aggressive female sexuality in public contrasts strongly with the normatively submissive demeanor and seclusive lives of cisnormative women. But the main reason hijras are not-women is that they cannot give birth.

With the arrival of Muslim rulers from Persia in the eleventh and twelfth centuries, eunuchs had important social roles as slaves and guardians of the harem. Hijra is an Urdu word with Turkish roots, and it was widely used after the Mughal invasion to refer to someone who "is sterile, impotent, castrated, a transvestite, a man who has oral sex with other men, who has anal sex, a man with mutilated or defective sexual organs, a hermaphrodite, or a man who only produced female children."[22] In the British colonial period (from the eighteenth century to 1947), the understanding of hijras as eunuchs predominated. The British were determined to eliminate the hijra community by delineating their gender as a criminal caste with a reputation for breaking the law by kidnapping and castrating children, practicing sodomy, and dressing and performing as women in public places.[23]

By the mid-twentieth century—defined by India's independence from British rule, the expansion of global communication systems, and the rethinking of nonnormative sex, gender and sexuality—changes began to occur in hijra identity, practice, and definition. In contemporary India and Bangladesh, many hijras now identify as gay—not in the Western sense of being homosexual but rather, as in much of the world, referring to their strong sexual desire to being anally penetrated by men.[24] This sexual desire, emphasizing performance rather than anatomy, now serves as the central axis of identity for many hijras on the Indian subcontinent.[25]

Other societal shifts of the late twentieth century, which include rising international human rights activism, nongovernmental organizations proliferation in South Asia, and changes in medical and scientific thought, also influenced how hijras are seen: they are now incorporated into the global category of transgender. They have thus been granted many civil, legal, and social welfare benefits. India, Bangladesh, and Pakistan now legally recognize hijras as a third gender; India has decriminalized sodomy (that is, gay sex); and individuals seek gender-affirming medical and surgical interventions in increasing numbers.[26]

As hijras expanded their global communications—appearing in popular American and British press—they became politically active and powerful advocates for their community, claiming rights to define themselves in non-traditional and positive ways. Today, hijras construct their identity and authenticity not only through the lens of gender and sexuality but also by establishing the importance of hijra kinship and community.

BISSU AND WARIA

Southeast Asia, which includes the nation-states of Malaysia, Myanmar, Thailand, Cambodia, Laos, Vietnam, and Indonesia, is known for its widespread acceptance and positive ideology regarding the many transgender roles that are part of its indigenous and contemporary cultures. A wide range of nonnormative sex/gender roles and individuals are not only tolerated and accommodated but also accorded legitimacy and even prestige, though there are significant regional cultural differences.[27]

A religious role similar to India's hijras exists in Indonesia, a multicultural nation that traditionally accommodated diverse nonnormative sex/gender roles. Indonesian culture was significantly influenced by Hinduism and Buddhism, which spread throughout the archipelago from the seventh to the fourteenth centuries; contact with mystical Shia Islamic philosophy in the thirteenth century was also an important influence. Beginning in the sixteenth century, the impact of Dutch colonialism and Christianity largely undermined this widespread Indonesian sex/gender pluralism. By the seventeenth century, the political, economic, and religious influence of Sunni Islamic traders who brought sharia law resulted in the suppression of nonnormative sex/gender roles and practices throughout Indonesia. The reign of a conservative Islamic government after Indonesian independence in 1947 continued to suppress traditional Indonesian cultures until the end of the twentieth century, when a more liberal Islamic government took power. This new government promoted Indonesian national unity partly through promoting cultural revitalization, including traditional nonnormative sex/gender roles and rituals.[28]

A central alternative sex/gender role revived in Indonesia is the *bissu*, a prestigious and sacred role with roots in Indian and Tantric Buddhist practices. The bissu exist as part of the traditional culture of the Bugis, the largest ethnic group in South Sulawesi. In early modern times (roughly the fifteenth to eighteenth centuries), Bugis was a hierarchical chiefly state. During this period, the bissu safeguarded royal regalia and sacred, royal texts; they were also responsible for performing rituals that insured the well-being of the state and the cosmos. The bissu role was mainly occupied by individuals assigned male at birth who engaged in cross-gender practices and same-sex relations; they also had close contact with the spiritual world.[29] In Bugis culture, most human beings are divided into male and female before birth, but bissu are regarded as androgynous, which is central to their identity, as well as to many Bugis origin myths. The bissu are spiritually called to their sacred role, which is confirmed by undergoing a consecration ritual still performed today. Even in the late twentieth century, according to Bugis culture, bissu who took a cisgender male husband also had supernatural spouses, usually one male and one female.

In 1957, the Indonesian Islamic government of President Suharto destroyed the Bugis kingdom, undermining its traditional culture, which included outlawing the bissu. They were forced to conduct their rituals covertly, if at all. In the 1950s and 1960s, Muslim fundamentalist groups violently persecuted and massacred Bugis in large numbers. In 1998, when Suharto's New Order government lost power, Indonesia witnessed a revival of traditional Indonesian cultural practices, with the Bugis embracing the bissu as a way to reassert their ethnic identity. While some Muslims still consider the bissu sinful, their rituals grew increasingly popular with cisnormative people. Today, their most important role is to bestow blessings for good harvests, protect society against natural disasters, bless people before they undertake a journey (including the pilgrimage to Mecca), heal the sick, and officiate at life-cycle rituals (for instance, births, deaths, and marriages). They are also encouraged to perform in Indonesian cultural festivals at home and abroad.[30] The current Indonesian government's emphasis on reviving local traditions, as part of its effort to expand Indonesian national unity, has vastly improved and expanded bissu status and power.

The Indonesian bissu and the Indian hijra are examples of the religious basis for many nonnormative sex/gender roles in Southeast Asia. This regional sex/gender pluralism also includes many roles that are not sacred but rather primarily revolve around sexuality, public performances, and gender, as described below in Indonesia and Thailand.

The nonnormative religious role of the bissu in Bugis culture contrasts with another valued Indonesian nonnormative sex/gender role: the *waria*, also called *calabai*. Waria are assigned male at birth and express their identities by dressing and comporting themselves as women, professing exclusive sexual desires for heterosexual men, and rejecting heterosexual marriage.[31] In the nineteenth century, they were labeled hermaphrodites, and they have also been referred to as transvestites. Up until the takeover by the reform government in 1988, waria frequently dressed as men during the day to avoid the stigma of their identity. Today, waria almost universally and publicly enact feminine roles through their dress, accessories, and comportment, though like hijras, they may also be rude and aggressive, a cultural expectation for cisnormative men.[32]

In the mid-ninth century, dominant waria roles included city dock workers, sex workers, and low-class popular entertainers. After Indonesian independence (1945) and during the period of conservative Islamic dominance, waria avoided public places, but by the late 1960s, their position changed for the better. In addition to performing sex work, waria also entered—and dominated—the beauty salon business, readying brides and grooms for traditional weddings.[33] Furthermore, beauty remains a central feature of the waria role and waria performances,[34] and beauty contests are now widespread in the media and as public entertainment. This role not only added to the economic status of the waria but also gave them an important place in modern Indonesian society. The reformist Islamic government promoted public recognition of the waria as human beings and citizens of the nation, stressing their important contributions to national Indonesian culture.

Almost all waria are self-declared Muslims and regularly perform Muslim rituals. They are aware of the conflict between their role and strict Muslim ideology, and they try to mitigate the "sin" of their feminine identity and behavior by doing good deeds for their families and the nation.[35] Waria differentiate themselves from gay men by seeking only heterosexual male sexual partners. They enlarge their breasts with silicone injections and feminizing hormones, but few undergo surgical transition, in part because of the expense but also because it is forbidden under Islamic law.[36] Unlike the hijra, genital alteration is not central to waria identity, and in fact, according to their interpretation of the Muslim faith, such changes offend God. While some Indonesians believe waria are genitally deformed or sexually impotent, most share the waria's view about waria identity, that is, it is related to their desire to take the receptive sexual positions for pleasure. Their refusal to marry alienates them from their families, and many waria migrate to Europe, although some return to Indonesia and marry cisgender women.[37] In Indonesia, waria seek long-term relationships with their boyfriends and support them financially in return for love and romance.

While the Indonesian government legally and ideologically accepted—and even publicly praised—the waria for their contributions to Indonesian society and national culture, the same is not true for gay men and lesbians. In contrast to Thailand and the Philippines, homosexual relationships are largely concealed, as they are negatively sanctioned and surveilled, as happens in other Islamic societies. Recently, the Indonesian government has taken a repressive role in restricting many kinds of sexual activities, including gay and lesbian sexual practices.[38]

KATHOEY

In Thailand today, the discourse on sex, gender, and sexuality, as well as transgender individuals, has changed to include variable and evolving identities and roles. In traditional Thai culture, sexual orientation and sexual practice were not the basis of a personal or social identity. The modern Western opposition of homosexual/heterosexual did not exist, and Buddhism and ancient Thai law did not outline injunctions against homoeroticism.

The most public nonnormative sex/gender role in Thailand is the *kathoey*. Referred to in Buddhist origin myths as a third gender, kathoey are defined as males who act like females, appropriate feminine attributes and behaviors, and dress in women's clothing. Traditional Thai sex/gender discourse understood male and female homoeroticism as sex/gender inversion or "psychological hermaphroditism—having a woman's mind in a man's body." Today, the Thai attitude toward kathoey is ambivalent; kathoey face stigma as effeminate homosexuals who are "like women but are also not women," leading some to identify themselves, like waria, as a biological male who has the soul of a woman.[39]

Like waria, kathoey are also closely associated with the entertainment and beauty industries. They are highly visible and found in all but the highest social strata, working openly in cities and rural areas at ordinary jobs, with some even owning their own businesses. Many kathoey perform in transvestite revues or gay bars and theaters, and their beauty contests are well attended by locals, government officials, and tourists. Kathoey are viewed as entertaining and humorous and associated with feminine elegance and grace. Their reputation as sex workers, however, contributes to their derided social position, as upper middle-class urbanites critically stereotype them for being loud, lewd, and vulgar—all particularly un-Thai like behaviors.[40]

In the 1950s, Thailand was privy to the rise of a Western scientific, biomedical, and psychological discourse on sex and gender, leading to a stigmatized view of homosexuals as psychological perverts. Before the 1950s, private same-sex eroticism was not stigmatized in Thailand, and traditionally, the kathoey were considered biological hermaphrodites, a karmic condition preordained at birth and unalterable. While some still hold this view, the diffusion of the Western biomedical model negatively affected social attitudes toward sex/gender/sexual diversity, including cultural perception of the kathoey. Congruent with Thai patriarchy, the devalued status of cisgender women further stigmatizes effeminate men and transgender women. A cisgender Thai man who acts like a man and fulfills his social obligations to marry and father a family is still considered a man, even if his preferred sexual partner is male.

When the term *gay* entered Thai discourse in the 1970s, it referred mainly to effeminate, homosexual males, as was true in the United States. By the 1990s, the ideal gay man became increasingly masculinized. Today, the gay man in Thailand is identified by his enlarged biceps, accentuated body and facial hair, and claims to a strongly masculine identity; the perception of gay men is thus disassociated from the current transfeminine status of the kathoey.[41] This new gay identity also blurs opposing masculine/insertive and feminine/receptive roles in same-sex erotic practices. A Thai gay person no longer has defined gender roles, whereas clear gender roles remain a central feature of the Indonesian waria, the Indian hijra, and the Brazilian travesti. Like much of Southeast Asia and Polynesia, Thai society prioritizes the conventionality of one's public acts rather than the nonconformity of one's private emotions or behaviors. Erotic practices in Thailand are merely seen as personal preferences. Coming out, or the public expression of one's true self, is not valued in Thailand and Southeast Asia as it is in the United States.

The emergence of gay men as masculine men, alongside the emergence of kathoey as transgender homosexuals (rather than biological hermaphrodites) in the public eye, increased the social stigma and violence the kathoey experience in contemporary Thailand. As in Western cultures, by the 1980s, the categories of homosexual men and transgender women were considered psychological disorders and regarded as social problems by Thai academics and the upper middle class. Attempts to root out these "perversions" are part of official government rhetoric, which concurrently urges compassion. Thailand's acceptance of sex/gender diversity and nonnormative sexuality has its roots in Thai culture and history, and although ambivalent, its relative openness helps sustain the thriving business of gender-affirming surgical care in the world market and an international tourist economy known for its reputation as "pink chic."[42]

TRAVESTI

In contrast to Thailand, Brazilian culture views sex/gender diversity through its relationship to sexual practice, a theme that characterizes much of Latin America,[43] though some indigenous Mexican cultures view androgyny as a sacred symbol of the cosmos.[44] In spite of contemporary sex/gender diversity in Latin America, its cultures have a shared understanding: men and women are opposed in all ways, with males clearly superior.[45] Spanish and Portuguese roots in the region, specifically the influence of the Catholic Church and the culture of early Portuguese colonizers, contributed to a dominant, patriarchal ideology that stresses control over women.

This binary opposition—male and female, man and woman—affects differences in bodies, social status, rights and responsibilities, psychological characteristics, politics, and work. Cisgender men are characterized by their superiority and strength; masculinity manifests as aggressive sexuality, having many children, and the ability to control the sexuality of a man's wives and daughters. Cisgender women are defined as inferior and weak, though also beautiful and sexually desirable, a view reflected in the identities of the nonnormative sex/gender role of the *travesti*. The Catholic Church typecasts women as either virgins, mothers, or whores, emphasizing the importance of virginity; prostitutes and unfaithful wives are thus a threat to the honor and masculinity of cisgender men, as well as society.

Unlike the predominant Western sex/gender binary (homosexual/heterosexual and man/woman), the Brazilian gender binary assumes man and not-man, a dichotomy based not on anatomy but rather sexual practices—not on genitals themselves but instead on how those genitals are used, specifically the position taken in sexual intercourse.[46] This opposition between the active masculine (atividade)—those who penetrate—and the passive feminine (passividade)—those who are penetrated—is reflected in language: *comer* (to eat) describes male penetration and domination, and *dar* (to give) describes female submission. Men are thus identifiable as men by their role as the penetrating partner during sexual intercourse.

In Brazil, the travestis are an example of a nonnormative sex/gender role: effeminate males who take the passive role in sexual relations with men. Only if a male is known publicly to have "given" in sexual relations does he assume the position of a travestis rather than that of a man. Furthermore, while travestis readily self-identify as homosexual, the term *homosexual* is traditionally not applied to the penetrating partner in a same-sex sexual relationship. Thus, a male who enters into a sexual relationship with another cisgender male is still considered heterosexual so long as he performs the penetrative role in sexual intercourse.

Travestis, sometimes called *bichas*, or bugs, are expected to dress, sound, and act like women, and many also transform their bodies.[47] Young boys who self-identify as travestis may ingest or inject feminizing hormones to develop breasts and use silicone implants so their bodies reflect the Brazilian concept of feminine beauty: fleshy thighs and prominent buttocks. But unlike Western transgender women, travestis do not believe they are women or could ever be one because "God created them male and their sex can never be changed."[48] Travestis do not wish to remove their penises, in part because they believe that without a penis, semen will be trapped in their bodies, reach their brains, and cause madness. They will tuck their penises between their legs in deference to their boyfriends' manhood and to enhance their appeal as sex workers.[49] Travestis identify themselves not *as* women but rather *like* women, particularly in their sexual desire to be anally penetrated by men. Thus, travestis are both not-man and *like* woman, adopting a heterogender identity.

As in Thailand, Brazil faced the same pathologizing European view of binary sex/gender relations, which could not accommodate its traditional, pluralistic understandings of sex/gender. Notably, the European framework emphasized that both partners in a same-sex sexual relationship were homosexual and that such relationships were detrimental to society.[50] This view remains widespread, but by the twenty-first century, the homosexual/heterosexual divide lost much of its pejorative meaning for both participants in a same-sex sexual relationship, particularly among the wealthy and educated classes. The traditional Brazilian model of gender and sexuality—man, woman, and travesti—still holds true in the less educated, rural, and poorer classes, particularly in the Northeast, defining Brazil's sex/gender ideology as pluralistic, complex, and sometimes contradictory.

Public perception of travestis is ambivalent, although by and large, travestis still face discrimination in public life. Cross-dressing is a positive, iconic component of Brazilian culture during Carnival, where cross-dressing and gender inversion are prominent for travestis and gender-conforming men, yet travestis themselves are generally demeaned for their nonnormative sex/gender expression.[51] Travestis often step into the public spotlight on television soap operas. Television star and travesti Roberta Close, who subsequently transitioned to female, is widely admired as the most beautiful woman in Brazil. Such adoration is not the norm, though, as most travestis face harassment and discrimination in the workplace and the street. As a result, many stay indoors during the day, only appearing in public at night.

These negative public perceptions of travestis contrast with the leadership roles they (and cisgender women) hold in the Afro-Brazilian religion of Candomblé.[52] Candomblé's spirits and rituals are based on the West African Yoruba religion in which male possession priests perform transvestism, feminine gestures, and feminine occupations. During the possession trance, which authenticates Candomblé priesthood, male and female Yoruba priests are called brides of the god, and they wear women's clothing, jewelry, hair styles, and cosmetics. Candomblé spiritual powers provide their practitioners—both travestis and women—with cultural and financial rewards. While the Brazilian government formerly outlawed the Candomblé and practices, today, many upper-class Brazilians seek out the magical services of Candomblé, while tourists enjoy the practices as a cultural attraction.

In Candomblé, meanings of penetration and possession amplify the association between women and *passivos* (male priests who are seen as submissive to the gods). Penetration of females by males offers a metaphor for the relationship between the gods and their followers. The term describing possession is *dar santo*—to give saint. In possession, the priest "gives" or submits to the god, with the god mounting the priest as a male rides his female partner.[53] The possessed Candomblé priests are called horses of the gods, symbolizing the passive role of women in sexual relations. From this belief, it follows that men who are ridden by the gods become passive, for they are renouncing their masculine atividade in *dando santo*—giving saint. Humans are thus female in relation to all Candomblé spirits.[54] This understanding explains the prominence of women and passivos in Afro-Brazilian possession religions, despite their inferior roles in the patriarchal Brazilian society.

LEITI

Since its discovery by Europeans, Polynesia has existed in the Western imagination as a romanticized place of unrestricted and casual sexuality, including a tolerant acceptance of gender diversity, a view almost diametrically opposed to European culture. Similar to Southeast Asia, Polynesian attitudes toward sex, gender, and sexuality rely on contrasting cultural understandings, specifically the controlled and uncontrolled aspects of human social existence: good behavior, characterized by restraining personal impulses, conforms to social roles; bad behavior, considered selfish and disgusting, is motivated by personal desire, impulsiveness, and self-gratification, particularly in matters of sexuality.

The many islands comprising Polynesia contain multiple, deep-rooted traditions of liminal or transgender roles for men and women. Gender relations in Polynesia are complementary, with men and women having their own spheres of work, sociality, and behavioral norms, though the intensity of gender role differentiation varies among the many islands. Two important Polynesian norms are widespread: (1) respected relationships between brothers and sisters and (2) divided roles for women, between the positively valued virginal girl and the less valued mature wife (who has had at least one child).[55]

Traditional gender diversity in Polynesia involves males who take on feminine characteristics. These individuals may be referred to as "in the way of a woman," "half man-half woman," or "lady." The roles are not consistently or precisely defined, and a man may move in and out of the feminine role. The most important signs of this liminality are engaging in women's work and almost exclusively in female social circles, as well as adopting feminine dress, speech, nonverbal gestures, and dance styles. With few exceptions,[56] scholars have rarely studied female liminal roles in Polynesia, and these roles remain in the shadows. Polynesians view liminal or transgender individuals as an inevitable aspect of society; however, while accepted and even admired for their creativity and modernity, gender liminal individuals are also marginalized from the cultural mainstream. As a diaspora, their numbers are increasing in Western societies, an indication that these roles and Polynesian gender liminal ideologies are changing.

One of the many Polynesian sex/gender variations involves the *leiti* of Tonga.[57] Tongan liminality is primarily a matter of gender: males who appear less virile are expected to desire straight men, act feminine, and assume a feminine sexual role. Tongans refer to transgender women as leiti, or woman, and sometimes as *fakaleiti*, in the way of a woman. They are a small but visible minority whose numbers appear to be growing each year.

The leiti feminine role directly contrasts with the culturally valued, hypermasculine Togan identity. This persona is a performance of virility and carries significant implications for one's social and political rank. Numerous characteristics define this role: controlled emotionality, a grounding of the self in local culture, competition between brothers, exclusively male friendship groups and networks, and relations with women, which are almost exclusively sexualized.

In contrast to Tongan men, leiti are emotionally demonstrative and impulsive; they are also concerned with beauty, domesticity, and creativity. Leiti worry about their body image, seek out the friendship of women, and try to engage with the cosmopolitan and modern world outside their island. If they have female siblings, they are also expected to fulfill their role as brothers, which includes guarding their sisters' reputation and respect.

Notably, leiti is a gendered role—feminine, in this case—rather than primarily a sexual role, and the Western idea of nongendered gay men is puzzling in Tonga. Leiti define straight men as the object of their erotic desires, and they act as the receiving partners in oral and anal connection throughout Polynesia. They are culturally obligated to provide gifts of money, alcohol, or entertainment to their male partners, a custom that emphasizes they are not real women but rather in the way of a woman. While they do have sexual relationships with cisgender Tongan men, this connection is emphatically denied by their male partners. Tongan men often flirt with leiti, taking the inserter role in sexual intercourse; they say a man has sex with a leiti because he cannot attract a "real woman." This relationship does not jeopardize heterosexual masculinity, and Tongan men are not stigmatized, although this response is changing with increasing Western influence, which disparages homosexuality. Tongans scorn the priority to define leiti along sexual lines, and many appear scandalized at the thought of same-sex sexuality, pointing out that God created man and woman.

Another significant component of contemporary leiti identity is their appropriation of modernism and globalism, which is not characteristic of many Tongans and key to understanding the leitis' place in Tongan society. Leiti actively associate with foreign men in urban bars, and they frequently work in occupations that involve the global economy. This cosmopolitan spirit is also central to the defining leiti cultural event, the Miss Galaxy beauty contest. The annual event's name conveys a global orientation and underscores leiti stereotypes: projecting an international glamour, appearing in the national costumes of other countries, donning extravagant and campy costumes, and adopting female stage names (either English or foreign but never Tongan). Leiti are seen as assured and brash individuals who know no shame, and their contest performances are generally exhibitionistic and often outrageous, as expected by their audiences. The dominant language for the contest is English, which many leiti do not speak well but which reinforces the prestige and worldliness of their preferred identities. The use of English also calls attention to the leitis' generally superior command of English compared to most Tongans. It also increases their identification with women, who are known in Tonga to speak better English than men. This association is partly because women are assumed to be more talkative, and partly because in reality, English proficiency supports leiti upward social mobility. As a result, Tongan men who speak "too much" English risk compromising their masculinity, especially since their prescribed gender role relies on deep local roots.

There is no early historical record of transgender individuals in Tonga, and some Tongans today claim this role is the result of Western influence, though the leiti description as in-between, and their performative, feminine identity is most likely traditionally Tongan. Western influence is changing in Tonga (and some other Polynesian societies), partly because of an increasing diaspora of gender-liminal individuals to the United States and Australia. Their participation in the new global discourse of sex/gender liminality, similar to that of the kathoey in Thailand and the bakla of the Philippines,[58] also impacts their status in their local societies. Some Polynesian migrants have redefined themselves as gay or lesbian, an identification that does not match their home islands' gender ideology; this alignment with Western modes of identification is considered socially disruptive. (Although Europeans first censured the sexual behavior of Polynesian gender-liminal individuals, specifically those in Tahiti, homoerotic desire and behaviors do not define Polynesian gender liminality.) Conversely, where there was strong colonial impact, such as in Hawaii, reasserting traditional transgender roles represents a positive aspect of precolonial culture; individuals and political activists are reclaiming these roles as a way to distance themselves from the postcolonial culture.

THE EFFECTS OF WESTERN COLONIALISM

Sexual and gender binaries, so deeply rooted in the mind-body split of Western philosophy, falsely legitimated a naturalized realm of biological difference. This ideology ignores other non-Western cultures, which not only acknowledge people who do not fit into the Western sex/gender/sexuality binary but also often elevate them to important cultural and religious roles.[59] For the most part, Western colonialism, Christian missionaries, the spread of Islam, and the adoption of Western medical and psychological science in the twentieth century had a negative impact on these nonbinary concepts of sex, gender, and sexuality—and in many cases, almost led to their extinction. An extensive and detailed study of this impact emphasizes the time frame from 1750 until 1918, which incorporates pre-Enlightenment and post-Enlightenment Europe, a period in which Western colonialism, missionary activity, and contact with Islam was at its height in the non-Western world.[60]

The effect of Western colonialism was complicated, sometimes contradictory, and affected different societies in diverse ways. Western interests, research, and writings focused mainly on sexuality, particularly male-to-male sexual behavior; however, they also noted nonbinary sex/gender roles, which were often (but not always) related to male-to-male sexual practice. This attention and the resulting literature included positive and negative views, as expressed by ethnographers, medical practitioners, sexologists, writers, and travelers in scientific and popular contexts. Although scientific impact is often seen as liberating, in this case, it had the negative effect of fixing identities based on erotic behavior and considering these identities and behaviors a psychological disorder. Classifying these cultural, moral values and behaviors as negative or even dangerous produced what was, for the most part, a highly Eurocentric, controlling doctrine in the colonies. As Edward Said noted in his attempt to unpack this Western position in his influential study *Orientalism,* colonial possessions were not only sources of economic benefit to Europe and useful places to send European undesirables but the Orient "was [also] a place where one could look for sexual experience unobtainable in Europe."[61] Earlier travel narratives from India, Africa, and the Middle East described sodomy, eunuchs, men who dressed like women, and hermaphrodites, which tickled the European imagination. Sodomy, in particular, was for centuries associated with the colonial "other."

Colonial European ideology emphasized that the sexual otherness of non-Western cultures was an inherent difference and incompatibility between people with different skin color—a long-held association between racial inferiority and sexual lasciviousness. This position was disputed by black writers such as Aliyyah I. Abdur-Rahman who noted that within the "peculiar institution" of slavery, white people had unchecked personal authority of the bodies of enslaved people, which engendered and concealed "all manner of sexual perversion."[62] The practice of slavery further served to feminize men by virtue of their subjugation, regular use of castration, and denial of patriarchal and citizenship rights.[63] In response to the psychoanalytical view of homosexuality as a neurosis, black writers denounced male-to-male sexuality as alien to their culture, a view still held today and illustrated by the controlling and sometimes violent action against male-to-male sexual relations found in many contemporary African and Muslim societies.[64] Non-Western colonial subjects perceived male-to-male sexual relationships (both in Africa and elsewhere) as central to the colonial project: the intentional construction of the other as feminine or effeminate and the subsequent, justifiable power imbalance between Europe and its colonies based on this gendered narrative. Thus, colonial subjects came to see homosexuality as a foreign import from Europe or the Arabic world, both of which feminized colonized nations and degraded them as perverse, regarding not only sexuality but also nonbinary sex/gender roles.

In contrast to this colonial ideology, many anthropological ethnographies stressed the healthy sexual patterns of tribal societies and explained away same-sex behavior as part of rites of passage, which transformed boys into men among the *sambia* of Melanesia and among many Native American societies.[65] However problematic this perspective was in relation to a diverse cultural reality, an influential result of this new approach and research orientation was that sexuality was no longer viewed strictly as a biological matter but instead was defined by culture.[66] It also led to new efforts to examine sex/gender and sexuality from a historical perspective, emphasizing the impact of Western colonialism, Western medical science, Western psychology, and Western culture on non-Western societies.

Accompanying the new global discourse of sex/gender/sexuality in which gay and lesbian identities have become accepted and sometimes embraced, there may paradoxically be a rejection of contemporary Western understandings as a form of neocolonialism. In parts of Polynesia and Africa, the growing global acceptance of same-sex relationships and gay marriage has had a negative impact; gay men may be arrested and even killed, LGBTQ communities must go underground, and many individuals seek asylum in the United States.[67]

With the decline of Western colonialism in the mid- to late twentieth century and the reversal of homosexuality as a perversion in American psychological ideology, many cultures and communities have resurrected nonbinary sex/gender roles, albeit altered from their traditional forms. Today, transgender individuals engage in local and international activism aimed at reviving these diverse, cultural sex/gender traditions; they also generate positive actions regarding their rights, such as the legalization of third gender status in India, Pakistan, and Bangladesh.

Furthermore, the changes in the twenty-first century make it clear that societal transformations regarding sex/gender diversity are nonlinear and include reversals and counterflows. The rapid, global reach of communication (for example, internet, tourism, social media, NGOs, human rights activism, migration) has led non-Western societies to adopt aspects of contemporary Western sex/gender roles, ideology, and practice, including medical and psychological therapy. In a positive twist, this influence has provoked Western nations to reexamine the assumptions and practices of their own cultural patterns, leading to greater responsiveness to transgender individuals in the United States. These reexaminations of sex/gender and sexuality reflect an essential goal of cultural anthropology: seeing other cultures from the inside. This practice offers the tremendous benefit of being able to view one's own culture more objectively, and in this case, it also offers transformation: greater compassion for and more inclusive treatment of transgender individuals who have long suffered on the margins of US society.

NOTES

1. Geertz, "Common Sense as a Cultural System," 10.
2. Kessler and McKenna, *Gender: An Ethnomethodological Approach*, vii.
3. King, *Gods of the Upper Air*, 269–71.
4. Besnier, "Gender and Sexuality: Contested Relations," 1, 4.
5. Butler, *Gender Trouble*, 6–7.
6. Nanda, *Gender Diversity: Crosscultural Variations*, 1–9.
7. Hubbard, *Homosexuality in Greece and Rome*, 1–20; Nanda, *Gender Diversity: Crosscultural Variations*, 87–94.
8. Bleys, *The Geography of Perversion*, 266–70; Ryan, *Trans Lives in a Globalizing World*, 266–70.
9. Winter, "Transgender," 1388–39.
10. Knudson et al., *Position Statement on Medical Necessity of Treatment, Sex Reassignment, and Insurance Coverage in the U.S.A.*
11. Karkazis, *Intersex, Medical Authority, and Lived Experience*, 265–69; Bolin, "Transcending and Transgendering," 453–54.
12. Besnier and Alexeyeff, *Gender on the Edge*, 5–10.
13. Nanda, *Gender Diversity*, 27–43; Reddy, *With Respect to Sex*; Hossain, *Beyond Emasculation*, 13–14; Goel, "India's Third Gender Rises Again."
14. Peletz, *Gender Pluralism*, 32–33.
15. O'Flaherty and Doniger, *Siva: The Erotic Ascetic*, 318.
16. Zwilling and Sweet. "The Evolution of Third Sex," 100.
17. Clark, "Representing the Indus Body," 304.
18. Hossain and Nanda, "Globalization and Change Among the Hijras of South Asia," 35–37.
19. Reddy, "The Bonds of Companionate Marriage," 178–79.
20. Cohen, "The Pleasures of Castration," 178–79; Reddy, "Crossing 'Lines' of Difference," 133–35.
21. Peletz, *Gender Pluralism*, 32–33.
22. Reddy, *With Respect to Sex*, 21.
23. Hinchy, *Governing Gender and Sexuality in Colonial India*, 1–17; Hossain and Nanda, "Globalization and Change," 39–41; Biswas, "How Britain Tried to 'Erase' India's Third Gender"; Hunter, "Hijras and the Legacy of British Colonial Rule in India."
24. Hossain, *Beyond Emasculation*, 141.
25. Hossain, "De-Indianizing Hijra," 327.
26. Nanjundaswamy and Gangadhar, *Transgender Challenges in India*, 80–82 and 224; Schultz, "Fighting for Equality in India," A14.
27. Peletz, *Gender Pluralism*, 264.
28. Boellstorff, "Between Religion and Desire," 576; Blackwood, "Gender Transgression in Colonial and Postcolonial Indonesia," 859–60, 864–67, and 871–72.

29. Pelras, *The Bugis*, 82–85.
30. Davies, *Challenging Gender Norms*, 93.
31. Boellstorff, "Playing Back the Nation," 167–68 and 175.
32. Hossain, *Beyond Emasculation*, 127.
33. Boellstorff, "Playing Back the Nation."
34. Toomistu, "Embodied Notions of Belonging."
35. Toomistu, "Thinking through the S(k)in," 74–75.
36. Toomistu, "Thinking through the S(k)in," 86–89.
37. Noor, "Transnational Love, Migration, and Kinship."
38. Paddock and Suhartono, "Indonesians Protest Bills," A7.
39. Costa and Matzner, *Male Bodies, Women's Souls*, 134.
40. Jackson, "Kathoey><Gay><Man," 177.
41. Jackson, *Dear Uncle Go*, 265–68.
42. Fuller, "Thais Cast a Wide Net for Diverse Tourists," A12.
43. Murray, *Latin American Male Homosexualities*, 243.
44. Marcos, "Beyond Binary Categories," 111.
45. Brandes, "Like Wounded Stags," 217–19; Gilmore, *Manhood in the Making*, 216–39.
46. Kulick, *Travesti*, 141–43.
47. Kulick, "The Gender of Brazilian Transgendered Prostitutes," 575–76.
48. Kulik, *Travesti*, 193ff.
49. Kulick, "The Gender of Brazilian Transgendered Prostitutes," 577.
50. Parker, "'Within Four Walls,'" 256–58.
51. Nanda, *Love and Marriage*, 49–50.
52. Matory, *Sex and the Empire*, 171.
53. Wafer, *The Taste of Blood*; Fry, *Para Ingles Ver*.
54. Wafer, *The Taste of Blood*; Fry, *Para Ingles Ver*.
55. Nanda, *Love and Marriage*, 86–88.
56. Elliston, "Negotiating Transitional Sexual Economies," 234–37.
57. Besnier, *On the Edge of the Global*, 125–59; Besnier, "Polynesian Gender Liminality through Time and Space," 285–328; Shore, "Sexuality and Gender in Samoa," 208–10.
58. Manalansan IV, *Global Divas*, ix–xi.
59. Ellingson and Green, *Religion and Sexuality in Cross-Cultural Perspective*, 111–35; Nanda, *Gender Diversity*, 28.
60. Bleys, *The Geography of Perversion*, 1–12.
61. Bleys, *The Geography of Perversion*, 3.
62. Abdur-Rahman, "'The Strangest Freaks of Despotism,'" 229.
63. Abdur-Rahman, "'The Strangest Freaks of Despotism,'" 230.
64. Murray and Roscoe, *Islamic Homosexualities*, 88–90; Chutel, "A Writer's Account of Transitioning"; Collins, "The Splendor of Gender Non-Conformity in Africa."

65. Herdt, *Guardians of the Flutes*, 318–20.
66. Foucault, *The History of Sexuality*, "Part 1: We Other Victorians."
67. Corey-Boulet, *Love Falls on Us*, 39–41.

WORKS CITED

Abdur-Rahman, Aliyyah I. "'The Strangest Freaks of Despotism': Queer Sexuality in Antebellum African American Slave Narratives." *African American Review* 40, no. 2 (2006): 223–37.

Besnier, Niko. "Gender and Sexuality: Contested Relations." In *The International Encyclopedia of Anthropology*, edited by Hilary Callan, 1–7. New York: Wiley, 2018.

———. *On the Edge of the Global: Modern Anxieties in a Pacific Island Nation*. Stanford, CA: Stanford University, 2011.

———. "Polynesian Gender Liminality through Time and Space." In *Third Sex, Third Gender: Beyond Sexual Dimorphism in Culture and* History, edited by Gilbert Herdt, 285–328. New York: Zone/MIT, 1996.

Besnier, Niko, and Kalissa Alexeyeff, eds. *Gender on the Edge: Transgender, Gay and Other Pacific Islanders.* Honolulu: University of Hawai'i, 2014.

Biswas, Soutik. "How Britain Tried to 'Erase' India's Third Gender." *BBC News*, May 31, 2019. Accessed May 31, 2019. https://www.bbc.com/news/world-asia-india-48442934?intlink_location=live-reporting-correspondent.

Blackwood, Evelyn. "Gender Transgression in Colonial and Postcolonial Indonesia." *Journal of Asian Studies* 64, no. 4 (2005): 849–79.

Bleys, Rudi. *The Geography of Perversion: Male-to-Male Sexual Behavior Outside the West and the Ethnographic Imagination, 1750–1918.* New York: New York University, 1996.

Boellstorff, Tom. "Between Religion and Desire: Being Muslim and Gay in Indonesia." *American Anthropologist* 107, no. 4 (2005): 575–85.

———. "Playing Back the Nation: Waria, Indonesian Transvestites." *Cultural Anthropology* 19 (2004): 159–95.

Bolin, Anne. "Transcending and Transgendering: Male to Female Transsexuals, Dichotomy and Diversity." In *Third Sex, Third Gender: Beyond Sexual Dimorphism in Culture and History*, edited by Gilbert Herdt, 447–86. New York: Zone, 1996.

Brandes, Stanley. "Like Wounded Stags: Male Sexual Ideology in an Andalusian Town." In *Sexual Meanings: The Cultural Construction of Gender and Sexuality*, edited by Sherry Ortner and Harriet Whitehead, 216–39. Cambridge: Cambridge University, 1981.

Butler, Judith. *Gender Trouble: Feminism and the Subversion of Identity*. London: Routledge, 1990.

Chutel, Lynsey. "A Writer's Account of Transitioning and Transcending Gender Shows Being Trans Is Not Un-African." *QuartzAfrica*, January 21, 2018. Accessed August 22, 2022. https://qz.com/africa/1184861/a-writers-account-of-transitioning and-transcending-gender shows-being-trans-is-not-un-african/.

Clark, Sharri R. "Representing the Indus Body: Sex, Gender, Sexuality, and the Anthropomorphic Terracotta Figurines from Harappa." *Asian Perspectives* 42, no. 2 (2003): 304–28.

Cohen, Lawrence. "The Pleasures of Castration: The Postoperative Status of Hijras, Jankhas and Academics." In *Sexual Nature, Sexual Culture*, edited by Paul R. Abramson and Steven D. Pinkerton, 276–304. Chicago, IL: University of Chicago, 1995.

Collins, Shanna. "The Splendor of Gender Non-Conformity in Africa." *Medium*, October 10, 2017. Accessed August 22, 2022. https://medium.com/@janeland_62637/the-splendor-of-gender-non-conformity-in-Africa-f894ff5706e1.

Corey-Boulet, Robbie. *Love Falls On Us: A Story of American Ideas and African LGBT Lives.* New York: Zed Books, 2019.

Costa, LeeRay, and Andrew Matzner. *Male Bodies, Women's Souls: Personal Narratives of Thailand's Transgendered Youth.* New York: Haworth Press, 2007.

Davies, Sharyn Graham. *Challenging Gender Norms: Five Genders Among the Bugis in Indonesia.* Belmont, CA: Wadsworth, 2007.

Ellingson, Stephen, and M. Christian Green, eds. *Religion and Sexuality in Cross-Cultural Perspective.* New York: Routledge, 2002.

Elliston, Deborah A. "Negotiating Transitional Sexual Economies: Female Mahu and Same-Sex Sexuality in 'Tahiti and Her Islands.'" In *Female Desire: Same-Sex Relations and Transgender Practices Across Cultures*, edited by Evelyn Blackwood and Saskia E. Wieringa, 230–52. New York: Columbia University, 1999.

Fanon, Franz. (1952). *Black Skin, White Masks*. Translated by Charles Lam Markmann. New York: Grove Press, 1967.

Feldman, Douglas. "Gay Marriage: The Struggle Is Far from Over." *Huffington Post,* July 15, 2013. Accessed August 4, 2020. http://www.huffingtonpost.com/American-anthropological-association/gay-marriage-the-struggle-is-far-from_over_b_3573685.html/.

Foucault, Michel. *The History of Sexuality: An Introduction*. Vol. 1. New York: Vintage, 1990.

Fry, Peter. "Male Homosexuality and Spirit Possession in Brazil." In *The Many Faces of Homosexuality: Anthropological Approaches to Homosexual Behavior*, edited by Evelyn Blackwood, 137–54. New York: Haworth Press, 1986.

———. *Para Ingles Ver: Identidade e Politica na Cultura Brasileira*. Rio de Janeiro: Zahar Editores, 1982. Quoted in Wafer, *The Taste of Blood*, 18.

Fuller, Thomas. "Thais Cast a Wide Net for Diverse Tourists: Courting Gay and Muslim Travelers." *New York Times*, August 4, 2013, A12.

Geertz, Clifford. "Common Sense as a Cultural System." *Antioch Review 33*, no. 1 (1975): 5–26.

Gilmore, David D. *Manhood in the Making: Cultural Concepts of Masculinity.* New Haven, CT: Yale University, 1990.

Goel, Ina. "India's Third Gender Rises Again." *Sapiens/Anthropology*. Accessed September 26, 2019. https://www.sapiens.org/body/hijra-india-third-gender.

Hayes, Kelley. "*Meu Querido Viado:* Gender and Possession Trance in Candomblex." Unpublished manuscript, last modified 1996.

Herdt, Gilbert. *Guardians of the Flutes: Idioms of Masculinity.* New York: McGraw-Hill, 1981.

———. *Same Sex, Different Cultures: Exploring Gay and Lesbian Lives.* London: Routledge, 1997.

Hinchy, Jessica. *Governing Gender and Sexuality in Colonial India: The Hijra, c. 1850–1900.* Cambridge: Cambridge University, 2019.

Hossain, Adnan. *Beyond Emasculation: Pleasure and Power in the Making of Hijra in Bangladesh.* Cambridge: Cambridge University, 2021.

———. "De-Indianizing Hijra: Intraregional Effacements and Inequalities in South Asian Queer Space." *Transgender Studies Quarterly* 5, no. 3 (2018): 321–31. https://doi.org/10.1215/23289252-6900710.

Hossain, Adnan, and Serena Nanda. "Globalization and Change Among the Hijras of South Asia." In *Trans Lives in a Globalizing World: Rights, Identities, and Politics*, edited by J. Michael Ryan, 34–49. New York: Routledge, 2020.

Hubbard, Thomas K. 2003. *Homosexuality in Greece and Rome: A Sourcebook of Basic Documents.* Berkeley: University of California Press.

Hunter, Sophie. "Hijras and the Legacy of British Colonial Rule in India." LSE Engenderings, June 17, 2019. Accessed May 31, 2019. https://blogs.lse.ac.uk/gender/2019/06/17/hijras-and-the-legacy-of-british-colonial-rule-in-india/#:~:text=The%20colonial%20state%20relied%20upon,diversity%20(Reddy%2C%202010).

Jackson, Peter. *Dear Uncle Go: Male Homosexuality in Thailand.* Bangkok: Bua, 1995.

———. "Kathoey><Gay><Man: The Historical Emergence of Gay Male Identity in Thailand." In *Sites of Desire: Economies of Pleasure: Sexualities in Asia and the Pacific*, edited by Lenore Manderson and Margaret Jolly, 166–90. Chicago, IL: University of Chicago, 1997.

Karkazis, Katrina. *Intersex, Medical Authority, and Lived Experience.* Durham, NC: Duke University, 2008.

Kessler, Suzanne, and Wendy McKenna. *Gender: An Ethnomethodological Approach.* New York: Wiley, 1978.

King, Charles. *Gods of the Upper Air: How a Circle of Renegade Anthropologists Reinvented Race, Sex, and Gender in the Twentieth Century.* New York: Doubleday, 2019.

Knudson, Gail, Vin Tangpricha, Jamison Green, et al. *Position Statement on Medical Necessity of Treatment, Sex Reassignment, and Insurance Coverage in the U.S.A.*

World Professional Association for Transgender Health, 2016. Accessed August 21, 2022. https://www.wpath.org/newsroom/medical-necessity-statement.

Kulick, Don. "The Gender of Brazilian Transgendered Prostitutes." *American Anthropologist* 99, no. 3 (1997): 574–85.

———. *Travesti: Sex, Gender and Culture among Brazilian Transgendered Prostitutes*. Chicago, IL: University of Chicago Press, 1998.

Magerl, Gabriela. "Waria: A Third Gender in Indonesia." MA diss., University of Vienna, 2000.

Manalansan IV, Martin F. *Global Divas: Filipino Gay Men in the Diaspora*. Durham, NC: Duke University, 1995.

Marcos, Sylvia. "Beyond Binary Categories: Mesoamerican Religious Sexuality." In *Religion and Sexuality in Cross-Cultural Perspective*, edited by Stephen Ellingson and M. Christian Green, 111–36. New York: Routledge, 2002.

Matory, Lorand J. *Sex and the Empire That Is No More: Gender and the Politics of Metaphor in Oyo Yoruba Religion*. Minneapolis: University of Minnesota Press, 1994.

Murray, Stephen O. *Latin American Male Homosexualities*. Albuquerque: University of New Mexico, 1995.

Murray, Stephen O., and Will Roscoe. *Islamic Homosexualities: Cultures, History, and Literature*. New York: New York University, 1997.

Nanda, Serena. *Gender Diversity: Crosscultural Variations*. Long Grove, IL: Waveland Press, 2000.

———. *Love and Marriage: Cultural Diversity in a Changing World*. Long Grove, IL: Waveland Press, 2019.

———. *Neither Man nor Woman: The Hijras of India*. 2nd ed. Belmont, CA: Wadsworth, 1999.

Nanjundaswamy, S., and M. R. Gangadhar. *Transgender Challenges in India*. New Delhi: AAYU Publications, 2016.

Noor, Basittanti. "Transnational Love, Migration, and Kinship: Gay and Transgender Indonesians in the Netherlands and Belgium." MA diss., University of Amsterdam, 2012.

O'Flaherty, Wendy Doniger. *Siva: The Erotic Ascetic*. New York: Oxford University, 1973.

———. *Women, Androgynes and Other Mythical Beasts*. Chicago, IL: University of Chicago, 1980.

Paddock, Richard C., and Muktita Suhartono. "Indonesians Protest Bills that Would Limit Rights." *New York Times*, October 1, 2019, A7.

Parker, Richard. "'Within Four Walls': Brazilian Sexual Culture and HIV/AIDS." In *Culture, Society, and Sexuality*, edited by Richard Parker and Peter Aggleton, 253–66. London: UCL Press, 1999.

Peacock, James. *Rites of Modernization: Symbols and Social Aspects of Indonesian Proletarian Drama*. Chicago, IL: University of Chicago Press, 1988.

Peletz, Michael G. *Gender Pluralism: Southeast Asia Since Early Modern Times.* New York: Routledge, 2009.

Pelras, Christian. *The Bugis.* Oxford: Blackwell, 1996.

Reddy, Gayatri. "The Bonds of Companionate Marriage and the Desire for Intimacy Among Hijras in Hyderabad, India." In *Modern Loves: The Anthropology of Romantic Courtship and Companionate Marriage*, edited by Jennifer Hirsch and Holly Wardlow, 174–92. Ann Arbor: University of Michigan, 2006.

———. "Crossing 'Lines' of Difference: Transnational Movements and Sexual Subjectivities in Hyderabad, India." In *Everyday Life in South Asia*, 2nd ed, edited by Diane P. Mines and Sara Lamb, 132–43. Bloomington: University of Indiana, 2010.

———. *With Respect to Sex: Negotiating Hijra Identity in South India.* Chicago, IL: University of Chicago Press, 2005.

Ryan, J. Michael, ed. *Trans Lives in a Globalizing World: Rights, Identities, and Politics.* London: Routledge, 2020.

Said, Tanti Noor. "Fantasising Romance Overseas." *Inside Indonesia: The Peoples and Cultures of Indonesia.* October 5, 2013. Accessed August 6, 2024. https://www.insideindonesia.org/fantasising-romance-overseas.

Schultz, Kai. "Fighting for Equality in India While Nursing an 'Ache for Love.'" *New York Times*, November 23, 2019, A14.

Shore, Brad. "Sexuality and Gender in Samoa: Conceptions and Missed Conceptions." In *Sexual Meanings: The Cultural Construction of Gender and Sexuality*, edited by Sherry B. Ortner and Harriet Whitehead, 192–215. Cambridge: Cambridge University, 1981.

Toomistu, Terje. "Embodied Notions of Belonging: Practices of Beauty among Waria in West Papua, Indonesia." *Asian Studies Review* 43, no. 4 (2019): 581–99.

———. "Thinking through the S(k)in: Indonesian Waria and Bodily Negotiations of Belonging Across Religious Sensitivities." *Indonesia and the Malay World* 50, no. 146 (2022): 73–95.

Valentine, David. *Imagining Transgender: An Ethnography of a Category.* Durham, NC: Duke University, 2007.

Wafer, James. *The Taste of Blood: Spirit Possession in Brazilian Candomble.* Philadelphia: University of Pennsylvania, 1991.

Winter, Sam. "Transgender." In *The International Encyclopedia of Sexuality*, edited by Patricia Whelehan and Anne Bolin, 1385–89. New York: John Wiley and Sons, 2015.

Zwilling, L., and Michael Sweet. "The Evolution of Third Sex Constructs in Ancient India: A Study in Ambiguity." In *Constructing Ideologies: Religion, Gender, and Social Definition in India*, edited by Julia Leslie, 99–133. Delhi: Oxford University, 2000.

2

THE RISE OF SEXOLOGY IN EUROPE

Clayton J. Whisnant

Modern researchers of sexuality can trace an intellectual lineage that predates the anatomical work of the late Renaissance; these older debates among physicians focused on the role of men and women in procreation. By the seventeenth century, books and cheap pamphlets giving sex advice began to circulate in the market.[1] Although some of this literature could come off as celebrating sexual desire, much of it warned about the threat of venereal disease and the dangers of nonprocreative sexuality. The Dutch clinician Hermann Boerhaave counseled that excessive sexual activity could lead to the weakening of the body, including fevers, aches, bodily decay, and even blindness. The German physician Friedrich Hoffman suggested that masturbation, in particular, harmed the nervous system and could lead to memory loss. Even more famously, the Swiss physician Samuel-Auguste Tissot suggested in his influential book *L'Onanisme* (*Onanism*, 1760) that masturbation and all other forms of nonprocreative sex (including homosexuality) robbed the body of fluids necessary for the health and energy of the male body. The results included a long list of grim symptoms: coughs, fevers, headaches, pimples, constipation, impotence, and madness.[2]

This early medical work, in short, was very much part of a larger culture that exalted procreation as the only acceptable expression of sexuality on both health and moral grounds. It would take over a century for scientific ideas about sexuality to extricate themselves from the prevailing religious and moral assumptions on the topic. Many doctors, researchers, and psychiatrists during the nineteenth and early twentieth centuries harbored deep concerns about the dangers lurking in sexuality—particularly nonprocreative sexuality—as suggested by much of the language they used: contagion, seduction, degeneration, neurological weakness, perversion, and mania. Nevertheless, over time, lead researchers in the medical field made positive advances: they differentiated sexuality from procreation; they increasingly distinguished the psychic from the physical; and above all, they increasingly understood that what was perceived as unusual was not necessarily indicative of a diseased or unnatural person. Such advances emerged in the late nineteenth and early twentieth centuries alongside the field of sexology, which gradually separated itself from psychiatry. This newer field became an important contributor to international discussions about two phenomena that many sexologists considered synonymous: sexuality between members of the same sex and gender nonconformity.

EARLY MEDICAL WORK ON SODOMY AND CONTRARY SEXUAL FEELINGS

Some of the first physicians to concern themselves with men who had sex with other men were forensic experts. Beginning as early as the seventeenth century, medical experts in France and the German states were sometimes called on by courts to offer their opinion about whether disorderly sexual conduct had taken place, that is, rape and sodomy. In the case of sex between men, they focused on examining the anus of the defendants for signs that anal intercourse had taken place.[3] Ambroise Tardieu was one notable doctor still working in this tradition in Paris in the 1850s; *Étude medico-légale sur les attentats aux mœurs (Forensic Study on Offenses against Morals)*, 1857—one of his most prominent publications—chronicled two hundred such cases that he claimed to have examined. Like earlier doctors, Tardieu drew attention to signs of anal penetration, but he broke new ground when arguing that sodomy also changed the shape of the active partner's penis, leaving it long, thin, and often tapered, not unlike a dog's penis.[4]

By the latter half of the nineteenth century, though, there were also signs in Germany of a changing medical perspective toward sodomy. Another forensic expert, Johann Ludwig Casper, director of Brandenburg's School for State Medicine and senior medical counsel for the city of Berlin, took to task the older forensic manuals for disseminating largely useless information, particularly as it related to identifying a pederast.[5] Part of the issue was that many pederasts did not practice anal intercourse at all, instead preferring mutual masturbation or oral intercourse. In cases of sodomy, he suggested that a peculiar shape of the buttocks was often a better sign of anal penetration than the evidence on which many experts had been relying. What made his essay different from earlier works, though, was his reliance on a diary the city police had confiscated from one of Berlin's so-called pederasts, who Casper referred to as Count Cajus. This journal gave some insight into Berlin's gay milieu, which Casper described with "a picturesqueness that is lacking in the earlier forensic studies," as the historian Scott Spector observes. During this discussion, he made the off-hand comment that pederasty was perhaps in many cases inborn, the result of a pathological constitution that one could sense in the "feminine-childlike nature" supposedly on display in Count Cajus's diary.[6]

Casper was not alone in beginning to link what some would soon be calling *homosexual activity*—at least after the Hungarian writer Karl Maria Kertbeny coined the term in 1868—with an underlying psychological disposition. In a broader sense, many psychiatrists were seeking to tie psychological illness to a known origin. Since the Enlightenment, psychiatrists had been divided over these root causes. Scholars posited that a mental disorder was triggered by an emotional event; was the sign, perhaps, of a disordered or immoral lifestyle; or alternately, was the result of an illness of the nerves that might be eventually explained through anatomical investigations of the human brain.[7] By the middle of the nineteenth century, the latter school of thought was winning out, at least among many of the research and teaching institutions. The dominant figure was Wilhelm Griesinger, director of the University of Berlin's polyclinic and an outspoken advocate of the belief that brain abnormalities or other issues with the nervous system caused mental illnesses.[8]

In 1869, one of Griesinger's assistants at the polyclinic, Carl Westphal, published what is widely considered one of the most important early medical works on homosexuality, entitled *Contrary Sexual Feeling: Symptom of a Neuropathic (Psychopathic) Condition*. Westphal reported on two individuals he had treated: Miss N., who had been brought to the polyclinic by her sister in 1864, and Ha., a man the police arrested in 1868 while wearing women's clothing at a local train station.

From today's perspective, these two sad cases appear different in many ways. Miss N. strikes readers as a deeply depressed lesbian who had been grappling with her sexuality unsuccessfully since an early age. As she grew up, she frequently developed infatuations with young women who could not return her affection, creating awkward social situations and at times attracting cruel abuse from the people around her. Not surprisingly, she experienced horrible mood swings and occasional fits of rage. Her family was confused and unsure about how to handle her; eventually they took the step of sending her for treatment in a mental asylum.[9]

Westphal's second case involved someone who might identify today as a male-to-female transgender person. Ha. had operated at least some of his adult life as a thief and a con artist, and Westphal observed that it was hard to know how much to trust anything he said.[10] Nevertheless, Westphal concluded Ha. was not lying when he said he had felt a compulsion to dress as a woman since childhood. Biologically, his body was no different from other men: hairy, with a "greatly protruding larynx" and traces of a beard on his close-shaven face. Nevertheless, Westphal observed that Ha. exhibited an "almost feminine behavior," tinged perhaps with a certain aristocratic affectation, and he spoke "mostly with a lisp in feminine tone."[11] While staying in the hospital, he was "continually busy with women's handicrafts."[12] Over the years, he seemed to have developed relationships primarily with women, sometimes with the women for whom he worked as a domestic servant but also at times with prostitutes who taught him the ins and outs of living on the street. Ha. insisted he had "never let a man touch him and has never had sexual intercourse with one, although he had many offers in that respect."[13] It seems unlikely that Ha. completely avoided sexual relations with men since he made a living for a time as a street prostitute, accepting as many gifts as possible from his lovers and taking any opportunity that came along to rob his clients. Given that Westphal's physical exam turned up no signs of anal intercourse, perhaps Ha. meant that he never had been sodomized by a man but had performed other sexual acts with men.[14] Or perhaps he lied, not wanting to confess to something that was against the law and that Westphal might find abhorrent.

Westphal felt that both Ha. and Miss N. suffered from a pathological condition: a moral insanity, indeed "a congenital inversion of the sexual feeling" that led a man to "feel like a woman, and a woman like a man."[15] Drawing a parallel conclusion based on these two cases seems a little surprising. Miss N. sometimes dreamed of being a man and reported playing boys' games when she was younger, but otherwise she did not report a compelling sense of actually being a man in the way Ha. felt he was a woman. And Ha. stated several times that he didn't feel sexual desire for men, whereas Miss N. was almost overwhelmed by her desire for other women. Through the lens of a present-day perspective, Westphal's diagnosis clearly conflates two separate issues, namely sexual desire for a member of one's sex and the feeling of having a gender identity different from the sex one is born into.

Why did Westphal nonetheless believe he was dealing with the same condition? At some level, as the classicist and queer theorist David Halperin once suggested, he was no doubt influenced by his wider culture: "Westphal, like many of his contemporaries, did not distinguish systematically between sexual deviance and gender deviance, and an identification with the opposite sex sometimes expressed itself as a feeling of sexual attraction to members of one's own sex."[16] Westphal also knew about Casper's earlier essay, which had intimated a possible connection between male same-sex attraction and femininity. A close reading of Westphal's text suggests that he was especially influenced in his thinking by a booklet[17] written by a certain Numa Numantius. This name was a pseudonym famously used by Karl Heinrich Ulrichs, remembered today as the world's first gay activist.

Karl Heinrich Ulrichs wasn't a scientist, but his work would ultimately have an enormous impact on sexology. Ulrichs had started a promising career as a civil servant in the North German kingdom of Hannover in the 1850s, but his prospects had been cut short by a rumor that he had been having sexual liaisons with lower-class men. In the early 1860s, he began to publish a series of studies on "the riddle of male-male love,"[18] first under the pseudonym Numa Numantius. In 1867, he was arrested for participating in demonstrations against Prussia, which was taking the lead in uniting Germany underneath its monarch. During the search of his house, his books were discovered and his identity as Numa Numantius exposed. Ulrichs didn't give up writing, though; he went on to publish another seven books under his own name over the next decade, with the last, *Critische Pfeile (Critical Arrows)* appearing in 1879.[19]

Ulrichs's small books were wide ranging, encompassing legal arguments, historical reflections, ethnographic descriptions, discussions of current events, reproductions of letter exchanges he had had with other homosexual men, and even philosophical meditations on issues connected with same-sex desire.[20] He is most remembered, however, for his argument that same-sex desire manifested in some people as the result of blending masculine and feminine qualities during embryonic development. The Urning (as he called a man who loved another man) was a kind of feminine being not simply because he felt sexual desire for other men, but because this femininity affected "his entire organism"—his behavior, his interests, his talents, and his attitude toward the world.[21] Famously, he described the Urning as a third sex, a female psyche (or soul) contained in a male body. The Urning (and also the Urningin, as he called a woman who loved another woman) reflected the original hermaphroditism of the entire human species, an early stage of embryonic development that most people outgrew, yet through an accident of nature occasionally left traces in some individuals' psyche. The embryonic development that produced an Urning was not a disability or a physical illness, Ulrichs insisted, but simply a natural variation.

THE FOUNDATION AND GROWTH OF SEXOLOGY

By the time Ulrichs published his last work in 1879, same-sex desire was beginning to attract attention, not only among psychiatrists but also from a wider public of educated readers. What Westphal had called *contrary sexual feeling* was translated into Italian in 1878 as sexual inversion and from there rendered into French, English, and many other languages.[22] Well into the twentieth century, this term jockeyed with *homosexual* for being the most popular term to describe same-sex desire, with the latter only really winning out in the 1920s.

For a time, sexual inversion (along with contrary sexual feeling, which didn't entirely disappear in Germany) carried with it the idea advocated by Casper, Ulrichs, and Westphal that same-sex desire was the manifestation of a larger gender inversion. By the turn of the twentieth century, notable authors (such as the German writer Hans Blüher) insisted that effeminate homosexuals might only be a subcategory of sexual inverts. Only in the 1920s did medical writers begin to more clearly differentiate sexuality from other behaviors associated with gender roles.

The growing influence of Freudian psychoanalysis was no doubt important in allowing people to differentiate sexual object choice from sex role, but significant transformations in the wider culture also played a part.[23] In Germany, the emergence of a visible homosexual rights movement after World War I, led by men who would publicly challenge stereotypes of the effeminate fairy (*Tunte*, literally aunt), might have impacted medical thinking.[24]

The interest in sexual inversion turned out to be one aspect of a larger preoccupation with sexuality during the 1890s. Arguably, this preoccupation was more prominent in the German-speaking world than elsewhere. A complex interaction between worries about the consequences of modernization and urbanization, on the one hand, and an explosion of reform-minded political activism on the other helped fuel a sort of political intervention to reify the meaning of sex for the nation. Moral purity groups organized to protect a traditional conception of the family and to keep sexuality restricted to procreation and married relationships. They were opposed by organizations such as the Scientific-Humanitarian Committee, the German Society for the Fight against Venereal Disease, and the League for the Protection of Mothers and Sex Reform that sought to free understandings of sexuality from a traditional religious framework and, in most cases, to fundamentally change relations between the sexes. These latter groups proved to be an important instrument for disseminating some of the new ideas being produced by physicians, psychiatrists, and other researchers about sexuality. Furthermore, they also allowed a number of people who lacked the usual academic pedigree, including a growing number of women, to contribute to sexological debates.[25]

White male professionals generally dominated sexology, though, especially once the field began to coalesce just before World War I. In Germany and Austria, a century of generous state and private investment into various institutions of scientific research (universities, hospitals, professional organizations, research institutes, and journals) bolstered the sociocultural authority of science. Simultaneously, such investment yielded an army of underemployed physicians who often got creative when it came to establishing "niches where they could claim specialized knowledge and authority," as historian Kirsten Leng has recently put it.[26] The rapidly emerging profession of sexology was a clear beneficiary in Germany and Austria, acquiring an academic legitimacy unparalleled in other areas of Europe.

The first generation of sexologists targeted so-called sexual perversity as their primary topic of interest. Widely considered as the father of sexology, Richard von Krafft-Ebing was one of the most influential psychiatrists in the world by the 1890s, known for his vast taxonomy of different kinds of "perversions." For a time, he became one of Austria's most famous exponents of the theory of degeneration, which held that the demands of modern civilization were producing a deterioration of the nervous system. His most important work was *Psychopathia Sexualis*, which outlined his whole catalog of sexual disorders and degenerative diseases.[27]

First published in 1886, *Psychopathia Sexualis* included descriptions of a vast number of cases Krafft-Ebing observed in years of practice, beginning in an asylum in the 1860s and ending with a prestigious university professorship and a private psychiatric practice in Vienna. *Psychopathia Sexualis* grew drastically in length over the years as more and more cases were added to its ever-growing taxonomy; the text eventually came out in its twelfth edition shortly after Krafft-Ebing's death in 1902.

When it came to sexual desire between two people of the same sex, by the 1889 edition Krafft-Ebing was differentiating between inborn and acquired forms of homosexuality. He also acknowledged that there were men and women whose sexual drive was aimed at members of the same sex but who otherwise showed no signs of gender inversion—a departure from the early understandings of sexual inversion, which conflated same-sex desire with absolute gender inversion. He also described several cases of "psychic hermaphrodites," individuals identifiable today as bisexuals.[28]

Looking at his talk of perversions and degeneration, historians of sexuality have tended to demonize Krafft-Ebing as one of the foremost scholars to pathologize sexuality, a view that held sway between roughly 1860 and 1970. However, the historian Harry Oosterhuis has recently suggested a more complicated understanding of Krafft-Ebing's work and influence. The lengthy case histories included in *Psychopathia Sexualis* were read avidly by many people of his time who in the present day might identify as sexual or gender nonconforming; they often found the diverse perspectives and voices in the book immensely comforting. Krafft-Ebing listened attentively and sympathetically to these voices, as demonstrated by his gradually shifting theories and taxonomy to account for information that didn't fit into his early system. While he continued to believe homosexuality was rooted in an abnormal nervous system, Krafft-Ebing developed a surprisingly eclectic range of methods in his private practice to help his patients work through their emotional difficulties. By the end of his life, he was coming around to the idea that contrary sexual feeling might not be a disease, but simply a condition. Ultimately, Krafft-Ebing came to oppose Europe's laws punishing homosexuality, an opinion informed not just by his own research but also by Karl Heinrich Ulrichs's extensive scholarship and writings.[29]

Psychopathia Sexualis was immensely influential. The content resonated strongly at the turn of the century in an intellectual climate of avant-garde writers, artists, and philosophers. These visionaries were preoccupied with uncovering the irrational impulses of mankind, criticizing the hypocritical values of institutional religion and bourgeois society, and championing the sexual drives that seemed to embody vitality, nature, and spirit. When it came specifically to sexual inversion, the avant-garde sometimes found the theory's association with blurred gender lines useful. This connection allowed them to resurrect the centuries-old symbol of the androgyne, with united masculinity and femininity symbolizing the healing of a fractured world. Or, alternately, gender fluidity could reflect a world in transition, a central theme of much fin-de-siècle literature and art.[30]

Under such intellectual influence, many works of the time explored a concept of sexual intermediaries. An important one was Otto Weininger's 1903 *Geschlecht und Character* (*Sex and Character*), which imagined masculine and feminine as psychological ideals that could be found in different proportions in all people. Describing both almost as metaphysical principles, Weininger identified femininity with sexuality, emotionality, and reproduction as well as chaos. Masculinity, on the other hand, was supposedly rational, achievement oriented, ordered, and creative. He argued that all people possessed aspects of both ideals, though some people exhibited more of an affinity for one element. Most women, not surprisingly, possessed more femininity than masculinity, but so did male homosexuals and Jews. All people, he thought, had an instinct toward balance that led them to fall in love with individuals whose proportion of masculinity and femininity complemented their own.[31]

From a twenty-first–century queer perspective, this idea of blended genders might sound modern. On a personal level, though, Weininger—being both homosexual and Jewish—was clearly haunted by the femininity he sensed within himself. Not long after his book was published, he shot himself in the chest and passed away in one of Vienna's hospitals.[32]

Weininger's work had no real scientific foundation. Nonetheless, it was widely read and discussed by an educated public, further promoting a discourse related to the genetics of sexuality. Not a few found it intriguing that much scientific research involving heredity and hormones seemed to verify the idea that sexual intermediaries might represent a natural state and that everyone in fact might carry traces of an original biological and perhaps also psychological hermaphroditism.

One such scientist who attracted public attention was Eugen Steinach, an endocrinologist who taught at the University of Prague before becoming a research director at Vienna's prestigious Academy of Science. During the 1910s and 1920s, a flurry of research into hormones took place, and Steinach played a prominent role, thanks in part to his penchant for self-promotion. In 1912, the year he moved to Vienna, he reported on a study with guinea pigs that involved transplanting a female ovary into a male animal. When the rodent developed milk-producing nipples and failed to experience further physical development or penis growth, Steinach had demonstrated a difference between the male and female sex hormones. A subsequent experiment on a female rat that received a male testis had a similar result: the rat seemed to develop a penis and its bark became noticeably more masculine. Steinach also noticed changes in behavior. The male animal that received an ovary acted like a mother and tried to suckle babies. The female with a testis responded to a female in heat and pursued her.[33]

Naturally, it didn't take long for sexologists to suspect that Steinach had finally uncovered the biological cause of homosexuality. Steinach himself suggested this claim in a series of studies. In one case, he examined the testicular tissue of a homosexual and claimed to have found abnormalities: atrophied tissue, degeneration in certain areas, and large cells (so-called F cells) not normally present.

A urologist from Vienna asked Steinach to assist him with what was essentially an early version of hormone conversion therapy involving the transplant of a donor testis into the body of a homosexual whose own testes had to be removed because of tuberculosis. Afterward, the man told the doctors his homosexual tendencies disappeared, and he experienced a heterosexual sex drive.[34] Hormone therapy (made easier in 1930s when hormones could be synthetically produced) would remain a popular medical recommendation through the 1950s, despite growing evidence since the 1930s that hormone therapy—at its best—could dull the sex drive but not fundamentally change someone's sexual orientation.[35]

Steinach's research received broader public acclaim during the early 1920s thanks to the wide release of a film dramatizing his work. One of the so-called enlightenment films of Weimar Germany—cinema that purported to have educational purposes for discussing sexuality but was often highly sensationalist and sometimes even slightly pornographic—the *Steinachfilm* (*Steinach Film*) explained the basics of endocrinal biology and suggested some of the possible effects of hormonal imbalances. It juxtaposed images of guinea pigs that Steinach had operated on with an intersex individual who had both breasts and a penis. It also included a scene in which Steinach assisted with transplanting a testis into the abdomen of a homosexual patient.[36] The public took notice, but interestingly, many psychiatrists were surprisingly slow to acknowledge Steinach's research, a fact that might be explained by the disciplinary divisions and professional rivalries that existed between them and endocrinologists like Steinach. Sexologists, in contrast, who were just establishing their own professional institutions and authority, were immediately excited about the explanatory power and therapeutic possibilities suggested by Steinach's studies.[37]

Sexology was indeed rapidly developing as a profession, reaching a watershed moment as early as 1908 when Magnus Hirschfeld founded *Die Zeitschrift für Sexualwissenschaft* (The Journal of Sexual Science) and Max Marcuse established *Sexual-Probleme* (Sexual Problems), the first two journals of the profession. By this time, sexologists were making a concerted effort to broaden the themes that sexology addressed beyond "perversions."[38] Soon the sexological community would be also heavily engaged with issues connected to venereal disease, sexually fulfilling relationships, healthy reproduction, hereditary illnesses, eugenics, birth control, and sex roles.

Sexual inversion remained a focal point for much research and discussion, for instance, the continued debate about the criminalization of homosexuality, as well as increased visibility of gay men, lesbians, and other gender nonconforming individuals in many of Europe's major cities. Both topics remained controversial issues, especially in 1920s Germany where debate around sexual inversion was wrapped up with anxieties about national weakness after a lost war and an overthrown monarchy. Sexologists found themselves divided politically. Progressives aligned themselves with Magnus Hirschfeld and Iwan Bloch's Medical Society for Sexual Science and Eugenics and, by the end of the 1920s, with the World League for Sexual Reform. More politically conservative scientists, who saw themselves as defending scientific objectivity from political bias, joined Albert Moll and Max Marcuse's International Society for Sex Research.[39] In contrast with the progressives who tended to defend the idea that sexual inversion was natural and inborn, conservatives such as Moll and Emil Kraepelin worried about the role of seduction, especially in cities such as Berlin where gay scenes were more visible than ever and where gay publications were sold openly in kiosks.[40]

HAVELOCK ELLIS'S CONTRIBUTIONS: NONPATHOLOGICAL INVERSION AND EONISM

While sexology grew rapidly as a profession in Germany and Austria, in Britain it was much slower to take root. Ignored by most British psychiatrists as a dubious continental import that showed a morbid fascination for repulsive subjects, sexology was taken up initially by a group of amateur scientists motivated largely by progressive social and legal goals.[41] These early British sexologists were generally marginal figures or, like Havelock Ellis, just beginning their careers.

Ellis obtained his medical training during the 1880s while also writing for progressive journals, translating scientific works into English, and keeping up productive relationships with a small group of promising intellectuals and artists in London, nearly all of them free thinkers and socialist sympathizers.[42] In 1891, just as he was beginning his professional career, Ellis began exchanging letters with John Addington Symonds, a poet and writer who had made a name for himself with his study of Renaissance Italy. Symonds ascertained Ellis's views toward same-sex love by questioning Ellis's opinion of Walt Whitman; he eventually proposed a joint study of sexual inversion that would take advantage of Ellis's knowledge and physician's credentials and would also include a section on history that could draw on Symonds's study of "Greek Love." Ellis was interested in part because of his close friendship with the pioneering homosexual activist Edward Carpenter but also because his wife had, early in their marriage, confessed her love for another woman.[43] Unfortunately, Symonds died suddenly from the flu in 1893 when their work was only in its formative stage. Symonds's contribution was consequently minimal, but their book was nevertheless published, first in 1896 with a German publisher as *Die konträre Geschlechtsgefühl,* and then a year later in English as *Sexual Inversion.*[44]

In many ways, *Sexual Inversion* seems at first glance rather timid, as Ellis did not seek out controversy or opportunities for self-promotion as some of his German counterparts did. While he incorporated a large number of case histories, Ellis received many of them secondhand, with the result that the writing lacked the intimacy of Krafft-Ebing's stories in *Psychopathia Sexualis*. Moreover, as his biographer Phyllis Grosskurth observes, Ellis's tendency to trust his sources at face value meant his work fell short of the probing intensity or flashes of insight that made Sigmund Freud's case studies famous.[45] Much of *Sexual Inversion* was devoted to simply covering the theories of sexology currently circulating in Germany. In the end, Ellis clearly sided with the argument that, in most cases, sexual inversion was a congenital condition.

Over the course of their correspondence, Ellis and Symonds routinely traded ideas on the topic of sexology. Ellis made it clear that sexual inversion as a congenital condition offered a stronger argument for legal reform, even if there might also be, as Symonds seemed to believe, some subtle social and cultural factors at work in shaping sex and gender identity.[46] Symonds had also expressed doubts about whether most male sexual inverts were effeminate, but in this early text Ellis deferred to scientific consensus: "It must be said that there is a distinctly general, though not universal, tendency for sexual inverts to approach the feminine type, either in psychic disposition or physical condition."[47] Like the German sexologists he tended to rely on, he suggested that inversion could be explained by "the latent organic bi-sexuality in each sex."[48]

Despite these similarities between *Sexual Inversion* and other sexological studies of the time, two aspects make Ellis's research remarkable. First, no doubt because of Ellis's experience with his wife, he devotes much more attention to female homosexuality than any writer had at this point. Admittedly, it was a small chapter, including only four cases, but still, he was able to make a strong case that female homosexuality was more widespread than most people assumed, yet it remained hidden from the public eye by some combination of ignorance and indifference.[49] The second aspect worth mentioning is Ellis's insistence on denying that there is anything pathological about sexual inversion. Next to Magnus Hirschfeld, who also published his first work in 1896, Ellis was the only figure in the medical community at the time willing to take this stand. This stance is easy to miss today since he also used off-putting terms such as *abnormal, aberration,* and *deviation* in his research. He made it explicit that his use of the term *abnormality* did not signify disease (and certainly not degeneration, which he criticized at some length) but simply an unusual variation, "one of those organic aberrations which we see throughout living nature, in plants and in animals."[50]

Sexual Inversion turned out to be just the first installment in the massive series *Studies in the Psychology of Sex*, which Ellis published over the next thirty years. In these studies, he developed his core belief that even abnormal behavior was rooted in nature. In an 1897 essay, he developed the concept of autoeroticism by which he meant not simply masturbation but more broadly "the phenomena of spontaneous sexual emotion generated in the absence of an external stimulus proceeding from another person." It therefore also included spontaneous erections, erotic dreams, and nocturnal emissions.[51]

One gets the sense that with autoeroticism, Ellis believed he was dealing with sexual impulse in its most stripped-down form—the sexual drive before it had become attached to a particular object. Remarkable to him was how many activities could exhibit aspects of autoeroticism for certain individuals: dancing, urinating, finger sucking, and so on. Ellis subsequently concluded that sexual desires were highly individualized.[52]

Variation also marked courtship rituals, evidenced in nature among diverse animal species, but that took on increasingly complex forms when manifested in human society. Ellis proposed that displays of power and giving or experiencing pain (for example, when one animal bites another during copulation) might explain the origins of sadism and masochism.[53] The role of symbolism in courtship might explain cases such as fetishism, that is, when an object or act becomes the central focus of sexual attraction.[54] The radical conclusion that one can draw from this study is easy to miss yet quite astounding when put simply: as Ivan Crozier states, "all sex acts are artificial manifestations of the sexual impulse, and in such a way all sexual acts are as abnormal or as normal as the rest, once moral dogma and legal sanctioning are removed from the equation."[55]

Ellis was working at an extraordinarily interesting time. The turn of the century witnessed what some call the birth of sexual liberalism or even sexual modernity.[56] On a more fundamental level, it was a time when understandings of the mind underwent a radical reworking. As the historian H. Stuart Hughes once observed, a number of thinkers across a surprisingly diverse group of disciplines began to ask questions about the nature of knowledge and consciousness, probing the role irrational forces and social influences played in mental operations. American pragmatists, British anthropologists, Austrian psychoanalysts, German sociologists, and French philosophers and novelists all made contributions to our evolving view of the mind, and Ellis's lifelong tendency to read widely and avidly made him perhaps more able than some to participate in this conversation.[57] Already, with his essay on erotic symbolism, there was potential for Ellis to acknowledge that the mind could become radically unmoored from the body. Arguably, this line of thinking led to its radical conclusion in his 1920s work on *Eonism*, his suggested term for those today known as transgender people. As a term, *Eonism* would remain in use among some medical and psychiatric professionals through the mid-twentieth century.

Psychiatrists before Ellis had documented cases of individuals who identified with members of the opposite sex; however, they typically categorized these individuals as homosexuals, as seen with Westphal's early case involving Ha. in 1869. Only in 1910 did Magnus Hirschfeld begin to differentiate these individuals in his work *Die Transvestiten* (*The Transvestites*), which defined crossdressing as a distinct phenomenon from homosexuality, although still an aspect along a broader spectrum of sexual intermediaries. Hirschfeld inspired many other scientists to look at similar cases with fresh eyes, though they could not agree initially on what to call the phenomenon: transsensible, transmutist, psychic hermaphroditism, or simply the drive to cross-dress (*Verkleidungstrieb*).[58]

In 1913, Ellis offered his own initial suggestion: *sexo-aesthetic inversion*, a term he thought better captured "the main characteristic of these people—the impulse to project themselves by sympathetic feeling into the object to which they are attracted, or the impulse of inner imitation."[59] Over time, he began to reconsider this suggestion, fearing that using inversion in this instance might cause confusion with *sexual* inversion, which, both he and Hirschfeld agreed, was a distinct phenomenon. He found limited cases involving homosexuality, but he was unsure whether the homosexuality in these instances wasn't merely an accidental byproduct of the psychic state.[60] Actually, what he found most interesting was how many individuals reported experiencing a negligible sexual impulse throughout their lives.

By the 1920s, Ellis was leaning toward a second option, Eonism, which he took from the famous case of the Chevalière d'Eon, the eighteenth-century nobleman who "adopted feminine dress on his own initiative and became commonly regarded as a woman."[61] In one of his characteristic moves, Ellis tried to relate Eonism to natural phenomena by suggesting it "may possibly represent not, as we might have been tempted to suppose, a corrupt or over-refined manifestation of late cultures, but the survival of an ancient and natural tendency of more primitive man."[62] He offered the example of a chieftain's daughter living on an island in the Torres strait near New Guinea. Growing up, the daughter had played with boys and refused for a long time to wear girls' clothing. "She now works in the garden man-fashion," Ellis observed, "using heavy digging sticks, and carried burdens man-fashion."[63] Although expressing itself most conspicuously as cross-dressing, Eonism was not simply a variant of fetishism, as some other psychiatrists suspected. In its most complete form, "the subject so identifies himself with those of his physical and psychic traits which recall the opposite sex that he feels really to belong to that sex, although he has no delusion regarding his anatomical conformation."[64]

CONCLUSION

Michel Foucault famously wrote in 1976 that the "nineteenth-century homosexual became a personage, a past, a case history, and a childhood, in addition to being a type of life, a life form, and a morphology. . . . The sodomite had been a temporary aberration; the homosexual was now a species."[65] With the emergence of the modern homosexual identity, Foucault emphasized the importance of scientific writings (especially medical and psychiatric) on homosexuality.[66] Today, historians of sexuality don't place quite as much weight on sexology's power to shape understandings of sexual identity.

Medical works about sexual inversion no doubt played an important role in shaping how the broader public perceived issues connected with same-sex desire and gender nonconformity; however, historians have cautioned against exaggerating the power that these scientific works had on society. The wider public, influenced by some blend of religion, tradition, and prejudice, often approached the new science of sexuality with a fair degree of skepticism, if not hostility.[67] Even when reading the medical literature on sexuality, the public always contextualized what it read, meaning that wider social and culture changes were important. Furthermore, individuals were known to pick and choose what they understood and remembered based on their own experiences and needs.[68] Scientists were not writing in a vacuum either; their medical sources responded to particular sociocultural contexts or preexisting identities and subcultures, as seen in Casper and Westphal.

While much of the literature focuses on the broader societal impacts of the emergent sexology field, it would be remiss to omit the effects on people who were the object of study—those associated with the theory of sexual inversion. There are many known instances of people (who today would identify with the LGBTQ community) who read this scientific material and found their lives transformed by the experience.[69] J. R. Ackerley, a successful British writer of the 1920s and 1930s, was just one. After reading the works of Edward Carpenter and Otto Weininger, he remembered feeling that "I was now on the sexual map and proud of my place on it."[70] But despite the influence of this work, LGBTQ individuals had a range of sources—from ancient history to more recent Romantic literature and poetry—to draw on as they fashioned some sense of their selves and their sexuality.[71]

Ultimately, sexology was an important scientific development, and by the 1920s it boasted a remarkable set of achievements: new professional institutions and publications, a list of remarkably creative thinkers, and a body of ideas about sexuality that were becoming increasingly complex and refined. In the process, the medical and scientific community, as well as the broader public, increasingly understood two key concepts: first, sexuality played a distinct role in human life beyond procreation; and second, the psychic life, although still often linked in close ways to the body, possessed its own independent logic and development. And finally, thinkers like Havelock Ellis and Magnus Hirschfeld (who is a topic in the next chapter), asserted that unusual sexual desires and behaviors might not be pathological.

It would be some time before the majority of the medical and psychiatric profession came around to this position. Many sexologists during the 1920s remained conservative toward nonnormative forms of sexual and gender behavior and expression. From today's perspective, even the works of such progressive thinkers as Havelock Ellis and Magnus Hirschfeld can be off-putting and limited in scope, given their highly medicalized ways of discussing matters—not to mention their Darwinian thinking, fascination with eugenics, and racist assumptions.[72] After World War II, the ideas of Ellis and Hirschfeld would be eclipsed by psychoanalysis, which was only then entering its international heyday, and by the more sociologically based sexology pioneered by Alfred Kinsey in the United States.

NOTES

1. Clark, *Desire: A History of European Sexuality*, 103–04; Porter and Hall, *The Facts of Life*, 33–90.
2. Bullough, *Science in the Bedroom*, 19–21.
3. Oosterhuis, *Stepchildren of Nature*, 38.
4. Davidson, *The Emergence of Sexuality*, 119–20.
5. Müller, "Johann Ludwig Casper," 29–31.
6. Spector, *Violent Sensations*, 82–5.
7. Porter, "Mental Illness," 244–49; Shorter, *A History of Psychiatry*, 26–32.
8. Shorter, *A History of Psychiatry*, 73–6.
9. Westphal, "Contrary Sexual Feelings," 88–96.
10. I will use masculine pronouns in this passage since they are the pronouns that Westphal used in the source and also what most people at the time would have used to refer to Ha., even though there is reason to believe that Ha. might have preferred the feminine pronouns.
11. Westphal, "Contrary Sexual Feelings," 96.
12. Westphal, "Contrary Sexual Feelings," 102.
13. Westphal, "Contrary Sexual Feelings," 98. Westphal used the male pronoun in the original.
14. And as Casper had already pointed out, anal exams are not a reliable way to detect anal intercourse.
15. Westphal, "Contrary Sexual Feelings," 88, 107.
16. Halperin, *How to Do the History of Homosexuality*, 128.
17. Karl Heinrich Ulrichs, as Numantius, wrote and published twelve booklets between 1864 and 1879. See Ulrichs, *The Riddle of "Man-Manly" Love*.
18. *The Riddle of Male Male Love* is the subtitle of Ulrich's sixth book, *Gladius Furens*. See Ulrichs, *The Riddle of "Man-Manly" Love*, Vol. 1, 259.
19. Beachy, *Gay Berlin*, 3–41. For a recent thorough study that analyzes Ulrich's contribution in terms of its intellectual environment, see Leck, *Vita Sexualist*.
20. Ulrichs, *The Riddle of "Man-Manly" Love*.
21. Ulrichs, *The Riddle of "Man-Manly" Love*, vol. 1, 36. The German word *Urning* is sometimes rendered as "Uranian" in English.
22. Beccalossi, *Female Sexual Inversion*, 52.
23. The first and enormously influential essay that differentiated between object choice and sex roles for historians of sexuality was George Chauncey, "From Sexual Inversion to Homosexuality."
24. See Whisnant, *Queer Identities and Politics in Germany*, 162–202.
25. For more information on some of the important women in these organizations, see Leng, *Sexual Politics and Feminist Science*.

26. Leng, *Sexual Politics and Feminist Science*, 47.
27. The most important study of Krafft-Ebing is Oosterhuis, *The Stepchildren of Nature*. For a shorter summary of his life and work, see Whisnant, *Queer Identities and Politics*, 24–27.
28. An English version of the twelfth edition is available as Krafft-Ebing, *Psychopathia Sexualis*.
29. Oosterhuis, *The Stepchildren of Nature*, 152–73.
30. Whisnant, *Queer Identities and Politics*, 130–34.
31. Weininger, *Sex and Character*.
32. An excellent study of Weininger that analyzes his work as part of his historical milieu is Sengoopta, *Otto Weininger*.
33. Benjamin, "Eugen Steinach," 432–33.
34. Sengoopta, *Secret Quintessence of Life*, 78–80.
35. LeVay, *Queer Science*, 109–13.
36. Beachy, *Gay Berlin*, 173–74.
37. Sutton, *Sex Between Body and Mind*, 120–21.
38. Sutton, *Sex Between Body and Mind*, 5–6.
39. Sigusch, "The Sexologist Albert Moll," 193–95.
40. For more information on Berlin's gay scene in the 1920s, see Whisnant, *Queer Identities and Politics in Germany*, 80–120; Beachy, *Gay Berlin*, 187–219.
41. Porter and Hall, *The Facts of Life*, 158.
42. Grosskurth, *Havelock Ellis*, 48–71.
43. Grosskurth, *Havelock Ellis*, 154–55.
44. Crozier, "Introduction," 57–60.
45. Grosskurth, *Havelock Ellis*, 232–35.
46. Crozier, "Introduction," 50–52.
47. Ellis and Symonds, *Sexual Inversion*, 192.
48. Bisexuality, in this case, should be taken to mean possessing characteristics of both genders, as opposed to referring specifically to the orientation of the sexual drive. Ellis and Symonds, *Sexual Inversion*, 202.
49. Ellis and Symonds, *Sexual Inversion*, 161.
50. Ellis and Symonds, *Sexual Inversion*, 203. See also Bullough, *Science in the Bedroom*, 81.
51. Havelock Ellis, *Studies in the Psychology of Sex*, vol. 1, part 1, 161.
52. Crozier, "Introduction," 27.
53. Grosskurth, *Havelock Ellis*, 225.
54. Ellis, *Studies in the Psychology of Sex*, vol. 2, part 1, 1.
55. Crozier, "Introduction," 33.
56. For more information, see Leck, *Vita Sexualis*; Jeffrey Weeks, *Sexuality and Its Discontents*; Brecher, *The Sex Researchers*; Robinson, *The Modernization of Sex*.

57. The classic work on this evolving view of the mind is Hughes, *Consciousness and Society*.

58. Sutton, *Sex between Body and Mind*, 177. One noteworthy case was reported by the German sexologist Max Marcuse. His study told of a man who, having read about experiments on changing the sex of deer, inquired whether a sex change operation might be possible. See Marcuse, "Ein Fall von Geschlechtsumwandlungstrieb."

59. Ellis, *Studies in the Psychology of Sex*, vol. 2, part 2, 27.

60. Ellis, *Studies in the Psychology of Sex*, vol. 2, part 2, 101.

61. Ellis, *Studies in the Psychology of Sex*, vol. 2, part 2, 2.

62. Ellis, *Studies in the Psychology of Sex*, vol. 2, part 2, 33.

63. Ellis, *Studies in the Psychology of Sex*, vol. 2, part 2, 33.

64. Ellis, *Studies in the Psychology of Sex*, vol. 2, part 2, 36.

65. Foucault, *The History of Sexuality*, vol. 1, 43.

66. For another early work based on the Foucault thesis, see Weeks, *Coming Out*.

67. Lots of evidence of this skepticism can be found in Porter and Hall, *The Facts of Life*, 155–77.

68. Some important works that consider the limitations of the Foucault thesis are Oosterhuis, *Stepchildren of Nature*; Chauncey, *Gay New York*; Doan, *Fashioning Sapphism*; and Spector, Puff, and Herzog, eds. *After the History of Sexuality*.

69. Although there are many versions of this abbreviation that are currently circulating, LGBTQ (or sometimes LGBTQ+) seems to be the alternative that is becoming widely used in academia, so that is what I will use for this publication.

70. Ackerley, *My Father and Myself*, 118. For other examples, see Doan, *Fashioning Sapphism*; Marhoefer, *Sex and the Weimar Republic*; and Oosterhuis, *Stepchildren of Nature*.

71. See, for example, Whisnant, *Queer Identities and Politics*, 122–61.

72. For more on the information on the role of eugenics, racism, and social Darwinism in the works of Magnus Hirschfeld, see Herzer, *Magnus Hirschfeld*.

WORKS CITED

Ackerley, J. R. *My Father and Myself*. New York: Harcourt Brace Jovanovich, 1968.

Beachy, Robert. *Gay Berlin: Birthplace of a Modern Identity*. New York: Alfred A. Knopf, 2014.

Beccalossi, Chiara. *Female Sexual Inversion: Same-Sex Desires in Italian and British Sexology, c. 1870–1920*. Basingstoke: Palgrave Macmillan, 2012.

Benjamin, Harry. "Eugen Steinach, 1861–1944: A Life of Research." *Scientific Monthly* 61, no. 6 (December 1945): 427–42.

Brecher, Edward. *The Sex Researchers*. Boston, MA: Little Brown, 1969.

Bullough, Vern. *Science in the Bedroom: A History of Sex Research*. New York: Basic Books, 1994.

Chauncey, George. "From Sexual Inversion to Homosexuality: Medicine and the Changing Conception of Female Deviance." *Salmagundi* 58/59 (Fall 1982–Winter 1983): 114–46.

———. *Gay New York: Gender, Urban Culture, and the Making of the Gay Male World, 1890–1940*. New York: Basic Books, 1994.

Clark, Anna. *Desire: A History of European Sexuality*. New York: Routledge, 2008.

Crozier, Ivan. "Introduction: Havelock Ellis, John Addington Symonds and the Construction of Sexual Inversion." In *Sexual Inversion: A Critical Edition*, edited by Havelock Ellis and John Addington Symonds, 1–86. Basingstoke: Palgrave Macmillan, 2008.

Davidson, Arnold I. *The Emergence of Sexuality: Historical Epistemology and the Formation of Concepts*. Cambridge, MA: Harvard University Press, 2001.

Doan, Laura. *Fashioning Sapphism: The Origins of a Modern English Lesbian Culture*. New York: Columbia University Press, 2001.

Ellis, Havelock. *Studies in the Psychology of Sex*. 2 vols. New York: Random House, 1942.

Ellis, Havelock, and John Addington Symonds. *Sexual Inversion: A Critical Edition*, edited by Ivan Crozier. Basingstoke: Palgrave Macmillan, 2008.

Foucault, Michel. *The History of Sexuality, Vol. 7, An Introduction*. Translated by Robert Hurley. New York: Vintage, 1978.

Grosskurth, Phyllis. *Havelock Ellis: A Biography*. New York: Alfred A. Knopf, 1980.

Halperin, David M. *How to Do the History of Homosexuality*. Chicago, IL: University of Chicago Press, 2002.

Manfred Herzer. *Magnus Hirschfeld: Leben und Werk eines jüdischen, schwulen und sozialistischen Sexologen*. Frankfurt: Campus-Verlag, 1992.

Hughes, H. Stuart. *Consciousness and Society: The Reorientation of European Social Thought 1890–1930*. New York: Vintage Books, 1961.

Krafft-Ebing, Richard von. *Psychopathia Sexualis*. Translated by Harry E. Wedeck. New York: G. P. Putnam's Sons, 1965.

Leck, Ralph M. *Vita Sexualis: Karl Ulrichs and the Origins of Sexual Science*. Urbana: University of Illinois Press, 2016.

Leng, Kirsten. *Sexual Politics and Feminist Science: Women Sexologists in Germany, 1900–1933*. Ithaca, NY: Cornell University Press, 2018.

LeVay, Simon. *Queer Science: The Use and Abuse of Research into Homosexuality*. Cambridge: MIT Press, 1996.

Marcuse, Max. "Ein Fall von Geschlechtsumwandlungstrieb." *Zeitschrift für Psychotherapie und medizinische Psychologie* 6 (1916): 176–92.

Marhoeffer, Laurie. *Sex and the Weimar Republic: German Homosexual Emancipation and the Rise of the Nazis*. Toronto: University of Toronto Press, 2015.

Moll, Albert. *Libido Sexualis: Studies in the Psychosexual Laws of Love, Verified by Clinical Sexual Case Histories.* Translated by David Berger. New York: American Ethnological Press, 1933.

Müller, Klaus. "Johann Ludwig Casper." In *Homosexualität: Handbuch der Theorie- und Forschungsgeschichte*, edited by Rüdiger Lautmann, 29–31. Frankfurt: Campus-Verlag, 1993.

Oosterhuis, Harry. *Stepchildren of Nature: Krafft-Ebing, Psychiatry, and the Making of Sexual Identity.* Chicago, IL: University of Chicago Press, 2000.

Porter, Roy. "Mental Illness." In *The Cambridge History of Medicine*, edited by Roy Porter, 238–59. Cambridge: Cambridge University Press, 2006.

Porter, Roy, and Leslie Hall. *The Facts of Life: The Creation of Sexual Knowledge in Britain, 1650–1950.* New Haven, CT: Yale University Press, 1995.

Robinson, Paul. *The Modernization of Sex.* New York: Harper and Row, 1978.

Sengoopta, Chandak. *The Most Secret Quintessence of Life: Sex, Glands, and Hormones, 1850–1950.* Chicago, IL: University of Chicago Press, 2006.

———. *Otto Weininger: Sex, Science, and Self in Imperial Vienna.* Chicago, IL: University of Chicago Press, 2000.

Shorter, Edward. *A History of Psychiatry: From the Era of the Asylum to the Age of Prozac.* New York: John Wiley and Sons, 1997.

Sigusch, Volkmar. "The Sexologist Albert Moll: Between Sigmund Freud and Magnus Hirschfeld." *Medical History* 56, no. 2 (2012): 184–200.

Spector, Scott. *Violent Sensations: Sex, Crime and Utopia in Vienna and Berlin, 1860–1914.* Chicago, IL: University of Chicago Press, 2016.

Spector, Scott, Helmut Puff, and Dagmar Herzog, eds. *After the History of Sexuality: German Genealogies with and beyond Foucault.* New York: Berghahn Books, 2012.

Sutton, Katie. *Sex Between Body and Mind: Psychoanalysis and Sexology in the German-Speaking World, 1890s–1930s.* Ann Arbor: University of Michigan Press, 2019.

Tardieu, Ambroise. *Étude medico-légale sur les attentats aux mœurs* (*Forensic Study on Offenses Against Morals*. Paris: J.B. Baillière et Fils, 1857.

Tissot, Samuel-Auguste. *L'Onanisme.* Lausanne: Chez Marc Chapuis et Compagnie, 1760.

Ulrichs, Karl Heinrich. *Critische Pfeile: Denkschrift über die Bestrafung der Urningsliebe.* Leipzig: Commissions-Verlag v. Otto & Stadler, 1879.

Ulrichs, Karl Heinrich. *The Riddle of "Man-Manly" Love.* 2 vols. Translated by Michael A. Lombardi-Nash. Buffalo, New York: Prometheus Books, 1994.

Weeks, Jeffrey. *Coming Out: Homosexual Politics in Britain from the Nineteenth Century to the Present.* London: Quartet Books, 1977.

———. *Sexuality and Its Discontents: Meanings, Myths, and Modern Sexualities.* London: Routledge, 1985.

Weininger, Otto. *Sex and Character: An Investigation of Fundamental Principles.* Translated by Ladislaus Löb. Bloomington: Indiana University Press, 2005.

Whisnant, Clayton J. *Queer Identities and Politics in Germany: A History, 1880–1945.* New York: Harrington Park Press, 2016.

Westphal, Carl. "Contrary Sexual Feelings: Symptom of a Neuropathic (Psychopathic) Condition." In *Sodomites and Urnings: Homosexual Representations in Classic German Journals.* Translated and edited by Michael A. Lombardi-Nash, 87–120. New York: Harrington Park Press, 1996.

2.1. PROFILE: THE CHEVALIÈRE D'EON (1728–1810)

Clayton J. Whisnant

The Chevalière d'Eon is famous today for living nearly the last half of her life as a woman; in 1777, the French King Louis XVI even acknowledged her as a woman in all senses of the word. When she passed away, her closest friends were as surprised as anyone that d'Eon was anatomically male.[1]

The case of d'Eon is an extraordinary one, not least because she fought for a time to retain the right to continue wearing men's clothes even as she insisted on being recognized publicly as a woman. Intriguingly, this case was also one of public fascination. Even before d'Eon began to make her much publicized transition, her name was fairly well known to anyone who kept up with political matters. Few knew that she was a spy, but in the 1760s, she had made a name for herself as a decorated captain of the elite brigade of Dragoons at the end of the Seven Years War. After the war was over, d'Eon was assigned to England as a diplomat (and a spy), where she served for several months until she came under attack from rivals who accused her of overspending royal funds. When d'Eon refused an order to return to France, she became an outlaw and potentially a traitor. In a desperate bid to salvage her career and financial situation, she published much of the secret government correspondence she had in her possession, a work that turned her into a cause célèbre for a time. In private, she threatened to reveal her mission as a royal spy if the crown refused to pay her debts or restore her livelihood.[2]

D'Eon was already familiar to the public, then, when she began to live as a woman. As rumors began to spread in London that she was a woman masquerading as a man—rumors she probably helped spread herself—many began to make high-stakes wagers on her gender. All the public attention finally forced her to return to France, but not before she had secured public acknowledgment of being a woman in a British court case. She even received

Figure 2.1.1. The Chevalière d'Eon (1728–1810). *Source*: Courtesy of the Bibliothèque nationale de France, Paris. Public domain.

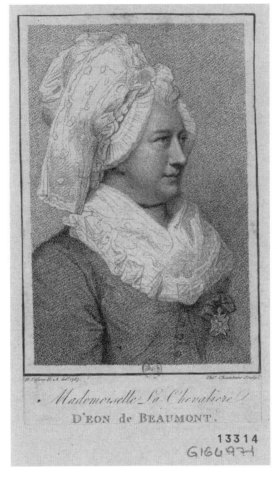

public recognition as a woman by Louis XVI, who had come to believe that his grandfather's employment of a woman in disguise as a diplomat and elite soldier was just one more piece of the mess left by his predecessor's reign.

After a brief period during which she tried to maintain the right to continue wearing masculine clothing and serving in government office, d'Eon consented to living the rest of her life in female attire in exchange for a pension. Over time she was forced to seek other means to supplement her income, including publishing books and performing in public exhibitions in which she fenced in female dress. In her autobiography, she insisted that she had been born a girl, but to claim an inheritance, her father had pretended she was a boy from birth.[3]

In 1785, d'Eon returned to London, where she spent the rest of her life. The French Revolution (1789–1799) left her without a pension or a country to which it was safe to return. In 1810 she passed away, having lived in poverty for the last years of her life with a good friend, the widow Mrs. Cole. While preparing the body, Mrs. Cole discovered that physically d'Eon was a man, a fact that so surprised her that she called in several doctors just to make sure.

NOTES

1. D'Eon's most thorough biographer, Gary Kates, presents a provocative argument that d'Eon's choice to publicly identify as a woman was at some level a daring yet calculated move to revive an endangered career, which raises some questions about d'Eon's actual gender identification. Doubts are also raised by the fact that d'Eon did her best to retain the right to wear masculine clothing, even after being publicly recognized as a woman. I have chosen to address her with feminine pronouns and titles, assuming that if she went to such great lengths to be recognized as a woman, she would have preferred it that way. While it is distinctly possible that her gender identification changed in the course of her life, the autobiography she wrote later insisted that she had always been a woman, so I will respect her wishes in this respect as well. Although I disagree with Kates, his biography is still by the far the best one, doing a much better job than some of the earlier, more sensationalist accounts at sorting fact from fiction. See Kates, *Monsieur d'Eon Is a Woman*.

2. Another recent work, a section of which focuses on d'Eon's public campaign to retain her job and financial position, is Burrows, 41.

3. An English version of her autobiography that includes a nice introduction is now available: Charles d'Eon de Beaumont, *The Maiden of Tonnerre*.

WORKS CITED

Beaumont, Charles d'Eon. *The Maiden of Tonnerre: The Vicissitudes of the Chevalier and the Chevalière d'Eon*. Translated and edited by Roland A. Champagne, Nina Ekstein, and Gary Kates. Baltimore, MD: Johns Hopkins University Press, 2001.

Burrows, Simon. *Blackmail, Scandal, and Revolution: London's French Libellistes, 1758–92*. Manchester: Manchester University Press, 2006.

Herzer, Manfred. *Magnus Hirschfeld: Leben und Werk eines jüdischen, schwulen und sozialistischen Sexologen*. Frankfurt: Campus, 1992.

Kates, Gary. *Monsieur d'Eon Is a Woman: A Tale of Political Intrigue and Sexual Masquerade*. New York: Basic Books, 1995.

3

PIONEERING SCIENTISTS
Hirschfeld, Benjamin, and Kinsey

Annette F. Timm and Jamison Green

Toward the end of the eighteenth century, in the waning years of the Enlightenment, the European medical community demonstrated extraordinary interest in sexual behavior and a growing conviction that what had previously been categorized only in religious terms—as various degrees of sin—should now be investigated using scientific methods. With some interventions from Italy, France, and Great Britain, it was primarily German, Swiss, and Austrian doctors who began to categorize human sexual desire and behavior and to formulate a discipline of sexual science in the mid-nineteenth century.[1]

Sexological findings arose out of the increasingly sexually tolerant atmosphere in cities such as Berlin, where thriving sexual subcultures became the incubators for sexual rights movements. This connection between sexological investigation and legal reform efforts was most evident in the work of Magnus Hirschfeld. Hirschfeld cofounded the Scientific Humanitarian Committee in 1897—often considered the world's first gay rights organization—and authored numerous influential books and articles about the spectrum of human sexual diversity. Historians Joanne Meyerowitz, Susan Stryker, and other scholars have pointed out that it was Harry Benjamin who provided the link between Hirschfeld and Alfred Kinsey, the scientist who had embarked on a quest to understand sexual behavior in the United States; Benjamin's professional experiences in Berlin acquainted him with the possibilities of gender-affirming surgeries and subsequently inspired him to cooperate with Kinsey's project of cataloguing all aspects of human sexual variation.[2] This scientific genealogy, from Hirschfeld to Benjamin to Kinsey, though more of an intertwining than a direct descendancy, would help shape emerging understandings of human sexuality and gender minorities on both sides of the Atlantic.[3]

Harry Benjamin, a young German physician, first traveled to New York in 1911 to conduct research on tuberculosis. Disappointed by the poor quality of research being done in the United States, he soon returned to Europe; however, he continued to travel between Germany and the United States until World War I, when travel back to Germany became impossible. By the time the war ended, he had chosen to reside permanently in the United States. In 1916, at Columbia University, Benjamin met Joseph Frankel, who was studying the function of glands about which little was then known. Frankel's discovery that the aging process began when the body ceased to produce sex hormones fascinated Benjamin, who began to treat aging patients with testosterone and estrogen. Blending his scientific interests in endocrinology, gerontology, and sexology, Benjamin serendipitously placed himself in a unique position, one that eventually launched the field of transgender medicine.[4]

Benjamin noted that it was as "a young student at the Berlin University" that he first met Hirschfeld, in 1906 or 1907.[5] After permanently relocating to the United States, Benjamin spent most of the summers between the two World Wars in Germany and often accompanied Hirschfeld on his research jaunts through Berlin's famously genderbending nightlife.[6] This pseudosocial, research-oriented connection between scientists, often in unorthodox settings, drove the early evolution of transgender medicine and healthcare, while also creating the only context outside of the psychoanalyst's offices where sexual behaviors would be safely discussed and cataloged for later scientific discussion and analysis. The traditional method of describing the transmission of knowledge about transgender people through formal academic/scientific conferences and peer-reviewed journal articles—all difficult for the general public to access—has produced a de-emotionalized and therefore somewhat inaccurate narrative that purposely underplayed the role of intimate relationships and the agency of those most affected by research in this field. Although motivated by an understandable attempt to preserve the privacy of marginalized and persecuted individuals, later historians sometimes unconsciously repeated the depersonalizing and quantifying tendencies of mid-twentieth-century medical researchers. Zeroing in on personal connections is therefore more than simply a strategy of engagement; it is critical to understanding how knowledge, particularly knowledge about sexuality, is created.

In the United States, Sexology (with a capital S) began with Kinsey. Though the United States, like any center of human activity, was full of sexual fascination and expression, the first half of the twentieth century was also dominated by sexual repression and moral panics about sexual abnormalities.[7] Responding to student questions that arose in the marriage course he had been asked to coordinate at Indiana University in 1938, Kinsey set out to scientifically examine—separately—human male and female sexual behavior to address a "severe disappointment"[8] in the available literature about sexual behavior. By July 1939, he had amassed 350 sexual histories from among his Indiana University students, and he was looking forward to collecting his "first thousand."[9] In 1940, in response to objections from clergy members and others in the Bloomington community, Kinsey was forced to choose between teaching the marriage course or his pursuit of case histories and his quest for scientific data about sexual behavior.[10] He chose the more challenging path.

There was no direct connection between Hirschfeld and Kinsey.[11] However, Kinsey's correspondence with Harry Benjamin reveals an entirely new story—one that Kinsey did not live long enough to tell—a story that revealed the active involvement and influence of trans individuals in his research. Through examining this record, it became obvious that a few highly motivated individuals, some of whom had their own personal connections to Germany, were responsible for bringing Benjamin and Kinsey together and for transforming their views on the diagnosis and treatment of individuals who wished to change their gendered self-presentation and their legal sex.

Kinsey studied Hirschfeld's research on transvestites. His library contained a growing collection of Hirschfeld's publications, and he relied on a German-speaking staff member, Hedwig Gruen Leser, to translate relevant passages, which he cited in his two monumental best-selling books, *Sexual Behavior in the Human Male* (1948) and *Sexual Behavior in the Human Female* (1953)—hereafter referred to as the *Male* and *Female* books.[12]

Kinsey generally dismissed this early German sexological work. It was only after he began collaborating with Benjamin that a significant German influence on Kinsey can be said to have taken hold—too late for Kinsey to have worked through the implications or to include this perspective in any published work. Although Kinsey did not live long enough to publish his research on transsexuality, how and why he even embraced the subject tells us much about the scientific study of sex in the twentieth century. Investigating precisely how he arrived at this subject turns out to be as interesting as what he might have written about it had he lived.

As we will see, Kinsey did not *find* "transsexuality" as a subject of scientific investigation; individuals who wanted to be investigated found him. They often found Kinsey by first finding Benjamin, who had himself come to the topic because trans individuals sought him out for his endocrinological expertise. In other words, to accurately track the transmission of knowledge about the transsexual experience, we must relinquish our tendency to view sex-related identities or experience as something "discovered" by medical experts and ask more focused questions about the life stories and desires of trans people. Even though the structure of what follows in this chapter still partially tracks the flow of ideas from one cisgender male expert to the next, the true agency lies elsewhere within the narrative—with trans people themselves.[13]

FROM HIRSCHFELD TO BENJAMIN

Histories of how trans individuals sought to live authentic lives in the twentieth century have generally been told through the lens of the work, writing, and private musings of medical experts.[14] There is a certain inevitability to this perspective, particularly in the first half of the century; it was most often the scientists and doctors who categorized and quantified, who made pronouncements about the need for legal reform, and who were consequently the targets of those who decried any change to the dominant social and cultural paradigm of cisnormativity. But as historians Edward Dickinson and Richard Wetzell have argued, we should not follow Michel Foucault in overemphasizing the "*Deutungsmacht* (interpretive authority) of bourgeois medical experts." Despite their power as self-appointed opinion leaders, they could not single-handedly produce sexual categories and identities without the participation of the patients they investigated.[15]

This *Deutungsmacht* still carries influence, as many people remain tempted to conflate sex, sexuality, and gender and to ignore the subjective experiences of individuals within their social settings and intimate relationships. As Foucault explained in his introduction to the tragic story of the nineteenth century "hermaphrodite" (a now objectionable word for what we today call *intersex*) Herculine Barbin,[16] the modern insistence that people only have one "true sex" arises from the eighteenth-century scientific conviction that there could be no such thing as a real mixture of the sexes. By the twentieth century, this meant that people who were identified as intersex were only considered "pseudo-hermaphrodites"—not *real* hermaphrodites or a true mixture of the sexes but imperfect versions of one sex or the other. As the subjects rather than the authors of this research, sexually categorized people certainly experienced an appropriation of their life stories, particularly due to the emotionless and often objectifying way they were presented in medical texts.

Meanwhile, anatomical investigations purported to determine which biological sex was predominant in the genitals; such analysis was read as ipso facto evidence that the opposite sex of the "true sex" should be the one the individual in question desired (was attracted to), thus preserving a heterosexual social order. Under this biopolitical regime, which still governs many public discussions and popular opinions about intersex and trans people, sexuality (the sexual desire of the individual) is secondary to biology and to heteronormative and cisnormative statutes. As will become apparent in the biographical discussion (in chapter 7) of Carla Erskine (a trans patient of Harry Benjamin's who underwent gender-affirming surgery in 1953 at the University of California San Francisco), these sociomedical structures make it imperative to pay attention to two taxonomical dichotomies and how they intersect: sex/sexuality (the match or mismatch between anatomy and choice of love object) and sex/gender (the match or mismatch between one's anatomy and one's social presentation and comportment). Even as these categories are manifestly blurred in lived lives, medical and psychological authorities—not to mention social mores and legal systems—have sought to keep them intact. As historians Gillian Frank and Lauren Gutterman argue, well into the 1970s and to some degree up to the present, "the messier realities of trans people's lives, including queer desires or gender queer identities, needed to be smoothed out for them to be accepted by physicians and a wider public."[17]

All of this sociomedical history helps explain the frequent erasure of intersex individuals within trans historical narratives, since the tendency to think about ourselves (and therefore also people of the past) as having one true sex persists. Even researchers like Kinsey and Benjamin, who accepted the potential mismatch between sex and sexuality (that is, that same-sex love was natural) or between sex and gender (the "transsexual phenomenon" in Benjamin's formulation), could not quite disregard that there might be one true sex.

Foucault's insistence on debunking a true sex theory made it clear that reductive readings of sexuality were unhelpful. As professor of economic and social history Franz Eder argues, the "positive and productive building of the 'sexual subject' and his [sic] 'desire'" has helped refine the top-down approach that a simplistic reading of Foucault produced.[18] In other words, we must pay attention to how various experts who sought to scientifically categorize sexual identity in the twentieth century were both operating within specific paradigms of scientific argument and being influenced by the subjects of their research. Dutch historian Harry Oosterhuis's study of Richard von Krafft-Ebing's professional and intellectual evolution is a model of this both/and approach because it emphasizes the degree to which the world's first sexologist deployed a dialogical methodology. Krafft-Ebing's *Psychopathia Sexualis*, first published in 1886, began as a list of sexual pathologies; but Oosterhuis argues that while this tactic "enabled medical treatment and other forms of restraint . . . it also opened up the possibility for the individuals involved to speak out, to find a voice, and to be acknowledged,"[19] making "both patients and doctors . . . agents of culture at large."[20] That the patients influenced the doctors in this earliest era of the medicalization of sexuality is made clear in Krafft-Ebing's increasing tolerance toward homosexuality, which he first viewed as a pathology, but later fought to decriminalize. He was one of the first signatories to Hirschfeld's petition for the abolition of section 175 of the German penal code, which outlined punishments for "unnatural" indecency or fornication (*widernatürliche Unzucht*) and which applied primarily to sexual acts between men.[21]

Sensitivity to the desires and needs of patients became a hallmark of sexological research, at least in Germany, where Hirschfeld's founding of the Institute for Sexual Science in Berlin in 1919 was motivated not only by the pursuit of medical knowledge but also by the larger effort to advocate for social tolerance and legal reform for sexual minorities. This activist role, however, meant that Hirschfeld and virtually all later researchers in the field of human sexuality were acutely sensitive to the public furor their work might produce, and they tended to rigorously conform to shifting norms of scientific argument. While the case-study approach dominated all forms of sexual science in the late nineteenth century—most famously in the work of Krafft-Ebing and Sigmund Freud—by the turn of the century, Hirschfeld became convinced that only statistical studies encompassing the broad spectrum of human sexual presentation, self-understanding, and behavior would convince the public to accept human sexual and gender diversity. In 1899, Hirschfeld began publishing the results of his Psycho-Biological Questionnaire, an approach to gathering information about sexual behavior that eventually collected information from approximately ten thousand individuals and was later emulated (with little attribution) by Kinsey.[22]

Hirschfeld also cultivated close relationships with anyone who conceived of themselves as sexually nonconforming and relied on detailed case histories to formulate his arguments about sexual diversity. This interpersonal approach is most apparent in his 1910 book *Die Transvestiten* (*The Transvestites*), which was based on the life stories of seventeen individuals who wrote to him about their desire to live in the clothing or the body of the other sex. These people might never have provided these candid accounts or made themselves known to medical authorities if they had not met Hirschfeld and been exposed to his sympathetic attitudes through their involvement in the trusted personal networks of Berlin's nightlife.[23] In the opening pages of *Die Transvestiten*, Hirschfeld admitted that the life stories of these individuals initially took him aback. Despite his openness to the idea of sexually mixed types (*Mischungsarten*, or what he also called *Zwischenstufen*—intermediary stages), he did not initially know what to make of these "strange people" (*seltsame Menschen*) who "despite totally normal sexual drives display strong physical tendencies of the other gender." In these cases, the individuals voluntarily contacted Hirschfeld, who then encouraged them to write autobiographies. He remained in contact with them for up to twelve years. While he had at first been convinced that these individuals were living in a state of "self-delusion," his personal connection to them eventually convinced him to supplement his "objective observation of large data sets" with more focused attention to a small group of individuals.[24] The objectified took on subjective agency, even within the eyes of a strict, scientific researcher like Hirschfeld.

Without detailing precisely how he met each individual, Hirschfeld noted that all but two of his contacts (who were referred by other doctors) came to him directly, either via writing or "orally" (*mündlich*). This vague description is likely an allusion to the fact that Hirschfeld spent considerable amounts of time visiting the various bars and cafés of Berlin's vibrant sexual subcultures.[25] This methodology for finding research subjects conflicted, of course, with the scrupulously scientific aura he sought to project to the world in the interest of presenting himself as an objective scientific voice. In other words, behind the scientific atmosphere projected in public lectures and other outreach activities, the research of the Institute for Sexual Science depended on the trust that sexually nonconforming individuals placed in Hirschfeld (who divulged his homosexuality only in intimate settings) and his colleagues.[26] This trust turned the Institute into something more than a venue for scientific research.[27] The picture in Figure 3.1 visually depicts how intimate contacts became central to the collection of information and the advocacy for individuals who could not conform to the heteronormative culture of early twentieth-century Germany.

Hirschfeld's ability to use intimate personal connections for his research would have been virtually unimaginable in almost any other city in Europe or North America. The degree to which early twentieth-century Germany, and particularly Berlin, represented a new form of tolerance for sexual diversity is clear if we investigate Hirschfeld's close cooperation with the police. As the German historian Jens Dobler has argued, there was an astounding degree of cooperation between the Berlin police, the Scientific Humanitarian Committee,

Figure 3.1. "Hirschfeld is holding hands with his partner Karl Giese. The elderly person in front is Karl's mother. We do not know when this picture was made nor what kind of event it was. We obtained this picture from the former housekeeper, who joined the Institute in the summer of 1928. She told us that it was taken before she came to the Institute. Some texts that have reprinted this photo call it a "transvestite ball," but to us, it looks simply like some kind of costume party. Source: Photo and caption courtesy of Ralf Dose, M.A., Managing Director, Magnus-Hirschfeld-Gesellschaft (Research Center for the History of Sexual Science), Berlin, Germany.

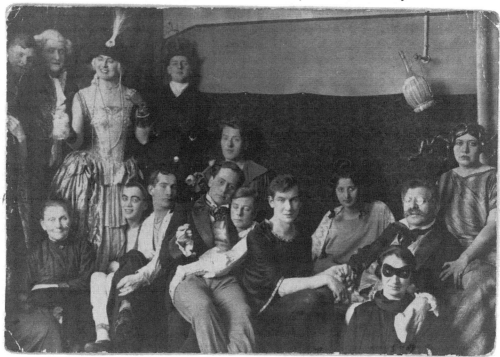

the publisher Friedrich Radszuweit's *Bund für Menschenrechte* (League for Human Rights, another organization campaigning for the repeal of section 175), and Hirschfeld himself.[28] In 1885, the Berlin police founded the Department for Pederasty (*Päderastenabteilung*) within its organization, and its four successive directors—Leopold von Meerscheidt-Hüllessem (1885–1900), Hans von Tresckow (1900–1911), Heinrich Kopp (1911–1923), and Bernhard Strewe (1923–1933)—displayed what historian Robert Beachy has called an attitude of "qualified toleration" for sexual minorities and their specific social and legal problems, right up to the beginning of the Nazi era.[29]

Throughout the late nineteenth and early twentieth centuries, the *Päderastenpatrouille* (pederast patrol) engaged ten to twelve constables whose official duties included the investigation of male prostitution and infringements against section 175. In this atmosphere, laws meant to undergird heteronormative understandings of acceptable self-presentation and sexual activity made individuals living a closeted sexual life of any kind vulnerable to a blackmailer's threat to turn them over to police. The relatively progressive impulses of the four successive directors of the *Päderastenabteilung* meant that police efforts tended to concentrate on prostitution and on protecting individuals from being blackmailed for their self-presentation or consensual relationships, which in practice created a remarkably tolerant atmosphere in the city.[30] This atmosphere fostered Hirschfeld's research, since it allowed for the flourishing sexual subculture that provided the venue for his encounters with a diverse spectrum of visitors to the restaurants and cafés frequented by "urnings" and other gender-questioning individuals in Berlin. (*Urnings* was a short-lived word for homosexuals or men "with feminine souls" and was coined in 1864 by German activist Karl Heinrich Ulrichs.) Hirschfeld estimated that there were already twenty or so of these establishments in Berlin in 1904,[31] and he often visited these places in the company of police constables. He later praised Meerscheidt-Hüllessem as a "champion of light and justice" who "with word and deed selflessly stood by hundreds and saved many of them from shame and death," and he described Hans von Tresckow as having "saved hundreds of homosexual men from despair and suicide" by prosecuting their blackmailers.[32] The close cooperation between sexologists, activists, and the police is best exemplified in Hirschfeld's creation of what he called "transvestite passes"—certified pieces of identification that the Berlin police department recognized and that therefore protected crossdressers from arrest under laws against "causing a public nuisance" or impersonation.[33]

Figure 3.2. A 1928 *Transvestitenpass* (transvestite pass). *Source*: Courtesy of the Magnus-Hirschfeld-Gesellschaft e.V.

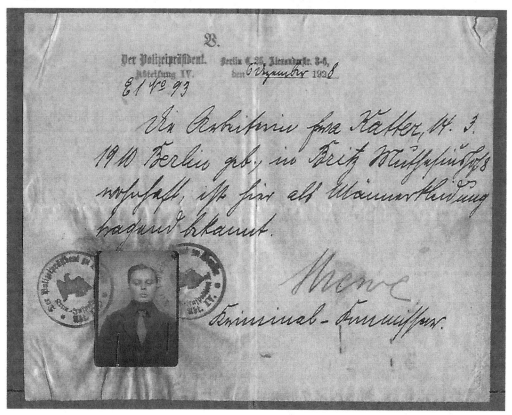

Hirschfeld's immersion in the nightlife of Berlin's sexual subcultures turns out to have been an important factor in transmitting knowledge about transsexuality from Germany to the United States: it created the conditions for Benjamin to learn from Hirschfeld. Benjamin was still a medical student in Germany when police inspector Heinrich Kopp, who was a mutual friend, introduced them. In his *Reminiscences,* written in 1970, Benjamin described Kopp as a "sympathetic and serious student of the homosexual and other sexual problems." Benjamin continued, "A couple of times, I was invited to accompany Hirschfeld and Kopp, who were good friends, on tours through a few gay bars in Berlin. The most famous was the Eldorado[34] where mainly transvestites gathered, and female impersonators performed."[35]

Benjamin started spending his summers in Berlin in 1921, visiting the Institute for Sexual Science and meeting with Hirschfeld and his colleagues on a yearly basis. Bemused that the "courageous" but famously grumpy and stingy Hirschfeld had earned the nickname *Tante Magnesia* (Aunt Magnesia) from the adoring patrons of these clubs,[36] Benjamin took mental notes on how scientific knowledge about sexual diversity could be gathered through unconventional personal contacts with gender-questioning individuals. Although Benjamin never denied the influence of his German mentors, he would later obscure Hirschfeld's impact on his own thinking by claiming to have invented the term *transsexuality*. Even Kinsey might have been exposed to Hirschfeld's terminology through his acquaintance with Benjamin because the word *transsexuality* appeared in the *Male* book in 1948, long after Kinsey and Benjamin met.[37]

But the critical point remains: none of these men discovered sexual diversity. Sexually diverse individuals instead sought out those who might help them, and the patients themselves taught these men what their personal experiences might mean for our larger understanding of the spectrum of human sexual and gender experience. After coining the word *transvestite*, Hirschfeld was forced to realize that the term could not fully describe many of the individuals who sought him out in Berlin's bars and nightclubs. (There is no direct German equivalent for the term *gender*.) It was these trans people, most of whom never became household names, who were also responsible for creating the networks of knowledge that began to span the Atlantic in the early twentieth century.

Figure 3.3. Harry Benjamin with Magnus Hirschfeld. *Source*: From the Collections of the Kinsey Institute, Indiana University. All rights reserved.

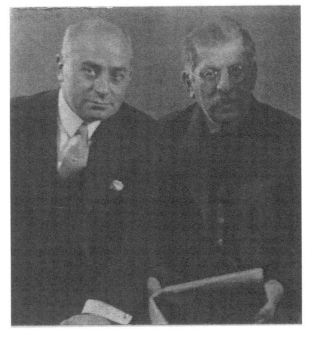

THE BENJAMIN–KINSEY COLLABORATION

Exploring the Benjamin–Kinsey collaboration helps us further understand the importance of personal networks in the history of sexology. After beginning to correspond with Kinsey in the spring of 1944, Benjamin finally met the famous biologist "sometime around 1945,"[38] and the two men began comparing notes about gathering sexual data through personal contacts and visits to bars and nightclubs.[39] Thus began a pivotal intellectual collaboration between the two men that would last the rest of Kinsey's life.

Although he left behind no definitive statements on the subject, the evidence strongly suggests that even Kinsey began to at least entertain the possibility that trans identities were within the spectrum of "normal."[40] By 1949, he and his primary collaborators—Wardell Pomeroy, Clyde Martin, and Paul Gebhard—explicitly tried to tear down preconceptions of normal human sexual development. They argued, for instance, that the term *crimes against nature* had no scientific grounding:

> [The law] proscribes [sexual acts which do no damage to property or to person] on the ground that they are crimes against nature—that is, abnormal or perverse behavior—and punishable because they are so rated. They are punishable without respect to the mutual desire of the parties involved to engage in such activities and irrespective of the fact that the persons immediately concerned may find satisfaction in their performance. In all the criminal law, there is practically no other behavior which is forbidden on the ground that nature may be offended, and that nature must be protected from such offense. This is the unique aspect of our sex codes.[41]

Given this line of argument and Kinsey's sympathetic reaction to the trans women he met through Benjamin in the early 1950s, it seems unlikely that he could have continued to reject the validity of their desires. Kinsey's fundamentally binary understanding of gender roles made it difficult for him to understand trans identities; however, the transition in his thought is visible in the few paragraphs he wrote about transvestism in the *Female* book. This second volume added to the *Male* book by providing at least a brief definition of transvestism (he notably did not use the word *transsexuality*), and it coyly alluded to research underway "to secure a sample which will ultimately allow us to estimate the number of transvestites in the United States."[42] The *Female* book was published in 1953, just before he and Benjamin started corresponding about the circle of trans women around Louise Lawrence in San Francisco (see chapter 7.1). It is not surprising, therefore, that Kinsey's understanding of the people he only called transvestites was dependent on his understanding of the fundamental difference between males and females and his assumption that "males are more liable to be conditioned by psychologic stimuli."[43]

We cannot know whether Kinsey's collaboration with Benjamin and his contacts with trans women would have changed his mind, but given their increasingly close personal and professional connection, Kinsey must have been affected—if not in his opinions, then at least in his methodology. In 1949, Kinsey referred an effeminate boy who wanted to become a girl to Benjamin,[44] and they began sharing files of people they generally referred to as transvestites. In September 1949, at precisely the same time Benjamin began to address his letters to Prok (Kinsey's nickname) rather than to Dr. Kinsey, the correspondence between the two men became more intimate, with frequent descriptions of the personal lives, medical quests, and intertwined social networks of the small but growing number of Americans who sought hormone treatment and surgery. Throughout the early 1950s, Benjamin reported to Kinsey on his frequent visits with the circle of intimates around Lawrence during his yearly summer residence in San Francisco (he ran a summer clinic on Sutter Street), and he forwarded information about his contacts to Kinsey.[45] Kinsey then traveled to take these individuals' histories, and he became intimately acquainted with a group of primarily trans women, mostly in San Francisco, Chicago, and New York.

Whenever Benjamin and Kinsey were in the same city, the two men went out to explore establishments they thought most likely to be "sexologically interesting." Benjamin led the way. Their common interest in this type of participant-observer research is apparent in their letters, such as the one dated September 1951, when Benjamin reported that he had taken a fascinating tour of the seedy bars of Mexico City and had seen "the lowest type of prostitution." Although his lack of Spanish skills and the extreme class divisions of the scene made it impossible for him to have a truly "sexciting" trip (as Albert Ellis, who was then working on his book *Sex without Guilt*, had wished him), he hoped Kinsey would join him on a return trip. In other words, Benjamin followed in the Hirschfeld tradition, and he found a kindred spirit in Kinsey, whose loitering in seedy areas of Chicago and other cities had already gotten him arrested (or nearly so) on several occasions.[46]

Kinsey's writing did not provide details about this methodology, which might be categorized as a type of anthropological fieldwork. He described his interview method in detail in various interviews and publications, but he said nothing about how he found many of his most "sexologically interesting" interview partners. As Donna Drucker, Elizabeth Stephens, and Peter Cryle have argued, Kinsey's self-perception was as a taxonomist—a gatherer of masses of data that could then be categorized and analyzed.[47] But the fact that he found so few trans individuals to investigate meant that his planned volume on transvestism, which might have included the few transsexual people he had interviewed, only could have been written with a less stringent reliance on statistics. He simply did not have the numbers for a reasonable sample. He clearly understood this shortcoming, but he was also eager to address the criticism he received for failing to investigate the significance of crossdressing in past publications;[48] he left it out of the *Male* book entirely and added only a few paragraphs on "transvestism" to the *Female* book.[49]

Despite the small pool of subjects, Kinsey's collection of material about trans cases was meticulous: he took detailed case histories and traveled long distances to meet with just one or two individuals. (For instance, he conducted a four-hour-long interview—double the usual length—with Carla Erskine who "found him to be a lovely and sympathetic man.")[50] Despite his antipathy for psychoanalysis, his methods of investigating transvestism were more personal than statistical, and in his early speculations about categorizing these individuals, he tended to opine that "no two of them are very much alike"—a judgment that would complicate any neat taxonomy.[51] This newly dubbed subject of transsexuality might even have forced him to somewhat revise his views on what Hirschfeld would have called the "intermediaries"—the various shadings between male and female.

In other words, his encounter with trans people was a difficult learning process that contradicted his instinctual reaction to gender difference. In the *Male* book, Kinsey rejected the idea of fixed sexual types. He particularly detested "unscientific" uses of the word *bi-sexuality*, indignantly objecting that it was "used to imply these persons have both masculine qualities and feminine qualities *within* their single bodies."[52] He refused to ever speak in terms of fixed sexual identities, writing only about "homosexual acts," never about "homosexuals," and despite his own creation of a scale of human sexual difference, he placed far more emphasis than Hirschfeld on social conditioning. Kinsey insisted that terms like *intersex* and *bisexual* could be used for humans only in ways analogous to biological descriptions of animals who possessed both male and female anatomical structures. Those who engaged in homosexual behaviors, then, were not physical or sexual intermediates but rather examples of the limitless human capacity for variety in sexual comportment. This position was a rejection of Hirschfeld's "theory of sexual transitions" (*Zwischenstufenlehre*), which posited that variations in sexual organs, physical build, sex drive, and emotional makeup produced a clearly categorizable—if also theoretically infinite—variety of sexual types.[53] Hirschfeld's insistence on this spectrum implied that the notion of solely male or female forms was illusory.[54]

Kinsey acknowledged Hirschfeld's pioneering efforts and was particularly respectful of the German sexologist's use of surveys (for instance, Hirschfeld's 1904 distribution of forms to 3,000 technical college students and 5,721 metal workers), but he ultimately dismissed all early studies on sexual behavior as failing to meet the sampling standards of scientific population analysis. Kinsey scoffed that much of Hirschfeld's information was "nothing more than gossip,"[55] and he seems to have ignored Hirschfeld's theory of sexual transitions altogether. Given what we know about Kinsey's rather selective reading habits,[56] his conclusions might merely have been a matter of failing to ask his translator to read the relevant works. As gender studies professor Heike Bauer has argued, Kinsey's reactions to Hirschfeld's work were almost certainly also influenced by the fact that "for Kinsey, Hirschfeld's own homosexuality disqualified the German from scientific authority."[57] It is nevertheless instructive that Kinsey cited, but did not comment on, Hirschfeld's 1910 book *Die Transvestiten*. Kinsey was clearly uncomfortable with any theories of sexual diversity that might threaten a gender order based on sexual dimorphism: the "natural" distinction between male and female. He acknowledged that men and women were "alike in their basic anatomy and physiology,"[58] but as sociology professor Janice Irvine has argued, his insistence on the "biological imperative" has the ring of someone desperate to justify the double standard.[59] As Kinsey put it in the *Female* book: "The human male's interest in maintaining his property rights in his female mate, his objections to his wife's extra-marital coitus, and her lesser objection to his extra-marital activity, are mammalian heritages."[60] Women, he insisted, had less sexual capacity and were less malleable to social conditioning; they had less "conditionability" than men and were therefore less likely to seek a variety of sexual experiences.[61] Kinsey had no problems finding ways of making the massive amount of data he collected fit these preconceptions. But as he and Benjamin began to collect information about transvestites and as they participated in long-term relationships with some of these individuals, Kinsey in particular faced dilemmas that challenged both his insistence on mass data collection and his sexually dimorphic worldview.

By the mid-1950s, only a handful of publicly acknowledged transsexual people lived in the United States. These individuals undoubtedly represented a tiny fraction of trans Americans. We can make this assumption because Christine Jorgensen and others who underwent public transitions received hundreds of letters from desperate people. (Jorgensen alone received "some twenty thousand" letters.)[62] Benjamin and Kinsey set out to find as many of these people as possible, and they believed they knew of all of the medically registered cases in the United States. But by the time of his death in 1956, Kinsey had collected only one hundred histories of trans women and eleven of trans men, and he knew of only ten cases where surgery had been performed.[63] This qualitative data was nothing like the dataset he relied on to write his *Male* and *Female* books, which were collectively based on 18,300 case studies and for which Kinsey developed a punch card system for data analysis.[64]

When it came to his research on the transsexual experience, Kinsey was forced to follow the theoretical, case-study approach more common to his German predecessors and their American followers, rather than maintaining the taxonomical rigor he pursued in his previous work. Given the much smaller sample size, and given his own sympathetic tendencies, he was forced to listen to the words of individuals and appreciate their self-representations in all of their complex and sometimes contradictory richness. Kinsey's interest in these individual cases and his undocumented reliance on them in the *Female* book indicate how important it is to understand the role of personal networks in the formulation of knowledge about sexuality. He depended on the social network between these people simply to find his research subjects, and both he and Benjamin inevitably became involved in the tensions, joys, and disappointments of people forced to live secretive and emotionally intense lives. Kinsey's extensive involvement with Benjamin, including their long correspondence about every aspect of the lives of trans women they knew in the early 1950s, makes it clear that this approach was a far more intimate and personal form of research than Kinsey had conducted in the past.

In 1951, Kinsey wrote to a person seeking surgery: "A male cannot be transformed into a female through any known surgical means. In other words, it would be very hopeless to attempt to amputate your male organs and implant a vagina." This assessment summed up his belief in the sexual binary and the fixity of sexual identity. "We humans," he continued, "are either heterosexual or homosexual."[65] While it is impossible to predict where his new research would have led him had he lived, there are hints from his correspondence with Benjamin—who already believed in human bisexuality and the benefits of surgical intervention in the 1950s—that Kinsey could not have easily sustained his conviction that transsexuality was just one more example of male/female sexual dimorphism.[66] At the very least, he would have been forced to acknowledge that his initial assumptions about the predominance of male-to-female transsexualism had been wrong. We now know trans people assigned female at birth likely existed in equal numbers to those assigned male,[67] but they were less likely to think they could be helped by medical science and therefore less likely to make themselves known to researchers like Benjamin and Kinsey.[68]

With a deeper look into the pages of the *Female* book, we can uncover the real-time transformation in Kinsey's approach to transsexualism and its implications for his understanding of the gender spectrum. In this book, as opposed to the first volume (*Male*), Kinsey felt compelled to address, although skeptically, the science of endocrinology, which was Benjamin's medical specialty and also provided the original basis for gender-affirming surgery through the experiments of Eugen Steinach.[69] While admitting that endocrinologists were among the "special consultants" for the project and that "hormones may have more effect on bodily functions than any other mechanism except the nervous system,"[70] Kinsey warned that popularized knowledge about the impact of hormones was "quite incorrect."

> Journalistic accounts of scientific research, over-enthusiastic advertising by some of the drug companies, over-optimistic reports from clinicians who have found a lucrative business in the administration of sex hormones, and some of the discussions among state legislators and public administrators who hope that hormone injections will provide one-package cure-alls for various social ills, have led the public to believe that endocrine organs are the glands of personality, and that there is such an exact knowledge of the way in which they control human behavior that properly qualified technicians should, at least in the near future, be able to control any and all aspects of human sexual behavior.[71]

Kinsey then went on to minimize the effect of hormones in general and to decry the common usage of distinguishing male and female hormones.[72] His purpose in fostering doubt in the science of endocrinology, however, became clear when he alluded to another of his ongoing research projects: "institutional sexual adjustment," in other words, sex in prisons, mental institutions, boarding schools, and the like. For Kinsey, the conviction that hormones drove sexual behavior led to the "unwarranted opinion that anything associated with reproduction must, ipso facto, be associated with an animal's sexual behavior, and it had justified intolerable abuses, such as the castration of sex offenders."[73] This skeptical approach to hormone treatment must have led to numerous debates with Benjamin. Given how central hormone preparations were to Benjamin's treatment of trans patients, it also meant that two of the five major projects Kinsey was working on when he died were on a collision course. (The other three projects were sexuality in art, sexual factors in marital adjustment, and the influence of drugs on sexual behavior.) It is of course difficult to say how this conflict would have played out. Would Kinsey have been persuaded by his intimate relationships with a relatively small number of trans people who were desperate for hormone treatment and who thrived once it was administered, or would he have insisted on maintaining his taxonomic and statistically rigorous methods until the birth control pill came to shatter his preconceptions about female sexual capacity?

By the mid-1950s, neither science nor society was yet able to parse sex, gender, and sexual orientation in such a way that transgender people might hope to find understanding, depathologization, destigmatization, or even reliable medical assistance from professionals. Trans people were forced to find their own ways to adapt to the society around them. And yet, like Jorgensen, a few of them were able to find the medical help they required. The crossdressers and transsexuals of the 1940s, 1950s, and 1960s were enmeshed in the same cultural structures that constrained the scientists, sexologists, and psychiatrists—like Benjamin, Kinsey, and others. Yet the motivation to innovate as well as investigate was driving people in all walks of life in the post–World War II era: soon civil rights, homophile equality, medical advancements, flights to the moon, and commercial expansion would grip the world's imagination. Innovative trans people would continue contributing to this evolution in many ways, including educating and empowering those whose services they needed to thrive.

NOTES

1. This is certainly not the place to rehearse the various stages of this history. For accessible summaries, see Mottier, *Sexuality*; Nye, *Sexuality*; Clark, *Desire*.

2. Meyerowitz, *How Sex Changed*, 45; Stryker, *Transgender History*, 38–40.

3. The link between Hirschfeld and Benjamin has now become well enough known to be recorded in textbook narratives. (See Haefele-Thomas, *Introduction to Transgender Studies*, 102–3.) While it is not quite correct to call Benjamin Hirschfeld's student, as Ardel Haefele-Thomas does (Benjamin was a fully qualified endocrinologist by the time he met Hirschfeld in Berlin), they accurately assess that Benjamin's success in being named the first person to study transgender or transsexual people has much to do with the accessibility of his work, in contrast to that of Hirschfeld or even Richard von Krafft-Ebing, who purposely obscured his most sensitive writings from the public by writing passages in Latin.

4. Ettner, *Gender Loving Care*, 11–13.

5. Benjamin, "Reminiscences," 3–4.

6. For a description of this nightlife, see Sutton, "We Too Deserve a Place in the Sun," 335–54; Beachy, *Gay Berlin*; and Smith, *Berlin Coquette*. On Benjamin's connections to researchers in Europe, Pfaefflin notes that Benjamin was "fully informed about Hirschfeld's work" and "eagerly soaked up every new finding of sexual endocrinology and sexual psychology years before he met the first transsexual patient." Pfaefflin, "Sex Reassignment, Harry Benjamin, and Some European Roots," 97–103.

7. Fone does an excellent job of documenting American social stress about improper sexual behavior, which relied on gender tropes and expectations as primary indicators of homosexuality, an overarching label for perversion and the lens through which all variation from normal could conveniently be seen. See Fone, *Homophobia: A History*, 355–421.

8. Pomeroy, *Dr. Kinsey*, 54.

9. Pomeroy, *Dr. Kinsey*, 54.

10. Pomeroy, *Dr. Kinsey*, 57–61.

11. This chapter is adapted from Bakker et al., *Others of My Kind*, with the kind permission of the author and publisher. We (Annette Timm and her colleagues working on *Others of My Kind*) expected that Kinsey must have somehow drawn on the research of Hirschfeld, and we expected to base our exhibition on a small archival treasure, the "Hirschfeld Scrapbook," which we knew was housed in the archives of the Kinsey Institute in Bloomington. We were disappointed to discover that the scrapbook (a scattered collection of letters, reports, and published documents from Hirschfeld's years as a researcher and gay-rights activist) had arrived at the Institute after Kinsey's death in 1956. (Someone had found it in Nice in 1959, long after Hirschfeld's own death in 1935.)

12. Kinsey's two books were an immediate sensation—the *Male* book had gone into its sixth printing ten days after it was released. See Pomeroy, *Dr. Kinsey*, 265. Although tracking down sales numbers is a daunting task, it is clear that the two books together sold hundreds of thousands of copies and were translated into many languages. See Suresha, "Properly Placed Before the Public"; Kinsey, Pomeroy, and Martin, *Male*; Kinsey et al., *Female*.

13. See chapter 7 in this volume.

14. Even the most well-known and influential trans and intersex memoirs of this period tend to emphasize the role of doctors or are narrated by others. The most obvious example is the biography of Lili Elbe, which is almost always called a memoir or an autobiography despite having been written by someone else; see Hoyer, *Man into Woman*. Another example of medical intervention in the authorship of trans/intersex memoirs (labeling oneself as intersex to account for one's gender diversity and desire to change physically) is Hirschfeld's influence in the publication by Body, *Memoirs of a Man's Maiden Years*.

15. See Foucault, *History of Sexuality*; Dickinson and Wetzell, "Historiography of Sexuality," 298–99.

16. Having lived her entire life as a female, Barbin was "discovered" to be male when she was twenty-two and forced to change her gender presentation to male. This prevented her from continuing a relationship with her female lover. She committed suicide in 1868. See Foucault, *Herculine Barbin*, vii–xvii.

17. Frank, Gillian and Lauren Gutterman, "Canary," at 11:25–11:40 in the recording.

18. Eder, *Kultur*, 17.

19. Oosterhuis, *Stepchildren*, 185.

20. Oosterhuis, *Stepchildren*, 12.

21. Oosterhuis, "Sexual Modernity," 137. See also Krafft-Ebing, "Neue Studien." Krafft-Ebing argued that homosexuality should not be thought of as an indication of degeneration (p. 2) and that it was more akin to a small physical deformity than to a depravity or sickness (p. 5).

22. An analysis of some of the questionnaires can be found in Hirschfeld's medical journal, the *Jahrbuch für sexuelle Zwischenstufen*, but the originals were mostly destroyed when the institute was plundered by Nazi students on May 9, 1933. See Herrn, Taylor, and Timm, "A Visual Sourcebook," 64. The estimate of ten thousand questionnaires is from Hirschfeld, *The Transvestites*, 11. In 1904, Hirschfeld conducted a survey of students and metal workers in Berlin seeking to establish the proportion of homosexual and bisexual individuals in the population to campaign against anti-homosexual laws. His work experienced a setback when he was fined 200 Marks for sending survey postcards asking about sexual identification through the mail. See Hirschfeld, "Das Ergebnis," 109–78. This is the only Hirschfeld questionnaire to which Kinsey refers. See Kinsey, Pomeroy, and Martin, *Male*, 691.

23. Hirschfeld, *Die Transvestiten*. This book was not translated into English until 1991.

24. Hirschfeld, *Die Transvestiten*, 4–5.

25. He describes some of these visits in detail in Hirschfeld, *Berlins*. Even in this book, which was clearly meant for a popular audience, Hirschfeld maintains the

voice of the objective (in other words, nonparticipant) observer, yet the inclusion of information about intimate relationships and festive rituals are indications that these visits were neither fleeting nor impersonal.

26. Trust is central to political organization of all kinds. See Frevert, "Does Trust Have a History?" (Prof. Timm thanks Katie Sutton for pointing her to this citation.) This is just one example of Frevert's work on the history of emotions, a subject that has recently gained more scholarly attention. See Biess, "History of Emotions"; Scheer, "Are Emotions a Kind of Practice."

27. See the various contributions in Taylor, Timm, and Herrn, *Not Straight*.

28. Dobler, *Zwischen*, 43–51.

29. Beachy, *Gay Berlin*, 55.

30. Dobler, *Zwischen*, 399–406.

31. Hirschfeld notes that it is difficult to give an exact number, because of the underground nature of these establishments. The estimate is from Hirschfeld, *Berlins*, 74.

32. Hirschfeld, *Die Homosexualität*, 1001–02.

33. Following advice from Hirschfeld, Berlin police officials issued this *Transvestitenpass* (transvestite pass) to Eva Katter (who called himself Gert and was a carpenter) on December 6, 1928. The card reads: "The worker Eva Katter, born on March 14, 1910, and residing in Britz Muthesisush of 8, is known here as someone who wears male clothing. Strewe, Police Commissioner." Katter was a patient at the Institute for Sexual Science and was occasionally presented to visitors as a "demonstration case" (medical specimen). While living in the former German Democratic Republic, he was one of the few institute patients to later establish contact with the Magnus Hirschfeld Society. In donating his records, Katter reclaimed his history and made it part of the Institute's archive. He died in 1995.

34. Photographs of patrons at the Eldorado may be seen at https://ghdi.ghi-dc.org/sub_image.cfm?image_id=4243.

35. Benjamin, "Reminiscences," 4.

36. Benjamin, "Reminiscences," 4.

37. Kinsey conflates various terms in a way that Benjamin would most likely have objected to: "The terms sexual inversion, intersexuality, transsexuality, the third sex, psychosexual hermaphroditism, and others have been applied not merely to designate the nature of the partner involved in sexual relation, but to emphasize the general opinion that individuals engaging in homosexual activity are neither male nor female, but persons of mixed sex." See Kinsey, Pomeroy, and Martin, *Male*, 612.

38. Benjamin notes that it was Robert Latou Dickinson who brought the two together. See Benjamin "Reminiscences," 9.

39. In a letter from August 24, 1946, Kinsey thanks Benjamin for "the splendid help you gave us while we were in the city. Your leads were valuable and it becomes

very apparent that we must get San Francisco started before you give up spending your summers there. You could do worlds for us in helping us to know people." Kinsey Institute Library & Special Collections, Harry Benjamin Collection (hereafter KILSC-HB), Correspondence, Folder 1.

40. Kinsey et al., "Concepts of Normality," 12. Kinsey argued that "Wherever one finds contradictory interpretations of what is sexually normal and abnormal, one should consider whether philosophic, moral, or social evaluations, or scientific records of material fact are involved."

41. Kinsey et al., "Concepts of Normality," 12.

42. Kinsey et al., *Female*, 681.

43. Kinsey et al., *Female*, 681.

44. Benjamin, "Introduction," 3.

45. The Health Information Portability and Accountability Act and its attendant regulations were only introduced in 1996. While there were general professional (and personally held) ethics that valued privacy, doctors routinely discussed patients. Real knowledge about LGBTQ+ health was particularly sparse, and as a result, specialists often exchanged information among trusted colleagues.

46. Albert Deutsch, "What Dr. Kinsey Is up to Now!" *Look*, May 8, 1951, quoted in Gathorne-Hardy, Wolfe, and Condon, *Kinsey*, 98–99.

47. Drucker, *Classification of Sex*, 1, 9; Cryle and Stephens, *Normality*, 336. On quantification in the life sciences and its influence on sexology more generally, see Chiang, "Liberating Sex," 50–52.

48. Simon, "Review of Judith," 91–93. Of course, this critique was by no means the loudest that Kinsey's books elicited. He immediately became and remains a favored subject of contempt for the Christian right, as exemplified particularly by the writings of Judith A. Reisman and Edward W. Eichel, which now exists only as a self-published e-book. William Simon has accurately described their assessment as nothing but a paranoid assembly of "innuendo, distortion, and selective representation of decontextualized 'facts.'"

49. Meyerowitz, "Sex Research," 77; Kinsey et al., *Female*, 679–81.

50. Carla Erskine (pseudonym) to Benjamin, 14 Oct 1953, KILSC-HB, Box 4, Ser. II C. On the usual length of Kinsey's interviews, see Paul A. Robinson, *The Modernization of Sex: Havelock Ellis, Alfred Kinsey, William Masters and Virginia Johnson* (Ithaca, NY: Cornell University Press, 1989), 44.

51. Meyerowitz, *How Sex Changed*, 85, citing correspondence from Kinsey to Lawrence, 10 Oct 1949, KILSC, Lawrence Collection.

52. Kinsey, Pomeroy, and Martin, *Male*, 656–57.

53. Herrn, Taylor, and Timm, "Magnus Hirschfelds, 173–96, 185. As Herrn points out, this notion of a spectrum did not protect Hirschfeld from privileging homosexuality over other intermediary variations. See also Hill, "Sexuality and Gender," 316–32, esp. 320.

54. Magnus Hirschfeld, *Geschlechtskunde*, vol. 1: Die körperseelischen Grundlagen (Stuttgart: Julius Püttmann, 1926), 599, cited in Herrn, Taylor, and Timm, "Magnus Hirschfelds," 185.

55. Kinsey, Pomeroy, and Martin, *Male*, 691, in reference to Hirschfeld, "Das Ergebnis," 109–78.

56. Drucker, *Classification of Sex*, 74. As Donna Drucker notes, Kinsey privileged works that relied on scientific rather than religiously inspired argument, on face-to-face interviews or survey data, and on large sample sizes. While Hirschfeld's work would have satisfied the first three criteria and certainly had the advantage of also exploring nonmarital sex, Kinsey would certainly have considered it insufficiently quantitative.

57. Bauer, "Sexology Backward," 133–49. Bauer provides a fascinating and instructive textual analysis of Kinsey to further excavate the links between the two men.

58. Kinsey et al., *Female*, 641.

59. Irvine, *Disorders of Desire*, 47–48.

60. Kinsey et al., *Female*, 412, quoted in Irvine, *Disorders of Desire*, 28.

61. Kinsey et al., *Female*, 412, quoted in Irvine, *Disorders of Desire*, 35.

62. Jorgensen, *Christine Jorgensen*, 189, cited in Meyerowitz, *How Sex Changed*, 92–93.

63. Meyerowitz, "Sex Research," 80.

64. The figure of 18,300 case studies comes from Frayser and Whitby, *Studies in Human Sexuality*, 103. Drucker cites the number of 18,000 case studies for both the *Male* and the *Female* volumes; see Drucker, *Classification of Sex*, 112. On Kinsey's punch card system, see Drucker, *Classification of Sex*, esp. 107–15.

65. Quoted in Jones, *Alfred C. Kinsey*, 622.

66. Meyerowitz argues that Kinsey's sustained contact and long campaign to change his mind about transvestism had "planted [the] seed of doubt" by the early 1950s. Meyerowitz, "Sex Research," 75.

67. Beemyn notes that the first female-assigned, nonintersexed person to have received hormonal treatment (in 1939) and genital surgery (in 1946) was the British physician Michael Dillon. (See chapter 4 for more on Dillon.) Meyerowitz points out that while the ratios of reported cases have been very skewed toward trans women in the past, "today some doctors in the United States find roughly equivalent numbers of male-to-females (MTFs) and female-to-males (FTMs)." See Meyerowitz, *How Sex Changed*, 9. See also the chapter "Have Female-to-Male Transsexuals Always Existed?" in Devor, *FTM*; Skidmore, *True Sex*; Mak, "Passing Women."

68. Beemyn, "Transgender History," 11.

69. See Chapter 14:1. Profile: Eugen Steinach.

70. Kinsey et al., *Female*, 90, 716.

71. Kinsey et al., *Female*, 721.

72. Kinsey et al., *Female*, 729.
73. Kinsey, Pomeroy, and Martin, *Male*, 727–28.

WORKS CITED

Bakker, Alex, Rainer Herrn, Michael Thomas Taylor, and Annette F. Timm. *Others of My Kind: Transatlantic Transgender Histories*. Alberta, Canada: University of Calgary Press, 2020.

Bauer, Heike. "Sexology Backward: Hirschfeld, Kinsey and the Reshaping of Sex Research in the 1950s." In *Queer 1950s: Rethinking Sexuality in the Postwar Years*, edited by Heike Baur and Matt Cook, 133–49. New York: Palgrave MacMillan, 2012.

Beachy, Robert. *Gay Berlin: Birthplace of a Modern Identity*. New York: Knopf, 2014.

Beemyn, Genny. "Transgender History in the United States: A Special Unabridged Version of a Book Chapter from *Trans Bodies, Trans Selves*," edited by Laura Erickson-Schroth, 501–36. Oxford: Oxford University Press, 2014. Accessed June 24, 2019. https://www.umass.edu/stonewall/sites/default/files/Infoforandabout/transpeople/genny_beemyn_transgender_history_in_the_united_states.pdf.

Benjamin, Harry. "Introduction." In *Transsexualism and Sex Reassignment*, edited by Richard Green and John Money, 1–10. Baltimore, MD: Johns Hopkins University Press, 1969.

———. "Reminiscences." *Journal of Sex Research* 6, no. 1 (1970): 3–4.

Biess, Frank. "History of Emotions." *German History* 28, no. 1 (2010): 67–80.

Body, N. O. *Memoirs of a Man's Maiden Years*. Translated by Deborah Simon. Philadelphia: University of Pennsylvania Press, 2009.

Chiang, Howard H. "Liberating Sex, Knowing Desire: Scientia Sexualis and Epistemic Turning Points in the History of Sexuality." *History of the Human Sciences* 23, no. 5 (2010): 42–69.

Clark, Anna. *Desire: A History of European Sexuality*. New York: Routledge, 2008.

Cryle, Peter, and Elizabeth Stephens. *Normality: A Critical Genealogy*. Chicago, IL: University of Chicago Press, 2017.

Devor, Aaron. (1997). *FTM: Female-to-Male Transsexuals in Society*. Bloomington: Indiana University Press, 2016.

Dickinson, Edward Ross, and Richard F. Wetzell. "The Historiography of Sexuality in Modern Germany." *German History* 23, no. 3 (2005): 291–305.

Dobler, Jens. *Zwischen Duldungspolitik und Verbrechensbekämpfung: Homosexuellenverfolgung durch die Berliner Polizei von 1848 bis 1933*. Frankfurt: Verlag für Polizeiwissenschaft, 2008.

Drucker, Donna J. *The Classification of Sex: Alfred Kinsey and the Organization of Knowledge* Pittsburgh, PA: University of Pittsburgh Press, 2014.

Eder, Franz X. *Kultur der Begierde: eine Geschichte der Sexualität.* Munich: Verlag C. H. Beck, 2002.

Ettner, Randi. *Gender Loving Care: A Guide to Counseling Gender-Variant Clients.* New York: W. W. Norton, 1999.

Fone, Byrne. *Homophobia: A History.* New York: Metropolitan Books, Henry Holt, 2000.

Foucault, Michel. *Herculine Barbin.* Translated by Richard McDougall. New York: Random House, 1980.

———. *History of Sexuality, Vol. 1, An Introduction.* New York: Pantheon Books, 1978.

Frank, Gillian, and Lauren Gutterman. "Canary." Podcast hosted and created by Gillian Frank and Lauren Gutterman. *Sexing History*, 2020, Season 2, Episode 4. Accessed August 5, 2024. https://www.sexinghistory.com/episode-24.

Frayser, Suzanne G., and Thomas J. Whitby. 1995. *Studies in Human Sexuality: A Selected Guide.* 2nd ed. Englewood, CO: Libraries Unlimited, 1995.

Frevert, Ute. "Does Trust Have a History?" *Max Weber Programme Lectures: Published Papers (2007–2016).* San Domenico di Fiesole: European University Institute, 2009. Accessed August 5, 2024. http://cadmus.eui.eu//handle/1814/11258.

Gathorne-Hardy, Jonathan, Linda Wolfe, and Bill Condon. *Kinsey: Public and Private.* New York: Newmarket Press, 2004.

Haefele-Thomas, Ardel. *Introduction to Transgender Studies.* New York: Harrington Park Press, 2019.

Herrn, Rainer. "Magnus Hirschfelds Geschlechterkosmogonie: Die Zwischenstufentheorie im Kontext hegemonialer." In *Männlichkeiten und Moderne: Geschlecht in den Wissenskulturen um 1900*, edited by Ulrike Brunotte and Rainer Herrn, 173–96. Bielefeld: Transcript Verlag, 2007.

Herrn, Rainer, Michael Thomas Taylor, and Annette F. Timm. "Magnus Hirschfeld's Institute for Sexual Science: A Visual Sourcebook." In *Not Straight from Germany: Sexual Publics and Sexual Citizenship since Magnus Hirschfeld*, edited by Michael Thomas Taylor, Annette F. Timm, and Rainer Hern, 37–79. Ann Arbor: Michigan University Press, 2017.

Hill, Darryl B. "Sexuality and Gender in Hirschfeld's *Die Transvestiten*: A Case of the 'Elusive Evidence of the Ordinary.'" *Journal of the History of Sexuality* 14, no. 3 (2005): 316–32.

Hirschfeld, Magnus. (1904) 1991. *Berlins drittes Geschlecht: Mit einem Anhang: Paul Näcke, Ein Besuch bei den Homosexuellen in Berlin*, edited by Manfred Herzer. Berlin: Verlag Rosa Winkel.

———. "Das Ergebnis der statistischen Untersuchungen über den Prozentsatz der Homosexuellen." *Jahrbuch für sexuelle Zwischenstufen* 6 (1904): 109–78.

———. *Die Homosexualität des Mannes und des Weibes.* Berlin: Louis Marcus Verlagsbuchhandlung, 1914.

———. *Die Transvestiten: Eine Untersuchung über den erotischen Verkleidungstrieb.* Berlin: Alfred Pulvermacher, 1910.

——— . *The Transvestites: The Erotic Drive to Cross-Dress*. Buffalo, NY: Prometheus Books, 1991.

Hoyer, Niels, ed. *Man into Woman: An Authentic Record of a Change of Sex*. Translated by H. J. Stenning. New York: E. P. Dutton, 1933.

Irvine, Janice M. *Disorders of Desire: Sexuality and Gender in Modern American Sexology*. Philadelphia, PA: Temple University Press, 2005.

Jones, James H. *Alfred C. Kinsey: A Public/Private Life*. New York: W. W. Norton, 1997.

Jorgensen, Christine. *Christine Jorgensen: A Personal Autobiography*, with an introduction by Harry Benjamin. New York: P. S. Eriksson, 1967.

Kinsey, Alfred C., Wardell R. Pomeroy, and Clyde E. Martin. *Sexual Behavior in the Human Male*. Philadelphia, PA: W. B. Saunders, 1948.

Kinsey, Alfred C., Wardell B. Pomeroy, Clyde E. Martin, and Paul H. Gebhard. "Concepts of Normality and Abnormality in Sexual Behavior." In *Psychosexual Development in Health and Disease*, edited by Paul H. Hoch and Joseph Zubin, 11–32. New York: Grune & Stratton, 1949.

Kinsey, Alfred C., Wardell R. Pomeroy, Paul H. Gebhard, Clyde E. Martin, and John Bancroft. *Sexual Behavior in the Human Female*. Philadelphia, PA: W. B. Saunders, 1953.

Krafft-Ebing, Richard von. "Neue Studien auf dem Gebiete der Homosexualität." *Jahrbuch für sexuelle Zwischenstufen* 3 (1901): 1–36.

Mak, Geertje. " 'Passing Women' in the Consulting Room of Magnus Hirschfeld: On Why the Term 'Transvestite' Was Not Employed for Crossdressing Women." *Österreichische Zeitschrift für Geschichtswissenschaften* 9, no. 3 (1998): 384–99.

Meyerowitz, Joanne. *How Sex Changed: A History of Transsexuality in the United States*. Cambridge: Harvard University Press, 2002.

Meyerowitz, Joanne J. "Sex Research at the Borders of Gender: Transvestites, Transsexuals, and Alfred C. Kinsey." *Bulletin of the History of Medicine* 75, no. 1 (2001): 72–90.

Mottier, Veronique. *Sexuality: A Very Short Introduction*. Oxford: Oxford University Press, 2008.

Nye, Robert A., ed. *Sexuality*. Oxford: Oxford University Press, 1999.

Oosterhuis, Harry. "Sexual Modernity in the Works of Richard von Krafft-Ebing and Albert Moll." *Medical History* 56, no. 2 (2012): 133–55.

——— . *Stepchildren of Nature: Krafft-Ebing, Psychiatry and the Making of Sexual Identity*. Chicago, IL: University of Chicago Press, 2000.

Pfaefflin, Friedemann. "Sex Reassignment, Harry Benjamin, and Some European Roots." *International Journal of Transgenderism* 1, no. 2 (1997). Accessed August 5, 2024. web.archive.org/web/20070427233344/http://www.symposion.com/ijt/ijtc0 202.htm.

Pomeroy, Wardell Baxter. *Dr. Kinsey and the Institute for Sex Research*. New York: Harper and Row, 1972.

Scheer, Monique. "Are Emotions a Kind of Practice (and Is That What Makes Them Have a History)? A Bourdieuian Approach to Understanding Emotion." *History and Theory* 51, no. 2 (2012): 193–220.

Simon, William. "Review of Judith A. Reisman and Edward W. Eichel's *Kinsey, Sex and Fraud: The Indoctrination of a People. An Investigation into the Human Sexuality Research of Alfred C. Kinsey, Wardell B. Pomeroy, Clyde E. Martin, and Paul H. Gebhard.*" *Archives of Sexual Behavior* 21 (1992): 91–93.

Skidmore, Emily. *True Sex: The Lives of Trans Men at the Turn of the Twentieth Century*. New York: New York University Press, 2017.

Smith, Jill Suzanne. *Berlin Coquette: Prostitution and the New German Woman, 1890–1933*. Ithaca, NY: Cornell University Press, 2014.

Stryker, Susan. *Transgender History*. Berkeley, CA: Seal Press, 2008.

Suresha, Ron Jackson. "'Properly Placed Before the Public': Publication and Translation of the Kinsey Reports." *Journal of Bisexuality* 8, nos. 3–4 (2008): 203–28.

Sutton, Katie. "'We Too Deserve a Place in the Sun': The Politics of Transvestite Identity in Weimar Germany." *German Studies Review* 35, no 2 (2012): 335–54.

Taylor, Michael Thomas, Annette F. Timm, and Rainer Herrn, eds. *Not Straight from Germany: Sexual Publics and Sexual Citizenship since Magnus Hirschfeld*. Ann Arbor: Michigan University Press, 2017.

3.1. PROFILE: LILI ELBE (1882–1931)

Carolyn Wolf-Gould

In 1933, Neils Hoyer published *Man into Woman*,[1] an edited autobiographical account of Lili Elbe's surgical transition, one of the first at Hirschfeld's Institute of Sexual Science in Berlin. Lili, born Einar Wegener in Denmark in 1882, attended the Royal Danish Academy of Fine Arts in Copenhagen and became an acclaimed landscape painter. At the academy, she met and later (1904) married Gerda Gottlieb, a painter, fashion illustrator, and illustrator of lesbian erotica. Around 1908, after the Danish actress Anna Larson missed her modeling session with Gerda Wegener, Gerda asked her spouse to pose in women's clothing, an event that led to Lili's awakening to her feminine gender identity.[2] After this, Lili frequently modeled for Gerda as a woman. In 1912, word got out that the exquisite woman in Gottlieb's paintings was Einar Wegener, the respected Danish painter—scandal ensued. The two moved to Paris, a more liberal environment, where they both continued to work. Elbe exhibited her work at the famed Salon d'Automne and lived more and more as herself over the following two decades. During this time, she became increasingly desperate to live as a woman and, in 1930, sought help from Magnus Hirschfeld at the Institute of Sexual Science, where she underwent four or five experimental gender surgeries, beginning that year.

Hoyer's widely published version of Elbe's autobiography established Western cultural expectations about transgender and gender-diverse people and justification for the transsexual experience. The accuracy of Hoyer's take is questionable, but he relayed Elbe's story with dignity and compassion; he described her experience with dysphoria, stigma, minority stress, and her emotional turmoil through her surgeries. After orchiectomy, Elbe, in physical and emotional pain, asked the questions that confounded not just herself but also the Western world: "Who am I? What am I? What was I? What shall I become?"[3]

Hoyer and Elbe's doctors justified Elbe's gender disturbance as an intersex condition, an early theory for transgenderism that embraced the popular concept of universal bisexuality—the belief that all humans contain male and female components.[4] Preoperatively, Elbe's surgeon speculated that she was born with ovaries hidden within her abdomen, organs that became "stunted and withered," yet still gave her a bigender soul. After surgery, Elbe's physician supposedly confirmed this finding (although no pathology report exists), and Elbe's wife Gerda spilled her heart, professing: "The secret of existing as a double being, hitherto divined by no doctor, has only been unveiled today, after Werner Kreutz had guessed at its existence in Paris, and like a wizard deciphered it."[5] Hoyer's tale presented Elbe's experience as a biological struggle between two distinct individuals—Einar Wegener and Lili Elbe—who coexisted within one body, competing for its possession, with Elbe increasingly in charge.

Elbe's first surgical procedure (an orchiectomy) reportedly led to a feminine transformation so complete that no one recognized her. Gottlieb gushed that Wegener was dead and Elbe's handwriting, voice, and expression were entirely changed. An orchiectomy does not effect a complete feminine transformation; however, without any precedent, Americans read stories and latched onto this magical thinking about medical transitions. Details about Elbe's whiteness, talent, and education launched cultural expectations later perpetuated by Christine Jorgensen about the "right kind" of transsexual. In addition, the trope of the gender physician as a man with life-changing power second only to God firmly took root in Hoyer's narrative: "Hitherto Lili has been like clay which others had prepared and to which the Professor has given form and life. . . . By a single glance the Professor awoke her heart to life, a life with all the instincts of woman."[6] Hoyer described Elbe's reaction to her surgeon: "A single glance of this man had deprived her of all her strength. . . . It was the first time her woman's heart had trembled before her lord and master, before the man who had constituted himself her protector, and she understood why she then submitted so utterly to him and his will."[7]

Eventually, Elbe parted with Gottlieb and became engaged to a cisgender man, conforming to the masculine-defined, socially enforced performative gender role expectations of the time. Her narrative helped establish the experience of white, heterosexual, educated, upperclass trans women as the transsexual standard, ushering in barriers for those with diverse intersectional identities who subsequently tried to access care. Elbe died in 1931 from complications of her last gender-affirming surgery. Her gripping story set the stage for American cultural debates on the appropriateness of gender-affirming medical interventions.

NOTES

1. Hoyer, *Man into Woman*.
2. Lamb, "Biography of Lili Elbe."
3. Hoyer, *Man into Woman*, 102.
4. See chapter 6 in this volume.
5. Hoyer, *Man Into Woman*, 40.
6. Hoyer, *Man Into Woman*, 30.
7. Hoyer, *Man Into Woman*, 128.

WORKS CITED

Hoyer, Niels, ed. (1953). *Man Into Woman*. New York: E. P. Dutton, Popular Library.
Lamb, Bill. "Biography of Lili Elbe, Pioneering Transgender Woman." Thought Co, 2020. Accessed September 28, 2022. https://www.thoughtco.com/lili-elbe-biography-4176321.

3.2. PROFILE: OTTO SPENGLER (1873–UNKNOWN)

Christopher Wolf-Gould

Otto Spengler, an early trans rights activist, was the first patient to seek feminizing hormones from Harry Benjamin, and one of the first trans individuals to collaborate with medical researchers and clinicians in the United States. Born in West Prussia, Germany, in 1873,[1] Spengler was assigned male at birth, but from a young age, he often cross-dressed beneath masculine clothing and wore his hair long.[2] He lived in Berlin as a child and emigrated to New York City at age nineteen.[3] Like Magnus Hirschfeld and Benjamin, Spengler served as an important networking link between the trans community and LGBT activists in Berlin and the United States in the early 1900s. His willingness to share his story with various groups of people in the United States and Germany, including the early sexologists, contributed to developing transcontinental understanding of what was then referred to as *transvestism*.

In Berlin, Spengler applied for the right to "transvest" (that is, cross-dress), but the police department turned down his request.[4] After arriving in the United States, he cross-dressed at home, at his business, and sometimes in public. He married and had three children. His youngest daughter, Hildegard, called him Papa-lady.[5] From a contemporary perspective, Spengler would likely have identified as a transgender woman, based on his "profound longing for female clothes," the wish to "be castrated to be more like a woman," and the desire to "live as a woman absolutely."[6] But during this era, he faced limited options for social transition and lacked accurate language for self-description.

Spengler made a name for himself after he opened the successful Argus Pressclipping Bureau in New York City in 1902.[7] His vast collection of World War I newspaper clippings is now in the Library of Congress collections.[8] He compiled a compendium of biographies of notable German-Americans[9] and pursued an interest in archeology, with travel to what was then known as the Orient and museums in Europe.[10] Spengler actively participated in the German-American community (which included clinicians and medical researchers) and served as a founding member of German immigrant associations in New York.[11]

In 1906, in New York, Spengler served as a director of the Scientific-Humanitarian Committee, the Berlin-based organization founded by Hirschfeld in 1897 and dedicated to research that supported the rights of homosexuals.[12] In May 1906, as part of his work for the committee, Spengler presented a well-received lecture entitled "Sexual Intermediaries" to the German Scientific Society of New York.[13] This talk was one of the first lectures on sexual intermediaries in New York.[14] In the committee's subsequent newsletter, Spengler described the discussion that followed his presentation:

> The debate was very lively. Representatives of all the professions were in the audience—ministers, lawyers, doctors. This was probably the

first such speech given in New York, and I managed to make some headway with my limited resources. You can deduce the inflexibility of some people from this incident: after the topic had been illuminated from all sides, a lawyer stood up and maintained that homosexuals belong in prison. This shows plainly what educational efforts are still required here, where such educated people are so stupid. . . . I hope there will be more understanding here. Now people just faint when the subject is broached.[15]

In 1914, Bernard Talmey, another member of the tight German-American community, published "Transvestism: A Contribution to the Study of the Psychology of Sex" in the *New York Medical Journal*;[16] it was one of the first articles in US medical literature that described people who might now be considered transgender.[17] Talmey, who knew Spengler socially, referred to him as case number 1, Mr. S, and included excerpts from letters written to Spengler by four individuals from the United States, England, and Germany, which revealed the extent of Spengler's network with cross-dressers on both continents.[18] One correspondent in the Talmey publication used the name Miss Othilie when addressing letters to Spengler.[19] Talmey viewed transvestism as pathologic; however, perhaps because of his long-term personal connection to Spengler, he wrote with compassion about his subjects and suggested that cross-dressing stemmed from the "esthetic sensibility" of a man who "harbors exalted ideas and is striving to secure artistic enjoyment in appreciation of the beautiful."[20] He concluded that cross-dressing was not necessarily connected to homosexuality and suggested that these "honorable and moral people"[21] should be allowed to wear clothes of the opposite sex in public. Whimsical photographs included with the article show Spengler dressed in female attire and posing as the Prussian Queen Louise from a celebrated painting.[22]

In 1928, the German pharmaceutical company Schering rolled out commercially available estrogens, including one labeled Progynon.[23] Spengler asked Benjamin for parenteral Progynon for breast development. After some investigation, Benjamin agreed to a treatment protocol, his first experience prescribing gender-affirming hormone therapy.[24] After a few months, Spengler developed small breasts, which pleased him and which Benjamin described as mild gynecomastia.[25] Spengler also underwent a modified Steinach procedure at age fifty-two, which involved radiation of the testicles to reduce the endogenous secretion of testosterone.[26] The date Benjamin treated Spengler is undocumented, but it was likely in the 1930s.[27]

Spengler developed close contacts with the transvestite population in Berlin and contributed several of his artistic photos for the 1931 issue of *Das 3. Geschlecht*, a German periodical focused on transvestites.[28] Leah Schaefer and Connie Wheeler, colleagues of Harry Benjamin, claimed that Spengler was the inspiration for Hirschfeld's seminal *Die Transvestities*, published in 1910.[29] Photos and mention of Spengler also peppered the Benjamin and Alfred Kinsey correspondence, as Benjamin was the source for most of Kinsey's knowledge about trans individuals.[30]

When interviewed by the psychiatrist and researcher George Henry, Spengler, at age sixty-four and under the pseudonym of Rudolph von H., had fallen on difficult times. He was living alone after marital separation, had medical problems, and had suffered an economic downturn in his business.[31] Henry diagnosed Spengler as a narcissist, dismissed his contributions as a historian, and attributed his desire to cross-dress to exhibitionism and vanity.[32] Spengler lived in relative obscurity these later years, and the date of his death is not documented. Posthumously, we now recognize that Spengler's contribution to the history of transgender medicine is rich and extensive.

NOTES

1. Smith, "George Ernest Otto Spengler."
2. Spengler's preference for pronouns is unknown, and the option to change pronouns was limited in this era. In historical documents, Spengler is only referred to with masculine pronouns. Given his unstated preferences, I refer to him in the pronouns publicly used at this time.
3. Timm, "I Am So Grateful," 89.
4. Zagria, "Otto Spengler."
5. Henry, *Sex Variants*, 493.
6. Talmey, "Transvestism," 364.
7. Timm, "I Am So Grateful," 89.
8. Library of Congress, *Collection: World War History*.
9. Spengler, *Das Deutsche Element*, 1–378.
10. Timm, "I Am So Grateful," 89.
11. Timm, "I Am So Grateful," 89.
12. Katz, *Gay American History*, 381.
13. Terry, *An American Obsession*, 111–12.
14. Zagria, "Otto Spengler."
15. Katz, *Gay American History*, 381.

16. Talmey, "Transvestism," 362–68.
17. Timm, "I Am So Grateful," 88.
18. Refer to profile of Louise Lawrence in chapter 7.1 in this volume for more information about early social networks.
19. Talmey, "Transvestism," 367.
20. Talmey, "Transvestism," 368.
21. Talmey, "Transvestism," 368.
22. Talmey, "Transvestism," 362; Thomas and Herrn, "Images of Otto Spengler," 13.
23. Foran, "A Tale of Two Hormones," 39.
24. Benjamin, "Introduction," 1–2.
25. Benjamin, "Introduction," 1–2.
26. Refer to profile of Eugen Steinach in chapter 14.1 of this volume for more information on the Steinach procedure.
27. Timm, "I Am So Grateful," 91.
28. Thomas and Herrn, "Images of Otto Spengler," 14.
29. Timm, "I Am So Grateful," 123.
30. Thomas and Herrn, "Images of Otto Spengler," 15–16.
31. Henry, *Sex Variants*, 489.
32. Timm, "I Am So Grateful," 91.

WORKS CITED

Benjamin, Harry. "Introduction." In *Transsexualism and Sex* Reassignment, edited by John Green and Richard Money, 9–10. Baltimore, MD: Johns Hopkins Press, 1969.A

Foran, Terri. "A Tale of Two Hormones." *Fertility and Reproduction* 1, no. 1 (2019): 39–42.

Green, Richard, and John Money, eds. *Transsexualism and Sex Reassignment.* Baltimore, MD: Johns Hopkins Press, 1969.

Henry, George W. *Sex Variants: A Study of Homosexual Patterns.* New York: P. B. Hoeber, 1948.

Katz, Jonathan. *Gay American History.* New York: Thomas Y. Crowell, 1992.

Library of Congress. *Collection: World War History: Newspaper Clippings, 1914 to 1926.* Accessed September 16, 2021. https://www.loc.gov/collections/world-war-history-newspaper-clippings/.

Santen, R. J., and E. Simpson. "History of Estrogen: Its Purification, Structure, Synthesis, Biologic Actions, and Clinical Implications." *Endocrinology* 16, no. 3 (2019): 605–29.

Simpson E, Santen RJ. "Celebrating 75 Years of Oestrogen." *Journal of Molecular Endocrinology* 55, no. 3 (2015): T1–20.

Smith, Ivy Jo. "George Ernest Otto Spengler." *Geni*, December 31, 2014. Accessed August 23, 2021. https://www.geni.com/people/George-Spengler/6000000008880051603.

Spengler, Otto, ed. *Das Deutsche Element Der Stadt New York*. New York: Spengler, 1913.

Talmey, B. S. "Transvestism: A Contribution to the Study of the Psychology of Sex." *New York Medical Journal* 99 (1914): 362–08.

Talmey, Bernard. *Love: A Treatise on the Science of Sex-Attraction. For the Use of Physicians and Students of Medical Jurisprudence*. New York: Practitioners' Publishing, 1908.

Terry, Jennifer. *An American Obsession: Science, Medicine, and Homosexuality in Modern Society*. Chicago, IL: University of Chicago Press, 1999.

Thomas, Michael, and Rainer Herrn. "Images of Otto Spengler." In *Others of My Kind, Transatlantic Transgender Histories*, edited by Alex Bakker, Rainer Herrn, Michael Taylor, and Annette Timm, 13–18. Calgary, Alberta: University of Calgary Press, 2020.

Timm, Annette. "'I Am So Grateful to All You Men of Medicine': Trans Circles of Knowledge and Intimacy." In *Others of My Kind, Transatlantic Transgender Histories*, edited by Alex Bakker, Rainer Hern, Michael Taylor, and Annette Timm, 88–89. Calgary, Alberta: University of Calgary Press, 2020.

Zagria. "Otto Spengler (1876?–194?) Businessperson." *zagriablogspot.com* (blog), November 18, 2016. Accessed January 15, 2021. https://zagria.blogspot.com/2016/11/otto-spengler-1876-194-businessperson.html#.YANl6C2ZPBK

3.3. ESTABLISHING NORTH AMERICAN CULTURAL NORMS: EARLY TRANSGENDER COLONISTS AND AMERICANS (1600–1930s)

Carolyn Wolf-Gould

A few recorded accounts of gender-nonconforming people in the New World offer a glimpse into developing norms that later informed the cultural response to medical interventions in the United States.

The story of Thomas Hall reveals the extent of a community and legal investigation about gender ambiguity during this period. Around 1627, Hall immigrated from England to Worrosquyoacke, Virginia (a settlement that bordered Jamestown), as an indentured servant.[1] Born Thomasine Hall in 1603, Hall was raised as a girl, but as a young adult, began alternating between male and female clothing and employment. After arriving in Virginia, Hall usually presented as male, but sometimes chose feminine clothing, unsettling the colonists who relied on gender norms to control the social order within their rapidly changing immigrant community. After rumors circulated that Hall conducted an affair with the governor's maid, Hall ran into legal troubles. If Hall was a man, Hall could be prosecuted for sexual congress with a servant. While Hall slept, several laypeople took it upon themselves to examine Hall's genitalia and agreed that, while puzzling, they believed Hall was male. Hall detailed a bigendered social history to the court, claimed to be both male and female, and admitted to the possession of a small, nonfunctional penis. Hall's case was heard in Quarter Court in 1629, with Governor John Pott presiding. The court ruled that Hall had a dual nature. In punishment for Hall's gender ambiguity and the chaos Hall brought to the colony, the court ruled that Hall must henceforth always dress in mixed masculine–feminine clothing.

A few other recorded snippets described gender-diverse individuals who lived within early colonial North America. In 1769, a Spanish missionary penned his loathing for some of the Indigenous people he encountered on his arrival to California:

> I have substantial evidence that those Indian men who both here and farther inland, are observed in the dress, clothing, and character of women—there being two or three such in each village—pass as Sodomites by profession (it being confirmed that all these Indians are much addicted to this abominable vice) and permit the heathen to practice the execrable, unnatural abuse of their bodies. They are called *joyas* and are held in great esteem. Let this mention suffice for a matter which could not be omitted—on account of the bearing it may have on the discussion of the reduction of these natives—with a promise to revert in another place to an excess so criminal that it seems even forbidden to speak its name.[2]

The Spaniards proceeded to execute the *joyas*; some Spaniards tossed Indigenous people to their mastiffs and greyhounds, which had developed a taste for human flesh.[3]

In 1771, a Boston newspaper advertised to capture a runaway: "A Negro Man Servant, named Cato . . . well known by the Name of Miss Betty Cooper,"[4] acknowledging Cato's feminine name, if not her humanity. Also in 1771, Queen Anne awarded Edward Hyde, Earl of Cornbury (1661–1723), the governorship of New York and New Jersey in return for his political loyalty.[5] During his seven-year reign in the colonies, the population distrusted him; various individuals accused him of embezzlement, accepting bribes, interfering in local governance, persecuting Presbyterians, and cross-dressing.[6] Two mysterious portraits of an androgynous-appearing person in a blue frock hang in the Dallas Museum of Art and the New York State Historical Society; some assert they are portraits of Lord Cornbury in drag.[7] While it's unclear if the charges of cross-dressing were true or an attempt to slander the Lord, the ridicule attests to early, negative cultural views regarding cross-dressing.

In 1776, Jemima Wilkinson (1752–1819), assigned female at birth, emerged from a near-death experience, transiting a mystical conversion that led to identifying as neither male nor female. He adopted masculine pronouns, dressed in androgynous attire, claimed the name The Public Universal Friend, and launched both a new religious sect in English-speaking America and the concept of nonbinary gender identity. Expelled from his Quaker meeting, The Friend became an itinerate prophet, claiming that a divine male spirit had taken possession of Wilkinson's female body. Many Americans viewed The Friend as an aberration; nevertheless, he traveled throughout New England with a retinue of twelve to twenty adherents, delivering apocalyptic sermons, attending to the bereaved, comforting soldiers, and attracting a considerable following of errant Quakers, women, and others who were moved by his ministry.[8]

THE ROLE OF THE POPULAR PRESS

Before the beginning of the twentieth century, the nation lacked a cohesive narrative to explain transgenderism and continued to learn about transgender and gender-diverse (TGD) people through personal encounters or press reports. There was plenty else to think about in a country reeling from the Civil War; ongoing racial tensions; mass migrations; suffrage; industrialization; urbanization; clashes with American Indians; the gold rush; and the growth of roadways, railways, and communication infrastructure. Yet nothing sells better than scandal and sex. In the absence of scientific inquiry, the US popular press stepped up to inform the American public about gender transgressions in sensationalized newspaper accounts, packed with editorial bias. These stories reflected and established existing cultural norms just before the arrival of European medical reports about gender transitions.

Historian Emily Skidmore culled newspaper reports to identify sixty-five transgender men who lived between 1870 and 1930.[9] These primarily white men tended to settle in rural American communities, preferring the tolerance and personal connections fostered by small-town familiarity over the hubbub of urban centers.[10] It was easier and safer to pass as male and blend into the established community. The press published accounts of discovery when these men were outed by life events. Stories generally followed a consistent template: the "true sex" of a person who had been cross-living in stealth was suddenly revealed by the discovery of genitals at odds with cultural assumptions . . . and everybody was shocked.

For the most part, these individuals conformed to the dominant white, masculine, heteronormative cultural expectations of the time: marrying and functioning as husbands, frequenting saloons, performing manual labor, and serving as contributing members to their communities. The discovery stories were designed to scandalize, but some accounts also validated the individual's masculine role and community's acceptance.[11] After the death of farmhand George Green in Ettrick, Virginia, in 1902, and the subsequent discovery that he was anatomically female, his widow buried him in male clothing in the Catholic cemetery and eulogized him thus: "The noblest soul that ever lived. He has worked hard through his life and has been all I had to cheer me. . . . He was a Christian and I believe he is now with Christ."[12] Other cross-living men received mixed reports; more than four hundred women cross-dressed during the Civil War to fight as soldiers on both sides of the conflict.[13] When discovered, they were summarily discharged and alternately described in the press as heroes and freaks.

On the Western Frontier from 1870 to 1920, TGD people colored daily life.[14] An 1880 *New York Times* obituary described the bravery of Charley Parkhurst (One-Eyed Charley), one of the "most dexterous and celebrated of the famous California stagecoach drivers," and the shocking discovery that he "was . . . a woman" by those who prepared him for burial.[15] The Wild West culture adhered to a binary two-sex/two-gender model, and without words for transgender embodiment, society referred to these individuals as cross-dressers or homosexuals or sex inverts or explained their behaviors as situational, that is, the only way for a woman to survive in the West (or serve in the war) was to masquerade as a man.[16] It was harder to rationalize male-to-female cross-dressers, whose existence ran counter to the pioneer image of the West; the culture othered these individuals, associating their TGD identity with non-white, non-Anglo races.[17]

While white transgender men received mixed renderings from the press, stories about transgender women, especially African American women—steeped in ridicule, derision, and censure—established and perpetuated the inextricable link between racism, classism, misogyny, and transphobia. In June 1836, two

New York newspapers reported on the case of Mary Jones, an African American sex worker outed as male during an investigation for picking the pockets of her johns.[18] In court, she stated that she "attended parties among the people of my own Color dressed this way—and in New Orleans, I always dressed this way."[19] She presented to the court "neatly dressed in female attire and his head covered by a female wig." A member of the audience snatched the wig from her head during the trial, to a roar of laughter from all assembled. The court sentenced Jones to five years of hard labor in Sing Sing Correctional Facility for grand larceny. Henry Robinson published a lithograph of Jones in feminine clothing with the title *The Man-Monster; Peter Sewally, alias Mary Jones*, cementing her place in history as a male freak—or effectively as a nonperson.[20]

Figure 3.3.1. Peter Sewally, "The Man Monster," 1836. *Source*: Harry T. Peters "America on Stone" Lithography Collection, National Museum of American History. Public domain.

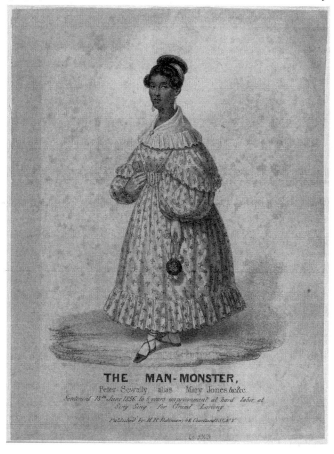

NOTES

1. Brown, "Changed . . . into the Fashion of a Man," 17–193.
2. Fages and Priestly, *An Historical, Political, and Natural Description of California*, 503.
3. Gutierrez, "Bar Chee Ampe and Beyond."
4. Hopkins, "'Well Known as Miss Better Cooper,'" 1.
5. Anonymous, "Portrait of a Lady."
6. Anonymous, "Portrait of an Unidentifed Woman."
7. Anonymous, "Portrait of a Lady"; Anonymous, "Portrait of an Unidentifed Woman."
8. Morris, "The Person Formerly Known as Jemima Wilkinson."
9. Skidmore, *True Sex: The Lives of Trans Men*, 43–67.
10. Skidmore, *True Sex: The Lives of Trans Men*, 43–44.
11. Skidmore, *True Sex: The Lives of Trans Men*, 43–67.
12. *Times*, "Mrs. Green's Secret A Life Sacrifice," 13.
13. Blanton, "Women Soldiers of the Civil War."
14. Boag, *Re-Dressing America's Frontier Past*, 1–187.
15. *New York Times*, "A Noted Old California Stage-Driver Discovered," 2.
16. Boag, *Re-Dressing America's Frontier Past*, 5–6.
17. Boag, *Re-Dressing America's Frontier Past*, 6–7.
18. Katz, "The 'Man-Monster.'"
19. Katz, "The 'Man-Monster.'"
20. Katz, "The 'Man-Monster'"; Robinson, *The Man-Monster*.

WORKS CITED

Anonymous. *Portrait of a Lady, Possibly Edward Hyde, Lord Cornbury in a Dress*. c. 1705–1750. Dallas Museum of Art. Accessed January 2, 2021. https://collections.dma.org/artwork/4278319.

Anonymous. *Portrait of an Unidentifed Woman*. ca. 1710, oil on canvas. New-York Historical Society Museum & Library. Accessed January 2, 2021. https://emuseum.nyhistory.org/objects/41409/portrait-of-an-unidentified-woman?ctx=5c6dce31e443efe2109e800def8b1057ad7d83b4&idx=7.

Blanton, Deanne. "Women Soldiers of the Civil War." *National Achives, Prologue Magazine* 25, no. 1 (1993). Accessed January 2021. https://www.archives.gov/publications/prologue/1993/spring/women-in-the-civil-war-1.html.

Boag, Peter. *Re-Dressing America's Frontier Past*. Berkely: University of California Press, 2011.

Brown, Kathleen. "Changed . . . into the Fashion of a Man: The Politics of Sexual Difference in a Seventeenth-Century Anglo-American Settlement." *Journal of the History of Sexuality* 6, no. 2 (1995): 171–73.

Fages, Don Pedro, and Herbert I. Priestly. *An Historical, Political, and Natural Description of California. Vol. 5. The Catholic Historical Review*, 488–509. Washington, DC: Catholic University of America Press, 1919.

Gutierrez, Jeanne. "Bar Chee Ampe and Beyond: Uncovering Two-Spirit Identity, Part 1." *New-York Historical Society Museum and Library.* November 13, 2019. Accessed September 28, 2021. https://womenatthecenter.nyhistory.org/two-spirit-identity-1/.

Hopkins, Caitlin. " 'Well Known as Miss Better Cooper' Gender Expression in 18th-Century Boston." *Public Seminar.* December 20, 2018. Accessed January 2, 2021. https://publicseminar.org/2018/12/well-known-as-miss-betty-cooper/.

Katz, Jonathan. "The 'Man-Monster.' " *Outhistory*, September 28, 2013. Accessed January 3, 2021. http://outhistory.org/exhibits/show/sewally-jones/man-monster.

Morris, Adam. "The Person Formerly Known as Jemima Wilkinson." *Los Angeles Review of Books*, March 26, 2019. Accessed September 29, 2021. https://lareviewofbooks.org/article/the-person-formerly-known-as-jemima-wilkinson/.

New York Times. "A Noted Old California Stage-Driver Discovered, After Death, to be a Woman." January 9, 1880, 2.

Robinson, Henry R. *The Man-Monster.* New York: Museum of the City of New York, 1836.

Skidmore, Emily. *True Sex: The Lives of Trans Men at the Turn of the Twentieth Century.* New York: New York University Press, 2017.

Times. "Mrs. Green's Secret A Life Sacrifice." March 23, 1902, 13–14.

4

INTERNATIONAL PIONEERS OF TRANS-SPECIFIC CARE

Alexander Boscia and Cecile A. Ferrando

Therapeutic approaches for patients who present with gender dysphoria include complex interdisciplinary interventions, tailored to meet the specific needs of individual people. While the treatment approach may vary, the goal is always the same: to alleviate the intense discomfort associated with gender dysphoria. In the early twentieth century, in direct response to transgender individuals who voiced their need for treatment, surgeons in Europe and Africa developed and performed the first gender-affirming surgeries and provided the first hormonal therapies. Three physicians pioneered contemporary medical and surgical practices: Sir Harold Gillies (1882–1960), a plastic surgeon in Britain; Dr. Georges Burou (1910–1987), an obstetrician–gynecologist in Morocco; and Dr. Christian Hamburger (1904–1992), an endocrinologist in Denmark. This chapter highlights the lives, perspectives, and techniques of these transformational pioneers.

While Burou, Gillies, and Hamburger were not the first to attempt gender reassignment through surgical or hormonal methods, they are the most renowned of their time. Gillies introduced gender-affirming genital surgical procedures for transmasculine and transfeminine people; he documented these techniques in his published texts. Burou independently developed his vaginoplasty technique, performing hundreds of these operations from the 1950s until his tragic death in 1987 in a boating accident. His sole publication included illustrations that influenced many later surgeons.[1] Hamburger orchestrated the medical and surgical transition of Christine Jorgensen, the first American woman to undergo sex reassignment surgery; Jorgensen achieved lasting fame in the subsequent newspaper coverage and sensationalism that followed her transition.

THE REMARKABLE SURGICAL INNOVATIONS OF SIR HAROLD GILLIES (1882–1960)

The year was 1939. The place was Rooksdown House, an abandoned building at Park Prewett Hospital in the small town of Basingstoke in Kent, England. It was here that Sir Harold Gillies, knighted in 1930 in recognition of his wartime medical work, established a plastic surgery clinic for victims of facial trauma sustained during World War II.[2]

As one of the world's most eminent plastic surgeons, Gillies was no stranger to such work. During World War I, British soldiers returned from the front "with their noses gone, jaws exploded, entire faces a mass of bone and bloody gristle."[3] Gillies first served as a volunteer for the Red Cross and developed an interest in facial reconstruction surgery through his work with the French American dentist, Auguste Valadier, who established a unit for jaw work at the 83rd General Hospital in Wimereux. Gillies continued to study the cases of facial repair in German surgical textbooks, and he later seized the opportunity to observe the French facial surgeon Hippolyte Morestin at work in Rouen.[4]

The field of plastic surgery was in its infancy, and, like other surgeons, Gillies invented his techniques as he worked, "smoking furiously, operating for a dozen hours a day, [and] sketching noses on the backs of envelopes."[5] According to his nurse, Gillies treated a "stream of wounded men with half their faces literally blown to pieces, with the skin left hanging in shreds and the jawbones crushed to a pulp that felt like sand under your fingers."[6] In 460 BCE, Hippocrates pronounced that war was the only proper school for surgeons. Dr. Gillies agreed: "Unlike the student of today, who is weaned on small scar excisions and graduates to harelips, we were suddenly asked to produce half a face."[7] Although colleagues described Gillies as difficult to work with and an "irrepressible and often rude master,"[8] he showed "always kindness itself to his patients."[9]

When his country was not at war, Gillies applied his techniques to the repair of cosmetic defects. On a fishing trip with friends, he noticed that the daughter of the house had "a nose which could be improved." He left proofs of his chapter on plastic surgery of the nose on his bedside table, so she would see them when cleaning his room. She requested his services shortly thereafter.[10]

An avid prankster, Gillies possessed an unrelenting sense of humor. At an awards ceremony, the announcer called Gilllies's name and directed the spotlight toward his table, but the beam illuminated only an empty chair—Gillies was under the table.[11] He tricked his own butler by showing up at his front door in disguise. He enjoyed telling the improbable story that he had grafted skin onto a patient's cheek using skin from her husband's bottom for which the husband thanked him profusely, saying, "Whenever my mother-in-law spends the weekend with us and kisses my wife goodbye, I always feel I'm getting my own back."[12]

In 1916, Gillies persuaded the British Army Surgeon-General to open a unit dedicated to facial reconstruction. He reasoned that "by concentrating casualties in one place, with an army of surgeons to deal with them, it would be possible to make real technical advances simply because of the scale of the problem." The facility, located in Sidcup, Kent, and named The Queen's Hospital, contained more than one thousand beds and brought together dozens of surgeons from all over the world. With more than five thousand case subjects, the new hospital provided an unrivaled teaching arena, and as predicted by Gillies, surgeons produced a number of significant technical advances, such as arterial flaps, the temporalis transfer, cartilage and bone auto- and allografts, and most importantly, the tubed pedicle.[13]

The significance of Gillies's tubed pedicle is best described by the American author Pagan Kennedy:

> In 1917, while he was peeling skin off a sailor's shoulder, Gillies noticed how the edges of the flap tended to curl inward, the way paper curls when it's held up to a candle. He realized that there was a much better way to move skin around the body: he would let the flap of skin curl in on itself and then sew it into a tube, sealing off the inner side from the air. These tubes of skin, or "suitcase handles," could grow on the patient's body for weeks at a time; they could be moved about, end over end across the body until they

reached their final destination; or they could stretch like stalks to wherever you needed the flesh. The "tube pedicle," as Gillies called it, revolutionized surgery; suddenly, the body had turned modular. A U-shaped handle of flesh could be grown on the chest and moved to the face to form a nose; an extra roll hanging off the stomach could become a penis.[14]

While Gillies is primarily remembered for his work in facial reconstruction, he spent a considerable portion of his time developing genital reconstruction procedures. In his book *The Principles and Art of Plastic Surgery*, he reported that "in no part of plastic surgery is the need for form and function more compelling than in that of the sex organs."[15] Gillies independently pioneered a vaginoplasty procedure several years before Burou even attempted it. During this time, British mayhem laws prohibited the "intentional mutilation of another person," specifically genital mutilation in the form of castration, so Gillies did not publish on vaginoplasty. Instead, he focused his academic work on phalloplasty—the creation of a new penis—a surgery that required no form of genital mutilation as defined by the law.

At first, Gillies worked with soldiers whose genitals had been mutilated in battle and with patients who had developmental anomalies, ranging from a congenital absence of the vagina or penis to common hypospadias.[16] He used the term *sex attitude* to describe how gender was assigned to those with ambiguous genitalia, now referred to as people with intersex conditions.[17] He observed that surgical correction of ambiguous genitalia did not always conform to the patient's inclinations or personality. Discussing the connection between genitalia and identity, Gillies asserted: "In all this welter of variants the predominating factor lies in the individual's own ego. It surely can be a complete mockery to have a male armamentarium and no male urge, or female organs and no desire. Social conventions, religious tenets, and legal directives all play a part in complicating such a problem."[18]

Gillies published case studies about individuals who he described as "[i]n the wrong sex pen." To cite a few examples: the maid, a young woman "with great lumbering strides" and "a hairy leg" who found herself rejecting the unwanted advances of the male butler while simultaneously falling in love with the laundry maid; the two sisters who "had gallantly served as women volunteers in the London Fire Brigade" before "realizing they were more male than female"; and the "women's international athletics champion." These cases all turned out to reflect people who had hypospadias, a fetal, developmental defect of the penis in a genetic male that misplaces the urethral opening at the base of the penis. This condition is sometimes severe enough that the genitalia appear like a vagina.[19]

In one of the earliest published reports on urethroplasty procedures, Gillies outlined his technique for hypospadias repair. In the case of the maid described above, he discovered that the shaft of the penis was of adequate size and that he needed only to construct a new urethra. For this task, he asked a general surgeon to collect the appendix during an exploratory laparotomy. Gillies then dissected the procured appendix down to a "long, slender mucosal tube," which he then inserted into the shaft as a urethra; however, the appendiceal graft was not quite long enough. A colporrhaphy (an operation that involves denuding and suturing the vaginal wall to narrow the vagina) "was in progress in the adjoining theatre . . . [and] a bit of homologous vaginal mucous membrane was stolen to finish off the urethral lining."[20] Unsurprisingly, the maid's body rejected this donated vaginal tissue, forcing Gillies to repeatedly catheterize the patient to maintain the patency of the urethra. He performed this surgery on both of the patients described above, but the results did not look much like a penis. He mused afterward that "there still remained the difficulty of changing over. The patient could not switch into trousers in his own village without giving the story away, so he moved to another under a new name."[21]

Gillies began work to develop a procedure for creating a surgical penis. In 1947, he published "Congenital Absence of the Penis," an article in which he described his new phalloplasty technique using the tubed pedicle graft that he had developed twenty years earlier.[22] His phalloplasty required three separate operations (stages) performed over approximately six months. In the first and second stages, he created a "three-in-one" skin flap on the abdomen. This single flap consisted of two adjacent rectangular skin flaps that shared a medial border (a smaller flap on the inner abdomen and a larger flap on the outer abdomen). In the first stage, he dissected the inner flap from the underlying subcutaneous tissue and rolled it into a thin tube. He then inserted a catheter to maintain patency of what was to become the new urethra. He allowed both the tubed pedicle and the larger, outer skin flap to lengthen for a period of three weeks. Next, he commenced stage two by dissecting the larger flap from the underlying subcutaneous tissue and wrapping it around the smaller, tubed pedicle to create a tube-within-a-tube structure, that is, a urethra-within-a-shaft. He filled the open space, surgically known as dead space, with cartilage from a rib. He allowed this three-in-one tubed pedicle (urethra, shaft, cartilage) to lengthen for an additional five weeks before moving to stage three: "The pedicle may be freed at its upper end and brought down to make a direct union with the existing urethral opening." He sutured the outer tube to the skin of the lower abdomen, creating the base of the penis. The cartilage served to "preserve shape and easy flow of urine down the new urethra." The final stage entailed tidying up the pedicle and fashioning the external meatus.[23]

This procedure was fraught with complications, including infections, urinary incontinence, and misalignment of the neourethra, which resulted in extravasation of urine into the penile shaft. Nonetheless, patients (and Gillies) expressed satisfaction with the results. Gillies's article included a number of images of his neophallus, including an action shot of a patient urinating into a pitcher with his new equipment.[24] He also described an eleven-year postoperative examination of a patient as follows: "The local condition was entirely satisfactory and gave no trouble. Urination was quite normal except for a small amount of dribbling. The patient has become a senior medical student . . . the penis is very normal to look at except for being narrow at the base, and the everted umbilical skin makes an excellent glans penis."[25]

In 1943, a London surgeon referred a young, bearded automotive garage worker Michael Dillon to Gillies, requesting help for a different problem: "He was trapped in the wrong body. And so, he needed to change that body. It was that simple."[26] The London surgeon first met Dillon in the hospital after Dillon was admitted for a hypoglycemic event. The surgeon—himself a mentee of Gillies—agreed not only to perform Dillon's double mastectomy but also assisted Dillon with the legal issues that he encountered while transitioning gender. Gillies was responsible for the surgical procedure to create a penis for the patient; he recruited the American surgeon Dr. Ralph Millard to be his assistant during the surgery. The two doctors had previously collaborated intellectually, as Millard contributed to Gillies's textbook *Principles and Art of Plastic Surgery*. Referencing Dillon's surgery, Millard explained, "We were excited . . . Gillies was undaunted. . . . He knew how to charter unknown waters without too much concern."[27] Gillies detailed Dillon's case in a chapter of his textbook with the heading, "Female with a Male Outlook."[28]

To assist Dillon, Gillies created a neophallus using a technique similar to that described in "Congenital Absence of the Penis." He improvised by stitching Dillon's clitoris into the base of his new penis to preserve erotic sensation. Gillies was proud of his work, recalling, "After initial difficulties, no trouble has been experienced with urination. . . . Provided thus with a new organ, the patient's life has been a social success; he has become an active and successful businessman and is anxious to have everything done that would make it justifiable for him to marry."[29]

Dillon described his experience in his autobiography, *Out of the Ordinary*.[30] In Kennedy's *The First Man-Made Man,* a biography about Dillon, she offers additional insights, notably a description of the love affair between Dillon and Roberta Cowell—a transgender woman and Gillies's first vaginoplasty patient.[31] Despite fear of litigation due to the mayhem statutes, Gillies published an account of Cowell's procedure in his case report, *Male with Female Outlook,* describing a technique similar to the one Burou would independently develop a few years later.[32] He referred to Cowell's testicular atrophy, a result of feminizing hormone therapy, to justify that his procedure did not cause genital mutilation.

> The body and shaft of the penis were slipped out of the loose hairless skin cover, the penis was discarded, and the skin envelope closed at its free end and invaginated into a prepared cavity. It was like a finger-stall and indeed was pushed into place on the surgeon's finger. As the new vagina was thereby walled with penile skin the principle of repair by like tissue was exemplified. The cavity was artificially produced by dilation and blunt dissection between the uro-genital membrane and the anterior rectal wall, and into its apex the tip of the skin finger-stall was fixed by suture.
>
> What to do with the corpora was the next problem. The spongiosum, complete with urethra, after division below the glans, was easily separated from the cavernosa, shortened, and its oval cut end sutured into the estimated position of the female meatus. So far encouraging—but what was to be done with the huge erectile corpora cavernosa surmounted by the blue glans? Here a mistake of design and surgical upbringing led to preserving them to be split longitudinally to surround the new vagina as erectile labia majora.[33]

Although Gillies is more renowned for his facial reconstruction work, his impact on genital reconstruction is undeniable—not only on the surgical field at large but also on his patients. A lifelong smoker, Gillies continued operating until his sudden death at the age of seventy-eight, likely as a result of arterial disease due to poor circulation.[34]

THE CASABLANCA CONNECTION: GEORGES BUROU (1910–1987)

The year was 1950. The place was the Clinique du Parc at 13 Rue Lapebie (now Rue Melouia) in Casablanca, Morocco. Burou had just finished building his five-story obstetrics and gynecology clinic. He and his wife Jeanne "Nanou" Boisvert lived in an apartment above the outpatient offices on the prestigious Avenue d'Amade (now Avenue Hassan II). On the fourth and fifth floors, the clinic maintained operating rooms, a surgical ward, a fifteen-crib nursery, and delivery rooms. The second and third floors housed patient rooms. Burou designed the clinic building so it attached in the rear to his private quarters and outpatient offices.[35]

Burou was born on September 6, 1910, in Haute Pyrénées, France; however, he spent much of his life abroad. His parents lived and worked as schoolteachers in Algiers, Algeria, where he was raised and went on to receive his medical degree from the Algiers University of Medicine. He specialized in obstetrics and gynecology at the Maternity of Mustapha Hospital in Algiers and became Chef de Clinique at Parnet Hospital in a small Algiers suburb. A copper plate at the entrance of his Casablanca office read: "Ex-Interne des Hopitaux d'Algier and Ex-Chef de Clinique Obstétricale."[36]

The reasons for Burou's exit from Algeria in early 1940 are unclear. While he claimed that he followed his wife-to-be to Casablanca, where her parents had a farm,[37] others asserted that he was banned from the French Order of Medicine for having performed abortions, a practice prohibited by French law.[38] Burou continued to perform abortions in Morocco, maintaining that a woman should not have to bring an unwanted child into the world and that, when performed discreetly, abortions hurt no one.[39]

The strategic location of Burou's new Casablanca clinic offered dual access to his offices and clinic—through the elegant entrance on Avenue d'Amade or via the less conspicuous entrance on Rue Lapebie.[40] Moreover, with his attached apartment, he strove "not to distance himself from his patients," ultimately positioning himself to deliver babies at night.[41] Thus, for all intents and purposes, Dr. Burou was a self-proclaimed "obstetrician-gynecologist no different than any other."[42]

That is, until one day in 1956. He described this day in a 1974 article in *Paris Match*:

A pretty woman came to see me. In reality, it was a man, I didn't know this until after, a sound engineer from Casablanca, dressed in women's clothes, behaving like a woman, with a lovely breast obtained courtesy of bites of hormones, very little hair, a shapely, feminine body. He told me of his problems, he wanted to kill himself, holding the deep conviction that his male body was a tragic, irreversible accident of nature. Like a lefty forced to use his right hand. Faced with this totally new problem which interested me enormously, I studied male and female pelvises for months and I hospitalized him in my clinic which is located next to my office and beneath my apartment. The operation lasted three hours. The patient remained for one month in recovery. She was satisfied beyond expression. I had made a real woman out of him.[43]

In the years to follow, Burou found fame in the worldwide transgender community and the phrase "going to Casablanca" became a popular colloquialism for "getting a sex change."[44] At the height of his sex-reassignment work, he performed five to six vaginoplasties per month, with each procedure lasting approximately one hour.[45] Over two decades, he performed approximately three thousand vaginoplasties for Americans, British, Italians, Japanese, and Germans. His patient roster included university professors, teachers, physicians, painters, writers, performers, transvestites, and prostitutes.[46]

Burou operated on a number of transgender celebrities, including French actress Coccinelle, British model April Ashley, and Welsh author Jan Morris. In her memoir *Conundrum*, Morris recounted her transition from male to female and described Burou on his rounds as "dressed for the corniche and looking in general pretty devastating."[47] She described how he would sit at the end of her bed "and chat desultorily of this and that, type a few very slow words on my typewriter, read a headline from the *Times* in a delectable Maurice Chevalier accent, and eventually take an infinitely gentle look at his handiwork."[48] The documentary *I am a Woman Now* profiled a subset of his patients through interviews conducted fifty years after their surgeries.[49]

Despite his fame in the transgender community, few academic gynecologic surgeons knew of Burou's work. He presented his techniques in scientific conferences only twice—first in 1973 at the Second Interdisciplinary Symposium on Gender Dysphoria Syndrome at Stanford University, almost twenty years

Figure 4.1 Surgical drawing used by Georges Burou at the Proceedings of the Second Interdisciplinary Symposium on Gender Dysphoria Syndrome, Stanford University School of Medicine, 1973. *Source*: https://archive.org/details/proceedings_gds, p. 193.

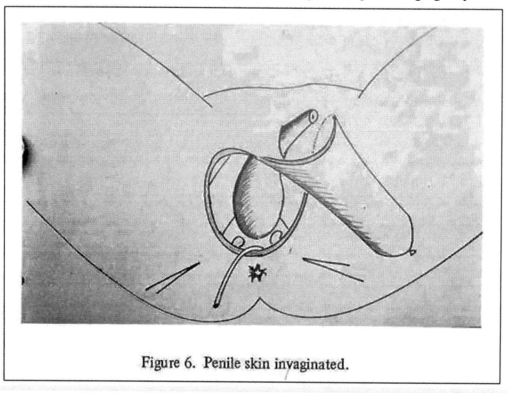

Figure 6. Penile skin invaginated.

after he completed his first vaginoplasty. He presented again that same year at the International Congress of Sexology in Paris.[50]

In proceedings from the Stanford symposium, Burou described his technique:

> The entire surgical operation is done in one stage, consisting of two successive steps . . . the goal of the first step is to create a space between the rectum and the prostate. The first incision is made posteriorly between the anal area and the scrotal ridge. This first part is extremely important, because you can determine at any time by intrarectal inspection that there is no lesion to the rectal wall. This is very important to avoid any further complications during the dissection in the rectum in the prerectal space . . . the cleavage is done when you admit easily two fingers of a vaginal retractor. One

can meet at the end of this new space a natural formation which makes you feel that you are really meeting the natural vaginal cul-de-sac, Douglas space. The first step is over.[51]

He described the second step as relatively easy, consisting of orchiectomy, revision of the urethra, and complete dissection of the penile skin from the shaft and erectile bodies, after which the skin was sutured and closed to become the neovagina. The surgeon then inserts the neovagina into the pre-rectal space (from step one).[52]

He also described postoperative care: "The management of the new vagina is being made by frequent and daily introductions of small vaginal retractors. In the next few days permeability of the urethra must also be maintained by daily introduction of the catheter and making sure that there is no stenosis and that it is completely patent."[53] Most patients spent approximately two weeks in his clinic to undergo and recover from the procedure. As a rule, Burou rarely conducted long-term follow-ups with patients, assuming, "I think most of them want to forget about having to undergo this operation, because these are men who have spent their whole life wanting to be a woman."[54]

Burou charged $5,000 for his transsexual operation which included "twelve to fifteen days hospitalization at our clinique, medical care and fees included, as well as the doctor's fee."[55] At the Stanford Symposium in 1973, he reported that "all of the patients who undergo surgery have been prepared, undergo psychiatric care, [are] on hormones, and made quite feminine."[56] His letters to preoperative patients contained explicit instructions to bring medical records and laboratory results, if available.[57] Morris later disputed Burou's claim to comprehensive care, stating, "Burou did not bother too much with diagnosis or pre-treatment."[58]

At the same symposium, Burou also presented his penile inversion vaginoplasty as "the first report on this new technique . . . utilizing the live graft which can be made from the penile skin when properly dissected."[59] Unbeknown to Burou, though, Gillies and Millard had already developed the penile inversion vaginoplasty in late 1952 or 1953[60] and published their reports in "The Principles and Art of Plastic Surgery."[61] The accepted view is that Gillies and Burou developed the penile inversion technique independently; despite the lag time between their respective reports, the current literature refers to the Gillies–Burou inverted penile tube technique.[62]

While Burou leaves a profound, professional legacy, the story of his death is equally as compelling. One December day in 1987, he set off in a boat with his friend's two adolescent children. When they were caught in a storm off the coast of Pont Blondin (a beach north of Casablanca), he gave the only two life jackets to his young guests, thereby sacrificing his own life to the sea.[63]

Although Gillies and Burou are remembered as pioneers of transgender surgery, neither was particularly interested in the medical management of transgender patients. Dillon, Cowell, and others approached them after already having taken hormones, and both surgeons reported that hormone therapy rendered their procedures less difficult. Other individuals and clinicians experimented with hormonal therapy for masculinization and feminization. Hamburger brought this treatment into the spotlight when he rose to fame as the physician to the first American transgender woman.

CHRISTIAN HAMBURGER (1904–1992): PHYSICIAN TO CHRISTINE JORGENSEN

The year was 1952. The place was Copenhagen, Denmark. It was here, only two years prior, that Christine Jorgensen (née George Jorgensen) met the Danish endocrinologist Hamburger and began her transition. Hamburger described this encounter in his article "Transvestism: Hormonal, Psychiatric, and Surgical Treatment."[64] He reported that the patient, a twenty-four-year-old tourist visiting a friend in Denmark, discovered and approached him requesting "to be relieved of the essential source of the detested masculine component of his body . . . he hoped with medical assistance to be able to obtain permission to live on 'as nearly a woman as possible.' "[65] Hamburger, an endocrinologist who had devoted his career to reproductive endocrinology, agreed to provide Jorgensen with medical assistance.

Hamburger began his work in endocrinology in 1930. In his doctoral thesis, he described the gonadotropic hormones released from the pituitary and placenta, as well as his more notable discovery: the placenta produced human chorionic gonadotropin, the hormone responsible for maintaining pregnancy.[66] He received clinical training at a number of Copenhagen hospitals, and, in 1934, became head of the Hormone Department of Statens Seruminstitut. In 1947, he cofounded the Danish Society for Endocrinology, initially serving as chairman and, in 1960, became chief editor of the journal *Acta endocrinologica*.[67] Armed with these credentials, he designed a treatment approach for Jorgensen that included intentional medical management, expanding the protocols established by surgeons such as Drs. Gillies and Burou. Hamburger first offered Jorgensen an extended course of hormone therapy with the expectation that, over time, she would begin to dress and live as a woman, change her gender on legal documents, participate in psychiatric evaluation, and finally, undergo surgical castration and "demasculinization."[68]

Hamburger developed core recommendations to tackle what he considered the all-dominant problem facing transvestites (or *eonists*[69])—that is, how to effectively "facilitate the eonist's life and existence." His recommendations included social transition (permission to wear women's clothes in public and legal recognition and registration as a woman); hormonal transition (administration of estrogenic substances); and surgical transition (castration, demasculinization, and formation of artificial vagina). Hamburger emphasized that his suggestions were guidelines, not rules, citing that "in this affection there can never be any standard and routine treatment." He explained the importance of understanding the patient's goals and emphasized that treatment recommendations should be based on individual needs.[70]

Interestingly, Hamburger discouraged surgery to construct a neovagina, calling the operation undesirable from an ethical point of view. He did not elaborate on his beliefs and stated only that most transvestites were sufficiently satisfied with the aesthetics rendered by castration and demasculinization, thus rendering the "technically difficult" neovagina procedure unnecessary. He also claimed that "the need of sexual contact is usually of very minor importance."[71] This position may have been the case for Jorgensen, but Gillies disagreed with this statement, as did thousands of transgender people.

Despite his aversion to surgical neovaginas, Hamburger advocated for the legalization of surgical castration: "The sex glands must, in the eyes of society, be protected at any price. It is not immediately evident with what right society compels persons to tolerate the presence of these organs if their presence is felt to be an intolerable burden, in some cases poisoning the patient's life from youth to old age."[72] He speculated that societal misunderstanding about the difference between homosexuality and "genuine transvestism" contributed to societal disapproval for castration: "It is possible that the authorities are afraid that a number of homosexual and otherwise sexually abnormal persons might attempt to obtain castration, pretending to be a transvestite."[73] Like Dr. Alan Hart,[74] he invoked the principles of eugenics to justify castration, declaring, "it would do no harm if a number of sexually abnormal men were castrated and thus deprived of their sexual libido."[75]

He also wrote about his fear of patient regret after irreversible surgical procedures, recognizing the weight of such a decision. Despite his reservations, though, Hamburger concluded that "[I]f an adult man of sound mind, after having been told the risks of the operation and after careful consideration, himself accepts the responsibility and persists in his wish, it is unreasonable that society should act as a guardian endowed with a superior wisdom." Citing the danger of patient regret, he also emphasized the importance of multi-pronged medical management during transition; prior hormonal treatment and psychiatric observation can affirm patient choice before undergoing surgery.[76]

Jorgensen underwent castration in the winter of 1952. News of her transition reached New York before she was discharged from Hamburger's clinic. "As far as is known, the press succeeded in tracing the contents of a private letter from the patient to his relatives in New York—and published the story without his knowledge or consent."[77] In the year after publishing his article on Jorgensen's transition, Hamburger received 1,117 letters from patients all over the world; of these, "465 patients appeared to have a genuine desire for alteration of sex."[78] (These patients authored 756 of the original 1,117 letters Hamburger received, representing more than two-thirds of patients who reached out to him.) In 1953, he published an article in *Acta Endocrinologica* entitled "The Desire for Change of Sex as Shown by Personal Letters from 465 Men and Women."[79] In this study, he performed a statistical analysis of these letters with regard to geographical distribution, age distribution, marital status, fertility, sexual libido, motivations governing the desire for change of sex, somatic development, and previous appeals for medical assistance. He published a small number of the letters and summarized his findings:

> These many personal letters from almost five hundred deeply unhappy persons leave an overwhelming impression. One tragic existence is unfolded after another; they cry for help and understanding. It is depressing to realize how little can be done to come to their aid. One feels it a duty to appeal to the medical profession and to the responsible legislature: do your utmost to ease the existence of these fellow-men who are deprived of the possibilities of a harmonious and happy life—through no fault of their own.[80]

Little information exists on the death of Hamburger, yet it is clear that over his lifetime, his contributions have left an important legacy. To this day, the medical professionals recognize him as a significant innovator in his respective field.

CONCLUSION

The extraordinary and brave work of these three men represents a fundamental catalyst for present-day surgical practices and innovations. Today, surgeons still perform the penile inversion vaginoplasty, albeit with personalized, procedural modifications. And Gillies's tube-within-a tube phalloplasty concept is still the gold standard among surgical techniques for performing this procedure. It is likely these pioneers of transgender surgery would be impressed with the advances made in the field and pleased that many of their methods are still in use today in various forms.

Almost seventy years later, though, the field of transgender surgery remains in its infancy. Transgender medicine centers are appearing throughout the United States, with the goal of providing holistic care to transgender patients (not unlike Hamburger's goals); however, these centers—and hospitals at large—urgently need more practicing surgeons. Data from TransHealthCare.org, the largest and most comprehensive database of gender surgeons, show that, as of August 2020, only approximately sixty-six surgeons offer male-to-female vaginoplasty in twenty-one states; fifty-two surgeons in twenty-seven states offer female-to-male phalloplasty procedures across the United States.[81] These numbers only continue to increase with the development of new, nationwide transgender surgery fellowship trainings, programs that Gillies, Burou, and Hamburger would certainly be proud to acknowledge.

NOTES

1. Burou, "Male to Female," 190.
2. Shastri-Hurst, "The Father of Modern Plastic Surgery," 182; Amar, "Casablanca."
3. Kennedy, *The First Man-Made Man*, 61.
4. Bamji, "Sir Harold Gillies," 149; Burou, "Male to Female," 192.
5. Kennedy, *The First Man-Made Man*, 62.
6. Kennedy, *The First Man-Made Man*, 82.
7. Alexander, "Faces of War."
8. Millard, "Gillies Memorial Lecture," 75.
9. Bamji, "Sir Harold Gillies," 150.
10. Bamji, "Sir Harold Gillies," 150.
11. Kennedy, *The First Man-Made Man*, 66.
12. Bamji, "Sir Harold Gillies," 151.

13. Bamji, "Sir Harold Gillies," 153.
14. Kennedy, *The First Man-Made Man*, 62–63.
15. Gillies and Millard, "The Principles and Art of Plastic Surgery," 369.
16. Gillies and Millard, "The Principles and Art of Plastic Surgery," 369.
17. Gillies and Millard, "The Principles and Art of Plastic Surgery," 370.
18. Gillies and Millard, "The Principles and Art of Plastic Surgery," 371.
19. Gillies and Millard, "The Principles and Art of Plastic Surgery," 371–72.
20. Gillies and Millard, "The Principles and Art of Plastic Surgery," 372.
21. Gillies and Millard, "The Principles and Art of Plastic Surgery," 372.
22. Gillies and Harrison, "Congenital Absence of the Penis," 13.
23. Gillies and Harrison, "Congenital Absence of the Penis," 14.
24. Gillies and Harrison, "Congenital Absence of the Penis," 14.
25. Gillies and Harrison, "Congenital Absence of the Penis," 16.
26. Kennedy, *The First Man-Made Man*, 60.
27. Kennedy, *The First Man-Made Man*, 79.
28. Gillies and Millard, "The Principles and Art of Plastic Surgery," 370.
29. Gillies and Millard, "The Principles and Art of Plastic Surgery," 372–73.
30. Jivaka, *Out of the Ordinary*, 173.
31. Kennedy, *The First Man-Made Man*, 96.
32. Gillies and Millard, "The Principles and Art of Plastic Surgery," 386.
33. Gillies and Millard, "The Principles and Art of Plastic Surgery," 385–88.
34. Bamji, "Sir Harold Gillies," 150.
35. Hage, Karim, and Laub, "On the Origin of Pedicled Skin," 724.
36. Hage, Karim, and Laub, "On the Origin of Pedicled Skin," 724.
37. Hage, Karim, and Laub, "On the Origin of Pedicled Skin," 725–26.
38. Amar, "Casablanca."
39. Amar, "Casablanca."
40. Hage, Karim, and Laub, "On the Origin of Pedicled Skin," 727.
41. Merlin, "L'homme qui change le sexe," 37.
42. Merlin, "L'homme qui change le sexe," 37–38.
43. Merlin, "L'homme qui change le sexe," 39.
44. Goddard, Vickery, and Terry, "Development of Feminizing Genitoplasty," 983.
45. Hage, Karim, and Laub, "On the Origin of Pedicled Skin," 727.
46. Merlin, "L'homme qui change le sexe," 38.
47. Morris, *Conundrum*, 131.
48. Morris, *Conundrum*, 165.
49. van Erp, *I Am a Woman Now*.
50. Merlin, "L'homme qui change le sexe," 37.
51. Burou, "Male to Female," 189.
52. Burou, "Male to Female," 190.
53. Burou, "Male to Female," 190–91.

54. Merlin, "L'homme qui change le sexe," 38.
55. Hage, Karim, and Laub, "On the Origin of Pedicled Skin," 725.
56. Burou, "Male to Female," 191.
57. Hage, Karim, and Laub, "On the Origin of Pedicled Skin," 726.
58. Morris, *Conundrum*, 121.
59. Burou, "Male to Female," 188.
60. Hage, Karim, and Laub, "On the Origin of Pedicled Skin," 725.
61. Gillies and Millard, "The Principles and Art of Plastic Surgery," 380.
62. Goddard, Vickery, and Terry, "Development of Feminizing Genitoplasty," 983.
63. Amar, "Casablanca."
64. Hamburger, Sturup, and Dahl-Eversen, "Transvestism," 368.
65. Hamburger, Sturup, and Dahl-Eversen, "Transvestism," 369–70.
66. Pedersen-Biergaard, "Christian Hamburger," S4.
67. Pedersen-Biergaard, "Christian Hamburger," S5.
68. Hamburger, Sturup, and Dahl-Eversen, "Transvestism," 372.
69. *APA Dictionary of Psychology*. Accessed 25 July 2021. dictionary.apa.org/eonism. A term for a male who adopts a female role (or vice versa). The term is a reference to Charles Eon de Beaumont, a French political adventurer who died in 1810 after posing as a woman for many years.
70. Hamburger, Sturup, and Dahl-Eversen, "Transvestism," 368.
71. Hamburger, Sturup, and Dahl-Eversen, "Transvestism," 368–69.
72. Hamburger, Sturup, and Dahl-Eversen, "Transvestism," 370.
73. Hamburger, Sturup, and Dahl-Eversen, "Transvestism," 371.
74. Refer to profile of Alan Hart in chapter 17.1 in this volume for more information.
75. Hamburger, Sturup, and Dahl-Eversen, "Transvestism," 372.
76. Hamburger, Sturup, and Dahl-Eversen, "Transvestism," 372.
77. Hamburger, "The Desire for Change of Sex," 372–73.
78. Hamburger, Sturup, and Dahl-Eversen, "Transvestism," 374.
79. Hamburger, "The Desire for Change of Sex," 374.
80. Hamburger, "The Desire for Change of Sex," 375.
81. TransHealthCare, *The Go-To Guide to Gender Surgeons*.

WORKS CITED

Alexander, Caroline. "Faces of War." *Smithsonian Magazine*, February 2007. Accessed August 10, 2024. https://www.smithsonianmag.com/arts_culture/faces-of-war-145799854.

Amar, Ali. "Casablanca, la mecque mythique des transsexuels." *Bab El Med*, January 11, 2016. Accessed July 28, 2020. http://www.babelmed.net/article/3666-casablanca-la-mecque-mythique-des-transsexuels/.

Bamji, Andrew. "Sir Harold Gillies: Surgical Pioneer." *Trauma* 8, no. 3 (2006): 143–56.

Burou, George. "Male to Female Transformation." In *Proceedings of the Second Interdisciplinary Symposium on Gender Dysphoria Syndrome*, edited by Patrick Gandy and Donald R. Laub, 188–94. Stanford, CA: Division of Reconstructive and Rehabilitation Surgery, Stanford University Medical Center, 1973. Accessed August 4, 2021. https://ai.eecs.umich.edu/people/conway/TS/Burou/Burou.html.

Gillies, Harold, and D. Ralph Millard. "The Principles and Art of Plastic Surgery." In *Genitalia*, 368–88. New York: Little, Brown, 1957.

Gillies, Harold, and R. J. Harrison. "Congenital Absence of the Penis with Embryological Considerations." *British Journal of Plastic Surgery* 1, no. 1 (1948): 12–28.

Goddard, Jonathan Charles, Richard M. Vickery, and Tim R. Terry. "Development of Feminizing Genitoplasty for Gender Dysphoria." *Journal of Sexual Medicine* 4, no. 4 (2007): 981–89.

Hage, J. Joris, Refaat B. Karim, and Donald R. Laub. "On the Origin of Pedicled Skin Inversion Vaginoplasty: Life and Work of Dr Georges Borou of Casablanca." *Annals of Plastic Surgery* 59, no. 6 (2007): 723–29.

Hamburger, Christian. "The Desire for Change of Sex as Shown by Personal Letters from 465 Men and Women." *Acta Endocrinologica* 14, no. 4 (1953): 361–75.

Hamburger, Christian, G. K. Sturup, and E. Dahl-Eversen. "Transvestism: Hormonal, Psychiatric and Surgical Treatment." *Journal of the American Medical Association* 152, no. 5 (1953): 391–96.

Jivaka, Lobzang (Michael Dillon). *Out of the Ordinary*, edited by Jacob Lau and Cameron Partridge. New York: Fordham University Press, 2016.

Kennedy, Pagan. *The First Man-Made Man: The Story of Two Sex Changes, One Love Affair, and a Twentieth-Century Medical Revolution*. New York: Bloomsbury, 2007.

Merlin, V. "L'Homme qui change le sexe." *Paris Match* (1973): 37–39.

Millard, D. Ralph. "Gillies Memorial Lecture: Jousting with the First Knight of Plastic Surgery." *British Journal of Plastic Surgery* 25 (1972): 73–82.

Morris, Jan. *Conundrum*. New York: New York Review Books, 2005.

Pedersen-Biergaard, K. "Christian Hamburger on the Occasion of his Sixtieth Birthday." *Acta Endocrinologica* 45, no. 4 (1964): S3–S7.

Shastri-Hurst, Neil. "The Father of Modern Plastic Surgery." *Trauma* 14, no. 2 (2011): 179–87.

TransHealthCare. "The Go-To Guide to Gender Surgeons." 2020. Accessed August 12, 2020. https://transhealthcare.org.

van Erp, Michiel, dir. *I Am a Woman Now*. Produced by De Familie, 2011.

World Professional Association for Transgender Health. *Standards of Care for the Health of Transsexual, Transgender, and Gender Nonconforming People*, 7th vers. 2012. Accessed August 10, 2020. https://www.wpath.org.

4.1. PROFILES: MICHAEL DILLON (1915–1962) AND ROBERTA COWELL (1918–2011)

Alexander Boscia and Cecile A. Ferrando

> I, R.C. have, of my own free will asked and persuaded L.M.D., who I am aware is an unqualified man, a 5th year medical student, to perform an orchidectomy upon me.
>
> —Roberta Cowell, quoted in Pagan Kennedy, *The First Man-Made Man*

Roberta Cowell (née Robert Cowell) met Laurence Michael Dillon (née Laura Maud Dillon) for the first time in London in 1951, a few months before she signed the above affidavit, effectively releasing Dillon from responsibility in the event of surgical complications from the orchiectomy. She had read his book *Self: A Study in Ethics and Endocrinology*, and she appreciated his advocacy for surgical sex change procedures. After an exchange of letters, Dillon agreed to meet Cowell for lunch. During this encounter, Cowell was struck by Dillon's overt masculinity and "low opinion of women."[1] Nevertheless, she played along with the conversation, aware that if she wanted an orchiectomy, she would need his help.

In the 1950s, legal barriers to surgical transition for transgender people stemmed from Great Britain's mayhem statutes and male doctors' misogynist views about women's bodies. (Many male practitioners at the time considered ovaries and uteruses the root of frailty and hysteria, thus requiring monitoring or removal to treat a variety of ailments.) Men developed the field of gynecology to look after the "fairer sex," a population many physicians believed could not be trusted to look after themselves. For these reasons, Dillon faced minimal medical resistance and fewer legal obstacles when he entered the office of Sir Harold Gillies to request a hysterectomy and assistance in changing his gender and name on his legal documents. Urologists focused on care of the male genitalia, and doctors associated the testes with strength and virility; they did not routinely monitor or recommend removing men's parts. The process of obtaining a surgical sex change was decidedly more difficult for Cowell than for Dillon, necessitating the surgical assistance of Dillon, then an unqualified, though apparently capable, medical student.[2]

Cowell listened patiently to Dillon as he talked about surgical transitions, interrupting to ask who she should see for her operation and how she could legally change her sex. Dillon, drawn to this woman in distress, agreed to continue meeting. Over the next few months, he fell in love with Cowell and agreed to perform her orchiectomy. The operation was a success. She later met with Dr. George Dusseau, who on examining her declared Cowell intersex. Armed with this documentation, Cowell was able to legally change her sex. To complete her transition in 1951, she met with Gillies and became his first vaginoplasty patient.[3]

After Cowell transitioned, she shattered Dillon's hopes by turning down his marriage proposal. She published two autobiographies, claiming she had been born with an intersex condition. A decade later, she had fallen out of the public eye; however, she continued to be active in British motor car racing and in logging hours as a pilot, her two great passions. She died in 2011. Per her request, her death was not publicized, and the funeral was a private affair with few people.[4]

Unlike Cowell, Dillon preferred to avoid the spotlight. After obtaining his medical degree in 1951, he took a job on a merchant navy ship in 1952 as physician to the crew. He spent the next six years traveling the seas and visiting many countries. A sincere student of Eastern philosophical traditions, he decided in 1958 to pursue religious training in India. His retreat to a life of spiritual reflection coincided with the discovery of his transsexual history by the British tabloid press. Dillon had no intention of tangling with his younger brother over an Irish baronetcy to which he would have been entitled as the oldest male; he was loathe to publicly assert his identity in a court of law or to subject himself to further ridicule in the press.

Instead, Dillon became one of the first westerners that a Tibetan monk accepted as a novice, and he subsequently adopted the name Lobzang Jivaka. By 1960, still in India and suffering from malnutrition and typhoid fever, he devoted himself once again to writing—having published several books already in England. His first book *Self: A Study in Ethics and Endocrinology* presaged Harry Benjamin's hormonal theories and first publication about transsexual experience by two decades. He completed his autobiography, entitled *"Out of the Ordinary,"* on his forty-seventh birthday in 1962, just two weeks before he died.[5] The manuscript arrived at his agent's office a few months later, but it was not published until 2018.[6] Had it been released in his lifetime Dillon would have become the world's first public trans man.

NOTES

1. Kennedy, *The First Man-Made Man*, 4.
2. Kennedy, *The First Man-Made Man*, 87.

3. Kennedy, *The First Man-Made Man*, 6–7.
4. Cowell, A. "Overlooked No More."
5. Kennedy, *The First Man-Made Man*, 129–90.
6. Dillon/Jivaka, *Out of the Ordinary*, 2–3.

WORKS CITED

Cowell, Alan. "Overlooked No More: Roberta Cowell. Trans Trailblazer; Pilot and Auto Racer." *New York Times*, 2020. Access August 2024. https://www.nytimes.com/2020/06/05/obituaries/roberta-cowell-overlooked.html

Dillon, Michael. *Self: A Study in Ethics and Endocrinology*. London: William Heinemann Medical Books, 1946.

Dillon, Michael/Jivaka, Lobzang. *Out of the Ordinary*, edited by Jacob Lau and Cameron Partridge. New York, NY: Fordham University Press, 2016.

Kennedy, Pagan. *The First Man-Made Man: The Story of Two Sex Changes, One Love Affair, and a Twentieth-Century Medical Revolution*. New York: Bloomsbury, 2007.

4.2. PROFILES: COCCINELLE (1931–2006), APRIL ASHLEY (1935–2021), AND JAN MORRIS (1926–2020)

Alexander Boscia and Cecile A. Ferrando

April Ashley, who had been saving money for her operation by performing at Le Carousel, a nightclub in Paris, became the ninth patient of Georges Burou and one of the first British women to undergo his vaginoplasty procedure in the 1950s. Ashley described her initial encounter with "the Wizard of Casablanca": he showed pictures of the operation "in vehement technicolor . . . the gore, the blood, the knives," and he asked her to sign a release to absolve him of all responsibility should anything go awry.[1] As the anesthetic was administered, Ashley heard Burou murmur, "Au revoir, Monsieur." When she awoke, she heard "Bonjour, Mademoiselle."[2]

Prior to her transition, Ashley had been featured in *Vogue*, establishing herself as one of the most sought-after models in England. After a friend sold the story of her surgical transition to the newspapers, she was never able to work as a model again. Ashley gained critical fame when her husband won an annulment case against her. Filed in 1963 and decided in 1970,[3] it was the first British case to hold that postoperative transsexuals remained their sex at birth regardless of their transition status or how they may appear to be of the opposite gender. With this ruling, the British court effectively rendered Ashley male, which was grounds for granting her husband the requested annulment; at the time, same-sex marriage was illegal in the United Kingdom. Due to the harsh treatment she faced from within the legal system, Ashley became an outspoken advocate for transgender people. In 2012, she was appointed member of The Most Excellent Order of the British Empire for her work on transgender equality.[4]

Ashley was not the only celebrity to undergo surgical transition with Burou. Jacques-Charles Dufresnoy took the name Jacqueline Charlotte Dufresnoy, but she was better known as Coccinelle. Coccinelle—an actress, entertainer, and singer—became a sensation in France. She was known for her beauty and her extravagant performances, including one revue entitled *Cherchez la Femme* (*Look for the Woman*) at the Paris Olympia. Like Ashley, Coccinelle also served as an advocate for transgender rights. After her surgical transition in 1958, she married the French journalist Francis Bonne, a union that received official recognition from the French government. She founded the organization *Devenir Femme*, a transgender support and advocacy organization.[5]

Jan Morris, a Welsh author, was another famous patient of Burou's. Born James Morris, she described her 1972 surgical transition in her memoir *Conundrum*: "I was not going to change the truth of me, only discard the falsity." Morris's career as a writer spanned decades before and after her transition. In 1953, as a correspondent for *The Times* in London, she was the only journalist embedded in the team for Sir Edmund Hillary's and Tenzing Norgay's 1953 ascent of Mount Everest, and she reported their success from base camp at 17,900 feet through a coded telegram.[6] She wrote more than forty books, including a trilogy on the social history of the British Empire, *Pax Britannica* (1968), *Heaven's Command* (1973), and *Farewell the Trumpets* (1978). She also authored numerous essays based on her travels, from visiting Hiroshima after the bomb to living in a palazzo in the Grand Canal or on Field Marshal Bernard Montgomery's houseboat on the Nile.[7]

Morris married Elizabeth Tuckniss in 1949, just prior to her surgery. Sadly, British law forced their divorce after her gender-affirming procedure, but they remained together and raised their five children. In 2008, they underwent a civil union ceremony, reaffirming their mutual commitment, which endured until Morris's death in 2020 at the age of ninety-four. They were buried together with a gravestone that reads: "Here are two friends, at the end of one life."[8]

NOTES

1. Fallowell and Ashley, *April Ashley's Odyssey*, 84.
2. Fallowell and Ashley, *April Ashley's Odyssey*, 87.
3. Corbett v Corbett (Ashley).
4. Carter, "April Ashley."
5. Perrone, "Coccinelle."
6. Morris, *Conundrum*, 103.
7. Adams, "Jan Morris."
8. Adams, "Jan Morris."

WORKS CITED

Adams, Tim. "Jan Morris: You're Talking to Someone at the Very End of Things." *Guardian*, March 1, 2020. Accessed May 17, 2020. https://www.theguardian.com/books/2020/mar/01/jan-morris-thinking-again-interview-youre-talking-to-someone-at-the-very-end-of-things.

Carter, Helen. "April Ashley, Transgender Icon: Liverpool Exhibition Opens." *BBC News Online*, September 27, 2013. Accessed March 9, 2020. https://www.bbc.com/news/uk-england-merseyside-24271931.

Corbett v. Corbett (Ashley). 2 All ER 33 (1970, 1971).

DeKruif, Paul. *The Male Hormone.* New York: Harcourt Brace, 1945.

Dillon, Michael. *Self: A Study in Ethics and Endocrinology.* Portsmouth, NH: William Heinemann Medical Books, 1946.

Doctor, Richard F. *Becoming a Woman: A Biography of Christine Jorgensen.* Philadelphia, PA: Haworth Press, 2008.

Fallowell, Duncan, and April Ashley. *April Ashley's Odyssey.* London: J. Cape, 1982.

Horwell, Veronica. "Jan Morris Obituary." *Guardian*, November 20, 2020. Accessed May 9, 2021. https://www.theguardian.com/books/2020/nov/20/jan-morris-obituary.

Lyall, Sarah. "The Many Lives of Jan Morris." *New York Times*, April 25, 2019. Accessed May 9, 2021. https://www.nytimes.com/2019/04/25/books/jan-morris-in-my-minds-eye.html.

McQuiston, John T. "Christine Jorgensen, 62, Is Dead; Was First to Have a Sex Change." *New York Times*, May 4, 1989. Accessed January 22, 2020. https://www.nytimes.com/1989/05/04/obituaries/christine-jorgensen-62-is-dead-was-first-to-have-a-sex-change.html.

Morris, Jan. *Conundrum.* New York: New York Review Books, 2005.

Perrone, Pierre. "Coccinelle: Transsexual Entertainer." *Independent*, October 16, 2006. Accessed August 11, 2020. https://www.independent.co.uk/news/obituaries/coccinelle-6230828.html.

5

TWO SPIRIT HEALTH IN NORTH AMERICA

Trudie Jackson

> We don't waste people the way white society does. Every person has their gift.
>
> —Crow Elder

Y'aht'eeh. My name is Trudie Jackson.[1] I am an enrolled member of the Diné or Navajo Nation. My clans are of the Bitter Water on my mother's side and the Folded Arms people on my father's side. The Mexican people are on my maternal grandfather's side, and the Yucca-Strung-Out-In-A-Line are on my paternal grandfather's side. I grew up in a small community called Teec Nos Pos on the beautiful Navajo Nation, in Arizona. At age five, I began attending Indian Boarding School. There, I attended classes taught by nonnative teachers, was bullied for existing outside the gender binary, and was disciplined for speaking my Diné language. In junior high school, I moved to Utah to participate in the Indian Student Placement Program, which was sponsored by the Church of Jesus Christ of the Latter-day Saints. I lived in a Mormon foster home where I was indoctrinated with Mormon teachings and referred to as a Lamanite.[2]

My ancestors endured similar trauma when colonizers tackled the Indian problem by shipping them off to federal Indian boarding schools for forced assimilation into the dominant Christian culture. Like my ancestors, I was wounded by these events, and like them, I am resilient. I am an activist, a scholar, a life-long learner, and an advocate for my community. I am a proud, Diné Two Spirit transgender woman of color, and as such, I embody a number of exceptional, yet discounted, intersectional identities. It is with these experiences that I share this story about the health of Two Spirit people in North America.

Neither colonial histories nor contemporary queer theories accurately reflect my experience of race, nation, sexuality, or gender. Two Spirit bodies are not treated with the same respect as those of cisgender American Indian or nonnative individuals. Many of us do not engage in mainstream Two Spirit LGBT (2SLGBT) organizations because they tend to lump us into 2SLGBT taxonomy or with queer people of color—a process that effectively erases our stories and fails to recognize that their privilege often eclipses our right to exist. Growing up in border towns in the 1970s, I encountered verbal and physical homophobic attacks within my schools, family, and community. Thus, I chose to build my life in an urban environment. Now, I listen to the younger generation, and while many still leave the reservations for these reasons, some may remain and still openly embrace themselves as 2SLGBT—and ultimately walk in two worlds. As I listen, I feel the need to look back in time, for history is fluid and subjective, to tell the largely untold tale of our ancestors' experiences. My purpose in writing this chapter is to describe how Two Spirit people came to live as we live today and how our history continues to impact our collective health and wellness.

Most of our recorded history was compiled by nonnative colonists, scholars, and anthropologists. To decolonize this chapter, I centered it around the voices of American Indian people and their allies, those who were directly impacted by colonialism and are best able to articulate our vision to reclaim and embrace our own narratives to heal. To explore our undocumented history, I have tapped Indigenous ways of knowing. As nonnative American Indian scholar Will Roscoe wrote: "Rather than technology, Native societies emphasized knowledge, especially familiarity with the environment . . . intuitive forms of knowledge were highly developed . . . visions, dreams, and trance states were valued as sources of information, direction, ability and fortune. Ideals of balance, harmony, and integration between humans and nature were widespread."[3] Storytelling provides access to these rich cultural sources and supports the passage of wisdom from generation to generation. I fill the gaps in this chapter with cultural knowledge and teachings passed to me by my elders.

INDIGENOUS TERMINOLOGY: TRIBAL LANGUAGES AND TWO SPIRIT IDENTITIES

Historical, cultural, and anthropological evidence reveals that prior to colonialism and Christianity, Two Spirit people held accepted or even honored places within their tribal communities. These geographically and culturally diverse Indigenous communities had their own words to refer to those we now describe as Two Spirit, including terms such as *lhamana* or *katsotse* (Zuni), *winkte* (Teton/Lakota), *joya* (Chumash), *badé* (Crow), *nádleehí* (Diné), and *elha* (Cocopa).[4] English translations fail to capture the subtle meanings of these terms, which referenced varying roles, occupations, dress, and behaviors within the more than 350 documented tribes. In our early recorded histories, American Indian communities embraced these nonbinary concepts of gender.[5]

Early Spanish explorers and settlers made contact with Two Spirit people who they referred to as *berdache,* a term traced back to the 1600s in Persia, meaning young captive or slave.[6] The word *berdache* later became popular in Europe when referring to a passive, young partner in a male homosexual relationship. European settlers and anthropologists used this term to describe Indigenous people who cross-dressed, performed work associated with both masculine and feminine roles, or engaged in homosexual practices.[7] As colonization imposed new concepts about the nature of masculinity and femininity on Indigenous communities, widespread homophobia emerged. This phobia compounded the derogatory meaning of the word *berdache*, which is now considered inappropriate, as it fails to reflect the nuanced gender roles, identities, and sexualities as lived by American Indians.[8]

At the 1990 International Two Spirit Gathering in Winnipeg, Canada, a group of elders and activists who objected to the word *berdache* reintroduced the term *Two Spirit*. The words are "intentionally complex . . . meant to be an umbrella term for people who use words and concepts from their specific traditions to describe themselves . . . like *queer*, it is meant to be inclusive, ambiguous and fluid" and to challenge "white-dominated GLBTQ community's labels and taxonomies."[9] Two Spirit individuals may be male-bodied or female-bodied with either feminine or masculine characteristics. They cross social gender roles, embody diverse gender expressions and sexual orientations, and have been viewed as double blessed with the spirit of both man and woman. In many precolonial Indigenous communities, Two Spirit individuals were respected for their unique roles and responsibilities and were felt to possess a gift. Driskill noted, "The stance that Two Spirit people carry very *particular* medicine . . . is one rooted within Native worldviews . . . as part of larger practices of maintaining and continuing Native cultural practices."[10] While queer movements within the dominant, white culture often reject religion due to its heterosexist or transphobic stance, Native Two Spirit individuals historically held a prominent place within traditional religious life.[11] The term *Two Spirit* is not recognized at the tribal government level and not all people embrace or use it in day-to-day life.

Anthropologists often refer to Indigenous third or fourth genders, but American Indian scholar Wesley Thomas described five traditional gender categories in the Diné language. These terms referenced biological sex, sex-linked occupations, behaviors, and roles.[12] The primary gender was *adzáán*—women who served as decision makers and heads of households within the matrilineal and matrilocal center of Navajo culture. The second, *hastiin*, referred to the gender marker, but not the sexual marker for a male. A person of the third gender was *nádleehí*, a name with a complex and evolving meaning. Originally translated to English as *hermaphrodite, nádleehí* referred to males with standard anatomical parts who demonstrated social characteristics of the opposite gender. Under the same concept of nádleehí, Thomas referred to the fourth and fifth genders as *masculine females* and *feminine males*. In Navajo culture, the nádleehí functioned in dual roles as male and female and served as esteemed herbalists, shamans, warriors, peacemakers, storytellers, healers, matchmakers, couples' counselors, and guardians for orphans. Navajo language had no term for gender dysphoria but a rich understanding of gender diversity.[13]

An array of terms exists for those who could be described as transgender, but I caution readers to use this word carefully, as not all Indigenous people who fit this category from an outsider's perspective identify as transgender. In 2013, Irene Vernon and I published *Closing the Gap: A Research Agenda for the Study of Health Needs Among American Indian/Native Hawaiian Transgender Individuals*.[14] We conducted focus groups with forty-two gender-diverse Indigenous people from four major cities and asked: "What are your thoughts on the term Two Spirit or your own tribal word?" Only two participants identified as Two Spirit. The majority of participants chose transgender over Two Spirit, and several preferred the specific traditional words from their tribal language. Some used one term when on the Indian reservation and another in urban settings.

Contemporary Two Spirit people trace their heritage to diverse tribal communities across North America and have varied lived experiences. Some choose to live in traditional ways on the Indian reservation and others have assimilated into mainstream American culture without much awareness of their heritage. American Indian scholar Wesley Thomas devised a heuristic device[15] to categorize Two Spirit individuals based on their connection to or separation from traditional Navajo culture (Box 5.1).

> **Box 5.1**
> **Gender Diversity in Navajo Culture:**
> **Traditional-Assimilated Cultural Continuum**
>
> 1. **Traditional**: A traditional nádleehí lives matrilocally on the reservation. They are considered culturally wealthy and an anchor to the extended family. They are defined on the basis of their occupational preference or social role and are often involved in spiritual activities.
>
> 2. **Transitional**: A transitionalist lives on or off the reservation but maintains strong family ties. Transitionalists retain Navajo religious beliefs but are not as involved in traditional culture. Some transitionalists identify more with Western LGBT identities than they do with nádleehí. They are more exposed to Western culture and Western education.
>
> 3. **Contemporary**: A contemporary individual has some or little knowledge of Navajo culture, religious beliefs, and occupational positions and has some or little connection with reservation life. These people have a closer relationship to Western LGBT communities than to Navajo culture. Some contemporary individuals who identify as gay or lesbian might also identify as Two-Spirit.
>
> 4. **Acculturated**: An acculturated individual has lived away from the reservation for several generations and has little to no knowledge of Navajo language. They are aware of and acknowledge their Navajo tribal heritage.
>
> 5. **Assimilated**: An assimilated individual is not aware of their tribal heritage and does not acknowledge it.
>
> *Note.* From Thomas, Wesley. "Navajo Cultural Constructions of Gender and Sexuality." In *Two-Spirit People*, edited by Sue-Ellen Jacobs, Wesley Thomas, and Sabine Lang, 156–173. Urbana: University of Illinois Press, 1997.

While useful, I feel Thomas's device does not capture my Two Spirit trans experience as someone who lives off the reservation but is closely tied to my historical and cultural roots. Therefore, I propose a new category—inter-Indigenous—for those like me. My definition of *inter-Indigenous* stems from the work of scholar Kimberlé Crenshaw, who coined the term *intersectionality*, which refers to how an individual's multiple intersectional identities combine to create different kinds of oppression or privilege.[16] I have combined her ideas with Indigenous-centered identifying philosophies: (1) Pan-Indianism, a liberation philosophy and a political approach to promote unity among some American Indian people by synthesizing the traditions and wisdom of more than one nation;[17] and (2) Urban Indians, or American Indians who live in urban areas. My *inter-Indigenous* term refers to identities that may include different (1) tribal affiliations (with or without federal and state recognition) and cultures; (2) rural and/or urban status; and (3) approaches that may or may not embrace Two Spirit identification, either apart from or in addition to identifying as 2SLGBT within mainstream 2SLGBT movements. Inter-Indigenous incorporates age identities, including our awareness of the elders, who hold the stories and traditions that have been passed down through generations. As time passes, their wisdom will die with them unless the next generation preserves these teachings. Like all Two Spirit people, I have experienced varying degrees of oppression, privilege, and community acceptance or rejection on and off the reservation because of my inter-Indigenous identities.

THE CHANGING ONES: HISTORICAL FIGURES IN AMERICAN INDIAN CULTURES

Two Spirit mythology is still shared among contemporary American Indian and Two Spirit communities. Within some of these myths, Two Spirit characters are honored; in others, they are shamed, mocked, or killed. The Diné Origin Myth features the story of a nádleehí named Kay-des-tizhi, the Man-Wrapped-in-a-Rainbow, created as both man and woman by the God Begochiddy. Kay-des-tizhi served as a wealthy advisor and mediator.[18] Actual nádleehí often functioned as mediators by facilitating marriages and connections to and within the spiritual world.[19] *The Hermaphrodite*[20] (recorded in 1906) tells the story of a young man who had no interest in women. Even when a young woman lay with him, he had no desire for her and sent her away. The following day, he went to the springs for a bath. On returning home, he dreamt about Spider-Woman sitting with her legs apart and water gushing from within. Spider-Woman informed him that after bathing in the water, he would act like a woman, but the young man did not wish for this transformation. He sought help from a medicine man, but the healer was unable to locate the necessary medicine: green moss from the bottom of the stream. Spider-Woman had made all the green moss disappear so the young man could not be cured. Rejecting a life as half woman and half man, he committed suicide, in shame. Myths from many Indigenous nations include stories about the origins of Two Spirit people, men who became women, pregnant men, and violence against Two Spirit people.[21] These myths contain teachings that gave voice to Two Spirit beings.

Historical Indigenous people, including Osh-Tisch (Crow), We'wha (Zuni), Lozen (Chiricahua Apache), and Hastiin Klah (Diné) trailblazed today's Two Spirit movement. American Indian languages often lacked gendered pronouns, and I find no documentation of the expressed gender identity or pronoun preferences for any of these individuals.[22] For this reason, in this chapter I will refer to these people with the singular they/them/their pronouns.

Osh-Tish (1854–1929) was known as one of the last traditional Crow *badé*.[23] They were a powerful medicine person; as a youth, they had a vision where they were "taken underwater by water spirits" and "received the power to be a mediator of spiritual forces, an in-between person."[24] Assigned male at birth, Osh-Tish dressed in women's clothing, performed feminine tasks, and served as the leader of the *badé* in their community.[25] Occasionally, they dressed in men's clothing and fought as a warrior during raids. In 1876, they were given the name Osh-Tish, which means "finds them and kills them," after a successful raid against enemies during the Battle of the Rosebud.[26] In the late 1890s, an agent from the Bureau of Indian Affairs harassed the badé—arrested them, cut their hair, and forced them to wear masculine clothing. In a demonstration of support, Chief Pretty Eagle visited the Crow Agency and insisted that the agent leave the reservation.[27] A Baptist minister arrived in 1903; he condemned the badé and warned congregants to avoid Osh-Tish. Subsequently, no one else took on the role of badé, perhaps for this reason.[28]

We'Wha (1849–1896), a member of the Zuni tribe, was known as *lhamana* (Zuni Two Spirit).[29] Assigned male at birth, they developed skills as a weaver and potter (traditionally women's roles) and were also a hunter and spiritual leader. They were a prominent member of the tribe, accomplished in its secular and religious tribal history. We'Wha participated in male religious activities, managed the household of their adopted family, and earned money by washing clothes for whites and selling their artwork.[30] From their interactions with US military officers at the mission school where they worked and through their friendship with anthropologist Matilda Coxe Stevenson, who studied the Zuni, We'Wha learned English. Stevenson noted that We'Wha was "the most intelligent person in the pueblo . . . loved by all children to whom he was ever so kind."[31] In 1886, We'Wha accompanied Stevenson to Washington, DC,[32] where they lived for six months. Stevenson studied We'Wha's artwork and interviewed them about Zuni culture and religion. During this time, We'Wha also served as a cultural ambassador for their people, demonstrating their weaving techniques at the Smithsonian and meeting people of high society, including US President Grover Cleveland.[33] All received them as a Zuni priestess, princess, or maiden, and they achieved national celebrity during this visit.

Lozen (1840–1889), another prominent Two Spirit figure, was a member of the Chiricahua Apache and the sister of Victorio, a Warm Springs band chief. As a warrior, Lozen, assigned female at birth, accompanied Victorio and other Apache leaders in battles against the US Army. They "rode beside her brother as a warrior. She lives solely to aid him and her people. And she is sacred, even as a White Painted Woman. She is respected above all living women."[34] Lozen excelled in riding, fighting, roping, and stealing horses.[35] Victorio said, "She is my right hand. Strong as a man, braver than most, and cunning in strategy, Lozen is a shield to her people."[36] Lozen possessed extensive knowledge on the therapeutic properties of plants and minerals and was revered for their powers as a healer and prophet, particularly their ability to sense the locations of the enemy through ritual ceremonies.[37] In addition to traditional work of women, they also served on the Council of Leaders, joined men on the warpath to rampage against American settlers who had taken their homelands, and delivered a baby on the sidelines of battle.[38] After their brother died, they joined Geronimo's band where they met with Dahteste, a woman who had fought with Cochise's band against Western expansion.[39] Dahteste had negotiated peace treaties for her people, served as an English translator and, in 1835, helped Geronimo escape from detainment at the San Carlos Reservation.[40] Lozen and Dahteste became romantically involved and rode beside Geronimo until he surrendered in 1886.[41] They accompanied Geronimo and 498 other Apaches to a prisoner-of-war camp in Florida, where they were separated and suffered from loneliness, humidity, heat, tuberculosis, malaria, and smallpox.[42] Lozen died of tuberculosis after moving to a prisoner-of-war camp in Alabama, prior to the release of the remaining Apaches from their group. After twenty-seven years of internment, Dahteste was released to join the Mescalero Apache in New Mexico, where she reportedly possessed many sheep (a sign of wealth) and mourned Lozen to the end of her days.[43]

Hastiin Klah (1867–1937), the most famous nádleehí in Diné history, served as a religious leader, chanter, sand painter, politician, and weaver.[44] After recovering from a serious accident as a youth, they were confirmed as nádleehí, or "the one who is changing." They were expected to assist their mother and sister with weaving, typically women's work,[45] and developed the ability to weave smooth, finely patterned rugs. They were first recognized as a master weaver at the 1893 World's Columbian Exposition in Chicago and

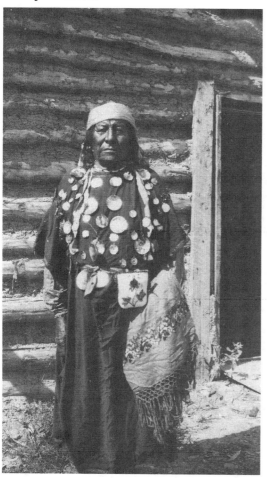

Figure 5.1. Photo of Osh-Tish. *Source*: National Museum of the American Indian, Smithsonian Institution (catalogue number N34256). Used with permission.

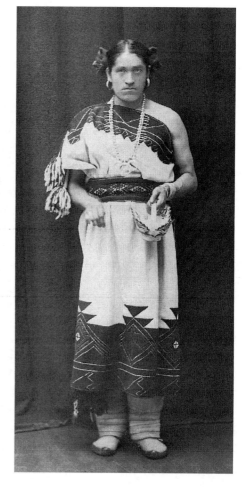

Figure 5.2. Photo of We'Wha, between circa 1871 and circa 1907. *Source*: National Archives and Records Administration. Public domain.

Figure 5.3 Photo of Hastiin Klah (1867–1937). *Source*: Wikipedia.org.

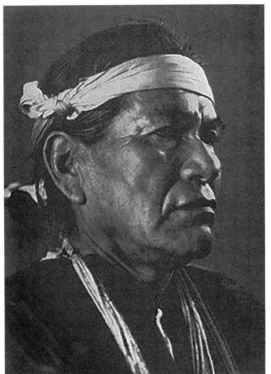

later formed a friendship with the heiress Mary Cabot Wheelwright after she purchased one of their tapestries. They also became a prestigious medicine man and ceremonial chanter, which were traditional male roles. As Klah aged, they recognized there were few apprentices to whom they could pass down their knowledge, and they feared Indigenous religious teachings would be lost. Thus, they began to weave images from traditional sand paintings and religious chants into their work, preserving history through artistry—a practice initially frowned on by the Diné people due to its religious content.[46] Klah proposed to Wheelwright that she help them safeguard their ceremonial knowledge, and the two of them spent ten years transcribing and cataloguing Klah's teachings. Wheelwright later decided to use her inheritance to establish a museum in Santa Fe devoted to Diné arts and religion, inviting Klah to assist with all planning, including architectural design and collections. Klah died a few months before the dedication of the Museum of Navajo Ceremonial Art (later named the Wheelwright Museum of the American Indian).[47]

THE COLONIZATION OF TWO SPIRIT PEOPLE

As settlers encroached on Indigenous territories, they imposed their thoughts and practices on these communities, demanding assimilation, acculturation, civilization, and erasure of the American Indian identity. The concept of Manifest Destiny, a term coined in 1845, promoted the belief that the white American settlers were ordained by God to expand dominion across the North American continent. This ethos sanctioned the imposition of Western dogma pertaining to gender, gender roles, and heteronormativity; the erasure of traditional cultures and the forced assimilation of American Indian youth through boarding schools; the spread of Christianity; and the establishment of governmental policies that codified Western expectations as law.

The result of these processes not only forced American Indian people to assimilate into colonial culture but also created a system of ethnic cleansing and genocide to ensure that individuals lost—if not their lives—their relationship to the land, their livestock, religion, communities, and identities. Historical trauma is "cumulative emotional and psychological wounding over the lifespan and across generations, emanating from massive group trauma experiences."[48] While all American Indian communities suffered (and continue to suffer), the historical trauma of American Indian Two Spirit people requires special attention as a unique, complex iteration of the trauma suffered by all.

Manifest Destiny was based on the belief that to be civilized one must first be Christianized. Richard Pratt, a boarding school superintendent, coined the phrase, "Kill the Indian, Save the Man,"[49] a concept that led to cultural genocide, including the rejection of Indigenous religious, spiritual, cultural, and medicinal practices. The introduction of Christianity as a system of power across North America in the fifteenth century not only regulated and erased the social and spiritual connections of Indigenous people but also led to the slaughter of gender-diverse Indigenous individuals. A sixteenth-century painting by Theodor de Bry depicts an episode in 1513, when Vasco Núñez de Balboa, appalled by the Two Spirit Indigenous people, threw forty-two of them to his greyhounds as food.[50] In the 1700s, Spanish missionaries exterminated the *joyas* (Two Spirit people in California) and practiced gendercide by disciplining, controlling, and punishing those who expressed gender diversity or whose sexuality challenged mainstream beliefs.[51]

The imposition of Christian values and morals on American Indian societies forced American Indian peoples to adopt Western notions of family, home, desire, and personal identity.[52] As traditional forms of sexuality disappeared, heterosexuality arrived as a colonial concept. Indians first became straight when heteronormativity became the framework for settler-state occupation and early settlers categorized queer Indigenous sexuality as savage, degenerate, and something that must be eliminated.[53] In many Native communities, gender-diverse behaviors that people once accepted as normal aspects of tribal life became viewed as deviant and immoral. Christian homophobic and transphobic doctrines altered American Indian cultures and stigmatized Two Spirit people.

Early Indigenous cultures focused on the knowledge, behaviors, and the complementarity of both genders—man and woman—and that of Two Spirit people. Many nations, such as the Diné, had matriarchal societies with matrilineal descent, inheritance, and ownership of wealth. Colonization introduced the concept of heteropatriarchy, as well as Western constructs of masculine identity and the gender binary, forcing Indigenous people to view men and women as distinct categories with prescribed gender roles. Colonists stripped Indigenous men of their role as warriors and imposed the Western expectation that they serve as heads of households and wage earners or as farmers. Western masculine roles were reinforced in residential schools, sports, and governmental policies. The settlers' heteropatriarchal world view promoted gendered colonization as a form of power to strip Indigenous people of their tribal identities, including Two Spirit .

The implementation of federal Indian policies also ensured the assimilation and acculturation of North American Indians into the Western, gendered culture. In Canada, the Gradual Civilization Act (1857) and Gradual Enfranchisement Act (1869) sought to assimilate First Nation people into the dominant culture by promising enfranchisement to men who were deemed by the Superintendent General of Indian Affairs to have "good moral character," based on their level of education and ability to communicate in English or French, to maintain sobriety, and to be free from debt.[54] The Indian Act of 1876 evolved to create a system for "Indian protection" that forced assimilation of First Nation people. This sweeping, paternalistic set of laws regulated the day-to-day life of registered First Nation Indians and their communities, including the imposition of governmental structures, control over land use, definitions for who qualified as an Indian for Indian status, and the rights to practice their culture and traditions.[55] Two Spirit people suffered especially under this new regime because their very nonbinary existence challenged gender and cultural norms championed by settler colonialists—in boarding schools and broader society. It's unlikely that a Two Spirit individual would have met the arbitrary standard for "good moral character" when their identity was rendered deviant.

This systematic legal violence had the outright intent to perpetuate the same ethnic cleansing begun generations ago. In 1920, Canadian Deputy Superintendent General Campbell Scott presented amendments to this legislation, remarking, "Our objective is to continue until there is not a single Indian in Canada that has not been absorbed into the body politic and there is no Indian question, no Indian Department, that is the object of this bill."[56] Similar legislation also persisted in varying forms in the United States until 1994, when Indian Affairs released the Tribal Self Governance Act[57] to codify the inherent right to self-government. Struggles around sovereignty rooted in these earlier, paternalistic policies persist to this day.

The intent of settlers to conquer and claim land was an ambition unknown to American Indian people, who did not view land as a commodity. Indigenous peoples' relationships, responsibilities, heritage, loyalties, and languages deepened with meaning as they extended through time and space.[58] Settlers pushed American Indian communities from their original homelands and hunting grounds; they then occupied this land for their sole use. By claiming ownership over the land, settlers attempted to sever Indigenous people from their connection to their ancestral and historical place in the world. Those Two Spirit people who participated in traditional religions and ceremonies in sacred spaces lost this connection. Two Spirit religious leaders were intimately connected to and dependent on the history of distinct places, which held cultural significance, as a means to continue their tribal traditions and uphold their sacred role. Ultimately, land occupation split all Indigenous people from their cultural past, as well as their means for survival—hunting, farming, harvesting—and sources of water.

Early American Indians suffered from a number of health problems and diseases but contact with Europeans introduced a host of new epidemics that decimated communities. These diseases included bubonic plague, measles, smallpox, and cholera.[59] Traditional healers and Two Spirit medicine people possessed knowledge about the plants and herbs for treating familiar illnesses but were unprepared to manage these new diseases. Regardless, Europeans destroyed, rejected, or prohibited such traditional medicine practices,[60] simultaneously undermining the leadership of Two Spirit healers. Governmental agents viewed tribal healing practices as a hindrance to the civilization of the Indians.[61] These social and cultural changes negatively impacted American Indian health and the role Two Spirit people played in tribal communities.

Between 1880 and 1930, North American federal governments removed American Indian children from their homes and enrolled them in Indian boarding schools—often hundreds of miles from their homes—to undergo a systematic process of assimilation. The schools, usually run by missionaries in conjunction with government agents, "enforced strict compliance with European and Christian standards of conduct, including prohibition of cultural practices and conformity to rigid gender roles."[62] Colonial gender norms made Two Spirit histories, traditions, and identities a specific genocidal target. Since it was also forbidden to speak tribal languages, children lost access to tribal, and specifically Two Spirit, histories. Those who disobeyed the rules were harshly punished and forced to deny their heritage, increasing their Two Spirit vulnerability.[63] One study found that Indigenous transgender youth who attended boarding school were more likely to have an alcohol use disorder, used illicit drugs more than once in the past year, and attempted suicide or had suicidal thoughts during their life.[64] The bones of these children litter the grounds of the boarding schools,[65] and their voices echo within our communities.

This institutional colonization persisted into the latter half of the twentieth century: the second era of forced removal of American Indian children occurred from the 1950s to 1978, when the child welfare departments stepped in. In Canada, "the sixties scoop" refers to a period of time when social workers removed children from reservations on various pretexts, including the social worker's perception of poverty, poor hygiene or nutrition, or inferior housing standards, without regard for the effect of this forced removal on the child, family, or reservation.[66] In the United States, the Bureau of Indian Affairs started its Indian Adoption Project within the Child Welfare League of America to promote the adoption of Indian children by nonnative families.[67] As evidenced by decades of legal violence that undermined the humanity of Americans Indians, North American governments manufactured the perception that Indigenous communities could not raise their own children. These child welfare procedures—themselves a form of patriarchal, political violence—did not acknowledge or account for the state's role in creating ethnocultural hierarchies that subjugated American Indians to the very substandard socioeconomic and health conditions from which the agency rescued children.

Another form of colonization has been conducted by researchers. In the late 1800s, nonnative anthropologists descended on American Indian communities to collect artifacts and data on the language and cultures of a vanishing race.[68] As they moved artifacts to museums and muddled cultural practices through translation, Two Spirit people lost sacred property and the true meaning of their traditions. Ultimately, nonnative scholars hijacked the fields of anthropology, queer studies, and Native American studies, interpreting data through a nonnative lens; scrambling the meanings of our languages, customs, and practices; and imposing colonial values on higher educational programs centered on Indigenous people.[69] While the field of Native American studies beckoned toward new possibilities, academic positions were filled with nonnative scholars. Most of the work was done within Western theories of knowledge, offering only a Western point of view.[70] The research highlighted settler colonialism and heteropatriarchy; scholars judged Indigenous people for not sharing the same goals and values of settlers. American Indian scholar and activist Elizabeth Cook-Lynn's 1997 seminal article, "Who Stole Native American Studies?" identified the ongoing influence of colonialism in academia, condemning this ideology that further dehumanized American Indians, discredited Indigenous scholars, and politicized research agendas. Nonnative scholars recorded contrived versions of Indigenous history. Cook-Lynn offered this analysis: "It was not just deconstruction, it was reconstruction."[71] Lacking the dominant Euro-American authority, the few Indigenous scholars within these institutions experienced isolation and discrimination reminiscent of colonial violence and cultural genocide.[72] Until recently, Two Spirit voices were absent entirely from the field of queer studies.

THE IMPACT OF COLONIZATION ON TWO SPIRIT HEALTH

The resulting stigma from colonization wreaks havoc on the self-confidence, self-worth, health, and well-being of Two Spirit individuals today. Facing the continued pressure of settler morality and social violence, reservations have become homophobic and transphobic environments. Fifty-seven percent of American Indian and Alaskan Native respondents to the *2015 United States Transgender Survey (USTS) Report on the Experiences of American Indian & Alaskan Native Respondents* reported that they had attempted suicide at some point in their lives, compared to forty percent in the USTS sample overall—a rate twelve times higher than that in the US population.[73] We lack data to compare suicide rates for Two Spirit people on and off the reservations but know that risks for those on the reservations are high. Tribal members criticize Two Spirit individuals in public settings on tribal sovereign land; some Two Spirit people try to blend in and avoid notice in public settings. Many Two Spirit people chose to relocate to urban areas for acceptance, only to find themselves isolated from mainstream society due to culture shock and racist cultural practices.

Historical trauma is embodied in depression, substance abuse, self-destructive behaviors, suicidal thoughts and gestures, anxiety, low self-esteem, anger, and difficulty recognizing and expressing emotion.[74] Cries from the Two Spirit community for healthcare services to address these problems echo within the hallways of policy makers, the federally funded Indian Health Services (IHS), and the 638 Tribal Health facilities that are owned by sovereign nations in tribal communities. To bring attention to our needs, we rely on statistics and the voices of those impacted by this trauma. It's been difficult to collect data in our community due to problematic racial and ethnic and gender and sexual orientation–related classification, poor data management, difficulty coordinating data between states and tribes, and the challenges of working with a population that is hesitant to identify themselves to researchers.[75] It is well known that 2SLGBT people face additional healthcare disparities, but a paucity of data exists to describe the health of contemporary Two Spirit individuals who face unique intersectional, sociocultural, and historical influences.

As coauthor of the *2015 United States Transgender Survey (USTS) Report on the Experiences of American Indian & Alaskan Native Respondents*,[76] I immersed myself in quantifying the impact of historical trauma on my community. This report focused on the specific experiences of the 319 USTS survey respondents who identified as American Indian and Alaskan Native, which accounted for just over one percent of the entire survey population.[77] The portrait of American Indian and Alaskan Native USTS respondents shows that they lived in forty-two states and were affiliated with more than one hundred corporations and tribes. The following statistics (see bulleted list below as well as tables 5.1 and 5.2) offer a snapshot of the social isolation and economic hardship.

- Fifty-five percent of these respondents had one or more disabilities.
- Eighteen percent did not have insurance.
- Twenty-one percent reported that a professional suggested conversion therapy.
- Ninety-two percent of those who were out had experienced mistreatment at school.
- Sixty percent had suffered a form of family rejection.
- Seventeen percent had been rejected by faith communities.
- Fifty-nine percent said they would feel somewhat or very uncomfortable asking the police for help.

- Thirty-five percent had participated in the underground economy, including sex work, drug sales, and currently criminalized work.

- Twenty-one percent experienced homelessness in the past year.

Such statistics are not only a reflection of a particular population but also an expression of the systems and institutions in play, which relies on trauma sharing. These statistics are useful for needs assessments, grant writing, and

Table 5.1. Key Findings from *2015 United States Transgender Survey (USTS) Report on the Experiences of American Indian and Alaskan Native Respondents* Compared with USTS Overall Sample

American Indian and Alaskan Native Respondents	USTS Overall Sample
Fifty-seven percent had experienced homelessness at some point in their lives.	Two times the rate of USTS sample
Twenty-one percent had lost a job because of being transgender.	Compared with thirteen percent of USTS sample
Sixty-five percent have been sexually assaulted in their lifetime.	Compared with forty-seven percent of USTS sample
Fifty percent who saw a healthcare provider in the past year reported at least one negative experience related to being transgender.	Compared with thirty-three percent of USTS sample

Table 5.2. Key Findings from *2015 United States Transgender Survey Report on Experience of American Indian and Alaskan Native Respondents* Compared with US Population

American Indian and Alaskan Native Respondents	US Population
Twenty-three percent were unemployed.	Five times the rate of US population
Forty-one percent lived in poverty.	Three times the rate of US population
Two percent were living with HIV.	Seven times the rate of US population
Forty-six percent experienced serious psychological distress in the month before completing the survey.	Nine times the rate of US population

programming, which potentially help secure funding for the Two Spirit/TGD community. Simultaneously, this damage-centered research also creates further oppression by portraying our entire community as depleted and defeated rather than rich and resilient. Deficit models further colonize us by voicing only our pain and ensuring that we speak from the margins. Furthermore, statistics like this do not capture nuanced inter-Indigenous identities. Scholar Eve Tuck recommends using desire-based research frameworks, which "can yield analyses that upend commonly held assumptions of responsibility, cohesiveness, ignorance, and paralysis within dispossessed and disenfranchised communities. Desire, yes, accounts for the loss and despair, but also the hope, the visions, the wisdom of lived lives and communities."[78]

In *Closing the Gap: A Research Agenda for the Study of Health Needs Among American Indian/Native Hawaiian Transgender Individuals*, we conducted focus groups to identify key health research needs, as defined by these communities.[79] Participants voiced the inability to access affirming care from healthcare professionals, which led to self-treatment with black market hormones. Many physicians who work for IHS clinics are fresh out of residency and their primary goal is to pay off student loans, not care for our people. Most of these clinicians are not familiar with transgender healthcare or how to work with the Two Spirit community. Furthermore, Two Spirit people cited they feared a lack of confidentiality in the community-based clinics. As a result, many of us seek care from nonnative providers who lack American Indian cultural competency but know about medical transitions. Two Spirit people often move off the reservation to live in cities with the hope of better healthcare and more respect for their gender identity and sexual orientation.

Focus group participants also reflected on their social status and reception more broadly. They spoke to the specific mental health issues (invisibility and isolation) of trans elders, who seldom lived beyond age sixty. Participants posited, "Where is our older generation?" and "When you feel that no one cares, then you don't care for yourself." They also spoke to the difficulty in their everyday lives: "We have so much against us, and you have to be strong or else you have no choice . . . I have no family, so I have to stand on my own two feet and fight for myself." Another commented specifically on how people received them, explaining, "You are in the world and your parents, family, church, and community are telling you, 'What the hell are you wearing girls' clothes for? Are you fucking crazy?'"

A major theme of our study was resiliency in the face of adversity, a strength attributed to participants' lived experiences, culture, and history. Such resiliency stemmed from work to both support others and advocate together for change. Participants noted that helping others was a core cultural value rooted in history. One stated, "Our spirit is that I would not let them be on the streets. Although much has been lost, it is in our life to help take care of kids and be peacemakers. . . . We are caretakers of babies and elders, and still, this continues to be our role today." They also spoke to why understanding one's history was so valuable: knowledge of culture and history affirmed their personhood on individual and sociocultural levels. One respondent explained that "culture gives you an answer as to why there is a place for you. . . . This is the strength behind those who are transitioning." Another participant said, "Knowing the role of the nádleehí can save the culture and increase self-esteem." The power of these and other stories helps repair the damage of colonialism by inspiring our community members to seek social justice through collaborative social change.

THE MOVEMENT TO DECOLONIZE TWO SPIRIT HEALTHCARE

The process of decolonizing healthcare for Two Spirit people requires us to tell our stories and assert our importance within the cultural, ceremonial, and spiritual traditions of our communities. Decolonization refers to the "ongoing, radical resistance against colonization that includes struggles for land redress, self-determination, healing historical trauma, cultural continuance, and reconciliation."[80] Thus, decolonization is a movement for social transformation, one that embraces the work of our Two Spirit scholars, artists, authors, activists, and healers. Listening to these voices, we can create medical institutions that recognize and meet our unique healthcare needs.

To decolonize our healthcare, we first look to the Indigenous Two Spirit scholars and artists to contextualize theoretical and historical realities. They have championed a "uniquely Native-centered and tribally specific understanding of gender and sexuality as a way to critique colonialism, queerphobia, racism, and misogyny as part of decolonial struggles."[81] Scholar Jodi Byrd contended that queer scholars such as Judith Butler ignore Indigenous peoples in their theorization.[82] She described how Indigenous critical theory transforms queer theory and critical theory to interrupt the colonialist structures that support racialized and gendered oppressions. Scholar Qwo-Li Driskill acknowledged the diverse traditions and understandings of gender and sexuality among different nations but posited that "[The] shared experiences under heteropatriarchal, gender-polarized colonial regimes . . . give rise to critiques that position Native Two Spirit GLBTQ/genders as oppositional to colonial powers . . . and critique both the colonial nature of many GLBTQ movements in the United States and Canada and the queer-/transphobia internalized by Native nations."[83] Driskill urged us to reckon with our erasure not only within first wave colonialism but also within both white-dominated queer theory and queer people of color critiques. Such theories are not rooted in tribally specific traditions, and we may not be thoroughly conscious that colonialism is an ongoing process.[84] Modern, sociocultural colonialism compounds historical trauma and requires Indigenous-led theoretical and activist leadership to disrupt our own erasure. Driskill, for example, applied the metaphor of double weaving (traditional double woven Cherokee baskets have independent inside and outside designs) to weave together the theoretical splints of queer and Indigenous studies. He asserted, "Taking these splints of Two Spirit critiques and doubleweaving them into a conversation with queer studies pushes queer studies in the US and Canada toward decolonial work that is responsible to the land and life it builds itself on."[85] Scholars like Byrd and Driskill ask us to embrace our desire, to radically reimagine our futures—for Two Spirit individuals and American Indians at large.[86]

To decolonize Two Spirit healthcare, we must also voice our lived experiences. Ma-Nee Chacaby's book *A Two Spirit Journey*[87] highlights her journey as a Two Spirit Cree and Ojibwa elder. She describes a critical period in her life when she focused on accepting her female lovers while juggling the needs of her two children. Her identity as a Two Spirit woman emerged after facing repeated setbacks around acceptance in mainstream Canadian 2SLGBT community; Two Spirit erasure within the 2SLGBT community is not just theoretical, as Byrd alluded to in her analysis, but the lived experience of people like Chacaby. This rejection forced her to reconnect with her Indigenous culture, traditions, and language and to learn to walk in balance as a Two Spirit woman in a settler state. Chacaby faced poverty, substance abuse, violence, and discrimination, yet she still demonstrated resilience. She survived in the local fishing industry, a competitive environment with low wages, long hours, and demeaning attitudes regarding her sexual orientation. Additionally, she engaged with her community and led the first American Indian gay pride parade in Thunder Bay. By asserting her own personhood, Chacaby addresses how to occupy space in the colonial arena, one that includes exclusive, mainstream 2SLGBT communities in Canada. Her personal reflection also includes lessons on how to cope with depression—a critical point to amplify Two Spirit people's capacity for resilience and individual self-determination.

Kent Monkman, a queer Two Spirit and First Nations artist, challenges the structures of museums by viewing them as colonial spaces that must be decentered and decolonized. Through artwork, performance, film, photography, and objects, he explores themes of colonization, sexuality, loss, and resilience, as well as the complexities of historic and contemporary Indigenous experiences.[88] His images include references to the impact of residential boarding schools, forced relocation, land and resource dispossessions, sexual and gender violence, genocide, and the parental authority imposed by colonists. Monkman explains that the history of art in Canada is a living document of colonization from the viewpoint of the Europeans who eyed the First People. He challenges us to question whether or not Indigenous people are in these paintings, and if so, how are we perceived? In his work, Monkman juxtaposes oppressive and suppressive views of gender and sexuality under Christian beliefs with a "trickster—a time-traveling, shape-shifting, gender-fluid alter-ego named Miss Chief Eagle Testickle."[89] This trickster challenges Western beliefs by subverting viewer expectations. Miss Chief Eagle Testickle exposes the Christian piety and the sexual and racist hypocrisy of the colonizers, yet the proffered, alternative narrative—one infused with humor, nakedness, flamboyant dress, and high heels—also metaphorically reclaims history for Miss Chief Eagle Testickle and the American Indians embodied by the persona.

In his 2016 painting *The Daddies* (Figure 5.4),[90] Monkman placed images reminiscent of the old master paintings of the Founding Fathers alongside Miss Chief Eagle Testickle, whose naked, spread-eagle pose usurps the gaze. The title refers to the tools of colonial patriarchal violence, including the role of the Great Father, which implied that American Indians were children requiring governmental supervision and discipline. The eyes of the Founding Fathers are fixed on Miss Testickle's crotch, evoking the historical refusal of the "Daddies" to recognize Indigenous gender, sexual, and social norms; the imposition of their colonial perceptions of a gender binary; and the hypocrisy of those who proclaimed disgust with Indigenous sexual and gender norms but who appear titillated by the person before them.

Two Spirit activism is a decolonizing force that positions academic theory and artistic expression within grassroots practices to transform our world. Two Spirit activists and allies contest tribal policies that refuse to recognize gay marriage, including the controversial Diné Marriage Act of 2005 for the Navajo Nation. While the US Supreme Court sanctioned same-sex marriage in

Figure 5.4. Kent Monkman, *The Daddies*, 2016. Acrylic on canvas, 60 in. × 112½ in. *Source*: Image courtesy of the artist.

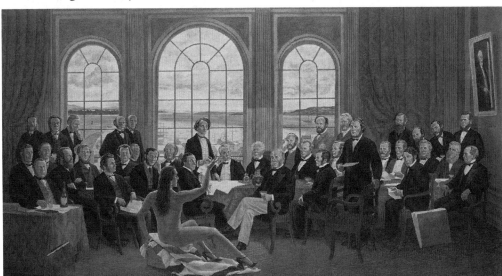

2015, all but a handful of American Indian Nations exercise sovereignty by perpetuating oppressive, Christian colonial practices to undermine the legality and morality of same-sex relationships. Several Nations, however, preceded the Supreme Court's ruling. The Coquille Tribe in Oregon became the first tribe to legalize same-sex marriage for tribal members in 2008.[91] The Suquamish Tribe in Washington accepted the Marriage Equality Act on August 1, 2011.[92] During the 2015 Navajo Studies Conference at Northern Arizona University, Delegate Krotty expressed her support for Navajo Two Spirit members and vowed to bring back the cultural teachings regarding the spiritual role of the nádleehí in Navajo ceremonies.

We also find many additional examples of Two Spirit activist leadership, reflecting their broader spiritual and cultural roles within American Indian Nations. Two Spirit individuals received recognition for establishing a camp at Standing Rock to protest the Dakota Access Pipeline and supporting the effort to protect sacred land, tackle climate change, and assert our relationship to the earth, water, sky, and other living animals.[93] The International Council of Two Spirit Societies includes seventeen North American Two Spirit organizations;[94] this advocacy group brings together diverse, regional representatives across Turtle Island.[95] Two Spirit individuals contributed to the development and success of the Tribal Training and Technical Assistance Center, part of the Substance Abuse and Mental Health Services Administration of the US Department of Health.[96] The Indigenous Ways of Knowing program of Lewis & Clark College in Portland, Oregon, engaged the Two Spirit community and legal community-based organizations to create the Tribal Equity Toolkit, a resource for Nations seeking legislative change in support of Two Spirit people.[97]

Even with the renewed leadership of Two Spirit individuals, there remains the unmet need—the unrealized desire—to decolonize the healthcare system to address the health needs of Two Spirit individuals adequately and respectfully. As specified in treaty obligations with the US federally recognized tribes, the federal government must provide healthcare services for American Indians. The IHS is an agency within the Department of Health and Human Services that claims to provide a comprehensive health service delivery system for approximately 2.2 million of the nation's estimated 3.7 million American Indian and Alaskan Native people.[98] Their mission is to partner with American Indian and Alaskan Native people "to raise physical, mental, social, and spiritual health to the highest level."[99] Their goal is to "ensure that comprehensive, culturally acceptable personal and public health services are available and accessible to all IAN people."[100] Historically, IHS has not fulfilled its mandate. While other health and human services programs responded to the AIDS epidemic by developing access to transgender healthcare, the IHS lagged.

IHS continues to fall short when providing care to 2SLGBT individuals. Significant provider-based and patient-based struggles intersect to create insurmountable barriers to care.[101] I am personally aware that transgender women receive general medical care from IHS clinics but are reluctant to ask for hormone therapy due to the lack of trained providers and the absence of affirming policies and procedures. They complain of being misgendered and harassed, and they experience invisibility and violations of privacy within these facilities. The focus groups from the previously cited *Closing the Gap* study support these claims. IHS also does not support inclusive intake forms or electronic health records, nor do they collect data to document our unique health needs.

Notably, at the time of this writing, most IHS clinics do not offer transition-related services. Two Spirit elders might say that no one needs to medically or surgically transition because, traditionally, the tribal communities embraced Two Spirit people, valuing their personhood, bodies, and roles. Modern Two Spirit individuals often do not feel embraced by their communities however, and many choose medical transitions to feel at peace in their bodies. For those who wish to medically or surgically transition, they must seek healthcare resources outside of the community—itself a kind of forced displacement and dispossession. Internalized transphobia, a relic of colonization and manifested as absent care, continues to haunt Two Spirit individuals who desire medical transitions.

On July 27, 2015, the IHS finally conducted a listening session with twenty-eight Two Spirit people from six IHS areas to advance and promote the health needs of the American Indian and Alaskan Native 2SLGBT community.[102] Five themes emerged from this session: services and eligibility, clinical services, behavioral health, youths' needs, and organizational strategies. Since then, the IHS has created a web page devoted to 2SLGBT health education, but this site lacks links to connect patients to affirming clinicians.[103] In 2019, the Cherokee Nation laid down the foundation for other Nations by developing the Cherokee Nation Health services, the largest tribally operated healthcare system in the United States.[104] This system offers a wide array of specialty services and boasts the first tribally associated medical school in the country. While services for Two Spirit people are not yet included, I believe this center is well positioned to fully manifest the calls of our resistance: We are not just reimagining but also actualizing our desire: a future for ourselves that includes holistic, culturally responsive, and gender-affirming healthcare.

CONCLUSION

While considering how to conclude this chapter, I traveled to Dine' Bikeyah and met with Wesley Thomas, an enrolled member of the Navajo Nation and a scholar of American Indian Two Spirit history. As we sat together at a flea market, we discussed how the term *Two Spirit* has evolved over the past three decades. While embraced in urban 2SLGBT spaces (and often by non-Indian people), the term remains controversial on Indian land and within colonized environments.

Thomas and I reflected on contemporary transphobia in tribal communities—another painful legacy of colonization. For Two Spirit people to reclaim their space within our tribal communities, we must reach out to the traditional members who remain connected to our cultural beliefs. But over the course of generations, as tribal members assimilated to colonial thought and processes, we lost many traditions, and we continue to lose them. Our Two Spirit elders have died off, taking their teachings with them. As recently as thirty years ago, medicine men still led traditional ceremonies, rites that connected us to our past. It takes decades for a medicine man to master these practices, and today they are hard to find. We are left with assimilated beliefs in place of our historical legacy. Most children of the current generation remain unaware of their culture, identity, and relationship to Mother Earth. As they assimilate into mainstream society, they leave their true native identity behind.

As a result, Two Spirit individuals, once revered, now face rejection. Transgender American Indian women suffer from violence, as exemplified by the murder of Fred Martinez, a Navajo youth from Cortez, Colorado, in 2001, and Jamie Wounded Arrow, from the Oglala-Lakota tribe, in 2017.[105] No specific laws exist to protect transgender people who reside within sovereign nations. Transphobic thought and practices drive gender community members, especially trans women, away from tribal land and into urban areas where they may find more acceptance. Two Spirit transgender men face erasure, as their specific problems and needs receive little to no attention in Indian country.

As a transgender woman and American Indian scholar, I often felt like I was the only one of my peers in a colonial, institutionalized educational system. I challenged existing scholarship to discover that my critiques were not well embraced. Like many transgender scholars, I felt defeated while pursuing higher education, but I also felt and still feel the need to advocate for my community. If not me, then who will speak for my people? This chapter attests to my work.

Today, my practice when entering any space is to acknowledge that my ancestors are with me and support me. I am grateful for their presence and thankful to share this chapter with you. I hope that by reading my words you will understand the impact of federal Indian policies on the education, religion, and health of Two Spirit people and the precariousness of our existence within our tribal communities. I hope to plant a seed in your mind. May that seed grow and flourish as you begin to understand the resiliency of Two Spirit individuals, despite colonial acts of erasure. We Two Spirit people remain a presence on Mother Earth, guided by our ancestors as we traverse hardship, stigma, discrimination, and hate. We decolonize colonial thinking and rhetoric to reaffirm that all Indigenous people are equal in the Great Spirit's eyes.

Ahe'hee. Walk in beauty.

NOTES

1. My sincere appreciation to Carolyn Wolf-Gould for providing support throughout the chapter from reading, revising, recommendations, and listening to my feedback.

The overwhelming support helped me get through the chapter as it kept me motivated as I saw the light at the end of the tunnel. Wesley Thomas, PhD, was also instrumental throughout the chapter, as I referenced a lot of his scholarship as well as the opportunity to sit down with him for a one-on-one conversation. Ahe'hee for sharing your knowledge, and I hope this chapter will inspire many future generations of American Indian Two-Spirit individuals to learn our history as we remain resilient as our ancestors. I would like to acknowledge these three individuals for taking the time to read and provide feedback on rough drafts of the chapter: Irene Vernon, PhD, Emeritus Professor, Colorado State University, Fort Collins; Grazia Cunningham, MPH, Northwest Portland Area Indian Health Board; and Wesley Thomas, PhD, Emeritus Professor, Navajo Technical University.

2. The Book of Mormon describes the Lamanites as a group of people descended from two Israelite brothers, who the Lord said would "come to the knowledge of their Redeemer" in the latter days, as part of God's covenant people. Mormons considered the American Indians Lamanites and focused their missionary work on Western Tribes. The stated goal of the Indian Student Placement program was to "provide Lamanite children with educational, spiritual, social, and cultural opportunities that would contribute to their leadership development." This program served as yet another organized system of cultural erasure and assimilation for American Indian youth (Indian Placement: The Three Most Common Questions, 1976; Lamanites Identities, n.d.)

3. Roscoe, *Changing Ones*, 6.
4. Roscoe, *Changing Ones*, 6–7, 213–22.
5. Roscoe, "North American Tribes," 48–76.
6. Roscoe, *Changing Ones*, 7.
7. Roscoe, *Changing Ones*, 7–8.
8. Jacobs, Thomas, and Lang, "Introduction," *Two-Spirit People*, 1–8.
9. Driskill, "Doubleweaving Two-Spirit Critiques," 69–72.
10. Driskill, "Doubleweaving Two-Spirit Critiques," 85–86.
11. Driskill, "Doubleweaving Two-Spirit Critiques."
12. Thomas, "Navajo Cultural Constructions of Gender and Sexuality," 156–73.
13. Thomas, "Navajo Cultural Constructions," 156–73.
14. Vernon and Jackson, "Closing the Gap," 37–58.
15. Thomas, "Navajo Cultural Constructions," 156–73.
16. Crenshaw, "Mapping the Margins," 282–313.
17. Robbins, "A Short History of Pan-Indianism."
18. Klah and Wheelwright, "The Story of the Emergence," 15–69; White-Sun and Dorsey, "The Hermaphrodite," 101–02.
19. Roscoe, *Changing Ones*, 41.
20. White-Sun and Dorsey, "The Hermaphrodite," 101–02.
21. Elledge, *Myths from the Arapaho to the Zuni*, 15–69.

22. Roscoe, *Changing Ones*, 17.
23. Roscoe, *Changing Ones*, 35.
24. Roscoe, *Changing Ones*, 23–38.
25. Roscoe, *Changing Ones*, 33–76.
26. Roscoe, *Changing Ones*, 33–76.
27. Roscoe, *Changing Ones*, 35.
28. Roscoe, *Changing Ones*, 33–76.
29. Roscoe, *The Zuni Man Woman*, 22.
30. Roscoe, "Strange Country This," 33–76.
31. Roscoe, *The Zuni Man Woman*, 46.
32. Gutierrez, "Bar Chee Ampe and Beyond."
33. Roscoe, *The Zuni Man Woman*, 70–71.
34. Ball, *In the Days of Victorio*, 14.
35. Wise, "What Everyone Can Learn."
36. Ball, *In the Days of Victorio*, 15.
37. Roscoe, *Changing Ones*, 90–91; Roscoe, "Strange Country This," 33–76; Wise, "What Everyone Can Learn."
38. Roscoe, *Changing Ones*, 90–91; Roscoe, "Strange Country This," 33–76; Wise, "What Everyone Can Learn."
39. Wise, "What Everyone Can Learn."
40. Wise, "What Everyone Can Learn."
41. Roscoe, *Changing Ones*, 90–91; Wise, "What Everyone Can Learn."
42. Wise, "What Everyone Can Learn."
43. Wise, "What Everyone Can Learn"; Roscoe, *Changing Ones*, 90–91.
44. Roscoe, *Changing Ones*, 39–65.
45. Roscoe, *Changing Ones*, 39–65.
46. Roscoe, *Changing Ones*, 39–65.
47. Roscoe, *Changing Ones*, 39–65.
48. Brave Heart, "The Historical Trauma," 7–13.
49. Pratt, "'Kill the Indian, and Save the Man,'" 46–59.
50. Miranda, "Extermination of the Joyas," 253–84; Gutierrez, "Bar Chee Ampe and Beyond."
51. Miranda, "Extermination of the Joyas."
52. Rifkin, *When Did Indians Become Straight?*, 8.
53. Rifkin, *When Did Indians Become Straight?*, 3–44.
54. Hanson, "The Indian Act"; Nitotemtik, "The Gradual Civilization Act."
55. Hanson, "The Indian Act"; Canada Justice Laws, "Indian Act."
56. National Archives of Canada, Record Group 10, Volume 6810.
57. US Congress, Tribal Self-Governance Act of 1994; Moreton-Robinson, "Introduction: Locations of Engagement in the First World," 3–19.
58. Moreton-Robinson, "Introduction," 10.

59. Martin and Goodman, "Health Conditions Before Columbus," 65–68.
60. Shelton, "Legal and Historical Basis of Indian Health Care," 15.
61. Shelton, "Legal and Historical Basis of Indian Health Care," 15.
62. Evans-Campbell et al., "Indian Boarding School Experience," 421–27.
63. Evans-Campbell et al., "Indian Boarding School Experience."
64. Evans-Campbell et al., "Indian Boarding School Experience."
65. Austen and Bilefsky, "Hundreds More Unmarked Graves."
66. Benson, *Children of the Dragonfly*, 12; Johnston, "The Sixties Scoop," 23–64.
67. Benson, *Children of the Dragonfly*, 12.
68. Buckley, "The Impact of Anthropology on Native American Culture."
69. Champagne, "Is American Indian Studies for Real?" 77–90; Cook-Lynn, "Who Stole Native American Studies?" 9–28. Here is an example of this form of colonization. My intent for this chapter was to center the work of Two Spirit Native American scholars and thus included references to the work of Qwo-Li Driskill. During the final edits for this chapter, I learned that Driskill's Indigenous heritage has been called into question by the Tribal Alliance Against Frauds (TAAF) who refer to Driskill as a "pretendian." According to TAAF, Driskill claimed Cherokee, Lenape, and Osage heritage, but Driskill's genealogy revealed no ancestry from an American Indian tribal nation (Constantino, Tribal Alliance Against Frauds Case Report, Subject "Paul Edward" Qwo-Li Driskill). I elected to keep Driskill's references in this chapter as I feel their work supports Two Spirit people, and as yet, I have seen no formal response from Driskill to TAAF's claim. Not all Native American scholars will agree with this decision, and I am still trying to parse how I feel about this development.
70. Champagne, "Is American Indian Studies for Real?"
71. Cook-Lynn, "Who Stole Native American Studies?" 16.
72. Tallbear, "Dear Indigenous Studies," 71–82.
73. James, Jackson, and Jim, *2015 U.S. Transgender Survey*, 19–20.
74. Brave Heart, "The Historical Trauma Response."
75. Vernon and Jackson, "Closing the Gap."
76. James, Jackson, and Jim, *2015 U.S. Transgender Survey*.
77. This publication was one of several that highlighted the experiences of communities of color within the larger *United States Transgender Survey* of the broad US TGD community. While surveys like this can offer a representative snapshot, there may be shortcomings, that is, diminished participation of marginalized populations for a host of reasons, including lack of survey access, fear, distrust, and skepticism. The report also mentioned that the 319 American Indian and Alaskan Native respondents did not include people who identified as multiracial/ethnic thus excluding an important intersectional identity that speaks to the American Indian and Alaskan Native trans experience. Researchers who identify with the community spearheaded this survey, which allowed participants to engage more openly.

78. Tuck, "Suspending Damage," 409–28.
79. Vernon and Jackson, "Closing the Gap."
80. Driskill, "Doubleweaving Two-Spirit Critiques," 69.
81. Driskill, "Doubleweaving Two-Spirit Critiques," 69.
82. Byrd, *The Transit of Empire*, 80.
83. Driskill, "Doubleweaving Two-Spirit Critiques," 69.
84. Driskill, "Doubleweaving Two-Spirit Critiques."
85. Driskill, "Doubleweaving Two-Spirit Critiques," 86.
86. Driskill, "Doubleweaving Two-Spirit Critiques."
87. Chacaby and Plummer, *A Two-Spirit Journey*, 1–256.
88. Monkman, "Kent Monkman."
89. Bingman, "Kent Monkman."
90. Monkman, *The Daddies*.
91. Graves, "Coquille Same-Sex Marriage Law Takes Effect."
92. Yardley, "A Washington State Indian Tribe Approves Same-Sex Marriage."
93. Jackson, "Identity, Gender, and Sexuality."
94. Ridings and Edmo, "Supporting Two-Spirit/Native American LGBT People."
95. Turtle Island includes Canada, the United States, and Mexico.
96. Ridings and Edmo, "Supporting Two-Spirit/Native American LGBT People."
97. Native American Program of Legal Aid Services of Oregon, *Tribal Equity Tool Kit 2.0*.
98. Department of Health and Human Services, "Indian Health Service: A Quick Look."
99. Department of Health and Human Services, "Indian Health Service: A Quick Look, "1.
100. Department of Health and Human Services, "Indian Health Service: A Quick Look," 1.
101. Angelino, Evans-Campbell, and Duran, "Assessing Health Provider Perspectives."
102. Department of Health and Human Services, "Indian Health Service Meeting."
103. Indian Health Services, "Lesbian, Gay, Bisexual, Transgender, Questioning."
104. Cherokee Nation, "Health Services."
105. Binkley, "Hate Crimes, Media and Two Spirits"; Reynolds, "Jamie Lee Wounded Arrow."

WORKS CITED

Angelino, Allessandra, Teresa Evans-Campbell, and Connie Duran. "Assessing Health Provider Perspectives Regarding Barriers American Indian/Alaska Native Transgender and Two-Spirit Youth Face Accessing Healthcare." *Journal of Racial and Ethnic Disparities* 7 (2019): 630–42. Accessed May 10, 2021. https://link.springer.com/article/10.1007%2Fs40615-019-00693-7.

Austen, Ian, and Dan Bilefsky. "Hundreds More Unmarked Graves Found at Former Residential School in Canada." *New York Times*, June 24, 2021. Accessed August 4, 2024. https://www.nytimes.com/2021/06/24/world/canada/indigenous-children-graves-saskatchewan-canada.html.

Ball, Eve. *In the Days of Victorio: Recollections of a Warm Springs Apache.* Tucson: University of Arizona Press, 2015.

Benson, Robert. *Children of the Dragonfly: Native American Voices on Child Custody and Education.* Tuscon: University of Arizona Press, 2001.

Bingham, Russell. "Kent Monkman." *Canadian Encyclopedia*, February 15, 2013. Accessed May 6, 2021. https://www.thecanadianencyclopedia.ca/en/article/kent-monkman.

Binkley, Gail. "Hate Crimes, Media and Two Spirits." *Huffpost*, March 18, 2010. https://www.huffpost.com/entry/hate-crimes-media-and-emt_b_334566. Accessed August 11, 2024.

Brave Heart, Maria Yellow Horse. "The Historical Trauma Response among Natives and Its Relationship with Substance Abuse: A Lakota Illustration." *Journal of Psychoactive Drugs* 35, no. 1 (2003): 7–13.

Buckley, Christine. "The Impact of Anthropology on Native American Culture." *UConn Today*, August 19, 2011. Accessed August 4, 2024. https://today.uconn.edu/2011/08/the-impact-of-anthropology-on-native-american-culture/.

Byrd, Jodi. *The Transit of Empire: Indigenous Critiques of Colonialism.* Minneapolis: University of Minnesota Press, 2011.

Canada Justice Laws. "Indian Act (R.S.C, 1985, c 1-5)." August 15, 2015. Accessed August 31, 2021. https://laws-lois.justice.gc.ca/eng/acts/i-5/.

Chacaby, Ma-Ne, and Mary Louisa Plummer. *A Two-Spirit Journey: The Autobiography of a Lesbian Ojibwa-Cree Elder.* Winnepeg, CA: University of Manitoba Press, 2016.

Champagne, D. "Is American Indian Studies for Real?" *Wicazo Sa Review* 23, no. 2 (2008): 77–90.

Cherokee Nation. "Health Services." Accessed December 2020. https://health.cherokee.org/.

Constantino, Lianna. "Tribal Alliance Against Frauds, Case Report, Subject: 'Paul Edward' Qwo-Li Driskill." Accessed August 11, 2024. https://img1.wsimg.com/blobby/go/cb8c60c3-bb00-4f8f-a887-209c14754737/downloads/TAAF%20Report%20on%20Paul%20Qwo-Li%20Driskill.pdf?ver=1721857832075.

Cook-Lynn, E. "Who Stole Native American Studies?" *Wicazo Sa Review* 12, no. 1 (1997): 9–28.

Crenshaw, Kimberlé. "Mapping the Margins: Intersectionality, Identity Politics, and Violence against Women of Color." In *Violence Against Women: Classic Papers*, edited by R. K. Bergen, J. L. Eldeson, and C. M. Renzetti, 282–313. New Zealand: Pearson Education, 1994.

Department of Health and Human Services, Indian Health Services. "Indian Health Service: A Quick Look." January 2015. Accessed August 4, 2024. https://www.ihs.gov/sites/newsroom/themes/responsive2017/display_objects/documents/factsheets/QuickLook.pdf.

Department of Health and Human Services, Indian Health Services. "Indian Health Service Meeting on American Indian/Alaska Native Lesbian, Gay, Bisexual, and Transgender Health Issues." July 27, 2015. Accessed December 2020. https://www.ihs.gov/sites/newsroom/themes/responsive2017/display_objects/documents/IHS_LGBT_ListeningSessionJuly27_Report.pdf.

Driskill, Qwo-Li. "Doubleweaving Two-Spirit Critiques: Building Alliances between Native and Queer Studies." *GLQ: A Journal of Lesbian and Gay Studies* 16, no. 1–2 (2010): 69–92.

Elledge, Jim, ed. *Gay, Lesbian, Bisexual, & Transgender Myths from the Arapaho to the Zuni.* New York: Peter Lang, 2002.

Epple, Carolyn. "A Navajo World View and Nádleehí: Implications for Western Categories." In *Two-Spirit People*, edited by Sue-Ellen Jacobs, Wesley Thomas, and Sabine Lang, 174–91. Urbana: University of Illinois Press, 1997.

Evans-Campbell, Teresa, Karina Walters, Cynthia Pearson, and Christopher Campbell. "Indian Boarding School Experience, Substance Use, and Mental Health among Urban Two-Spirit American Indian/Alaska Natives." *Americal Journal of Drug and Alcohol Abuse* 38, no. 5 (2012): 421–27.

Graves, Bill. "Coquille Same-Sex Marriage Law Takes Effect." *The Oregonian*, May 21, 2019. Accessed May 6, 2021. https://www.oregonlive.com/news/2009/05/coquille_samesex_marriage_law.html.

Gutierrez, Jeanne. "Bar Chee Ampe and Beyond: Uncovering Two-Spirit Identity, Part 1." *New-York Historical Society*, November 13, 2019. Accessed May 6, 2021. https://womenatthecenter.nyhistory.org/two-spirit-identity-1/.

Hanson, Eric. "The Indian Act." Indigenous Foundations, 2009. Accessed August 31, 2021. https://indigenousfoundations.arts.ubc.ca/the_indian_act/.

Indian Health Service. "Lesbian, Gay, Bisexual, Transgender, Questioning, (LGBTQ) and Two-Spirit Health: Transgender." Accessed May 10, 2021. https://www.ihs.gov/lgbt/health/transgender/.

Indian National Advisory Council. *An Act for the Gradual enfranchisement of Indians, the better management of Indian affairs, and to Extend the Provisions of the Act 31st Victoria, Chapter 42, S. C., 1869, c.6.* Accessed August 11, 2024. https://www.sac-isc.gc.ca/eng/1100100010204/1618939577385.

Jackson, Trudie. "Identity, Gender, and Sexuality: Two Spirit People Presence at the Dakota Access Pipeline Camo." Unpublished manuscript, Fall 2018.

Jacobs, Sue-Ellen, Wesley Thomas, and Sabine Lang. "Introduction." In *Two-Spirit People*, edited by Sue-Ellen Jacobs, Wesley Thomas, and Sabine Lang, 1–8. Urbana: University of Illinois Press, 1997.

James, Sandy E., Trudie Jackson, and Mattee Jim. *2015 U.S. Transgender Survey: Report on the Experiences of American Indian and Alaskan Native Respondents*. National Center for Transgender Equality, November 2017. Accessed December 2020. https://transequality.org/sites/default/files/docs/usts/USTS-AIAN-Report-Dec17.pdf.

Johnston, Patrick. "The Sixties Scoop." In *Native Children and the Child Welfare System*, 23–64. Toronto, Ontario: Canadian Council on Social Development, 1983.

Kgontarc. "Navajo Cultural Constructions of Gender and Sexuality." *Trans Bodies Across the Globe*, December 17, 2010. Accessed December 2020. https://transgenderglobe.wordpress.com/2010/12/17/navajo-cultural-constructions-of-gender-and-sexuality/.

Klah, Hasteem, and Mary Wheelwright, recorder. "The Story of the Emergence (1942) (Navajo)." In *Gay, Lesbian, Bisexual, & Transgender Myths from the Arapaho to the Zuni*, edited by Jim Elledge, 15–69. New York: Peter Lang, 2002.

Martin, Debra, and Alan Goodman. "Health Conditions Before Columbus: Paleopathology of Native North Americans." *Western Journal of Medicine* 176, no. 1 (2002): 65–68.

Miranda, Deborah. "Extermination of the Joyas: Gendercide in Spanish California." *GLQ: A Journal of Lesbian and Gay Studies* 16, no. 1–2 (2010): 253–84.

Monkman, Kent. "Kent Monkman." Accessed May 6, 2021. https://kentmonkman.com/.

Monkman, Kent. *The Daddies*. 2016. Acrylic on canvas. Collection of Christine Armstrong and Irfhan Rawji, Toronto. https://www.kentmonkman.com/painting/2017/1/9/the-daddies.

Moreton-Robinson, Aileen. "Introduction: Locations of Engagement in the First World." In *Critical Indigenous Studies*, edited by Aileen Moreton-Robinson, 3–16. Tuscon: University of Arizona Press, 2016.

National Archives of Canada. Record Group 10, Volume 6810, File 4702-3, Volume 7, 55 (L-3) and 63 (N-3) .

Native American Program of Legal Aid Services of Oregon, the Indigenous Ways of Knowing Program at Lewis & Clark Graduate School of Education and Counseling, the Western States Center, the Pride Foundation and Basic Rights Oregon. *Tribal Equity Tool Kit 2.0: Tribal Resolutions and Codes to Support Two Spirit and LGBT Justice in Indian Country*. November 21, 2013. Accessed August 4, 2024. https://graduate.lclark.edu/live/files/15810-tribal-equity-toolkit-20.

Nitotemtik, Tansi. "The Gradual Civilization Act." University of Alberta Law (blog), October 4, 2018. Accessed August 31, 2021. https://ualbertalaw.typepad.com/faculty/2018/10/the-gradual-civilization-act.html.

Parliament of Canada. "AANR Committee Meeting." March 2002. Accessed December 2020. https://www.ourcommons.ca/DocumentViewer/en/37-1/AANR/meeting-43/evidence.

Perdue, Theda, ed. *Sifters: Native American Women's Lives.* Oxford: Oxford University Press, 2011.

Pratt, Richard H. "'Kill the Indian, and Save the Man.'" In *Official Report of the Nineteenth Annual Conference of Charities and Correction*, 46–59. Fairfax, VA: George Mason University, 1892.

Reynolds, Daniel. "Jamie Lee Wounded Arrow Is Second Trans Woman Killed in 2017." *Advocate*, January 8, 2017. Accessed August 11, 2024. https://www.advocate.com/crime/2017/1/08/jamie-lee-wounded-arrow-second-trans-woman-killed-2017.

Ridings, A,. and S. Edmo. "Supporting Two-Spirit/Native American LGBT People." Center for American Progress. October 17, 2016. Accessed August 4, 2024. https://www.americanprogress.org/issues/lgbtq-rights/news/2016/10/17/144818/supporting-two-spiritnative-american-lgbt-people-2/.

Rifkin, Mark. *When Did Indians Become Straight? Kinship, the history of Sexuality, and Native Sovereignty.* New York: Oxford University Press, 2011.

Robbins, Dorothy. "A Short History of Pan-Indianism." Native American Information Service. July 30, 1997. Accessed May 5, 2021. http://www.hartford-hwp.com/archives/41/119.html.

Roscoe, Will. *Changing Ones: Third and Fourth Genders in Native North America.* New York: St. Martin's Press, 1998.

———. "North American Tribes with Berdache and Alternate Gender Roles." In *Living the Spirit*, edited by Will Roscoe, 217–23. New York: St. Martin's Press, 1988.

———. "Strange Country This: Images of Berdaches and Warrior Women." In *Living the Spirit*, edited by Will Roscoe, 48–76. New York: St. Martin's Press, 1988.

———. *The Zuni Man Woman.* Albuquerque: University of New Mexico Press, 1991.

Shelton, Brett. "Legal and Historical Basis of Indian Health Care." In *Promises to Keep: Public Health Policy for American Indians and Alaska Natives in the 21st Century*, edited by Yvette Roubideaux and Mim Dixon, 1–28. Washington, DC: American Public Health Association, 2001.

Tallbear, Kim. "Dear Indigenous Studies, It's Not Me, It's You: Why I Left and What Needs to Change." In *Critical Indigenous Studies*, edited by Aileeen Moreton-Robinson, 71–82. Tucson: University of Arizona Press, 2016.

Thomas, Wesley. "Navajo Cultural Constructions of Gender and Sexuality." In *Two-Spirit People*, edited by Sue-Ellen Jacobs, Wesley Thomas, and Sabine Lang, 156–73. Urbana: University of Illinois Press, 1997.

Tuck, Eve. "Suspending Damage: A Letter to Communities." *Harvard Educational Review* 79, no. 3 (2009): 409–28.

US Congress, House of Representatives. Tribal Self-Governance Act of 1994. HR 3805. 103rd Cong. Introduced in House November 15, 1993. Accessed August 4, 2024. https://www.congress.gov/bill/103rd-congress/house-bill/3508.

Vernon, Irene, and Trudie Jackson. "Closing the Gap: A Research Agenda for the Study of Health Needs among American Indian/Native Hawaiian Transgender Individuals." *Ethnic Studies Review* 36, no. 1 (2013): 37–58.

White-Sun and George A. Dorsey, recorder. "The Hermaphrodite (1906) (Pawnee)." In *Gay, Lesbian, Bisexual, and Transgender Myths from the Arapaho to the Zuni*, edited by Jim Elledge, 101–02. Austria: Peter Lang, 2002.

Williams, W. *The Spirit and the Flesh; Sexual Diversity in Native American Culture.* Boston, MA: Beacon Press, 1986.

Wise, Eryn. "What Everyone Can Learn About Women's History from this Two-Spirit Love Story." *Bustle*, March 29, 2019. Accessed May 22, 2021. https://www.bustle.com/p/lozen-dahtestes-two-spirit-love-story-is-the-womens-history-month-narrative-that-needs-to-be-told-16996854.

Yardley, William. "A Washington State Indian Tribe Approves Same-Sex Marriage." *New York Times*, August 11, 2011.

5.1. PROFILE: ASHLIANA HAWELU (1969–)

Ashliana Hawelu

Aloha. My name is Ashliana Hawelu. I was born on the island of Oahu, but my lineage is from the Big Island—Hawaii. My great-great-grandfather was a *kia manu*, a bird catcher, who made feather capes and headdresses for the *Alii* (chiefs).

In Hawaii, *aloha* is used as a greeting, but to Indigenous Hawaiian people, the word holds deeper meanings: love, hello, and farewell. It also refers to living in harmony with respect and kindness. Before the colonization of Hawaii in the 1800s, Indigenous Hawaiian people referred to those who lived in the spiritual–mind–body space between male and female with the all-inclusive word *mahu*. In ancient times, everyone had a role, regardless of what they wore, how they identified, or with whom they slept. We were judged by our *kuleana*—our contribution to the community—not our assigned sex at birth or gender identity. Many mahu were caregivers, *kahuna* (shamans), canoe builders, healers, hula instructors, or lei makers.

Like aloha, mahu has had multiple meanings over time. It describes the steam coming from a pot boiling on the stove or the smoke off the top of a volcano. When you stand on the beach and see the ocean sparkling under the midday sun and the beautiful blue sky, the in-between shadow or line that separates the sky and the ocean is also known as mahu. Historically, mahu referred to individuals, usually assigned male at birth, who occupied a third gender and held traditional social and spiritual roles.

The Hawaiian language is unique, created to send out only positive vibrations. We are unable to swear or call anyone names, only to identify and address negative actions and behaviors. The Hawaiian proverb, *I ka olelo ke ola, i ka olelo ka make* translates as, "In language there is life, in language there is death." Hawaiians believe we can wish blessings on someone or curse them to death through our words. Colonizers manipulated our language, using mahu to mean homosexual, someone who commits sodomy or behaves like a homosexual or hermaphrodite. They said it was a sin to be mahu. This teaching brought shame and hatred on members of our community and their families, a legacy that still threatens mahu today.

In 2001, members of our mahu community met to reclaim our place in society. We coined the word *mahuwahine* for transfeminine persons and *mahukane* for transmasculine persons to reclaim our cultural terms, restore their positive meaning, and embrace ourselves with respect and aloha. We began to rebuild our community through hula, storytelling, cultural disciplines, and healing. Through this restoration, many members of our community (statewide, outer islands) no longer felt ashamed of being mahu and worked toward building healthier and more productive lifestyles. Mahu is now used as an umbrella term for those with a variety of sexual and gender identities.

I am the oldest of five brothers and a sister who died at age three. My parents separated when I was seven years old, and I helped my mother raise my brothers. I grew up fast and always knew I was different because I mainly did female work (that is, house cleaning, babysitting), hung with girls, and cared for elders. My family and classmates teased me, calling me a "fag" and a "homo." My uncle forced me to learn to defend myself, so I studied karate and street fighting. After mastering the roundhouse kick, nobody ever teased me again.

When I came out, the only place that accepted mahu was the red light district of Chinatown. In 1983, at the age of fifteen, I started feminizing with hormones, and at sixteen I started sex work. I received my hormone shots from a doctor who did not bill for office visits, just charged fifteen dollars for a full shot and eight dollars for a half shot. At nights, I engaged in sex work to pay for my hormone treatment, feminization surgeries, and day-to-day survival expenses.

Sex work gave me a sense of community—something like church, if you will. It created a place where I was accepted for being me: mahu. We mahuwahine congregated and shared tricks of the trade; we discussed gender transitions, the best gender surgeons, sting operations, who got arrested, who was a cop, and tips on tricks and dates. Yes, it was dangerous, but the men or tricks who I dated made me feel womanly, paid for my time, and validated my transition. I felt like I had my own business until I got raped, hit over the head with a crowbar, forced to jump out of moving vehicles, and held at knifepoint and gunpoint. After all that torture, I also got arrested. Ugh, my life in high heels. Finally, I played it smart and found three sugar daddies who helped pay my rent, bills, and car note and gave me an allowance. I didn't need to work the streets anymore. If I did go out, it was to hang out with the girls—I missed my friends. Like the saying goes, "You can get the girl off the streets, but you can't get the streets out of the girl."

I was not the only person struggling with gender identity; there were many other women like me, and we gave each other guidance and support. In 1993, my friend and I, knowing we were at risk, sought HIV testing. I tested negative and was quickly dismissed, but my friend tested positive. We both wept, and I promised to help her find support and treatment. This event helped me define my life's purpose: to develop the first trans-led agency in Hawaii committed to advocacy and to establish an HIV prevention program for Hawaii's mahuwahine.

Opportunity for this work soon arrived at my door. In 1994, I was asked to speak at a conference in Honolulu on transgender people and sex work in Hawaii. There I met Carol Odo, a writer who described the hardships and injustice that we face and struggle with daily. We worked together to create proposals and grants for programs to assist disadvantaged transgender women.

From 1997 to 1998, I served as an outreach worker for Ke Ola Mamo, one of the five Native Hawaiian Health Care Systems created under the Native Hawaiian Health Care Act of 1988. Ke Ola Mamo's mission is to empower, educate, and promote the health and well-being of our Native Hawaiian community in O'ahu. Here, I conducted outreach, led social gatherings, and developed programs that empowered sex workers to participate in community-wide HIV prevention efforts. We distributed condoms, offered HIV prevention services, and re-instilled cultural values and disciplines through the community practice of *hula*. I also served as the transgender representative on the board of the Hawaiian Department of Health's HIV prevention, community, and planning group and collaborated with the National Native American AIDS Prevention Center. In 2000, we produced our first transgender pageant, *Diva of Polynesia*, intended to connect mahu with the broader community and help mend broken families who reject their transgender children.

In 2000, my peers and I identified the need to start a trans-led nonprofit to serve Hawaiian transgender women; we named the fledging organization Kulia Na Mamo (To Strive). Initially, we were denied a 501(c)(3) license. I flew to Washington, DC, carrying letters from Hawaiian senators Daniel Akaka and Daniel Inouye and the former governor of Hawaii, Neil Abercrombie, who praised our efforts to serve Hawaii's disenfranchised transgender people. With this support, Kulia Na Mamo was born in 2001. Our members prioritized the need to tell our own stories and build community. During our first year, a book published by Andrew Matzner titled *O Au No Keia (This Is Me)* captured the voices of Hawaii's mahuwahine, younger members of the mahu community, and transgender advocates, inspiring us to strive (*kulia*) for our highest potential. We helped create a documentary film titled, *Ke Kulana He Mahu: Remembering a Sense of Place*. By sharing our stories, we reconnected our broken paths to that of our elders and their vibrant historical culture. Kulia Na Mamo later formed an organizational network by gathering mahuwahine from all islands to unite and relearn cultural disciplines, pride, and practices rooted in the hula and chant.

Kulia Na Mamo also continued to provide needed services directly to the community, and I completed a course in nonprofit organizational management, which helped me further mobilize our community. We partnered with the Substance Abuse and Mental Health Services Administration, the Centers for Disease Control, and the National Native American AIDS Prevention Center to create a model for HIV prevention for transgender Hawaiians. In 2005, we obtained funding from the Kosasa Foundation to open a transition house for transgender individuals released from prison and whose families had rejected them. In 2007, we implemented a preemployment training program to assist transgender people—both masculine and feminine—in pursuit of job training and employment, higher education, and skills to enable them to leave sex work and enter mainstream society. I proudly watched as our trainees obtained GEDs, associate degrees, and master's degrees or found part- and full-time employment in social services, fast-food restaurants, banks, or as parking attendants and telemarketers. Others pursued degrees in cosmetology or taught English/Hawaiian language.

Our organization went on to achieve national and international recognition. In 2008, I presented the model for Kulia Na Mamo at the US Conference on AIDS in San Francisco, California. The following year, I served as a board member for the Center of Excellence for Transgender Health, working toward redefining the term *gender dysphoria* in the Diagnostic and *Statistical Manual of Mental Health Disorders, 5th edition*, so transgender medical and surgical care would be eligible for insurance coverage. In 2010, I represented Kulia Na Mamo and attended the first World Transgender Conference held in Barcelona, Spain, and networked with transgender people from all over the world.

By 2011, though, Kulia Na Mamo fell victim to budget cuts—transgender people were no longer a priority—and we folded. I visited my spirit guide for answers and learned that I would be moving into a different area of work. I completed hula school and became a hula teacher and graduated from Pahu Drumming School to become a professional Hawaiian drummer. After two years, I found my new professional calling in the field of mental health, where I work today, educating service providers and stakeholders on trans sensitivity and ensuring that transgender people with severe mental health issues receive equitable healthcare and services.

Figure 5.1.1. Ashliana Hawelu. *Source*: Courtesy of Ashliana Hawelu.

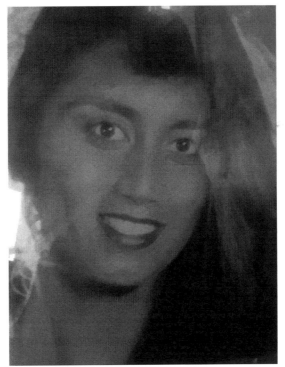

WORKS CITED

Abne, Brent, and Kathryn Xian, dir. *Ke Kaluna He Mahu: Remembering a Sense of Place.* Honolulu, Hawaii: Zang Pictures, 2001.

Matzner, Andrew. *O Au No Keia: Voices from Hawai'i's Mahu and Transgender Communities.* Bloomington, IN: Xlibris, 2001.

Section II

FROM THE MARGINS

Section II of this book explores the emergence of affirming medical practices in the United States. In chapter 6, anthropologist Tj Gundling recounts Christine Jorgensen's arrival home to the United States in 1953 after undergoing a medical and surgical transition in Denmark, the ensuing media blitz, and origins of transgender healthcare in the United States through the work of Dr. Harry Benjamin. This is followed by a short piece by Carolyn Wolf-Gould who describes first how Christine's publicity as a white, straight, educated, and middle-class trans woman established cultural expectations that led to barriers to care for trans women of color and then a description of the work of Monica Roberts, a Black American trans historian who searched for early stories of transgender and gender-diverse (TGD) people of color and uncovered only snippets about the lives of Carlett Brown, Avon Wilson, and Delisa Newton. In chapter 7, Annette Timm and Jamison Green focus on the work of two trans individuals, Carla Erskine (pseudonym) and Jude Patton, whose personal connections with early sexologists and members of the TGD community countered the existing narratives of shame and depravity that drove TGD people to the margins of society.

As medical care for TGD people evolved, so too did the field of psychiatry. In chapter 8, historians Dallas Denny, Jamison Green, and psychiatrist Hansel Arroyo chronicle the etiologic and treatment paradigms promoted by psychiatrists in the early to mid-1900s, scholarship that continues to pathologize and stigmatize TGD individuals today. This chapter is followed by two short commentaries on the cultural response to the rise of transgender healthcare during this era; the first profiles Dr. David O. Cauldwell, who left patient care in 1946 to become the editor of the question-and-answer section of *Sexology* magazine, publishing extensively on transsexuality, transvestism, and hermaphroditism over the following decade, creating a more liberal climate for discussion; the second explores how faith communities across the United States reacted to the visibility of transgender health care in the middle of the twentieth century and grappled with how the new medical practices could be reconciled with existing religious texts and tenets. In chapter 9, physician and educator Kyan Lynch reveals the hidden costs of medicalization with stories of those denied care from Carolyn Wolf-Gould and Dallas Denny and a description of a cultural practice that promotes access to care—the house ballroom culture, by LGBT scholar and activist Jennifer Lee.

Profiles highlighted in section II include Louise Lawrence and Virginia Prince, both of whom developed networks of TGD correspondents who began to form supportive communities by mail and, later, to educate medical professionals and researchers and connect these professionals to empowered TGD community members; Sharon Stuart, who described encounters with Prince and Benjamin; Roberta Cowell and Robert Allen, who attributed their gender-diversity to errors in nature; Joseph Lobdell, whose story served as the first published case study in an American academic journal of a person who today would be understood as transgender; and Lou Sullivan, who encouraged sexologists to recognize the experiences of gay and bisexual transgender men.

6

THE BEGINNINGS OF TRANS-AFFIRMING CARE IN THE UNITED STATES

Tj Gundling

Following the jubilation that accompanied the Allied victory in World War II, the United States entered a period of national anxiety, a psychosocial, cultural shift instigated by the emerging Cold War and renewed armed conflict on the Korean peninsula. This pervasive unease manifested in countless ways, perhaps most notoriously in 1945 with the reemergence of the House Committee on Un-American Activities,[1] designed to confront threats to democratic society posed by Communist political philosophy. Communism became the bugaboo of a generation, weaponized to rally nationalist spirit, champion science positivism and, perhaps most germane to this chapter, maintain tight messaging on what constituted a good family. The latter was steeped in rigid heteronormativity that demanded adherence to binary gender norms and demonized homosexuality.[2] Despite this socially conservative climate, the medical profession began to grapple with a newly proposed diagnostic category—transsexualism—distinct from existing diagnoses related to biological sex, gender, and sexuality.[3]

With the positivist outlook in the wake of World War II, societal consciousness linked science with progress, which would inexorably enhance everyday life in countless ways. New medical advancements contributed to this progress, yet providers struggled to reach consensus on how to treat people who insisted that, despite a preponderance of anatomical and physiological evidence to the contrary, they were truly members of the opposite sex. Even in the absence of consensus, numerous discoveries and technologies paved the way for the development of an inchoate field of transgender medical care, including the application of new and existing medical interventions for people experiencing what is now called gender dysphoria. For example, researchers developed methods to synthesize and safely administer human sex hormones in large quantities.[4] Further, doctors modified existing plastic surgery procedures, adapting them for genital sex conversions and for breast implants for those assigned male at birth.[5] They rarely attempted genital surgery for those assigned female at birth, due to the complexity of available procedures and resulting history of unsatisfactory outcomes. Nonetheless, these medical interventions allowed people to externalize, to a degree, their internal sense of authentic self.

In the mid-twentieth century, two individuals rested at the center of this discourse and medical advancement. Christine Jorgensen, the first well-known American woman to undergo sex reassignment surgery, and German-born, but New York City–based, physician Harry Benjamin, who was carefully following the Jorgensen story as it rapidly emerged in the popular press. Benjamin's relationship with Jorgensen inflected his professional activities exclusively toward advocacy for the acceptance and integration of trans people into larger society.[6] Together they ushered in the concept of what became known as a sex change to mainstream society in the United States.

Previously published transgender[7] histories have described the profound impact Jorgensen and Benjamin had on the medical profession and on attitudes and beliefs about sex, gender, and sexuality in postwar America.[8] For example, historian Joanne Meyerowitz provided an analysis of medical practitioners' confused discourse, which conflated biological sex, sexuality, and psychological sex[9] into weak hypotheses of causation that allowed ample space for widely divergent treatment plans. These pseudoscientific debates ran the gamut, generalizing from the experience of one individual to eliding individual phenomenological detail completely, but ultimately depicting the trans experience as monolithic.[10] Jorgensen's story contributed to new attitudes about and treatment for transsexualism, and Meyerowitz examined the media's role in creating an accessible narrative for mainstream consumption about gender dysphoria that still resonates today.[11]

Other focused commentary on Jorgensen specifically analyzed how she garnered public attention and, in some instances, approval. Historian Emily Skidmore described Jorgensen as a "good" transsexual who displayed a host of respectable, nonthreatening, intersectional identities and personal qualities.[12] She was white, middle class, a military veteran, heterosexual in her new role as a woman, and gender normative in presentation with an inclination toward domesticity. Jorgensen, poised and articulate in dealing with an insatiable, often contentious, and occasionally hostile media, quickly adapted to her celebrity status, deftly negotiating the vagaries of societal mood swings. Trans activist, organizer, and author Dallas Denny rightfully describes Jorgensen as "a woman of fierce resolve, and wondrous determination."[13] Communications professor David Serlin placed Jorgensen in the cultural context of postwar America by focusing on her personal narrative. In particular, Serlin examined the role of the media in situating Jorgensen within the broader trope of the soldier's story in which members of the military returned home from the battlefield, beleaguered heroes who had earned the respect and sympathy of a grateful nation. In Jorgensen's case, the Ex-GI turned Blonde Beauty returned to her homeland after two years of similarly challenging, although completely different circumstances.[14]

In this chapter, given that much has already been written about these transformative figures, only abbreviated biographical sketches of Jorgensen and Benjamin are included, predating their first meeting in 1953. The central focus highlights the dovetailing of their personal histories within a developing, yet recognizably modern, view of trans healthcare.[15] Specifically, I examine the advent of transsexualism as a diagnostic category, which emerged in response to confusing medical and public discourse surrounding Jorgensen's transition.

To wit, clinicians contextualized gender transition narratives within a vaguely defined *intersex* etiology[16]—a perplexing model as the term manifested two different meanings. Intersex could be broadly defined, describing variation along a male/female continuum existing throughout the body,[17] or its meaning could be restricted to variation in reproductive anatomy. Both of these intersex models emphasized a constitutional basis for gender diversity that involved some combination of genetic, glandular (hormonal), and anatomical components, in addition to environmental triggers. Despite their differences, however, each approach supported a similar underlying treatment model for transsexualism: the goal was to change the body to reflect the person's true, or at least dominant, biological sex.

To complicate things further, during this time sex change narratives began to shift away from anatomical and/or physiological causation toward one of misalignment of biological sex and psychological sex. This latter model, often distilled to the common trope of "born in the wrong body," decoupled what we would now refer to as gender identity from a normative soma, undermining the notion that a systemic or localized intersex condition affected both the body and the mind. This third conceptualization was favored by the psychological community who argued that transsexualism was a psychopathological condition—rather than a constitutional one—and often the result of family dysfunction during early social development. As a result, the appropriate treatment was to cure the subject through psychoanalysis or aversion therapy, in sharp contrast to that proposed by adherents of one or the other of the intersex models.[18] Many mental health practitioners considered sex change operations inimical to the Hippocratic Oath, as such procedures destroyed normative, functioning anatomy and offered only a simplistic solution for what they considered a complex psychological problem.[19] Against the backdrop of these competing models, Jorgensen entered a world that was not equipped on a social or medical level to comprehend, let alone accommodate, her appeal for understanding and assistance.

CHRISTINE JORGENSEN: EX-GI BECOMES BLONDE BEAUTY

Florence Jorgensen (*née* Hansen) gave birth to a baby on Memorial Day, May 30, 1926, in Bronx, New York. The infant displayed external genitalia prompting the attending medical personnel to confidently assign the child as male. The baby was given the name George, after her[20] father. For twenty-six years, George Jr. lived in a middle-class Lutheran household among a family deeply connected to their native Denmark through a tightly knit community of local Danish expatriates.[21] By all accounts, Jorgensen spent a largely unremarkable childhood growing up with her older sister Dolly, although instances of inscrutable feminine desires and behavior emerged from about age five. Attractions to dolls, dresses, and jump rope strongly contrasted with her rejection of short hair and distaste for rough-and-tumble play.[22]

In 1945, a family friend hired young Jorgensen to prepare newsreels for RKO-Pathe News in New York City, a job that aligned with Jorgensen's interest in photography, in part inspired by George Sr. But only a few months later,

Jorgensen was unexpectedly drafted into the military despite two previous wartime rejections for being under weight. For the next fourteen months, Jorgensen attended basic training at Camp Polk in Louisiana and assisted with the administrative reentry of returning soldiers into civilian society at the Fort Dix Separation Center in New Jersey. After being honorably discharged in December 1946, Jorgensen returned to RKO-Pathe News as a chauffeur and inquired about a possible future making movies in Hollywood. She contacted a friend living in Hollywood and boarded a Greyhound bus to California, with dreams of breaking into the film industry. However, her lack of success in landing even an entry-level position and emotionally hobbled by distracting thoughts about her sexuality and her gender quickly became discouraging. She exhausted her limited budget, and the sojourn ended with a miserable trip back home to New York.

After a brief period of recovery and reassessment, Jorgensen completed a photography degree in Connecticut under the G.I. Bill, yet the same internal distress that plagued her in Hollywood intensified, making it difficult for her to function. She developed a romantic attraction to a male friend, an event that triggered an internalized homophobia and fear of social opprobrium from the "lavender scare."[23] As she tried to reconcile this attraction, Jorgensen began to develop the sense that homosexuality was not her core issue.

She reconceptualized her sexual fantasies as the attraction a heterosexual woman felt for a man, and a nascent impression that her developmental path had gone askew began to take shape. She searched for any material that might help explain her experience and was influenced by a book called *The Male Hormone*, a highly deterministic volume that reduced men and masculinity to the action of testosterone on their brains and bodies.[24] The book recommended testosterone as a salutary elixir to "rescue broken men" from the ravages of aging. Although Jorgensen rejected this possibility in resolving her own dilemma, she seized on the connection between biological sex, sexual virility, and hormones. She read the book through the lens of someone not only struggling with a distressing sexuality but also navigating a troubling disconnect between who she was supposed to be, according to her family and society at large, and her emerging sense of self. These persistent experiences strengthened her conviction that she suffered from a glandular problem expressed in both mind and body, a belief that developed into her personal narrative of possessing a weak masculinity consistent with a vague intersex etiology. Throughout her life, Jorgensen stayed on message, citing her slight physique, scant body hair, underdeveloped sex organs, and the presence of feminine emotions and interests as evidence of this condition.

In 1949, while pursuing a second degree as a medical technician in Manhattan, Jorgensen revealed her internal struggle to a fellow student named Gen Angelo. Gen was the wife of a medical doctor, "Dr. Joe" Angelo, and thought that perhaps her husband could help. The doctor provided Jorgensen with medical reports that described sex transformation experiments being conducted in Europe. Although opinions vary on how Jorgensen obtained the estradiol tablets she self-administered, it's possible this doctor provided them.[25] Upon completing her studies that December, in an extraordinarily courageous display of self-actualization, Jorgensen decided to pursue conversion treatment[26] in Scandinavia with the hope of alleviating her internal anguish and fulfilling her desire to live as a heterosexual woman, both in body and in mind.[27]

On May 1, 1950, only weeks before her twenty-fourth birthday, Jorgensen set sail from New York, telling her parents and friends that she intended to visit extended family in Denmark and create a cinematic travelogue for American audiences. Her primary motivation for traveling overseas—to seek medical help—was a closely held secret shared only with Gen and Dr. Joe. She arrived in Copenhagen on May 11, and after traveling with friends throughout northwest Europe for several weeks, she had her first meeting with Danish endocrinologist Christian Hamburger. As a result of discussing her case with Hamburger, Jorgensen homed in on an intersex model. She recounted Hamburger saying, "Outwardly you have many of the sex characteristics of a man . . . inwardly, it is quite possible that you are a woman. Your body chemistry and *all of your body cells*, including your brain cells, may be female."[28] [Emphasis added.]

Hamburger explained that if he accepted her as a patient, he would not charge for his services, but he would impose a rigorous treatment plan, including the administration of hormones, monitoring of hormone levels, and ongoing psychiatric assessment. He evaluated Jorgensen, accepted her as a candidate for what was an experimental protocol, established baseline physiology, and then prescribed a short course of high-dose injectable estrogen, followed by a lower oral maintenance dose. This regimen, which Hamburger referred to as chemical castration, lowered Jorgensen's endogenous testosterone levels. Evaluation of Jorgensen's psychological state following the hormone treatment's success was required before considering irreversible surgical interventions. In September 1951, a mental health colleague of Hamburger's deemed Jorgensen fit to continue treatment, and she underwent the first of two surgical procedures: removal of the testes. Later, reflecting on this procedure, Jorgensen recalled, "I was not yet wholly a woman, but I had taken another major step along the way."[29] This quote reifies the linear transition narrative so common throughout subsequent decades.

In 1952, while waiting to undergo her second surgical procedure, Jorgensen busied herself with several important orders of business. She filmed her travelogue, which she hoped would afford her a "small source of income."[30] Anticipating her return to the United States in time for Christmas, Jorgensen petitioned for and successfully acquired a new passport with her chosen name.[31] In June 1952, she wrote to her parents to reveal the true nature of her trip abroad and justify her actions with her now fully articulated intersex model. In her letter she explained, "Among the greatest working part of our bodies are the glands. Several small, seemingly unimportant glands, and yet our whole body is governed by them. An imbalance in the glandular system puts the body under a strain, in an effort to adjust that imbalance. . . . Along with many other people, I had such an imbalance."[32] Responding to an encouraging reply from her parents in July she wrote, "I had a bit of a chemical war going on within me, one trying to outdo the other."[33] In the fall of 1952, Jorgensen underwent the "final plastic surgery [that] was necessary to give my body

Figure 6.1. Christine Jorgensen, 1954. *Source*: Photo by Maurice Seymour. Public domain.

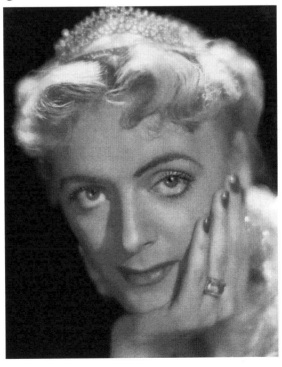

the complete outward appearance of a woman. . . . I also knew that . . . I never would be able to bear children."[34] Jorgensen later described this second surgery in her autobiography as the "removal of the immature sex organs."[35] According to her Danish medical team, they performed a penectomy and labiaplasty using scrotal tissue. By mutual agreement with Jorgensen, they stopped short of vaginoplasty.[36]

While she recovered, an American reporter was tipped off and came to visit her for an exclusive interview with the *New York Daily News*.[37] On December 1, 1952, this paper published the now infamous front-page headline and article, complete with before and after photographs, that introduced Jorgensen to an astounded American public. The story featured a transcript of the letter she previously sent to her parents explaining her internal conflict and its resolution.[38] The *Daily News* continued their coverage the following day, with quotes from her parents including her father's statement, "[Christine] deserves an award higher than the Congressional Medal of Honor. She volunteered to undergo this guinea pig treatment for herself and to help others."[39]

FROM STARLET TO ALTERED MALE

When the Jorgensen story broke in the United States, the medical community turned to existing diagnostic categories that described sexual pathologies. The term *transvestite* described anatomically normative individuals who expressed a compulsive desire to dress as the opposite sex. The term *homosexual* referred to those people attracted to members of the same biological sex. Both terms referred to individuals who were closeted within mainstream society and considered to possess deviant forms of sexuality. The term *hermaphrodite* referred to a third group of people—those born with ambiguous genitalia (pseudohermaphrodites) or, comparatively rare, "true" hermaphrodites displaying elements of both biological sexes, typically ovotestes. In these cases, doctors routinely recommended immediate corrective surgeries to normalize the anatomical appearance of these individuals, who we now identify as intersex.[40]

Jorgensen, her doctors, and the general public considered her an anomaly. Her presentation could not be accommodated by existing nosology, and this confusion was reflected within media reporting. According to philosopher C. Jacob Hale, "The first articles in December 1952 suggested that Jorgensen had been a physically normal male who became, through a miracle of medical science a white American ideal; a beautiful, glamorous, graceful, blonde woman with a tightly knit middle-class family, and a face and figure fit for the silver screen!"[41] The lay audience came away with the notion that Jorgensen had been literally transformed from a typical male into a typical female. After members of the media consulted US medical professionals, albeit with no direct information on the Jorgensen case, they reported that some experts believed she was a pseudohermaphrodite. Others suggested that a true change of sex was impossible.[42] These reports conflicted with Jorgensen's self-conception. She and her Danish doctors asserted that her case differed from transvestism, hermaphroditism, or homosexuality, as defined by the mostly heterosexual, white, male sexologists.[43] They attributed her distress to in utero glandular tissue that manufactured abnormal levels of feminizing hormones, and Jorgensen repeatedly described her dilemma as occupying a no-man's land of sex, rejecting any existing labels put on her by the media.

From December 1952 through March 1953, the press and public treated Jorgensen as a celebrity. While there were certainly skeptics, when she returned to the United States on February 13, 1953, most reporters cast her story in a positive light. The public accepted her transformation at face value, despite the fact that reporting revealed scant detail about her treatment with hormones and surgery. As an exemplar of American individualism, Jorgensen voiced respect for the wonders of modern science on one hand and her belief in the beneficence of God on the other.

As her story swiftly became common knowledge, Jorgensen contracted with the Hearst Corporation before leaving Denmark for an exclusive interview series with *American Weekly*, a supplement to the Sunday newspapers published by Hearst. The series, simply titled "The Story of My Life," ran for five consecutive Sundays beginning on February 15, 1953, to coincide with her return to the United States. The first part of this series reinforced the overly simplistic idea of a complete and literal transformation. "Now, after two and a half years of medical and surgical treatment, I had been changed from an apparent man to a woman."[44] Jorgensen characterized her condition as similar to a congenital defect by excerpting a letter she sent to her parents: "I am the same Brud, but, my dears, *nature made a mistake* which I have had corrected and now I am your daughter."[45] [Emphasis added.] In vague, superficial terms, she elaborated on her experience growing up, noting, "My doctors later told me that my physical system and body cells were attuned to feminine reactions in matters of affection as well as in my ability to adapt to many social situations."[46]

In the second part of this series, Jorgensen added, "I was distressed that my physical system and my emotions were . . . becoming attuned to feminine reactions. . . . I did not then understand the true nature of my glandular disturbance."[47] She noticed that despite eating large amounts of food "my chemical imbalance had already begun to prevent my normal physical growth."[48] In part three, she explained that she was "burdened by an ever-growing physical and emotional problem that seemed to so often far outweigh my slight, undeveloped body."[49] In the penultimate installment of "The Story of My Life," she included Hamburger's conclusion after their first visit in 1950: "What you tell me of your emotions and physical make-up leads me to believe that you may be a victim of a condition called transvestitism."[50]

As recounted by Jorgensen, Hamburger told her: "A one-hundred percent man, or a one-hundred percent woman does not exist. We all have rudiments of the hermaphrodite (dual sex) state within us."[51] He described intersex individuals as "those extremely unhappy persons in who male and female sex characteristics are *mixed* to a greater or lesser extent. The closer a person is placed towards the middle . . . the more likely it is that he, or she, will be a victim of sexual difficulties, such as . . . transvestitism."[52] [Emphasis added.] He viewed intersex conditions as a diffuse, broadly systemic phenomenon, in contrast to hermaphroditism, which then, as now, was typically restricted to reproductive anatomy.

Hamburger advanced his working hypothesis, citing the research of geneticist Richard Goldschmidt that all intersexes are chromosomally female and were born female although with normal male organs and glands due to extreme intrauterine disruption. Hamburger acknowledged that his hypothesis could not be tested, as "we cannot count the chromosomes in the cells with absolute certainty," but he believed it explained Jorgensen's case and others like it. Jorgensen internalized this message, reiterating throughout her life that all people were, to varying degrees, both female and male.[53]

In a recorded interview titled "Christine Jorgensen Reveals," Jorgensen captured her understanding of the distinction between the terms *hermaphrodite* and *intersex* by paraphrasing her doctor (presumably Hamburger): "[T]he hermaphrodite tends more to the actual genital organs of both sexes. If one person has the genital organs of both sexes then that was called a pseudo-hermaphrodite, whereas intersexuality, which was another term he used, means that there is a preponderance of one sex but there's also the other sex. So, every person is basically an intersexual but a hermaphrodite deals mainly with the genitalia and not the genetics nor the hormonal nor the psyche."[54]

The lack of specific details about Jorgensen's transition in "The Story of My Life" series and her vague discourse about everyone being part female and part male muddied the waters for the lay public, which started to realize

Jorgensen's transformation was not as simple as it had first appeared. Her honeymoon with the press ended abruptly in April with the publication of a multipart hit piece published in the socially conservative *New York Post*. Reporter Alvin Davis traveled to Denmark to meet with Jorgensen's medical team, concluding that "physically, if not mentally, Jorgensen was a normal male before 'treatment' . . . [Jorgensen] had no underdeveloped female sex organs that could be corrected by surgery . . . the surgery performed on him[*sic*] consisted of little more than castration."[55] As a result, members of the press and the medical community began to characterize Jorgensen as an altered male, undermining her oft-repeated narrative of being a person whose body defied simple categorization as male or female. Local newspapers and national periodicals spread the story throughout every part of the country. In April, *Time* magazine cited the *New York Post* article and provided a photograph of Jorgensen under which the caption reads "No she, he."[56] *Newsweek* followed suit in May, bluntly stating that "latest medical testimony seems to indicate that the now celebrated Christine Jorgensen is not hermaphrodite, not a pseudohermaphrodite, and not a female. The former George Jorgensen is a castrated male."[57]

PERSPECTIVES FROM ACROSS THE POND

Jorgensen was neither the only individual experiencing a deep sense of gender incongruity in the mid-twentieth century nor was she the only one who had the ability to access hormonal and surgical treatment. When her story broke, there were others in the United States who were keenly interested in the possibility of undergoing what became known as a sex change, or conversion, and who quickly followed in Jorgensen's footsteps.[58] Beyond the United States, contemporary reaction from England notably involved two people who had a similar experience yet were dismissive of Jorgensen, although for quite different reasons. These individuals were also at pains to demonstrate that they were authentic, in the sense that nature had made an error; they gathered anatomical or physiological evidence to prove that the condition did not exist solely in their minds.[59]

PROFILE: ROBERTA COWELL (1919–2011)

Roberta Cowell was born and raised in England and, upon reaching adulthood, became an avid car enthusiast, later joining the Royal Air Force as a fighter pilot for the allied forces during World War II. In her 1954 autobiography describing her own transition, and despite clear parallels with that of Jorgensen, she nonetheless concluded that their conditions were fundamentally different: "[B]ecause so many of the news stories were misleading, Christine's Danish physicians disclosed many of the details of her case. She had never been a pseudo-hermaphrodite, or a person possessing two sets of sexual characteristics, one *dormant* and one active. She was scientifically classified as a transvestite, a person with an irresistible urge to wear the clothing of the other sex." [Emphasis added.][60] In arriving at this diagnosis, Cowell focused exclusively on the genitalia and not any measurable systemic intersex condition. Cowell further explained, "Transvestitism indicates a high degree of *psychological* intersexualization; physical attributes are normal . . . it is far more difficult to deal with than malfunction of the mechanism of sex determination."[61] Cowell then disparaged transvestites in the harshest pathological terms. In contrast to her condemnation of Jorgensen, Cowell provided a truly tortuous explanation for how she was a female all along, despite being the biological parent of two daughters. According to Cowell, her true self slowly emerged over the course of many years while Jorgensen's conversion "had apparently been induced entirely through artificial means, no spontaneous changes having taken place at all (as they did in my case)."[62] Her argument would appear specious, given that she underwent hormonal therapy with estrogen and surgical removal of the testes in 1950, followed by a vaginoplasty a year later.

To further legitimize her own transition, Cowell invoked the narrow intersex definition, likening her experience to that of Danish painter Lili Elbe two decades earlier: "Examination revealed that his [sic] body had undoubted female conformation. He underwent a series of operations. The presence of rudimentary ovaries was established[63] . . . I did not hear of Lili's case until my own treatment was well under way. When I read the book about her life I noticed many similarities between her history and mine."[64]

PROFILE: ROBERT ALLEN (1914–1997)

Assigned female at birth, the childhood and early adulthood of "Joyce" Allen was filled with torment as a result of expressing a seemingly deep-seated masculine sensibility. With the support of loving parents and a handful of friends who would prove invaluable, Robert Allen emerged in his thirties after relocating to London from his provincial place of origin. Although details are not publicly available, it seems probable that this was the result of an intersex[65] condition that prevented the development of typical male reproductive anatomy in utero; however, later testimony of virility by medical doctors suggests that such anatomy eventually emerged.

Allen's story is an interesting one considering the dearth of firsthand accounts of atypical sex development from this time; he was ultimately inspired to write his memoir, which was published in 1954. The dust cover flap reads, "For years, the author refused all publicity about his unique experience, and it is partly to counter the sensational treatment of some recent cases that he has at last decided to write his autobiography." Given the timing, there can be little doubt that this passage refers to the publicity surrounding Jorgensen, although she is not mentioned by name.

Allen wrote that "whereas in the ordinary run of humanity men and women are a unity in body and soul, I was apparently split—or so it seemed at the time—with the twin halves of my personality at war with each other."[66] Apparently addressing Jorgensen, albeit indirectly, he concluded:

> I may appear dogmatic, but I state emphatically that a child who at birth was to be female can develop into a male, but no child identified as a male can develop into a female. There are those who speak of a man becoming a woman with a facile assumption of its possibility. I say it is an impossibility. When in 1944 I was privileged to have my identity changes, it was done upon the physical evidence which my body revealed at the time. Here I would like to make it quite clear that *no surgery or hormone treatment was necessary in my case*. The certificate of the Registrar General was granted not upon evidence that I was not a male but because I had been a male from the day of my birth. There is no such miracle known as a natural "change of sex." Any man who sets out to change his sex must necessarily rely on the knife and hormone injections. A Roman philosopher many years ago enunciated these words: "Take nature as your guide, for so reason bids you and advises you; to live happily is to live naturally." [Emphasis added.][67]

In this passage Allen again hints at his own intersex condition, while dismissing individuals assigned male at birth who made claims of being female.[68] Since Allen rejected out of hand the very idea of a genuine sex change, any transformation that necessitated medical intervention was deemed unnatural. Cowell may have shared this same impulse, and despite undergoing extensive medical treatment, she labored to distance herself from Jorgensen and argue that she was female all along.[69] As for etiology, while Jorgensen made the case that the root cause of her distress was glandular, and therefore systemic, Cowell and Allen focused on delayed emergence of their "real" biological sex. No mention is made of being on a male/female continuum, let alone what became known as psychological sex/gender identity. Yet at the end of the day, it's probable that Jorgensen, Cowell, and Allen felt very secure in their target gender, despite having differing explanations to account for their dilemma.

Cowell—and by extension Elbe—and Allen insisted that their transformations were the result of some intersex/hermaphroditic condition that profoundly impacted what should have been their normal sexual development. The case of Allen, although details are only hinted at, seems to present an example of something that may be akin to 5-alpha-reductase deficiency, although as an autosomal recessive trait, this outcome seems unlikely since both parents would have had to have been carriers.

Cowell's, and by extension Elbe's, narratives were less compelling than Allen's in suggesting they suffered from some form of arrested development or true hermaphroditism that nonetheless required surgical and hormonal intervention. In other words, all three made the case that they had been their target sex all along, whereas to them, Jorgensen was appropriately assigned male at birth, only later being transformed into an ersatz woman at the hands of overzealous surgeons and endocrinologists.

A REJOINDER FROM DENMARK

Jorgensen's relatively rapid fall from grace—from blonde beauty to altered male—reinforces the argument that in the 1950s, there was no distinction between what we now refer to as biological sex and gender. In fact, *gender* was a term that was rarely used due to the uncontested assumption that one could confidently predict an individual's gender identity and expression, as well as their sexual attraction, simply by knowing their biological sex assigned at birth based on a cursory examination of the external genitalia. Although Jorgensen had been taking estrogen for more than two years, had undergone two surgeries, and had received almost universal approval of her feminine presentation, she didn't possess the sine qua non of womanhood: the ability to bear children.[70] Hence, the medical community and public reviewed the available diagnostic categories and concluded that she was a transvestite who had undergone hormonal and surgical treatment but was nonetheless a male despite appearances.

In response to the conflicting press coverage of Jorgensen, her Danish medical team published a paper in the prestigious *Journal of the American Medical Association* in May 1953 to counter the inaccurate or plainly fabricated information contained in the US popular press. They maintained that "eonists[71] are persons with a fundamental feeling of being victims of a cruel mistake—a consequence of the female personality in a male body."[72] This quote foreshadows the aforementioned shift from the intersex model to the born-in-the-wrong-body trope that would manifest more fully over the next decade. The authors later complicated this relatively straightforward narrative by suggesting that "physical factors may play a decisive role, as evidenced by the frequent appearance of more or less pronounced feminine physical appearance. On the other hand, there are eonists having completely normal masculine habitus."[73] The Danes referred to the former, which included Jorgensen, as *genuine transvestites*, or *psychic hermaphrodites*, terms that did nothing to clarify the situation and were unintelligible in the United States. They further elaborated that "the eonist's feeling of being a woman is so deeply rooted and irresistible that it is tempting to seek deeper somatic causes of the disease. We have considered the possibility that some of the most pronounced transvestites might be intersexes (sex intergrades) of the highest degree . . . according to Goldschmidt's intersex theory. . . ."[74] The possibility of the existence of human [intersexes] can by no means be disregarded."[75]

What is clear from this historical discourse is that the medical community and the public at large were wrestling with a phenomenon that had no precedent as far as they were concerned. Yet Jorgensen was by no means the first person to experience what we now refer to as gender dysphoria or even the first person to undergo medical treatment. However, she was the first person who became a celebrity for doing so. It is also evident that existing medical jargon was inconsistent among Danish and American physicians. The distinction, or not, between the terms *intersex* and *hermaphrodite* is one important example of such inconsistency. As will be seen, the considerable efforts of Benjamin beginning in 1953 went some way toward providing clarity.

WHEN HARRY MET CHRISTINE

Benjamin was an endocrinologist originally from Germany but became a longtime resident of New York City although he also established an office in San Francisco, California. The sensationalized and shifting reporting on Jorgensen intrigued Benjamin, leading him to focus his considerable experience and empathy on a marginalized community in a professional and increasingly public way. Over the next few decades, Benjamin played an enormous role in the development of early modern transgender medical care in the United States, with Jorgensen as his muse.[76] According to psychologists Leah Schaeffer and Christine Wheeler, who knew Benjamin well, his work with gender dysphoric patients from 1948 until 1978 was "an accident for which he was totally prepared."[77] Jorgensen was not the first gender-nonconforming person Benjamin treated, but she was his most famous. In 1952, after the story broke, Benjamin wrote to one of his patients that he would "probably see [Jorgensen] when she gets home." The two first met in April 1953, after which Jorgensen became Benjamin's seventh patient.[78]

Benjamin was born in Berlin, Germany, on January 12, 1885, just as gender-diverse people first fell under the medical gaze. At the time, they were often mistakenly interpreted as extreme cases of homosexuality or, to use the lexicon of the time, inverts.[79] As a young adult he came into contact with Magnus Hirschfeld, one of the most important figures in early sexological history. Benjamin accompanied Hirschfeld to Weimar-era establishments frequented by homosexuals and transvestites, the latter becoming the eponymous subject of a book authored by Hirschfeld and published in 1910.[80] Thus, Benjamin gained familiarity with, and perhaps some level of empathy for, this group of people.

After completing his medical degree in Tubingen, Germany, in 1912 where he studied tuberculosis, Benjamin sailed to the United States to assist with the treatment of a wealthy patient who had contracted the disease. Unimpressed with American treatment protocols, he attempted to return to Berlin in 1914, but he was forced to head back to New York due to the outbreak of World War I. Although the United States became his permanent home, he frequently traveled to Europe after the war to visit colleagues, including the Austrian scientist Eugen Steinach. Steinach's experiments on rodents employed a novel method of redirecting sex hormones to nonreproductive targets throughout the body that rejuvenated aging individuals. As with Hirschfeld, this experience left a lasting impression on Benjamin, no doubt informing his later medical practice involving geriatric and transsexual patients.[81]

As a geriatric endocrinologist, Benjamin focused on the restorative power hormonal treatment afforded older people. Only once in his practice, in 1938, Benjamin prescribed hormone therapy to a transvestite.[82] At a 1966 lecture, Benjamin described this individual as "turning toward transsexualism." He added that it was a dangerous thing in New York City in the 1930s for this person to underdress in public and to fully dress as a woman at work.[83] Later, this same person was hit by a car and taken to a hospital with a broken leg, where medical staff discovered his feminine undergarments. Benjamin went to see him at the hospital and found him described in the medical chart as a degenerate. It would be another ten years before Benjamin encountered his next transgender patient.

In 1948, renowned sexologist Alfred Kinsey referred a twenty-three-year-old male who had an intense, internal sense of being a woman to Benjamin for consultation.[84] Benjamin recommended sex change surgery, but the procedure was blocked by the attorney general of Wisconsin, who invoked the mayhem statutes of that state, which criminalized surgery on healthy reproductive anatomy.[85] This decision and the subsequent legal obstacles elicited this trenchant response from Benjamin: It would be "wiser and more constructive to 'treat' society, educationally, so that logic, understanding and compassion might presvail [sic]."[86]

It was at this time that Benjamin began developing an intentional and ultimately exclusive practice for transsexual people. His letter of February 16, 1953, was received by Jorgensen shortly after she returned to the United States. As Jorgensen herself explained, "I didn't return from Europe until March of 1953 [sic], and I encountered a mountain of mail . . . many of which were from people who had problems that were similar to mine—and it was incredible and in that mountain of mail was a letter from Harry Benjamin who I had never heard of before and he told me he was guiding people . . . concerning transsexuality."[87] Each asked the other for support in responding to the thousands of pleas for help they both received.[88] Soon after becoming acquainted, Benjamin began monitoring Jorgensen's hormone therapy, and in 1954 he referred her to Dr. William Barbarito of Jersey City, New Jersey, for vaginoplasty.

Benjamin published his first professional paper on transgender people in August 1953, before the Danes published their paper on eonism.[89] His short article, similarly written in reaction to the intensive media coverage of the Jorgensen case, was interesting for at least two reasons. First, he proposed a new diagnostic category, transsexualism, for the more severe cases of transvestism: "[T]he desire of a certain group of men to dress as women, or of women to dress as men . . . can be powerful and overwhelming, even to the point of wanting to belong to the other sex and correct nature's anatomical 'error.' For such cases the term Transsexualism seems appropriate."[90] To further differentiate transsexualism not only from transvestism, he continued: "The infinite diversity of the *male-female scale* is strikingly and often tragically illustrated not only by hermaphroditic abnormalities, but also by transvestism and transsexualism as well as homosexual behavior."[91] [Emphasis added.] Benjamin's conceptualization of transsexualism resonated with that of the Danes' genuine transvestism, as did his characterization of sex existing on a scale. Exploring the scope of sex further, he added, "We are accustomed to decide a person's sex in accordance with anatomical characteristics principally by the presence of testes or ovaries. However, there may be more or less pronounced irregularities in the genetic and endocrine development with resultant 'intersexes' of varying character, degree and intensity." Here, too, Benjamin's use of the term *intersexes* aligned with his Danish colleagues.

The second notable conclusion to be drawn from this short paper is his continued rebuke of the psychological community for asserting that such transsexuals could be cured through psychotherapy. Drawing on his own expertise, he cited, "In thirty years of practice, this writer has never had the good fortune of having seen a pronounced case of homosexuality or transsexualism cured by psychoanalysis in spite of persistent regular treatment continued over years." Benjamin articulated this point repeatedly over the ensuing decades. A year later he reiterated, "All therapy, in cases of transsexualism—to the best of my knowledge—has proved useless as far as any cure is concerned. I know of no case where even intensive and prolonged psychoanalysis had any success."[92]

On December 18, 1953, Benjamin presented a paper before the Association for the Advancement of Psychotherapy. He expanded on his brief paper from earlier in the year and parsed his classification of gender-variant people to include three gradations along a continuum.[93] His first two gradations referred to male individuals who desired to *enact* the role of a woman without medical intervention beyond psychotherapy (transvestites), while his third gradation was distinguished from the first two as it referred to those who wanted to *become* women through hormonal and surgical means (transsexuals).[94] He mentioned Jorgensen as an example of this latter category: "This type is well represented by the case of Christine Jorgensen who published the facts of her own case frankly and with a well-conceived self-analysis."[95]

While Benjamin perpetuated the hypothesis of an underlying, yet only vaguely defined congenital predisposition, his etiology allowed for details of socialization to shape individual outcomes. Nonetheless, he again challenged his psychiatric colleagues. Benjamin argued that the etiology of transsexualism was not psychosomatic but rather a somatopsychic problem, emphasizing an underlying constitutional condition. He was careful to add that although psychotherapy could not effect a cure, especially in the more severe cases of transsexualism, he believed therapists should assist treatment by helping individuals adjust to the many changes associated with a social and medical gender transition. Benjamin accepted that the "problem" was not transsexualism, it was the fact that transsexuals had to live in a society that rejected them.

DISCUSSION AND CONCLUSION

This chapter contributes to a historiography that contextualizes current medical practice vis-à-vis individuals of trans experience. It captures an ethnographic moment when the existence of a distinct transsexual demographic entered the public consciousness in the United States and the healthcare system took its initial, furtive steps to attend to a stigmatized population that had been woefully underserved.[96] Like all significant culture change, this discourse was characterized by the frequent appearance of neologisms, as new language emerged to capture what was a previously concealed human experience.[97]

Benjamin and Jorgensen played pivotal public roles in establishing transsexualism as a condition distinct from other contemporary nosological entities, including transvestism and homosexuality. Although Benjamin did not introduce the term *transsexual*, he was an early adopter.[98] Mass media disseminated a variety of perspectives to the mainstream culture, initially through their coverage of Jorgensen in the 1950s.[99] Her unflappable demeanor, conventional femininity, and consistency in articulating her experience, coupled with Benjamin's authority as a man of science, placed them firmly in the vanguard, initiating an ongoing process of fostering empathy if not quite normalization of a phenomenon that teetered on the threshold of science fiction. They wrested professional control from a skeptical and aggressively contrarian mental health community that viewed transsexualism, like other conditions related to sex and sexuality, as psychopathology and therefore refused to abide hormonal or surgical interventions. These debates continue, although now to a lesser degree.

Jorgensen, despite formidable cultural opposition, succeeded in accessing experimental medical care while only in her twenties, in Europe at first, but later in the United States under Benjamin's care. Yet hers was a cautionary tale in that she served as the exception that proved the rule. Then, as now, alarming disparities in healthcare access for transgender people abound, attributed to a number of potentially compounding factors including socioeconomic status, race, gender, and sexuality. As a white ex-GI hewing closely to affirmed gender conventions of the day, Jorgensen's privileged sociocultural position improved her odds of achieving her goals of living an authentic life on her terms. As already noted, Jorgensen was not the first person to pursue medical treatment to live as the opposite sex.[100] While this assertion is true, and it is important to situate her in this historical context, there is no denying that Jorgensen's celebrity status placed her in a category all her own, then and since.[101] How many other people of her generation were unable to obtain the medical care they so deeply desired, due to their membership in additional marginalized groups?[102]

However, as a result of her celebrity and an insatiable press, Jorgensen found it impossible to lead a typical life beyond the public gaze. She gave up her dreams of making travel films and assembled a stage act in which she sang, told stories, and danced. Despite mostly positive reviews, it was clear that her audiences were drawn to her performances in part for titillation and to witness this mythic figure in person. She published her autobiography in 1967, with a film adaptation following in 1970;[103] subsequently joined the college speaking circuit; and appeared on television talk shows with the intent to educate as many individuals as she could. Later in life, Jorgensen suffered from alcoholism, a somber reminder of the price she paid to live publicly and authentically. Her human foibles aside, those who come after Jorgensen owe her a debt of gratitude. She died in San Clemente, California, on May 3, 1989.

Thanks to Benjamin and his peers, academics, activists, and members of the trans community now possess a vocabulary that was more than one hundred years in the making. In the late eighteenth and early nineteenth centuries, anthropologists in the United States engaged in rescue ethnography of rapidly disappearing indigenous societies. While trying to preserve the languages, rituals, and material culture of these groups, anthropologists also made incidental observations of sex/gender systems that contained elements that were profoundly disturbing to Western schemas. In some cases, they used terms such *hermaphrodite, transvestite,* and *homosexual* to describe the same individual, or even the same behaviors, highlighting yet another example of the conflation of biological sex, gender identity and expression, and sexuality.[104] As has been already documented, Western clinicians were equally culpable in propagating this overly simple model in which gender identity, gender expression, and sexuality were dependent variables of biological sex. Scholars have since isolated these concepts as distinct analytical categories and developed associated terminology to reflect this change. If Hirschfeld had shone daylight between the lives of homosexuals and transvestites, Benjamin further broadened this study of sex and gender diversity by advocating for transsexualism as a distinct experience.

Although Benjamin initially adopted the intersex trope as described by Jorgensen's Scandinavian medical team in the 1950s, he later came to accept a different, preexisting model that conceptualized transsexualism as a misalignment of psychological sex in people with normative physiology and anatomy. Both models justified surgical and hormonal intervention. Over time, the medical community began to view transsexuals as individuals possessing a gender identity that did not align with their anatomical sex rather than as individuals with an ill-defined intersex condition that pervaded the entire body.

This born-in-the-wrong-body narrative exists into the present.[105] Benjamin's shift was necessary as it became increasingly clear that no abnormal morphology or physiology consistently appeared in what the Danes referred to as true transvestites. However, this perception complicated matters in that it gave the impression of corroborating the psychological community's argument that transsexualism was a mental illness that needed to be cured. Nonetheless, Benjamin stridently asserted that psychiatric or psychoanalytic treatment could not alter one's gender identity; therefore changing the body was the only recourse to alleviate distress.

Sociologist Richard Ekins argued that Benjamin adopted this stance not because he lost faith in his initial perspective that men and women existed on a continuum of sex and gender akin to Kinsey's sexuality scale but because it allowed him to provide effective treatment for his suffering patients.[106] The American gender clinics of the 1960s functioned as gatekeepers, championing the gender binary—a central component of a broader heteronormative model that tightly controlled sex and gender. Benjamin himself, in paraphrasing the perspective of one male-to-female transsexual, stated, "I'm a woman, unfortunately in the wrong body."[107]

With the financial assistance of the Erickson Education Foundation, Benjamin and his colleagues established the Harry Benjamin Foundation in the mid-1960s to bring medical professionals together to conduct research into the transsexual phenomenon. In 1979, this developing group and others founded the Harry Benjamin International Gender Dysphoria Association, which developed and published medical standards of care that have been periodically updated during the ensuing decades.[108] As with Jorgensen, Benjamin's tireless efforts dramatically improved the lives of countless individuals who would have otherwise suffered in silence. Eight years after his retirement, Benjamin died in New York City, on August 24, 1986, at the age of 101.[109]

NOTES

1. Schultz, "House Un-American Activities Committee."

2. Importantly, at this time, medical professionals, academics, and others across society did not differentiate between biological sex and socially constructed gender, a critical distinction for second-wave feminists a decade later. Terms describing biological sex (female, male), gender expression (feminine, masculine), and gender identity (woman, man) were used more or less interchangeably. In fact, while hints at these distinctions appear now and again in the source material used in this chapter, from the late 1940s into the 1950s, the term *gender* appears only rarely.

3. While Benjamin took to this term quickly, it would not become widespread for another decade. As a neologism, *transsexualism* sought to clarify existing terminology, most specifically to distinguish it from *transvestism*, a term that had existed for decades.

4. For a useful overview of the history of endocrinology, including its use in justifying contemporary racist, sexist, heterosexist, and classist ideologies of the early twentieth century in the United States, see Serlin, *Replaceable You*. Most relevant to this study, Serlin describes the relatively rapid shift from comparatively crude organotherapy in which hormones were distilled directly from nonhuman gonads and adrenal glands to the synthesis of hormones from a variety of plentiful organic sources.

5. The visibility and increasing demand for sex change operations has been sometimes interpreted as meaning that these technological, medical advances *invented* transsexualism, in a sense analogous to Butler's argument that performativity of gender roles created a person's gender. Butler, *Gender Trouble*; see Billings and Urban, "Socio-Medical Construction," and Hausman, *Changing Sex*. While it is true that the term *transsexual* emerged in part as a result of existing medical treatments being repurposed to treat this "new" demographic, gender–nonconforming individuals, including those who would have likely been considered transsexual, have been documented throughout history and across many non-Western cultures.

6. Ekins, "Science, Politics, and Clinical Intervention"; Haeberle, "100th birthday"; Ihlenfeld et al., "Memorial for Harry Benjamin"; Person, "Creative Maverick"; Schaefer and Wheeler, "First Ten Cases"; Serlin, "Cold War Closet."

7. Like *gender*, the term *transgender* was a later addition to the lexicon and only took on its current meaning as an umbrella term in the 1990s.

8. Beemyn, "Transgender History"; Bullough, "Transsexualism in History"; Bullough and Bullough, *Cross Dressing*; Denny, "Methods of Coping and Treatment"; Docter, *Becoming a Woman*; Feinberg, *Transgender Warriors*; Gil-Peterson, *Histories of the Transgender Child*; Green and Money, *Transsexualism and Sex Reassignmen*; Heidenreich, "A Historical Perspective"; Ihlenfeld et al., "Memorial for Harry Benjamin"; Jorgensen, *A Personal Autobiography*; Meyerowitz, *How Sex Changed*; Meyerowitz, "Transforming Sex"; Meyerowitz, "Trangender Sweetheart"; Reay, *Trans America*; Reicherzer, "Evolving Language"; Rudacille, *Riddle of Gender*; Serlin, *Replaceable You*; Skidmore, "Good Transsexual"; Snorten, *Black on Both Sides*; Stryker, *Transgender History*.

9. The latter is what we would now refer to as gender identity.

10. cf. Cauldwell, "Psychopathia Transexualis"; Hamburger et al., "Transvestism." The latter interpretation quite likely influenced early academic gender clinics a decade later. To be considered eligible for treatment, the clinics demanded the articulation of a tightly circumscribed narrative that aligned with providers' perception of a singular trans experience."

11. Meyerowitz, *How Sex Changed*; Meyerowitz, "Transforming Sex."

12. Skidmore, "Good Transsexual."

13. Denny, "Methods of Coping and Treatment," 40.

14. Serlin, *Replaceable You*. Jorgensen served on the home front after the war ended (1945–1946) in an administrative capacity as thousands of soldiers were formally separated from the military and reintegrated into civilian life; her two-and-a-half years abroad (May 1950–February 1953) were spent transitioning in Denmark.

15. It is of course undeniable that other significant changes occurred later, most especially the recognition of the biocultural diversity of sex, gender, and sexuality human beings experience throughout their lives. From the last decade of the twentieth century to the present, it has become increasingly clear that no facile binary sex/gender system is equipped to contain such diversity.

16. This etiological schema has been called the hermaphroditic model by Kaufman, "Trans-representation," but I believe a better term would be the intersex model—not based on the current meaning of intersex (largely considered a less stigmatizing synonym for hermaphrodite) but in reference to its lexical use in the mid-twentieth century.

17. The European medical community, in particular, accepted intersex as some amorphous combination of male and female traits and behaviors.

18. See the preface in Cauldwell, *Transvestism*, for a brief but useful discussion of the prevailing etiological hypotheses to explain transvestism in the mid-1950s.

19. See Worden and Marsh, "Psychological Factors."

20. In her memoir, Jorgensen claims that she did not adopt a feminine name and pronouns or present as a woman until after she had been in Denmark and undergone

medical treatment. Given her eventual understanding of her gender identity in her twenties, feminine pronouns for her are used throughout this chapter.

21. With the exception of her maternal grandmother who hailed from Germany, Jorgensen's grandparents emigrated from Denmark to the United States. George Jr.'s maternal grandfather died in 1918, and although she knew her maternal grandmother, the influence of her paternal grandparents was much greater.

22. Jorgensen, *A Personal Autobiography*.

23. What later became known as the lavender scare in the 1950s (a riff on the red scare/communism) actually began in the late 1940s in part as a reaction to Kinsey's 1948 book on male sexuality. Adkins, "These People are Frightened to Death." See also chapter 12 in this volume.

24. De Kruif, *The Male Hormone*.

25. Docter, *Becoming a Woman*.

26. What is now referred to as gender confirmation surgery.

27. Jorgensen, *A Personal Autobiography*, 95. "I suppose I was living in a fool's paradise. I was going to Europe on the basis of a few scattered medical reports."

28. Jorgensen, *A Personal Autobiography*, 102.

29. Jorgensen, "My Life, Part 4," March 8, 1953, 11.

30. Jorgensen, "My Life, Part 5," March 15, 1953.

31. Although Jorgensen had considered other names, she chose Christine in honor of Dr. Christian Hamburger. Significantly, as pointed out by Docter, *Becoming a Woman*, in 1952 there was no sex marker on US passports, so there was no change of sex indicated on her documentation. Nonetheless, the change of name and her unambiguously feminine appearance obviated any need for a sex marker.

32. Jorgensen, *A Personal Autobiography*, 124.

33. Jorgensen, *A Personal Autobiography*, 130.

34. Jorgensen, "My Life, Part 4," March 8, 1953, 21.

35. Jorgensen, *A Personal Autobiography*, 135.

36. Hamburger et al., "Transvestism."

37. There is some dispute about who outed Jorgensen to the press, with several individuals speculating that she did it herself (see Denny, "Black Telephones"). Docter, *Becoming a Woman*, provides an intriguing alternative: as a result of a minor court appearance in 1952, a reporter had allegedly published an article about her in Denmark. Although Docter was unable to locate the article, it's possible that its contents were later recognized for their significance.

38. For some writers, Jorgensen's letter to her parents appeared to have been composed for public consumption, supporting the idea that she intended to reveal her story. It's therefore interpreted as the beginning of her controlling her media image and engaging in self-promotion. If true, her intentions might best be captured by the adage, "Be careful what you wish for."

39. Quoted in Serlin, *Replaceable You*, 168.

40. The term *disorder, or difference, of sex development* has begun to supersede intersex among medical providers. Given the history of the term *intersex*, a less ambiguous term is welcome, although the term *disorder* is ill-advised. The revision of the *Diagnostic and Statistical Manual* category of gender identity disorder to gender dysphoria is a useful parallel. Serlin, *Replaceable You*.

41. Docter, *Becoming a Woman*, xvi.

42. Terry, "Christine Jorgensen and the Media."

43. Sørensen and Hertoft in "Sexmodifying" make the salient observation that although Jorgensen underwent surgery in 1951 and 1952, it wouldn't be until a year later that the terms *transsexualism* and *genuine transvestism* appeared in professional publications about the case. Instead, "From the available documents it appears unmistakably, however, that in 1951 . . . the patient was considered a suffering homosexual who, because of mental scruples over own [*sic*] sexual inclinations, was not capable of living out his sexuality." Sørensen and Hertoft, "Sexmodifying," 62. It's also possible that a diagnosis of homosexuality was used to meet an established legal threshold in Denmark permitting the 1951 surgical castration to take place.

44. Jorgensen, "My Life, Part 1," February 15, 1953, 5. The impression that Jorgensen was now a woman in a literal sense would soon lead to some members of the public feeling duped once the details of her treatment, particularly the surgical interventions, became known.

45. Jorgensen, "My Life, Part 1," February 15, 1953, 6.

46. Jorgensen, "My Life, Part 1," February 15, 1953, 6.

47. Jorgensen, "My Life, Part 2," February 22, 1953, 5.

48. Jorgensen, "My Life, Part 2," February 22, 1953, 5.

49. Jorgensen, "My Life, Part 3," March 1, 1953, 12.

50. Jorgensen, "My Life, Part 4," March 8, 1953, 8. This quote was recounted in 1953, just months before the term *transsexualism*, distinct from *transvestism*, began to enter the medical lexicon, largely stimulated by Benjamin. Thus, it is unsurprising that Hamburger would have used an extant diagnostic term in putting a name to Jorgensen's experience in 1950. Jorgensen, "My Life, Part 4," March 8, 1953, 8.

51. Jorgensen, "My Life, Part 4," March 8, 1953, 11.

52. Jorgensen, "My Life, Part 4," March 8, 1953, 11.

53. Stating that *everyone* was both male and female, even if the details or the intensity differed, was a rhetorical flourish Jorgensen frequently used to generalize her predicament and garner sympathy.

54. Four years earlier, in the final installment of Jorgensen's *The Story of My Life* series, she paraphrased Hamburger who "has reviewed my case from a medical standpoint, especially in light of Goldschmidt's intersex theory. He has pointed out the possibility that some cases of transvestitism might be a manifestation of a high

degree of intersexuality" Jorgensen, March 15, 1953, 13. Jorgensen, "Christine Jorgensen Reveals."

55. Davis, "The Truth About 'Christine' Jorgensen."

56. *Time*, "The Case of Christine," 83.

57. *Newsweek*, "Boy or Girl?," 91n.

58. Tamara Rees and Charlotte McLeod are two of the better known cases, although they never achieved the celebrity nor were subjected to the accompanying scrutiny that Jorgensen endured.

59. They both considered Jorgensen to be a normative male, hence, the rationale for her conversion was purely to alleviate *psychological* distress. This perception would later emerge as the born-in-the-wrong-body narrative.

60. Cowell, *Roberta Cowell's Story*, 165.

61. Cowell, *Roberta Cowell's Story*, 171.

62. Cowell, *Roberta Cowell's Story*, 166.

63. In Elbe's autobiography, edited posthumously by a close friend, one physician speculated that this might be the case: "I think you possess both male and female organs, and that neither of them has sufficient room to develop properly." Hoyer, *Man Into Woman*, 27–28. It must be noted that no conclusive evidence to confirm this suspicion was included in the book.

64. Cowell, *Roberta Cowell's Story*, 168–69. For more information, see Hoyer, *Man Into Woman*.

65. In its current usage.

66. Allen, *But for the Grace*, 3.

67. Allen, *But for the Grace*, 126.

68. Note also, the casual switch between terms related to biological sex and those related to what we now call gender, considered more or less synonymous at the time.

69. The reader cannot help but wonder how a conversation between Allen and his compatriot Roberta Cowell might have gone.

70. To this day, biological females who are unable or unwilling to reproduce have their "womaness" called into question. This emphasis on reproduction as the most important role a woman can play in society is a reflection of the sexism that informs the heteronormative nuclear family mentioned in the introduction to this chapter.

71. *Eonist* was English physician Havelock Ellis' preferred alternative to Hirschfeld's term *transvestite*. See Ellis, *Studies in the Psychology of Sex*.

72. Hamburger et al., "Transvestism," 391.

73. Hamburger et al., "Transvestism," 392.

74. The theory referred to here was based on the study of insects, which displayed gynandromorphism in which male and female phenotypic traits were expressed throughout the entire organism, not just in the reproductive anatomy (Goldschmidt, "Intersexuality"). It's quite possible that the Danish team was using the term *intersex*

in this sense. **NB**: This paper appeared just after Benjamin's first publication advocating for the use of the term *transsexual* vis-à-vis Jorgensen and those like her. It is likely, however, that the Danes had not seen it or only became aware of it after their paper went to press.

75. Hamburger et al., "Transvestism," 392.

76. Benjamin used Jorgensen as a well-known point of reference in his writings and during lectures. In the preface to his most important work, he conceded that "without Christine Jorgensen and the unsought publicity of her 'conversion,' this book could hardly have been conceived." Benjamin, *The Transsexual Phenomenon*, 4. Benjamin also provided a forward to Jorgensen's autobiography a year later, again acknowledging the importance of her highly publicized story: "As a physician and, I hope, a medical man of understanding, I salute the courage of Christine Jorgensen and the warm humanity of the Jorgensen family." Jorgensen, *A Personal Autobiography*, vii.

77. Schaefer and Wheeler, "First Ten Cases," 74.

78. Schaefer and Wheeler, "First Ten Cases," 74.

79. See Krafft-Ebing, *Psychopathia Sexualis*.

80. Hirschfeld, *Transvestites*.

81. Harms, "Forty-four Years."

82. It is likely that this person was Otto Spengler, a patient of Benjamin's in the 1930s. The story recounted here, and in Benjamin's 1966 book, is relevant to this chapter only in that Spengler was considered his first trans patient. See Schaefer and Wheeler, "First Ten Cases." It should be noted that Spengler was seeing Benjamin for other reasons, well before he began treating trans people almost exclusively. That Spengler was a transvestite was revealed incidentally.

83. Benjamin, "Dr. Harry Benjamin Lecture," File 1, starting at 24:15.

84. One reason why Kinsey may have referred this patient to Benjamin was that he didn't share the latter's notion that transvestism was constitutional at its root but rather was the result of rearing. "Together with many other psychiatrists and psychologists, he [Kinsey] believes that this sexual deviation is a psychologically conditioned inclination acquired after birth as a result of precise and specific environmental experiences. He disputes the theories of glandular causation and constitutional origin." Cauldwell, *Transvestism*, 7; Schaefer, in Ihlenfeld et al., "Memorial for Harry Benjamin," 11–15; Schaefer and Wheeler, "First Ten Cases."

85. Eventually, on Benjamin's recommendation, the patient had surgery in Europe in the early 1950s, before moving to Canada. Surgeons' apprehension about the legality of gender surgery created the single greatest obstacle TGD people faced while attempting to access care. Clinicians feared prosecution based on the mayhem statutes—rooted in sixteenth-century English Law—which prohibited the intentional mutilation of body parts that could handicap a soldier in combat. These statutes, systematically codified by legislators into law, justified culturally racist, homophobic,

misogynistic, and transphobic beliefs. Clinicians, who were deeply suspicious of gender surgeries for a problem they perceived as caused by mental illness, brought forth these legal statutes, adding the specter of litigation to their list of reasons for denying care. Only the wealthy and determined found surgical care, often by traveling overseas, and the American public learned it was "illegal" to surgically alter one's sex. Khan, "Transgender Health," 385–86; Coke, "Laws of England," 116–18.

86. Benjamin, "Transvestism and Transsexualism," 14.

87. Quoted in Ettner, *Gender Loving Care*, 16–17.

88. Hamburger also received hundreds of pleas for help after the Jorgensen story broke. Hamburger, "The Desire for Change of Sex."

89. Benjamin, "Transvestism and Transsexualism," 11.

90. Benjamin had a lengthy and in-depth epistolary relationship with one of his patients named Doris. In late 1952 or early 1953, he wrote regarding Jorgensen, "We lack a proper scientific term for it. I would describe it as an 'obsessive urge to belong to the opposite sex.'" Quoted in Schaefer and Wheeler, "First Ten Cases," 81. It has been well documented that Benjamin wasn't the first person to use the term *transsexualism*; see Cauldwell, "Psychopathia Transexualis." However, he was the individual who established specific, differential diagnostic criteria and a treatment protocol that would later develop into more detailed standards of care. Benjamin, "Transvestism and Transsexualism," 11.

91. Benjamin, "Transvestism and Transsexualism."

92. Benjamin, "Transsexualism and Transvestism," 226. Remarkably, reparative/conversion therapies aimed at curing LGBTQ+ individuals continue to be practiced in some states in the United States despite the nearly complete lack of positive outcomes. Several states have now made the practice illegal.

93. Benjamin, "Transsexualism and Transvestism." In his book *The Transsexual Phenomenon*, Benjamin adopted an analog of the Kinsey Scale of sexual orientation, which ranged from exclusively heterosexual (0) to exclusively homosexual (6). Benjamin referred to his version as the Sex Orientation Scale, ranging from any person of normal sex and gender orientation (0) to a high intensity transsexual (6). Note that he is making a clear distinction between biological sex and gender in this later publication, although stops short of calling it a *Gender* Orientation Scale, perhaps only to preserve the acronym."

94. Other terms on the scale were *transsexualist, transsexist*, and *psychic hermaphrodite*. These terms suggest that the terminology was still in flux at this point.

95. Benjamin, "Transsexualism and Transvestism," 225.

96. Reay, "The Transsexual Phenomenon," convincingly argues that although the period covered in this chapter was important, it was just the beginning of a cultural and medical shift that continues to the present day. The full integration of gender-diverse people is by no means a settled matter.

97. Reicherzer, "Evolving Language."

98. See Benjamin, "Transvestism and Transsexualism."

99. See Ihlenfeld et al., "Memorial for Harry Benjamin," 26. Ironically, in her remarks at a 1987 memorial for Benjamin, who had died the previous year at the age of 101, Jorgensen stated, "I never went along with the word transsexual because I think it's transgender, gender is who you are, sexual is who you sleep with. That's important, but I never mentioned that while Harry was living." This quote is doubly interesting, as the term *transgender* was only just coming into use at that time, underscoring the lexicon's continual development. It could be said that Jorgensen was an early adopter of the term; however, she was probably not using it in the umbrella sense that it subsequently took in the 1990s.

100. cf. Reese, *Reborn*.

101. Caitlyn Jenner's transition in 2015 is arguably of the same caliber; however, this is in large part because of her already established celebrity status. cf. Meyerowitz, "Transforming Sex," for a slightly different interpretation.

102. Skidmore, "Good Transexual."

103. Rapper, *The Christine Jorgensen Story*.

104. See Devereux, "Institutionalized Homosexuality"; Hill, "Status of the Hermaphrodite."

105. See Bettcher, "Trapped in the Wrong Theory," and Latham, "Axiomatic." More recently, under the influence of queer and trans theory from the 1980s onward, emphasis on social construction and a palpable increase in nonbinary identities and embodiments is challenging the born-in-the-wrong-body trope as the only model that accurately captures the trans experience.

106. Ekins, "Science, Politics and Clinical Intervention."

107. Benjamin, "Dr. Harry Benjamin Lecture," File 1, 53:00.

108. The Harry Benjamin International Gender Dysphoria Association later became the World Professional Association for Transgender Health, who publish revised standards of care based on the latest research.

109. Pace, "Harry Benjamin Dies at 101."

WORKS CITED

Adkin, Judith. "'These People Are Frightened to Death.' Congressional Investigations and the Lavender Scare." The U.S. National Archives and Records Administration. *Prologue Magazine*, 48 no. 2 (Summer 2016). Accessed August 13, 2024. https://www.archives.gov/publications/prologue/2016/summer/lavender.html#:~:text=Beginning%20in%20the%20late%201940s,the%20power%20of%20congressional%20investigation

Allen, Robert. *But for the Grace: The True Story of a Dual Existence*. London: W. H. Allen, 1954.

Beemyn, Genny. "Transgender History in the United States: A Special Unabridged Version of a Book Chapter from *Trans Bodies, Trans Selves*," edited by Laura Erickson-Schroth. Oxford: Oxford University Press, 2014. Accessed March 6, 2021. https://www.umass.edu/stonewall/sites/default/files/Infoforandabout/transpeople/genny_beemyn_transgender_history_in_the_united_states.pdf.

Benjamin, Harry. "Dr. Harry Benjamin Lecture, Los Angeles, 1966." *ONE Archives*, September 18, 1966. Accessed May 27, 2022. https://www.digitaltransgenderarchive.net/files/p5547r47r.

———. *The Transsexual Phenomenon*. New York: Julian Press, 1966.

———. "Transsexualism and Transvestism as Psycho-somatic and Somato-Psychic Syndromes." *American Journal of Psychotherapy* 8 (1954): 219–30.

———. "Transvestism and Transsexualism." *International Journal of Sexology* 7, no. 1 (1953): 12–14.

Bettcher, Talia Mae. "Trapped in the Wrong Theory: Rethinking Trans Oppression and Resistance." *Signs: Journal of Women in Culture and Society* 39, no. 2 (2014): 383–406.

Billings, Dwight B., and Thomas Urban. "The Socio-Medical Construction of Transsexualism: An Interpretation and Critique." *Social Problems* 29, no. 3 (1982): 266–82.

Bullough, Vern L. "Transsexualism in History." *Archives of Sexual Behavior* 4 (1975): 561–71.

Bullough, Vern L., and Bonnie Bullough. *Cross Dressing, Sex, and Gender*. Philadelphia: University of Pennsylvania Press, 1993.

Butler, Judith. *Gender Trouble*. London: Routledge, 1990.

Cauldwell, David, ed. *Transvestism: Men in Female Dress*. New York: Sexology, 1955.

Cauldwell, David O. "Psychopathia Transexualis." *Sexology* 16 (1949): 274–80. Reprinted in *The Transgender Studies Reader*, edited by Susan Stryker and Stephen Whittle, 40–44. London: Routledge, 2006.

Coke, Edward. "The Third Part of the Institutes of the Laws of England: Concerning High Treason, and Other Please of the Crown, and Criminal Causes." 1629. Wythepedia, William and Mary Law Library. Accessed June 25, 2022. http://lawlibrary.wm.edu/wythepedia/library/CokeThirdPartOfTheInstitutesOfTheLawsOfEngland1644.pdf.

Cowell, Roberta. *Roberta Cowell's Story: An Autobiography*. New York: British Book Centre, 1954.

Davis, Alvin. "The Truth about 'Christine' Jorgensen, Part 1." *New York Post*, April 6, 1953, 3 and 16. E-copy, PDF of hard copy or microfiche.

De Kruif, Paul. *The Male Hormone*. San Diego, CA: Harcourt Brace, 1945.

Denny, Dallas. "Black Telephones, White Refrigerators: Rethinking Christine Jorgensen." In *Current Concepts in Transgender Identity*, edited by Dallas Denny, 35–44. New York: Garland Publishing Group, 1998.

———. "Transgender: Some Historical, Cross-Cultural, and Contemporary Models and Methods of Coping and Treatment." In *Gender Blending*, edited by Bonnie Bullough, Vern L. Bullough, and James Elias, 33–47. Amherst, NY: Prometheus Books, 1997.

Devereux, George. "Institutionalized Homosexuality of the Mohave Indians." *Human Biology* 9, no. 4 (1937): 498–527.

Docter, Richard. F. (2013) 2019. *Becoming a Woman: A Biography of Christine Jorgensen*. New York: Routledge.

Ekins, Richard. "Science, Politics and Clinical Intervention: Harry Benjamin, Transsexualism and the Problem of Heteronormativity." *Sexualities* 8, no. 3 (2005): 306–28.

Ellis, Havelock. *Studies in the Psychology of Sex, Vol. 7, Eonism and Other Supplementary Studies*. Philadelphia, PA: F. A. Davis, 1928.

Ettner, Randi. *Gender Loving Care: A Guide to Counseling Gender-Variant Clients*. New York: W. W. Norton, 1999.

Feinberg, Leslie. *Transgender Warriors: Making History from Joan of Arc to Dennis Rodman*. Boston, MA: Beacon Press, 1996.

Gil-Peterson, Julian. *Histories of the Transgender Child*. Minneapolis: University of Minnesota Press, 2018.

Goldschmidt, Richard. "Intersexuality and the Endocrine Aspect of Sex." *Endocrinology* 1, no. 4 (1917): 433–56.

Green, Richard, and John Money, eds. *Transsexualism and Sex Reassignment*. Baltimore, MD: Johns Hopkins Press, 1969.

Haeberle, E. J. "An Interview with Harry Benjamin (b. January 12, 1885) On the Occasion of His 100th Birthday." *Sexualmedizin*, 14, no. 1 (1985). Accessed March 6, 2021. https://web.archive.org/web/20041227133920/http://www2.hu-berlin.de/sexology/GESUND/ARCHIV/TRANS_B5.HTM.

Hamburger, Christian. "The Desire for Change of Sex as Shown by Personal Letters from 465 Men and Women." *Acta Endocrinologica* 14, no. 4 (1953): 361–75.

Hamburger, Christian, Georg K. Sturup, Herstedvester, and E. Dahl-Iversen. "Transvestism: Hormonal, Psychiatric, and Surgical Treatment." *Journal of the American Medical Association* 152, no. 5 (1953): 391–96.

Harms, Ernest. "Forty-four Years of Correspondence Between Eugen Steinach and Harry Benjamin." *Bulletin of the N. Y. Academy of Medicine* 45, no. 8 (1969): 761–66.

Hausman, Bernice L. *Changing Sex: Transsexualism, Technology, and the Idea of Gender*. Durham, NC: Duke University Press, 1995.

Heidenreich, Linda. "A Historical Perspective on Christine Jorgensen and the Development of an Identity." In *Gender Blending,* edited by Bonnie Bullough, Vern L. Bullough, and James Elias, 267–75. Amherst: Prometheus Books, 1997.

Hill, Willard Williams. "The Status of the Hermaphrodite and Transvestite in Navaho Culture." *American Anthropologist* 37 (1935): 273–79.

Hirschfeld, Magnus. (1910) 1991. *Transvestites: The Erotic Drive to Cross-Dress.* Amherst: printed by author.

Hoyer, Nels. (1931). *Man Into Woman: The First Sex Change.* London: Blue Boat Books, 2004.

Ihlenfeld, C. L. "Memorial for Harry Benjamin." *Archives of Sexual Behavior* 17, no. 5 (1988): 3–31. E-copy, PDF of original.

Jorgensen, Christine. *Christine Jorgensen: A Personal Autobiography.* New York: Paul A. Eriksson, 1967.

———. (1957) 2005. *Christine Jorgensen Reveals.* Repeat the Beat Records. LP. Accessed January 17, 2021. https://www.youtube.com/watch?v=nZfVvLFdEqs.

———. "My Life: Parts 1–5." *American Weekly,* February 15–March 15, 1953.

Kaufman, J. "Trans-Representation." *Qualitative Inquiry* 16, no. 2 (2010): 104–15.

Khan, Liza. "Transgender Health at the Crossroads: Legal Norms, Insurance Markets, and the Threat of Healthcare Reform." *Yale Journal of Health Policy, Law and Ethics* 11, no. 2 (2011): 234–418.

Krafft-Ebing, Richard von. (1886) 2006. *Psychopathia Sexualis.* English excerpt from *The Transgender Studies Reader,* edited by Susan Stryker and Stephen Whittle, 21–27. London: Routledge.

Latham, J. R. "Axiomatic: Constituting 'Transexuality' and Trans Sexualities in Medicine." *Sexualities* 22, no. 1–2 (2019): 13–30.

Meyerowitz, Joanne. "America's Original Transgender Sweetheart." *Politico,* June 16, 2015. Accessed June 15, 2022. https://www.politico.com/magazine/story/2015/06/caitlyn-jenner-was-not-americas-first-transgender-sweetheart-christine-jorgensen-119080/#:~:text=The%20Post%20revealed%20that%20Jorgensen,to%20her%20with%20male%20pronouns.

———. *How Sex Changed: A History of Transsexuality in the United States.* Cambridge: Harvard University Press, 2002.

———. "Transforming Sex: Christine Jorgensen in the Postwar U.S." *OAH Magazine of History,* March 2006, 16–20. E-copy, PDF of original periodical.

Newsweek. "Boy or Girl?" May 4, 1953, 91–92. E-copy, photocopy of hard copy or microfiche.

Pace, Eric. "Harry Benjamin Dies at 101; Specialist in Transsexualism." *New York Times,* August 27, 1986, D18.

Person, Ethel. "Harry Benjamin: Creative Maverick." *Journal of Gay & Lesbian Mental Health,* 12, no. 3 (2008): 259–75.

Rapper, Irving. *The Christine Jorgensen Story*. Produced by Edward Small. 1970.
Reay, Barry. "The Transsexual Phenomenon: A Counter-History." *Journal of Social History* 47, no. 4 (2014): 1042–70.
———. *Trans America: A Counter-history*. Cambridge: Polity Press, 2020.
Reese, Tamara (a.k.a. Rees). *Reborn: A Factual Life Story of a Transition from Male to Female*. 1995. Accessed on June 15, 2021. http://transascity.org/files/history/Reese_Tamara_Reborn_1955.pdf.
Reicherzer, Stacee. "Evolving Language and Understanding in the Historical Development of Gender Identity Disorder Diagnosis." *Journal of LGBT Issues in Counseling* 2, no. 4 (2008): 326–47.
Reis, Elizabeth. *Bodies in Doubt: An American History of Intersex*. Baltimore, MD: Johns Hopkins University Press, 2009.
Rudacille, Deborah. *The Riddle of Gender: Science, Activism, and Transgender Rights*. New York: Pantheon, 2005.
Schaefer, Leah C., and Christine C. Wheeler. "Harry Benjamin's First Ten Cases (1938–1953): A Clinical Historical Note." *Archives of Sexual Behavior* 24, no. 1 (1995): 73–93.
Schultz, David. "House Un-American Activities Committee." *First Amendment Encyclopedia. Middle Tennessee State University*, 2009. Accessed June 20, 2021. https://mtsu.edu/first-amendment/article/815/house-un-american-activities-committee.
Serlin, David H. "Christine Jorgensen and the Cold War Closet." *Radical History Review* 62 (1995): 136–65.
———. *Replaceable You: Engineering the Body in Postwar America*. Chicago, IL: University of Chicago Press, 2004.
Skidmore, Emily. "Constructing the 'Good Transsexual': Christine Jorgensen, Whiteness, and Heteronormativity in the Mid-Twentieth Century Press." *Feminist Studies* 37, no. 2 (2011): 270–300.
Snorten, C. Riley. *Black on Both Sides: A Racial History of Trans Identity*. Minneapolis: University of Minnesota Press, 2017.
Sørensen, Thorkilm, and P. Hertoft. "Sexmodifying [sic] Operations on Transsexuals in Denmark in the Period 1950–1977." *Acta Psychiatrica Scandinavica* 61, no. 1 (1980): 56–66.
Stryker, Susan. *Transgender History: The Roots of Today's Revolution*. 2nd ed. New York: Seal Press, 2017.
Stryker, Susan, and Stephen Whittle, eds. *The Transgender Studies Reader*. London: Routledge, 2006.
Terry, Emylia N. "Christine Jorgensen and the Media: Identity Politics in the Early 1950s Press." Research paper, University of Nevada, Las Vegas, 2012. Accessed March 6, 2021. https://digitalscholarship.unlv.edu/award/9.

Time. "Medicine: The Case of Christine." April 20, 1953, 82–84. E-copy, PDF of original hardy copy or microfiche.

Worden, Frederick G., and James T. Marsh. "Psychological Factors in Men Seeking Sex Transformation." *Journal of the American Medical Association* 157, no. 15 (1955): 1292–98.

6.1. CONSTRUCTION OF THE "GOOD" TRANSSEXUAL AND THOSE WHO DID NOT FIT THE BILL

Carolyn Wolf-Gould

Post-World War II has been referred to as the "age of anxiety";[1] Americans struggled to find stability and meaning in a world traumatized by war. At home, civil rights efforts intensified with legislation to end racial segregation in schools and public accommodation. African American troops legally joined the armed services. American physicians performed the first kidney transplant, and researchers launched clinical trials for oral contraceptives.[2] As protection against supposed, politically destabilizing communist threats to the nation and world (for example, equality of the sexes), cultural and political groups promoted the importance of the nuclear family and the traditional expectations of women as homemakers and men as breadwinners. These views contextualized the arrival of transgender medical practices to America.

In 1952, Christine Jorgensen returned to the United States from Denmark after her successful medical and surgical gender reassignment. Her arrival, leaked to the press, inspired three hundred reporters to meet her plane at Idlewild Airport, and the ensuing media blitz brought the possibilities of gender transition to the forefront of American consciousness. For the first time, a celebrated transgender person took control of her narrative, describing first her unbearable existence as a man and then her gender transition. Fascinated by Jorgensen's refined manner and the sober, dignified way she presented herself, the American people stayed riveted by her story for years. Even Jorgensen was incredulous: "I pushed the hydrogen-bomb tests on Eniwetok right off the front pages. A tragic war was still raging in Korea, George V1 died, and Britain had a new queen, sophisticated guided missiles were going off in New Mexico, Jonas Salk was working on a vaccine for infant paralysis . . . Christine Jorgensen was on page one."[3] Indeed, the sensationalist headlines quickly garnered national attention: "Ex-GI Becomes Blond Beauty."[4] Jorgensen's story had a profound effect on the isolated transgender and gender-diverse (TGD) people in the United States who, until then, had no template to ground their experience. Suddenly, they found words to describe themselves, an inspirational figure to follow, and descriptions of a medical gender transition they might hope to replicate.

Transsexual women like Jorgenson (those returning from Europe after treatment, or living in the United States without treatment), who conformed to the prevailing cultural expectations of women as white, feminine, sexually attractive, domestic, respectable, and heterosexual fared better in American society than those who did not.[5] Jorgenson expressed the wish to find a husband and settle down, declared her repugnance for prostitutes and homosexuals, and described a pretransition sexual advance from a man at an event that caused her to "lean over the edge of the pier" to vomit.[6] News stories about her featured parental pride, familial love, and the performance of traditional feminine domestic rituals. Considered "good transsexuals," women like Jorgenson established for the American public that the trans experience included white women with binary, hyperfeminine transitions, and normative (feminine heterosexual) orientation.

While this narrative elevated Jorgensen, it subjugated or rendered invisible the stories of those who deviated from the norms, particularly transgender women of color or lower socioeconomic class who rarely received the opportunity to tell their own stories. Journalists published their own damning commentary, labeling these women as social deviants, exotics, laughable, or inauthentic and attacking their race, social class, sexuality, appearance, and behavior.[7] Only a few accounts described the experiences of transgender people of color—individuals who also attempted to or successfully accessed gender-affirming care during this time.

PROFILES: MONICA ROBERTS (1962–2020), CARLETT BROWN (1927–UNKNOWN), AVON WILSON (DATES UNKNOWN), AND DELISA NEWTON (1934–UNKNOWN)

Shortly after her transition in 1994, Monica Roberts, a contemporary African American historian, asked: "Where is the history of African American trans people? What did my forebears accomplish? What did they do to contribute to the advancement of trans human rights and knowledge of trans people while living their own complex trans lives?"[8] Roberts mused on how her life might have been different if she had had a "marquee transwoman," someone with star power like Jorgensen to serve as her role model.[9] She began to search through African American magazine archives and eventually discovered three stories about Carlett Brown, Avon Wilson, and Delisa Newton, which she retold in her blog, *Transgriot*.[10]

In 1953, *Jet* published a series on Brown, a twenty-six-year-old US Navy veteran, shake dancer, and professional female impersonator who planned to travel to Europe for "an operation that will make him [sic] female, so that he can marry Eugene Martin, 24, now stationed in Frankfurt, Germany."[11] The report stated that Brown would be the first "Negro transvestite in history to transform his sex." It further revealed that Brown suffered from a mental illness—a "passion to become a female"—and that she possessed "the abnormal existence in [his] symptoms of female glands."[12] To travel, the federal government forced Brown to renounce her American citizenship, citing that "after the Christine Jorgensen affair, the United states refused to give an American citizen permission to alter his sex."[13] She also suffered from financial troubles and sold her blood for five dollars a pint to pay rent and buy food.[14] Ultimately, the federal government refused to allow her to leave the country until she had paid her back taxes.[15] Brown had planned consultations with Dr. Christian Hamburger, hoping for hormone injections, electrolysis, and then plastic surgery, penectomy, and ovarian implants, with the expressed hope that she could one day bear children—but her hopes came to naught.[16]

While three hundred reporters had greeted Jorgensen's airplane in 1952, catapulting her to fame, just one year later Brown was jailed in Boston for "masquerading in female attire."[17] Jorgensen and a few other white "good transsexuals"[18] received respectful press coverage, but the press ridiculed Brown. One article described her trip to a store to buy a wedding gown with emphasis on the gaping jaw of the saleslady, an attempt by the store detective to find legal precedent to refuse service, and her ultimate ejection from the store by a policeman.[19]

Roberts unearthed two snippets of information that referenced Wilson, an African American trans woman who underwent "sex change surgery" at the Johns Hopkins Gender Clinic in Baltimore in 1966.[20] Despite the fact that she was reportedly the clinic's first patient, the press coverage about Wilson revealed only that she was a "stunning girl," a former New York City dancer who "underwent special treatment," and "became the bride of Warren Combs, a musician."[21]

In 1966, *Sepia* magazine published a two-part autobiographical series on Newton, who testified to her unique status with this statement: "On this crowded planet, where billions of people live, I am the one and only Negro sex change!"[22] Newton hailed from New Orleans. She was the child of a Haitian, "beautiful mulatto woman who speaks both French and English fluently, in her soft, musical voice" and "a Baptist minister I never knew well." She describes her early life: "I was a complete misfit—I had the mind and body of a girl and the body of a boy." The story details Newton's history, from her lonely life as a misfit boy, to the military, to her career as a nurse, through a series of perilous love affairs and, finally, to finding physicians who helped her medically transition. She voiced skepticism regarding information she received regarding the etiology of her condition, sharing, "The doctors say I had no father figure to pattern myself after, so I identified with my stern, no-nonsense mother. Maybe." Finally, she achieved surgical transition. "The operation was sheer torture of body and soul, but it was worth it," she concluded.

In her blog, Roberts mourned that she never knew "exactly who was our first [transgender woman to transition] and hear about how their lives progressed post-surgery."[23] She grieved the absence of documentation about the lives or early African American transgender people. Contemporary scholar and author of *Black on Both Sides* C. Riley Snorton cited actress and advocate Laverne Cox's use of the phrase "state of emergency"[24] in reference to the relentless systemic violence faced by transgender women of color. He further reflected that the "*[R]eal* state of emergency that surfaces as a matter of history . . . institutions and their emplacement within current biopolitical and necropolitical orders bear upon the problem of history as a mode of organizing time according to anti-black and anti-trans 'rule.' They perpetuate racialized gender as the norm and as the necessary and naturalized consequence of the current order of things."[25] To address the dearth of historical data, Snorton instead described events that brought "blackness and transness—into the same frame . . . not a history, per se so much as it is a set of political propositions, theories of history, and writerly experiments."[26]

In 1949, when David O. Cauldwell introduced transsexuality to the American public in the pages of the general distribution publication *Sexology Magazine*, entrenched cultural systems of racial oppression had long existed, resulting in the marginalization of Black TGD people. Compared to white counterparts, they faced additional barriers to care because of their race. Increased societal stigma, education and employment disparities, limited access to care—or lackluster care from clinicians trained by racialized medical institutions—all contributed to inferior health outcomes and healthcare disparities for TGD people of color.

Emphasizing her quest for histories and documentation, in her blog, Roberts quoted Carter G. Woodson. He warned that "[t]hose who have no record of what their forebears have accomplished lose the inspiration which comes from the teaching of biography and history."[27] She reminds us:

> Black trans history is also vitally important to point out to cis Black people, our allies, and our detractors we not only exist, but our lives are part of the kente cloth fabric of the African American community. We also need to pass this history down so that it serves to inspire the next generation of trans kids who are following in our footsteps and point out Black trans people have a legacy and possibility models they can be proud of.[28]

Roberts died on October 5, 2020, at age fifty-eight, but her blog, *Transgriot*, named in honor of the storytellers in West African traditions, lives on in cyberspace. In addition to finding these stories on early transitions of Black transgender individuals, she went on to collect a trove of stories about Black TGD people,[29] including those of trans opera singers, athletes, activists, and politicians.[30] Roberts also worked to identify transgender murder victims and solve crimes that were unexplained due to misgendering and deadnaming, a commemoration of and to those lost to violence. Ms. Willis, a transgender activist, remembered her thus: "Often, she was the only one who noticed and sang our praises."[31]

NOTES

1. Loftin, "Unacceptable Mannerism," 577.
2. Harvard Medical School, *Timeline of Discovery*.
3. Jorgensen, *A Personal Autobiography*, 144.
4. *Daily News*, "EX-GI Becomes Blonde Beauty."
5. Skidmore, "Constructing the 'Good Transsexual.'"
6. Jorgensen, *A Personal Autobiography*, 83.
7. Skidmore, "Constructing the 'Good Transsexual.'"
8. Roberts, "Black Trans History Inspirational."
9. Roberts, "Musing about Avon Wilson's Blended Life."

10. Roberts, "Black Trans History Inspirational."
11. *Jet*, "Male Shake Dancer Plans to Change Sex," 24–25.
12. *Jet*, "Male Shake Dancer Plans to Change Sex," 24–15.
13. *Jet*, "Male Dancer Becomes Danish Citizen," 26–27.
14. *Jet*, "Jail Male Shake Dancer for Posing as a Woman," 20.
15. *Jet*, "Tax Snag Halts Male Dancer's Trip," 19.
16. *Jet*, "Tax Snag Halts Male Dancer's Trip," 19.
17. *Jet*, "Jail Male Shake Dancer for Posing as a Woman," 20.
18. Skidmore, "Constructing the 'Good Transsexual,'" 272.
19. *Jet*, "Male Dancer Becomes Danish Citizen," 27.
20. Roberts, "Musing about Avon Wilson's Blended Life."
21. Roberts, "Musing about Avon Wilson's Blended Life."
22. Newton, "From Man to Woman," 8–10.
23. Roberts, "Who Was the First African-America Transwoman?"; Roberts, "Musing about Avon Wilson's Blended Life"; Roberts, "Black Trans History Inspirational."
24. Cox, Interview by Robin Roberts, quoted in Snorton, *Black on Both Sides*, vii. Snorton states: "In 2015, while garnering publicity for the feature film Grandma in a live interview with Robin Roberts on *Good Morning America*, actress, artist, and advocate Laverne Cox expressed a public grief." Laverne Cox describes the murder of several trans woman referring to it as "a state of emergency."
25. Snorton, *Black on Both Sides*, viii–ix.
26. Snorton, *Black on Both Sides*, 6.
27. Roberts, "Black Trans History Inspirational."
28. Roberts, "Black Trans History Inspirational."
29. Kurutz, "Monica Roberts."
30. Kurutz, "Monica Roberts."
31. Kurutz, "Monica Roberts," section B, 10.

WORKS CITED

Cox, Laverne. Interview by Robin Roberts. *Good Morning America*, August 18, 2015.

Daily News. "EX-GI Becomes Blonde Beauty." December 1, 1952, 1. Accessed August 6, 2024. https://www.gettyimages.com/detail/news-photo/daily-news-front-page-december-1-1952-headline-ex-gi-news-photo/119594722.

Harvard Medical School. "Timeline of Discovery." Accessed January 3, 2021. https://hms.harvard.edu/about-hms/history-hms/timeline-discovery.

Jet. "Jail Male Shake Dancer for Posing as a Woman in Boston." *Commie Pinko Fag*, July 9, 1953. Accessed January 17, 2021. https://commiepinkofag.org/post/123221396122/jail-male-shake-dancer-for-posing-as-woman-in-boston.

———. "Male Dancer Becomes Danish Citizen to Change Sex." *Google Books*, June 25, 1953. Accessed January 17, 2021. https://books.google.com/books?id=hUIDAAAA MBAJ&pg=PA26&dq=Carlett+Brown+Jet&hl=en&sa=X&ved=2ahUKEwjY07 ei6Y7qAhXElnIEHUx9D5YQ6AEwBHoECAAQAg#v=onepage&q=Carlett%20 Brown%20Jet&f=false.

———. "Male Shake Dancer Plans to Change Sex, Wed GI in Europe." *Google Books*, June 18, 1953 Accessed January 17, 20201. https://books.google.com/books?id=g0IDAAAAMBAJ&pg=PA24&dq=Male+shake+dancer+plans+to+change+sex-+Jet+Magazine&hl=en&sa=X&ved=2ahUKEwir9ai27Y7qAhWdmHIEHfw-A1IQ6 AEwAXoECAAQAg#v=onepage&q=Male%20shake%20dancer%20plans%20to%20 change%20sex%20Jet%20Magazine&f=fa.

———. "Shake Dancer Postpones Sex Change for Face Lifting." *Transgender Digital Archives*, August 6, 1953, 19. Accessed August 6, 2024. https://www.digital transgenderarchive.net/files/b8515n46z.

———. "Tax Snag Halts Male Dancer's Trip for Sex Change." *Google Book*, October 15, 1953. Accessed January 17, 2021. https://books.google.com/books?id=sEIDA AAAMBAJ&pg=PA1&dq=Jet+October+15+1953&hl=en&sa=X&ved=2ahUKE wjEmImbiaTuAhWLjVkKHYv1C54Q6AEwAHoECAAQAg#v=onepage&q=Jet%20 October%2015%201953&f=false.

Jorgensen, Christine. *A Personal Autobiography.* New York: Paul S. Ericksson, 1967.

Kurutz, Steven. "Monica Roberts, Transgender Advocate and Journalist, Dies at 58." *New York Times*, October 13, 2020. Accessed October 18, 2022. https://www.nytimes.com/2020/10/13/us/monica-roberts-dead.html

Loftin, Craig. "Unacceptable Mannerisms: Gender Anxieties, Homosexual Activism, and Swish in the United States, 1945–1965." *Journal of Social History* 40, no. 3 (2007): 577–808.

Newton, Delisa. "From Man to Woman." *Sepia Magazine.* 1996. Accessed August 6, 2024. https://www.digitaltransgenderarchive.net/downloads/kd17ct167.

Roberts, Monica. "Black Trans History Inspirational." *Transgender Law Center.* February 25, 2015. Accessed Januray 16, 2021. https://transgenderlawcenter.org/archives/11401.

———. "Musing about Avon Wilson's Blended Life." *TransGriot*, April 5, 2009. Accessed January 20, 2021. https://transgriot.blogspot.com/2009/04/musing-about-avon-wilsons-blended-life.html.

———. "Who Was the First African-America Transwoman?" *TransGriot*, May 26, 2009. Accessed January 20, 2021. https://transgriot.blogspot.com/2009/05/who-was-first-african-american.html.

Skidmore, Emily. "Constructing the 'Good Transsexual': Christine Jorgensen, Whiteness, and Heteronormativity in the Mid-Twentieth-Century." *Feminist Studies* 37, no. 2 (2011): 270–300.

Snorton, C. Riley. *Black on Both Sides.* Minneapolis: University of Minnesota Press, 2017.

7

TRANS CIRCLES OF KNOWLEDGE AND INTIMACY

Annette F. Timm and Jamison Green

PART 1: "I AM SO GRATEFUL TO ALL YOU MEN OF MEDICINE WHO HAVE BEEN SO GOOD TO ME."

These words of appreciation appear in a January 1954 letter[1] from a forty-nine-year-old trans woman Carla Erskine (pseudonym) to the German-born American endocrinologist Harry Benjamin, who had helped advise and treat her before and after her gender-affirming surgery at the University of California San Francisco in December 1953.[2] Between 1953 and 1956, Benjamin and Erskine exchanged close to one hundred letters, discussing every detail of her physical transformation and her relationships with other *transvestites* (the term she generally used) in California. She was friends with Louise Lawrence, known to historians as a central figure in the network of trans individuals in 1950s America.[3] The two of them were part of a close-knit group in the San Francisco Bay area, and they cooperated with Benjamin to find research subjects for Alfred Kinsey's planned book about transsexuality—a project interrupted by his death from a heart ailment and pneumonia in 1956.[4] Unlike Christine Jorgensen, who became a media sensation in late 1952 after her gender-affirming treatment in Copenhagen, Erskine purposely and successfully preserved her anonymity. She was one of very few transgender Americans to have procured surgery—some in the United States, but most abroad—in defiance of the rulings of state and district attorneys (in states like Wisconsin and California),[5] who relied on an obscure British common-law statute meant to prevent the self-maiming of soldiers by describing surgery on healthy tissue as "mayhem."[6] Erskine's desperation led her to take matters into her own hands—autocastration with a sharp knife—an act that ultimately eased her path to receiving reconstructive genital surgery.[7] Although she saw herself as a pioneer, she had no interest in fame. Having just visited Lawrence and another trans friend in October 1954, Erskine wrote to Benjamin: "Couldn't the news paper [sic] have made a sensation of the meeting of the three of us? If they'd have known. As near as we can figure we almost had a quorum. 3 out of 9 in the U.S. as near as we could think."[8]

Erskine later became a professional photographer, but she had no intention of sharing the stereoscopic slides that she took of her trans friends with the press. Hoping to help Benjamin and Kinsey with their collaborative effort to better understand what they were most commonly calling *transvestism*, Erskine sent her slides to Benjamin. It was the discovery of these beautifully evocative slides in a box of vacation photos in the Benjamin Collection at the Kinsey Institute that provided part of the inspiration for the exhibition *TransTrans*, which I (Annette Timm) curated with Michael Thomas Taylor and Rainer Herrn at the Nickle Galleries at the University of Calgary in spring 2016. The images led to Erskine—and Erskine, her friends, and their predecessors have much to tell us about the intimate, personal networks that provided the foundation for knowledge about trans identities and their medicalized definitions in the United States and Europe in the mid-twentieth century.

Erskine was one of Benjamin's first trans research subjects and a key source for his 1966 book *The Transsexual Phenomenon,* the book that would solidify his reputation as one of the foremost researchers of what we would today call transgender or trans identity. The distanced, medicalized, and sometimes judgmental tone of his book belies the warmth and understanding exhibited in Benjamin's correspondence with his trans patients. It is difficult to gaze on the photos of genitals or read the harsh captions describing individual self-presentation in Benjamin's book without feeling that his research subjects had been exploited or unwillingly placed in biological categories of someone else's devising. The title of the book alone is probably enough to raise the suspicions of readers who are today much more sensitive about terminology and to the necessity of allowing trans individuals to speak for themselves.[9] However, despite the depersonalized tone typical of 1960s medical writing, Benjamin's book and Kinsey's research must be understood as the culmination of a long history of trans people advocating for themselves and demanding help from medical science. Rather than focusing only on what these experts said about their subjects, we need to go behind the scenes of the texts themselves and ask what trans individuals *taught* medical researchers. What did Benjamin—and through him Kinsey—learn from Erskine and her friends? How did strategies for gathering information about trans identities arise from these relationships, which were by no means as clinical as the era's medicalized descriptions and taxonomies might suggest? In what follows, we will provide some justification for the argument that intimate and personal networks have always been a key feature of trans history.

Perhaps no other relationship better exemplifies how trans individuals themselves accelerated the learning curve for medical experts than that between Erskine and Benjamin. In an active correspondence of at least four years in the early 1950s, Erskine wrote to Benjamin with increasing trust but also with measured insistence that she be understood as a complete and rational human being. Benjamin wrote back somewhat more concisely but also with a degree of personal concern and engagement that exceeded the boundaries of most doctor–patient relationships. There are breaks in the correspondence during the summers, when Benjamin lived at the Hotel Sir Francis Drake in San Francisco and met with his Californian patients in person. For this reason, we do not have any letters discussing Erskine's self-performed orchiectomy in August 1953 since Benjamin would have seen her in San Francisco. When they picked up threads of correspondence in the fall, Erskine not only informed him of medical issues but also reported on the complex relationships between her and the close circle of friends around Lawrence.

Like Lawrence, Erskine viewed herself as "doing missionary work for our cause." She described how happy she was to speak to the "psychiatric interns [who] sometimes become well known and prominent psychiatrists" and who had flocked to her bedside after her 1953 surgery. "The more medical people sympathetically interested in transvestism the better," she wrote to Benjamin in 1954.[10] She regularly offered (through Benjamin) to put Kinsey in touch with any "transvestites" she had met,[11] and she even considered the idea of compiling a scrapbook (like the one Lawrence was working on for Kinsey) with which she hoped to be able to "furnish a small hit towards the understanding and acceptance of this problem."[12] But Erskine soon realized fame was not for her. "I see nothing in publicity for me except trouble," she wrote.[13]

On December 30, 1953, while recovering from the gender-affirming genital surgery that she received at the University of California Hospital, Erskine wrote to Benjamin complaining that "the newspapers have somehow got hold of the fact that I have had this surgery."[14] The gossip columnist Herb Caen tried to acquire information from Erskine's surgeon, Frank Hinman Jr., but Hinman quashed this effort, drawing on his influence in the larger medical community to convince him and other muckrakers to back off. In Erskine's words, Hinman argued it "was not to the best interests of medicine, the public or myself to publish and that this case was not enough like Christine's to have sensational news value," by which she likely meant that unlike Jorgensen, Erskine had no intention of becoming famous.[15] The resulting article was thus typically titillating but mercifully brief, with incorrect initials (for which Erskine thanked Hinman) and no promise of future information: "Medical Insidem: A successful "Christine-type" operation has been performed on a man (initials L. C.) at U. C. Hospital by one of the town's topmost surgeons, who wants anonymity. The transformed male is now living as a woman in Redwood City. 'A much truer case than Christine's' is all the doctor will say."[16] Since Erskine's story has remained hidden, Hinman's efforts to maintain confidentiality seem to have had a lasting effect. I suspect (but have been unable to verify) that her ability to keep her story a secret rested on personal relationships with Caen and other newspaper columnists.[17]

All trans people faced the decision about whether to seek publicity and the logistics necessary to avoid becoming the unwilling recipient of public attention, and in the United States, all trans people in this period lived under the cloud and glow of Jorgensen's fame. While some were eager to achieve something similar, they also knew publicity would make it impossible to lead the normal life that most trans people sought. Having first met Jorgensen through Lawrence in the spring of 1954, Erskine had enormous respect for Jorgensen's success and influence on public opinion. "She's changing public opinion greatly,"[18] Erskine wrote to Benjamin, and she was impressed that despite some "false polish" gained from a career in show business, Jorgensen was not being spoiled by fame and was generally having a salutary effect on their cause to garner public acceptance for sexual transition.[19] But Erskine was not a performer, and she realized that any publicity would destroy her plans to work as a nurse.[20] She was devastated when she lost a nursing job for no apparent reason, strongly (and realistically) suspecting that the secret of her past life had been exposed.[21]

Benjamin evaluated Erskine as an entirely rational person, unlike some of the other trans people he and Kinsey interviewed, who they assessed as unstable. In the tables of his trans patients, Benjamin categorized Erskine's "psychological health" as "very good," which placed her just below a few others, whom he described as being in "excellent" psychological health, but above the majority of his patients, whose health he described as "poor," "doubtful," "fair," or just "satisfactory." Despite Benjamin's general support for Erskine's view that seeking fame was not advisable, by the time he was compiling the data for his 1966 book, he accepted that even trans women who became entertainers, such as Jorgensen and Aleshia Crenshaw (who later became a successful—passing—actress under the name Aleshia Brevard) could be described as being in "excellent" psychological health.[22] But in the 1950s, Benjamin and Kinsey seemed particularly suspicious of those seeking fame, and they were more likely to link psychological health with some kind of respectable employment. Although Erskine's difficulty in keeping a full-time job and that she frequently complained to Benjamin about her money problems and her inability to budget likely contributed to his slight downgrading of her psychological health,[23] her desire to remain a private person met with his approval.

This desire for secrecy and privacy gives the historian—in other words me, the person reading and writing about Erskine's private correspondence—pause. I hope this enterprise is ethically justified as being the kind of enlightenment that Erskine sought. Perhaps detailing her story decades after her 1976 death will inspire those still struggling with obstacles to social and medical transition to find the courage to reveal to cisgender readers how these stories also affect them. The history of how Erskine came to receive treatment and how she was treated by medical science is both heartening and troubling. It is only by being precise about the details that we can understand how far we have come and how far we still have to go in honoring individuals' own sense of sexual and gender identity. That said, I will spend some time exploring the more intimate details of Erskine's life and her correspondence with Benjamin.

In the nine-page autobiography that Erskine composed for Benjamin, she outlined a troubled childhood and a difficult young adulthood.[24] In this document, she cited her birthdate as January 13, 1910, but census data (and subsequent pronouncements of her age) make it clear that she was actually born in 1905 in Casper, Wyoming.[25] Having been born with a genital anomaly (Benjamin later diagnosed this as *hypospadias*),[26] she was initially raised as a girl. Benjamin's diagnosis conflicts with the decision of the doctor who attended her birth to tell Erskine's parents that she should be raised as a girl. It also complicates our assessment of whether the baby would today be classified as intersex. We must therefore be careful not to discount this possibility since the tendency to erase the history of intersex people remains strong.[27] There is conflicting evidence about what Erskine herself thought. She consistently called herself a transvestite, but she also described the female physical characteristics that were present long before she received any hormonal treatment. Of her time serving in the navy during World War II, she said "Heavens knows [sic] my breasts were larger then than now."[28] Erskine grew up convinced she was a girl, and by the time she reached her fifties, she was calling herself a transvestite and was desperate to erase all signs of maleness from her body. In some sense, her story provides us with emotional insight for two experiences: that of an intersex child who was lied to about her body and that of a trans person who was eager to receive medical help to live authentically in her experienced gender. Erskine could only use the words available to her to express the various ruptures in her sexual and gender identity, underlining the importance of historically contextualizing all terminology related to the trans and intersex experience.[29]

At some point in her childhood (the timing is unclear), an accident on a staircase prompted her parents to take her to a doctor, who informed them that their little girl was in fact a boy. The doctor performed (unspecified) surgery. This event led to a traumatic deterioration of her relationship with her parents, particularly her mother, who seemed to think she now had a "monster" in her home. Erskine fled the family home and made her way to Galveston, Texas.[30] Working as a sailor for two years, she lived for a time in Tahiti and then made her way back to the United States "on an Australian cattle boat," arriving in San Francisco in July 1925. After landing a temporary job playing the cornet with the Ringling Brothers circus, she "decided to try to live as a girl" and fled to Mexico City, where she took the name Marie Ciel Campbell. Although she did not explicitly state this in her autobiography for Benjamin, it is likely that she chose Mexico for legal reasons. As sociology professor Clare Sears has documented, San Francisco and many other American cities where she might have been accepted by other trans women had passed laws against cross-dressing in the late nineteenth and early twentieth centuries. Fearing her ability to pass as a woman under the constant threat of police attention would have made Mexico a much more comfortable place for her to live.[31] She did successfully pass as a woman in Mexico City, even entertaining a proposal of marriage, until she was discovered by "a pawing drunk"[32] and fled back to the United States to avoid humiliation.

She moved to Milwaukee, where a brief marriage to a woman named Ruth ended in frustration despite the birth of a son. "God knows I tried to be a man," Erskine writes, "but even my best tries ended in embarrassment. Still when Jack was born I thought that perhaps I had succeeded once at least." (She later discovered she had always been sterile and could not have been Jack's father.) Ruth's alcoholism and serial adultery, but particularly her tendency to proclaim Erskine's sexual shortcomings loud enough for the neighbours to hear, led Erskine to divorce and move to California. Erskine then served in the US Navy between 1941 and 1943, where her "physical abnormalities," particularly her breasts, were overlooked, but where her preexisting and ongoing morphine addiction was discovered, leading to her discharge for fraudulent enlistment. Two brief relationships (with a more sexually tolerant woman and an apparently asexual man) were followed by suicide attempts and the eventual decision to medically affirm her feminine identity:

> Due to the facts of my birth and the upbringing and due to the development of my breasts and due to the lack of body hair and the female pattern of its distribution and due to my narrow shoulders and small bones, I have always thought that there was more wrong with me than just sexual impotence and I made up my mind that if this were the case and in the same category, I would find out and if possible I would have this done. It seemed that if it were a possibility it would open up life itself again to me.[33]

But Erskine's search for medical help was frustrated by doctors' reticence to undertake such a transition so late in life.

In 1953, she decided to take matters into her own hands. On August 19, 1953, the *San Francisco Examiner* reported on Erskine's desperate act under the headline "Sex Operation on Self Fails":

> The case of a Half Moon Bay man who masueraded [sic] for six weeks as a female nursing home attendant and performed a crude operation to change his sex was disclosed yesterday by Sheriff Earl Whitmore. The man, who gave his name as [Carla Erskine], 43,

attempted vainly to emasculate himself last Saturday. He explained to Palo Alto hospital attendants that "I wanted to be like Christine." He was treated for shock and loss of blood, and was released Monday, Whitmore said. Erskine, a former fisherman who declined to give his male forename, had worked for the past six weeks as a domestic in a Menlo Park home for elderly persons. An official of the home commented last night that "[Erskine] no longer is with us."[34]

Luckily for Erskine, the article did not ignite the flurry of press attention that she so feared. But her self-surgery was certainly known in the trans circles of the day.[35] She later tried to dissuade others from following her example and refused their requests to help them do so on the grounds that she almost bled to death.[36]

Erskine met Benjamin soon after this event. He would have been in California for his summer sojourn and, given that he kept a close watch on any newspaper articles about trans people, it is possible the *San Francisco Examiner* article motivated the contact and that it was Benjamin who introduced Erskine to Lawrence. Erskine's correspondence with Benjamin begins on July 1, 1953, with a mention of their meeting at Lawrence's house; it also included her exact physical measurements, demonstrating Erskine's desire to be both Benjamin's patient and his research subject.[37] Her case clearly influenced Benjamin, who later prided himself on being able to prevent "attempts at suicide or self-mutilation" through hormonal treatment and sympathy. He must have been referring to Erskine with these words, and he noted in the introduction to Richard Green and John Money's book *Transsexualism and Sex Reassignment* that the "few instances of attempted self-castration by definitely non-psychotic individuals impressed me greatly. Their desperation as well as the entire clinical history with their vain search for help, often from childhood on, made me realize that the medical profession truly treated these patients as 'stepchildren.'"[38]

Benjamin also repeatedly told Erskine that her case was different from others. "Yours is as unsimilar as can be" from the Jorgensen case, he told Erskine when they were discussing the Caen article about her surgery.[39] It is difficult to tell exactly what he meant by this assertion. He clearly did not believe Erskine was intersex, because he refused her request to describe her as a "pseudo-hermaphrodite" to patch up relations with her son, who could not accept her transition. Benjamin demurred, noting that one would have to add the term *psychic* to the term *pseudo-hermaphrodite* and that this "would be a very controversial diagnosis. You have had undescended testicles for which you were operated. They were then in a normal position, but not capable of forming sperm cells."[40] Erskine pushed back: "I think this [using the word *pseudo-hermaphrodite*] would be no falsehood, and it would settle questions in an uninformed and somewhat immature mind that he couldn't possibly understand otherwise—I realize my own condition perfectly but to quite some few people who have to know of this change, the idea of hermaphroditeism [sic] is easier to explain and understand than is transvestism."[41] By this time, the diagnosis of "intersexuality" (which was listed on Erskine's hospital admitting form in December 1953 and which she found "interesting terminology") had disappeared from the discussion.[42] Since the relationship with her son was permanently broken (there is no evidence that he ever wrote to Benjamin), we cannot know what Erskine decided to tell him.

There is also great uncertainty about how Erskine represented herself to nonmedical professionals. Even before her surgery, she volunteered to speak to the San Francisco branch of the Mattachine Society, a gay rights organization that had been founded in 1950 in Los Angeles. This choice was yet another indication of her desire to educate more tolerant portions of the public. Her talk was promoted with the following flyer, distributed only to members:

We have made special arrangements to have a true transvestite give a prepared lecture on this most interesting topic entitled:

WHAT IS TRANSVESTISM?

Our speaker has a fascinating story to tell, and we want you all to be there to enjoy this delightful personality. This talk will go into detail and be most revealing, not only from a physical but also from a historical standpoint, citing famous cases from history.

The meeting is under direction of Mac and will be held at: 516–55th Street, Oakland, Apt. B. on Thursday evening, December 10, at 8 PM.[43]

Erskine reported to Benjamin that the talk was well received and that she repeated it at least one other time, but sadly, she did not take him up on his offer to have it transcribed and published in the *International Journal of Sexology*, the journal in which Benjamin was to publish what he claimed was the "very first medical article on transsexualism."[44] Given the usage of the day, the language ("true transvestite") suggests Erskine was representing herself as someone who had been male but was transitioning to female. Leaving aside her congenital malformations and even her own physical self-description as having "more wrong with me than just sexual impotence,"[45] I believe that this is the way that we should describe and understand her. Erskine's friends also clearly understood her to be a male-to-female transsexual (though they did not use this terminology until later).

As I have mentioned, Erskine and her friends thought of themselves as a small group of pioneers. They openly compared surgeries,[46] and they communicated with other trans individuals across the world to discuss their social, medical, and cultural struggles.[47]

Some of these relationships ended in heartache. Erskine told Benjamin of her bafflement that two of her trans friends, Angela D. and Judy S. (pictured in Figure 7.1) had stopped speaking to her, and she was suspicious that they

Figure 7.1 Erskine sent this portrait to Benjamin for his "transvestite" files in the fall of 1954. From back row: Angela D., Lawrence, Judy S., Erskine. *Source*: Photo by Alvin Harris. Copyright © 2017, The Trustees of Indiana University on behalf of the Kinsey Institute. All rights reserved.

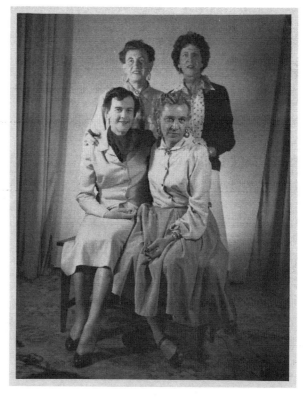

might have broken off the relationship to profit from their collaboratively developed idea to invent a new epilator.[48] Despite these disappointments, Erskine and Lawrence were constantly on the lookout for other trans women to refer to Benjamin and Kinsey. In some cases, this led them to individuals who were trying to emulate Jorgensen's path to fame. Erskine told Benjamin that she and her friends debated and ultimately rejected the idea of contacting Bunny Breckenridge. Breckenridge was a troubled actor and millionaire; his 1954 announcement that he planned to undergo a sex-change operation in Denmark appears to have been nothing but a publicity stunt, and he later served time in prison for committing "perverse acts" with two young boys.[49] Erskine quickly sensed Breckenridge's deception, calling him a "publicity seeking dilettante."[50] She had a much longer relationship with another troubled soul, Dixie MacLane, whom historian Susan Stryker describes as "a burlesque performer [who] tried to ride the wave of publicity about her surgery," succeeding to some small degree in the 1950s.[51] Erskine's letters to Benjamin detail her growing frustration with MacLane's emotionally demanding personality and desire for publicity. Benjamin described MacLane as "emotionally deeply unbalanced," and therefore unlikely to be able to obtain surgery.[52] Erskine complained that MacLane was "blowing her cork all over the place," threatening suicide, and displaying too much faith in the ability of surgery to transform personality. "She expects to be a woman and when she finds that the only thing gained will be the dubious legal right to dress in female attire, I am afraid for her."[53] Erskine broke off the friendship when MacLane forwarded her letters and those of Lawrence to a psychiatrist, Dr. Frederik Hartsuiker, in the Netherlands.[54]

Another incident that contributed to the breakup with MacLane involved the police, and it makes it clear just how important passing was for trans women in 1950s California. Having traveled to Los Angeles in the spring of 1955 for psychiatric testing with Frederic G. Wordon at the University of California Medical Center in Los Angeles, Erskine was apprehended by officers from the Los Angeles Police Department, an experience for which she blamed MacLane:

> As usual when I come in direct contact with Dixie, I got mad at her and, as usual about her ideas on publicity she expects and hopes to get when she gets home. I think it was because of the company I kept in Los Angeles (Dixie and [Karen] sure look "queen" letting their hair grow out etc.), but when they met me at the station a plain clothesman cornered me and told me he thought I was masquerading. I told him lets [sic] go to police Doctor and settle question [sic], which we did. Took only one minute and I was appologized

[*sic*] to an [*sic*] politely excorted [*sic*] to my hotel in style. The policeman wanted to be sure that I had no hard feelings as he said he was only doing his job—and that the two people (Dixie and [Karen]) who met me at the station were known homosexuals and because of my heighth [*sic*] and rather deep voice the "mistake" was an easy one to make. So everything ended nicely and this little episode has probably done a great deal to reassure me. I wonder if Dr. Kinsey might like a report of this incident? And I wonder if a written statement from you or Dr. Hinman might not save trouble and a bit of embarrassment if such an occasion should arise again. What do you think?[55]

In post–World War II Los Angeles, moral authorities viewed cross-dressing as a provocation that threatened the city's reputation and contributed to a cosmopolitanism that they viewed as threatening. As the collectively authored book *Lavender Los Angeles* explains, the Los Angeles Police Department therefore "relentlessly cracked down on LGBT expression . . . [They] raided gay bars, entrapped gay men, and arrested LGBT people who cross-dressed."[56] As Erskine's description of this episode demonstrates, trans people craved medical protection from this harassment (they would have been thrilled to have access to the kind of medical authorization that Magnus Hirschfeld's "transvestite passes," described in chapter 3, provided), and they quickly recognized genital surgery could offer some security. The tone of Erskine's letter to Benjamin and her concern about how MacLane and her other trans friend Karen might be endangering her cause by appearing disreputable in public makes it clear that she was desperately trying to appear deserving of medical treatment in Benjamin's eyes.

Another area of concern for trans patients was how their sex lives might be assessed by clinicians. Erskine told Benjamin that she thought MacLane was unsuitable for surgery because her friend "has and enjoys some kind of sex life and . . . would be very unhappy to give this up even tho [*sic*] she thinks it doesn't mean much to her now."[57] This one sentence hints at a sensitive subject that is rarely explicitly mentioned in their correspondence, perhaps for fear that it might fall into the wrong hands but likely also because of an awareness that stress on erotic desire could only harm the cause of increasing tolerance for transitioning individuals. Well into the 1990s, it was common for trans advocates to try to silence any discussion of erotic desire to avoid awakening a moral backlash.[58] During the 1950s, Benjamin was still describing trans women—people he was then calling "transsexualists"—as "the most disturbed group of male transvestites."[59] He thought their sexuality was largely "non-genital" and that the creation of an artificial vagina could aid the sexual satisfaction only of their male partners.[60] But he was also beginning to create a distinction between transvestites and transsexualists—the former, he insisted, derived sexual pleasure from their genitals, while the latter viewed these body parts with disgust.[61] This background, and the likelihood that Erskine and Benjamin discussed these theories, provides an additional twist to Benjamin's argument that Erskine was unlike Jorgensen and MacLane. There were clearly tensions surrounding trans eroticism during this era.

Sociology professor Richard Ekins has meticulously detailed how Benjamin's advocacy—his understanding of the "art of the possible"—led him to transform an early acceptance of human sexual variety (with Hirschfeldian undertones) into a more heteronormative categorization of surgery as a path to "normal" gender relations.[62] But this analysis crucially leaves out the influence of Kinsey and (more understandably) the sexual inclinations of those investigating trans lives. It is instructive that during a brief marriage to a heterosexual man, Erskine wrote to Benjamin about her surprise that she was achieving sexual satisfaction and was proud to be satisfying her husband, even without a vagina. She asked Benjamin to report on this experience to Kinsey.[63] She must have known that Kinsey initially disapproved of surgical intervention to remove the penis because he could not imagine why anyone would want to remove an organ of such orgiastic potential. This obsession with counting orgasms has not escaped the notice of those who have analyzed Kinsey's *Male* and *Female* books.[64] He defined sexuality as the potentially unlimited capacity for sexual release or "outlet"—a potential on whose fulfilment culture and society only acted as negative forces in the form of moral prescription and repression. But his own repressed childhood (his father railed against masturbation) and troubled early marriage (he and his wife needed medical advice to consummate their marriage) probably contributed to his valorization of the male orgasm as the most obvious (not to mention countable) manifestation of human sexual capacity.[65] These preconceptions were likely the origin of his initial reluctance to accept the existence of transgender individuals, especially because he (and initially Benjamin) assumed that the desire to change one's sex was an almost exclusively "male" (that is, male-to-female) phenomenon.

Kinsey's own sex life has been the subject of much fascination and was a key theme of the 2005 film about his life directed by Bill Condon. Benjamin has yet to receive the same biographical treatment, and we have only hints about how his own sexual practice might have influenced his views of the sexual lives of his trans patients. Aside from the discussions of nightlife that I have already mentioned, I have found only one cryptic yet revealing note from Benjamin to Kinsey that seems to be a description of sexual activity: "Did I tell you I have trouble with my girl?" Benjamin wrote in September 1951. "She has just reached the age of consent, and now she starts refusing. Any advice?"[66] We cannot know what Benjamin might have meant, and what appears to be an allusion to sex with an underage partner is certainly disturbing. There is also a hint in one of the interviews that Stryker conducted with Crenshaw that Benjamin might have had extramarital sexual relationships. Crenshaw, who began her transition as a female impersonator at Finoccio's bar in San Francisco,[67] describes herself as becoming one of Benjamin's "girls." Crenshaw met with Benjamin soon after receiving a diagnosis that would later allow her to have surgery. (From her biography, we can glean that she met Benjamin in 1958 and had surgery in 1962.) Crenshaw told Stryker that Benjamin "added me to his little list. You know how there are RGs—real girls? Well he always said there were RGs, and His—his girls."[68] Benjamin, Crenshaw noted to Stryker's nonsurprise, "had his own quirks. . . . He had a fetish for very thin girls with very long hair. He had a hair fetish. So that was his quirk." Stryker admitted to having heard this before, and Crenshaw responded with the reflection that "these are the sorts of things we don't want out. We try to build a mystique about transsexuals. I guess it's time to let the truth be out there though."[69] It is understandable that Benjamin's mystique has lasted this long, given the incredible service he provided for so many desperate individuals. But in our era of increasing understanding of the incredible plasticity and variability of human sexual identity, it strikes me as illogical to continue to try to cleanly separate scientific understandings of sexuality from the researcher's own emotional responses.

Everything I have said so far about the close personal relationship Erskine and Benjamin cultivated after 1953 helps us read the images that we displayed in the two iterations of the exhibition *TransTrans* in 2016 and 2019–2020. Between 1953 and 1955, Erskine sent Benjamin stereoscopic slides of her friends, most of whom were sitting on a couch in Lawrence's living room. This aspect of her "missionary work" was so important to her that she prioritized developing and mailing the slides despite a near-constant state of poverty.[70]

She and her friends hoped these photographs would portray their successful integration into everyday life. They wanted to convince Benjamin and Kinsey that their desires were valid and that medical intervention could be successful. Erskine's devotion to the cause of scientific inquiry is evident because she gave Benjamin permission to use her images to foster knowledge about transsexuality, including her willingness to have nude pictures of herself published in Benjamin's 1966 book (though Benjamin anonymized her and placed a black box over her eyes).[71] I would argue that the intrusion into Erskine's private life that republishing these pictures represents is justified by the fact that it helps us understand how adamantly Erskine and her friends tried to convince Benjamin of their own "normality." The slides from Louise's couch call out for us to accept the normality of those photographed. The images are personal, playful, and intimate, and they express the joy of transformation and personal fulfilment.

But it must also be said that the images are not professional quality portraits. Erskine's attempt to make a living with a portrait studio lasted a little over a year, collapsing in December 1955.[72] She had already been complaining to Benjamin about her renewed financial difficulties and how she had been thinking of making:

> a large selection of photomicrographs of biological specimens [from the oceanside near her home] and purvey them to the educational system as aids to teaching. . . . I have given up trying to conduct business for myself as I know from past experience that Im [sic] not able to manage the sales and business management end of it. . . . It always comes back to this basic problem, that I do not understand financial affairs and am not capable in realizing [sic] on my work. So here I am sitting with a brand new and beautiful life and dont [sic] know what to do about it. I am in a rut and life is passing me by. How does one break out of a rut?[73]

I have made several efforts to discover precisely the details of Erskine's "beautiful life" but have only been able to find a few tantalizing hints about how she turned this interest in microphotography into a successful career. In November 1972, Caen, the San Francisco gossip columnist who had first encountered Erskine when he wrote about her self-surgery in 1953, asked his readers: "You know the Avenue Theatre on San Bruno Avenue, which plays silent movies? Well, [Carla Erskine], who made her fortune in electronics, bought it because she's mad for that big organ. Quite a woman is [Carla]; not only does she own a gullwing Mercedes and a white Rolls, she just qualified—at age 68!—to fly solo in her Skyhawk plane."[74] From this, we can gather that

Erskine became wealthy in the decade after she stopped writing to Benjamin. "She came to the rescue," Vernon Gregory, the owner of Avenue Theatre told *Oakland Tribune* reporter Elinor Hayes in July 1969. "She is a living genius who has made a fortune in her own electronic business and has installed an organ in her home."[75]

How did she achieve this dramatic reversal in her economic fortunes? The details have been difficult to determine. The only extended description of her life that I have been able to uncover is in a blog post written by the plastic surgeon Donald R. Laub. On his website, "Many People, Many Passports," Laub provides entertaining stories about his illustrious career as a plastic surgeon in California. He served as the chief of plastic surgery at Stanford University School of Medicine between 1968 and 1980, and he was the founder of Interplast (now called ReSurge International), an international charity providing life-changing operations for people in countries too poor to offer such services. The entry about Clair Elgin (a slight misspelling of another name Erskine used) makes it clear that despite a few vaguely recalled details of personal history, Laub did indeed meet Erskine in 1963. She required surgery for a hernia, and she asked Laub, the still aspiring plastic surgeon, to "get that tattoo aligned exactly right when you do the suturing."[76] Laub later performed transgender surgeries himself,[77] and in his blog, he describes how this early encounter began a long-term friendship and collaboration with Erskine. Sadly, by the time I tracked down this story, I was told by a former secretary of Laub's that he was suffering from brain cancer, so I was unable to interview him.

Erskine had eventually found a new career. As Laub put it in his blog: "during the birth of Silicon Valley she was able to make microphotography negatives of the plans for a computer chip; the manufacturing process utilized silver salts in the negatives of her microphotos to etch silicon into chips." Having received shares in "one of the more prominent laser and computer companies in Silicon Valley," she had been able to build a beautiful Japanese-style home in the hills of Los Altos. Laub later encouraged her to invent three-dimensional television (which she apparently did), and when her personal nurse, a man with whom she lived in an apparently platonic relationship, told him that she was becoming depressed in retirement, Laub employed Erskine as a photographer for Interplast. By the 1970s, she was "worth several million" and had donated a large sum to Laub's research.[78] Sadly, in 1976, Erskine was diagnosed with metastatic cancer of the rib—a recurrence of a previous bout with lung cancer. On hearing that she likely had only six weeks to live,

Erskine asked the young medical student who had delivered the news to hand over her purse. She then swallowed the cyanide capsules that she had brought with her to the hospital and died twenty-four hours later.

I tell this story, despite being unable to confirm some of the details, because the letters to Benjamin trail off in 1955, leaving the impression that Erskine might not have been achieving a successful personal and professional life. (In his book, Benjamin misleadingly reproduces a picture of her working in a short-lived nursing job, although he certainly knew that she had become a "chemical" photographer by 1965.)[79] Laub's obvious affection for Erskine, and his sadness-filled respect for her decision to end her life, makes it clear that she had found peace. She had, writes Laub, "display[ed] more wisdom than any of us, perhaps abandoning her beautifully ornamented body. She may have elected not to try another life. [Carla] was a friend. Not in the sense of a friend I considered 'close' or a friend I would ask to dinner or a friend I would introduce at a party, but as a friend who was a co-worker, a valuable and essential member of the team, and therefore, an extension of myself."[80] It was only when he wrote this blog entry thirty years later that Laub forgave the medical student for being so rashly honest in providing Erskine with her cancer prognosis. In other words, she had continued to establish intimate networks of knowledge to the end of her life and beyond.

PART 2: WHAT ABOUT THE BOYS?

Exploring the history of Benjamin and Kinsey's work with trans women and the way that both thought of themselves as the pioneers of trans research can easily make it seem as if trans men were completely invisible or absent during this era. They were neither, but their stories have been more difficult to uncover, because doctors in the United States did not begin taking an interest in their medical care until the 1960s. The story of one man, Jude Patton, helps underline that trans men were not far behind trans women in establishing the kinds of connections to medical researchers that helped drive medical research and social tolerance forward.

Patton was adopted at seven months old. He was twelve years old, living with his mother and father in Alton, Illinois,[81] when Jorgensen made her 1952 debut before an American populace steeped in a Barnum & Bailey culture of sideshow freaks.[82] Patton's family had little money, and his father, a pipefitter, had a heart condition that kept him from working through much of Patton's childhood. His mother took on many jobs, including working for a year as a hairdresser, which was helpful when Patton saw Mary Martin's Peter Pan on national television in 1955 and begged his mother to cut his long hair to be like Peter's. His mother complied. Patton was five feet six inches tall, round-faced, and sweet looking, though he also appeared androgynous. He was shy, but he excelled in school. His smaller size and quiet demeanor masked a voracious appetite for learning, especially about anything having to do with animals, science, and nature. He even studied German for two years while in high school because of the language's association with scientific epistemology.

Patton was awarded an Illinois State scholarship upon graduation from high school in 1958, but he refused to go to college because he would be required to wear skirts and other feminine clothing. At age eighteen, he had had enough of that. Instead, he worked driving delivery trucks and in factories, eventually becoming a veterinary assistant, where he could wear masculine clothing, help animals, and continue to learn about science. He saw other masculine-appearing women around town, but he never initiated conversations with them. In those days, due to prejudice that associated homosexuality with pedophilia, adult lesbian, gay, or bisexual people avoided young people out of fear of being arrested. So, Patton kept to himself. He tried to earn money to help his parents and support his insatiable quest for knowledge, particularly information that would help him understand himself. He searched the local libraries for scientific literature about human sexuality. He assumed other masculine-appearing women felt the same way he did. He did not appreciate the variety of queer experience until he turned twenty-one and began frequenting bars in St. Louis, Missouri, where lesbians congregated.

In 1965, aware of the limitations he faced living in Alton, Illinois, Patton decided to move to Los Angeles, California, to join friends and look for work. He worked as a veterinary assistant for Bay Cities Dog and Cat Hospital in Venice, California. Soon thereafter, he was also offered the night attendant job at the clinic, which entitled him to live in an apartment on the premises. In 1966, he landed a position as a dog groomer at Personal Touch Grooming, owned and operated by an older couple, Henry and Lorraine Sudduth, both of whom took an immediate liking to Patton. In 1969, increased business necessitated a second groomer. The new employee—we'll call him D. F.[83]—took one look at Patton and told him about his sex change. Established circles of knowledge and intimacy were changing social mores, allowing such connections and the sharing of medical information, even at work.

D. F. told Patton that he had been one of the original six female-to-males at the Johns Hopkins clinic in 1965. He had been taking testosterone for several years, had undergone top surgery in Baltimore, and was hoping to have genital reconstruction with plastic surgeon Donald Laub, at Stanford University in Palo Alto. D. F. gave Patton a copy of Benjamin's book *The Transsexual Phenomenon* (which Patton devoured) and referred Patton to his endocrinologist, Gerald Leve, in Los Angeles. Patton began frequenting the university medical libraries in Los Angeles, trying to learn everything he could about transsexualism, gender, gender identity, and sexual expression. He started testosterone therapy in late 1970. Around this time, Patton also met another fellow, J. H., who planned to apply to the Stanford program for genital surgery. The three of them applied, and of the three, Patton was accepted first. Likely because of Patton's interest in medicine and willingness to share his warmth and humanity, he developed a strong and collegial rapport with Laub.

Benjamin included only one example of a transsexual man in his *The Transsexual Phenomenon*. He based his analysis of "female transsexualism" (as the condition was labeled at the time) on the twenty transmasculine patients he had seen in his career through 1964.[84] Trans men were thought to be rare, a tiny portion of the small minority of people who struggled with their gender identity, leading one prominent clinician and researcher, psychiatrist Ira B. Pauly, to postulate in 1968 that one in four hundred thousand females would identify as and seek treatment for transsexualism, while one in one hundred thousand males would do the same. Pauly wrote, "I have estimated that there are at least 2000 male and 500 female transsexuals in the United States."[85] Patton, who had started to meet more men like himself through the Stanford program, believed these estimates were low.

Patton underwent a series of four hospitalizations with Laub and his associates between September 1972 and September 1973, starting with chest reconstruction ("top surgery") and the first stage of phallus construction. In December 1972, he underwent top revision, a total hysterectomy, and an appendectomy, as well as further work on the phallus construction. In March 1973, Patton's surgeons completed his phallus construction, placed testicular implants, and performed a tummy tuck to remove excess abdominal tissue left from the phallus construction. Complications with the testicular implants necessitated a revision of that procedure in September 1973.

At Laub's request, Patton served in a caregiving role for other trans patients. He hosted one of Laub's patients from Denmark as he progressed through several surgeries, feeding him, tending to his postoperative care, and transporting him back and forth between Los Angeles and Palo Alto, driving over five hours each way. Throughout this period, Patton and Laub seized many opportunities to discuss various aspects of medical care for trans people.

In September 1973, Patton started taking classes at three different colleges. Based on his questions in class, his knowledge, and his willingness to discuss transsexualism, instructors began to invite him to speak on campus about his life and transition. Patton first spoke at a sociology class at California State University, Long Beach (CSULB) taught by Professor Howard Fradkin. Shortly thereafter, Fradkin introduced Patton to Bonnie Bullough, Dean of Nursing at CSULB and her husband Vern, an historian of medicine and sexuality professor at California State University at Northridge. The Bulloughs produced numerous books, including studies of homosexuality and cross-dressing. At CSULB, Patton also met sex therapists and researchers Bill Hartman and Marilyn Fithian ("the Masters and Johnson of the West Coast"[86]) who ran the Center for Sex Research in Long Beach, California. At that time, academic sexologists, as well as many psychiatrists, psychologists, and medical doctors, believed transsexuals were not fit to participate in the field; yet both couples and numerous professors encouraged Patton as a student, teacher, and investigator. They continued to refer him to other professors as a speaker and introduced him to the scientific literature and a broad cross-section of the community engaged in scientific sexual research.

Sexology attracted tremendous interest in the 1970s, and scholars examined virtually every subject through a sexological lens. The availability of the birth control pill in the 1960s and the legalization of abortion in 1973 made the idea of "free love" a mantra for many. Human sexuality–focused research and educational organizations proliferated across the country. The first, the Society for the Scientific Study of Sex, also known as Quad-S, was founded in 1957, with Benjamin among the six charter members. In 1964, Mary S. Calderone, a medical director at Planned Parenthood Federation of America, established the Sexuality Information and Education Council of the United States to focus on delivering accurate information about sexuality and sex education. In 1967, the American Association of Sex Educators, Counselors and Therapists was created. Sexologists, researchers, educators, and subject matter advocates from a wide range of professional disciplines across the country belonged to one or more of these associations, though trans-identified members were few and often closeted. Patton became certified as a sex educator and a sex therapist and was a member of all the professional sexuality associations, and at that time he was the only "out" trans man. Patton noticed that only Virginia Prince and Ariadne Kane were "out" as cross-dressers in academic and research circles during this period, belonging to some of the same professional groups. As more trans-identified individuals began to seek information or assistance with their transitions, many of the universities with programs in human sexuality launched "gender programs."[87]

In 1975, Laub organized the annual International Conference on Gender Identity, hosted for the first time in the United States at Stanford University. This and the previous three such conferences (all held in Europe) were supported by the Erickson Educational Foundation[88] for the purpose of bringing together surgeons, endocrinologists, psychiatrists, and psychologists who were interested in studying and working with transgender and gender-diverse people. Laub invited Patton to attend the meeting as his guest, which was a revolutionary step on Laub's part and could have earned him considerable censure had the other professionals known he had invited a "consumer" to a professional meeting. Patton wrote:

> I was simply thrilled to be invited by Dr. Laub to attend. At the time, I had very little college completed and felt very humble to be allowed to be present. The professionals attending were very knowledgeable. I did feel that most saw us as "mentally ill" and [they] objectified us, but [they also thought] that surgery was the "right" treatment for those they considered to be "true transsexuals." No one in the audience, except my treatment team, knew that I was trans. I did not speak up at all. I sat next to John Money during one of the [conference] days.[89]

Patton was confident he was the only trans person at the event.

Shortly after this conference, Patton began publishing *Renaissance News*, a quarterly newsletter intended to share medical and social information with other transsexual people. Similar support groups and newsletters, mostly for cisgender cross-dressing men, had begun to proliferate in urban areas throughout the United States, so with the help of his mother, Lillian, who served as a mother figure for attendees, Patton hosted one of the first such groups for trans men. During this period, Patton also met trans woman Joanna Clark, who later worked with him to create J2CP, an information service that took over the work of the Janus Information Facility in 1986.[90] Patton's community-creating and information-sharing efforts facilitated community among trans people and their providers.

In 1978, Patton completed a Bachelor of Art degree in social ecology at the University of California Irvine. In 1979, at the inauguration of the Harry Benjamin International Gender Dysphoria Association (HBIGDA) in San Diego,[91] Laub surprised everyone (including Patton) by nominating Patton for a seat on the new organization's board of directors. Many group members fiercely rejected the concept of a trans person as a full participant in their fledgling professional association. Ultimately, fourteen voted against and fourteen voted in favor of Patton's board membership; Laub cast the deciding vote, shattering the concrete ceiling restricting trans representation in professional organizations. Patton soon was appointed the HBIGDA board's Community Liaison.

Figure 7.2. Jude Patton (1940–) 2011. The photo was taken by Milton ("Mickey") Diamond, MD, at the World Professional Association for Transgender Health Biennial Scientific Symposium in Atlanta, Georgia. *Source*: Courtesy of Jude Patton.

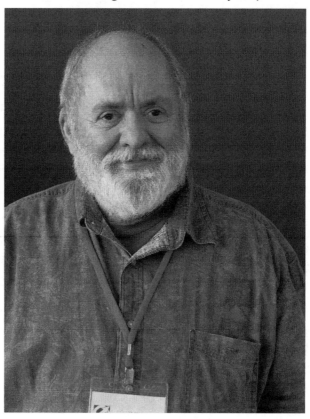

In 1980, Patton completed a Master of Arts degree in marriage and family therapy at Azusa Pacific University, and soon thereafter he became licensed to practice in that field. In 1982, Patton stopped publishing the *Renaissance News* because he began taking classes at the University of Southern California School of Medicine to become a physician assistant. Also in 1982, Patton joined with Clark, Diane Saunders, Joy Schaffer, Carol Katz, and Candice Brown in forming the first Transgender Rights Committee associated with the American Civil Liberties Union, Southern California.

In 1993, J2CP handed their source material for the Erickson pamphlets and other transsexual-related information over to Dallas Denny at the American Educational Gender Information Service. These efforts to sustain and increase information exchange were ultimately central to the development and growth of the transgender community in the 1990s. The collegial relationships between people like Reed Erickson;[92] Lou Sullivan; Rupert Raj of Toronto, Canada; and Patton—four very different yet pivotal individuals whose interests were broadly focused on education—were crucial to the advancement of the field of transgender medicine. Simultaneously, as seen in the example of Patton, trans people's efforts to penetrate the ranks of the medical community were just beginning—an important development as researchers and surgical innovators were building an institutional structure and medical approach around a controversial treatment.

CONCLUSION

The stories of Erskine and Patton make it clear that three aspects of trans history require more concentrated reflection than they have previously been accorded: international connections, personal (and even intimate) networks, and the sexual self-understandings and practices of the researchers and popularizers themselves. Historians have begun to insist that scholars attend to the way emotions and intimacy produce causal effects on trajectories of knowledge, political developments, and patterns of tolerance and prejudice.[93] Revealing intimate histories is not the same thing as voyeurism or sensationalism. Timm has alluded to the uncomfortable feelings she experienced while analyzing the intimate correspondence between doctors and patients, including the erotic and otherwise extremely private images that trans women in the 1950s shared with men like Benjamin and Kinsey—men in whom these individuals placed enormous faith and trust. Transgender and transsexual men have struggled with similar dilemmas in their attempts to validate their lives and their sexualities. As a trans man, co-author Jamison Green has also experienced the voyeurism and oversexualized interest of some researchers, particularly prior to the turn of the twenty-first century.

The ongoing social intolerance prevalent in many societies means that revealing intimate relationships or questioning the supposedly sterile and sometimes patronizing objectivity of scientific research may create unjustifiable risks for individuals. Yet secrets about sex or gender have never improved the lives of those persecuted for their desires and self-understandings. It has never truly helped anyone to act as if human sexual desire or subjective interpersonal relationships can be ignored without intensifying the mechanisms of repression.

We have tried to demonstrate that the respect Otto Spengler (see Chapter 3.2), Erskine, Lawrence, and others were accorded by scientists and medical practitioners like Benjamin, Kinsey, and Laub, as well as the varying degrees of happiness that these relationships produced, definitively overrules any objections that scientific objectivity was compromised when researchers took their trans patients' feelings seriously. The history of trans experience in Germany and the United States teaches us that intimate relationships are not necessarily inimical to scientific knowledge—provided these relationships are built on mutual respect and structured in ways that protect individual bodily integrity. Indeed, without the interpersonal trust that developed across the Atlantic over the course of several decades in the mid-twentieth century, the lives of trans people today would be immeasurably more difficult.

NOTES

1. Letter from Carla Erskine to Harry Benjamin, 22 January 1954, Kinsey Institute Library & Special Collections, Harry Benjamin Collection (hereafter KILSC-HB), Box 4, Ser. II C.

2. In this chapter, the authors describe the lives of two trans individuals who used their personal connections with sexologists and members of the transgender and gender-diverse community to lift the shroud of shame and misunderstanding that held trans people down. The first part of this chapter, focused on Carla Erskine, is written by Annette Timm and adapted by Jamison Green from Bakker et al., *Others of My Kind*; it is adapted here with the kind permission of the author and publisher. The second part, written by Green, introduces readers to the life and work of Jude Patton.

3. Lawrence's role as a pioneer was recently honored by the creation of an archive that carries her name—the Louise Lawrence Transgender Archive. The archive's website describes her "instrumental [work] in developing the trans community's connection to pioneering sex researchers such as Alfred Kinsey and Harry Benjamin." See https://lltransarchive.org/ (last accessed August 20, 2022) and chapter 7.1 in this volume.

4. Erskine describes her various friendships with Californian trans women in her letters to Benjamin. A letter to Benjamin in July 1953 makes it clear that they originally met at Lawrence's apartment in the early summer of 1953, likely at the beginning of his yearly sojourn in San Francisco. Erskine to Benjamin, 1 July 1953, KILSC-HB, Box 4, Ser. II C.

5. Erskine to Benjamin, 5 Oct 1954, KILSC-HB, Box 4, Ser. II C.

6. For a somewhat more detailed account of these rulings, see Meyerowitz, *How Sex Changed*, 47–48.

7. Erskine alludes to the fact that self-surgery had almost caused her to bleed to death in a letter to Benjamin on 5 Oct 1953, KILSC-HB, Box 4, Ser. II C.

8. Erskine was not including Louise Lawrence, who never underwent surgery. Erskine to Benjamin, 5 Oct 1954, KILSC-HB, Box 4, Ser. II C.

9. See Serano, *Whipping Girl*, 23–34. Serano provides a concise and sensitive discussion of debates over terminology that has influenced Dr. Timm's wording in this chapter.

10. Erskine to Benjamin, 4 Jan 1953, KILSC-HB, Box 4, Ser. II C.

11. Erskine to Benjamin, 18 Nov 1953, KILSC-HB, Box 4, Ser. II C.

12. Erskine to Benjamin, 9 May 1954, KILSC-HB, Box 4, Ser. II C.

13. Erskine to Benjamin, 19 Jan 1954, KILSC-HB, Box 4, Ser. II C.

14. Erskine to Benjamin, 19 Jan 1954, KILSC-HB, Box 4, Ser. II C.

15. Erskine to Benjamin, 10 Feb 1954, KILSC-HB, Box 4, Ser. II C.

16. Caen, "Baghdad-by-the-Bay," *San Francisco Chronicle*, n.d.

17. It seems otherwise inexplicable that Erskine's name would appear in San Francisco gossip columns years later, with no reference to her gender. See Caen, San Francisco: Herb Caen, November 18, 1972 (a syndicated column) and Rosenbaum, "Our Man on the Town."

18. Erskine to Benjamin, 18 Nov 1953, KILSC-HB, Box 4, Ser. II C.

19. Erskine to Benjamin, 3 Apr 1954, KILSC-HB, Box 4, Ser. II C.

20. Erskine to Benjamin, 22 Jan 1954, KILSC-HB, Box 4, Ser. II C.

21. Erskine to Benjamin, 15 May 1954, KILSC-HB, Box 4, Ser. II C.

22. Benjamin's notes in preparation for writing *The Transsexual Phenomenon*. See various copies of this table in KILSC-HB, Box 28 Series VI E. To Series VI. G.

23. See, for example, Erskine to Benjamin, 3 Dec 1953, KILSC-HB, Box 4, Ser. II C.

24. Typewritten document, titled only with "[Erskine], 1953," KILSC-HB, Box 4, Ser. II C.

25. Erskine apparently told Laub (a former doctor and later friend) she was born in "Arabia," but I have found no reliable confirmation of this fact. See Laub, "The Clair Elgin Story."

26. Benjamin, *The Transsexual Phenomenon*, 52. Based on his medical and personal relationship with Erskine, Laub diagnoses her as having had "grade 3 hypospadias, a birth defect in which the urine comes out just above the scrotum." Laub, "The Clair Elgin Story."

27. On the history of intersex and the ethics of speaking about it today, see Dreger, *Intersex in the Age of Ethics*; Dreger, *Hermaphrodites and the Medical Invention of Sex*; Reis, "Divergence or Disorder?"; Reis, *Bodies in Doubt*; Eder, The Volatility of Sex; and Davis, *Contesting Intersex*.

28. "[Carla Erskine], 1953," KILSC-HB, Box 4, Ser. II C.

29. See Davis, *Beyond Trans*. It also adds some fuel to current arguments that our obsession with gender classification in daily life has caused nothing but pain.

30. She claims that this occurred in 1923, which would have made her only thirteen had the birthdate of 1910 been correct. Given that she was really born in 1905, it seems more plausible that she would have run away at the age of eighteen.

31. See Sears, *Arresting Dress*. In a newspaper interview, Sears notes that these laws were primarily passed in frontier towns keen to attract newcomers by projecting a respectable image. This motivated a crackdown on prostitution that affected cross-dressers since "for a woman to dress as a man in some way communicated to other people that she was more adventurous, more sexually available." Tagawa, "When Crossdressing Was Criminal."

32. As a reminder, these quotations come from the autobiography Erskine wrote for Benjamin (see note 17).

33. See note 17.

34. *San Francisco Examiner*, "Sex Operation on Self Fails," 8. Census data tell me she was actually 48 at the time of this article, but she had begun lying about her age, perhaps to improve her chances of acquiring surgery.

35. In an interview with Stryker, Don Lucas (a founding member of the San Francisco chapter of the Mattachine Society), names Erskine as one of at least two individuals who had performed self-surgery.

36. Erskine to Benjamin, 5 Oct 1953, KILSC-HB, Box 4, Ser. II C.

37. Erskine to Benjamin, 1 July 1953, KILSC-HB, Box 4, Ser. II C.

38. Benjamin, "Introduction," 3. It is possible but unclear whether Benjamin was consciously alluding to Richard von Krafft-Ebing's use of the term *stepchildren of nature* to describe his patients. See Oosterhuis, *Stepchildren of Nature*.

39. Benjamin to Erskine, 25 Jan 1954, KILSC-HB, Box 4, Ser. II C.

40. Benjamin to Erskine, 25 Nov 1953, KILSC-HB, Box 4, Ser. II C. Benjamin is presumably describing the operation performed on Erskine as a child.

41. Erskine to Benjamin, 30 Nov 1953, KILSC-HB, Box 4, Ser. II C.

42. Erskine to Benjamin, 7 Dec 1953, KILSC-HB, Box 4, Ser. II C.

43. Erskine forwarded this announcement to Benjamin. KILSC-HB, Box 4, Ser. II C.

44. Benjamin, "Introduction," 4. In claiming this originality, Benjamin was certainly obscuring the inspiration he had received from the work of Magnus Hirschfeld. For the article itself, see Benjamin, "Transvestism and Transsexualism."

45. "[Carla Erskine], 1953," KILSC-HB, Box 4, Ser. II C.

46. Erskine thought Hinman's technique created a "far more natural" effect than that used for two of her friends. Erskine to Benjamin, 5 Oct 1954, KILSC-HB, Box 4, Ser. II C. However, according to Benjamin's table of surgeries, compiled for *The Transsexual Phenomenon*, this appears to be the only such surgery Hinman performed. See KILSC-HB 28.

47. In October 1954, Erskine attempted to make contact with the English trans woman Cowell, a former racing driver and World War II fighter pilot whose autobiography proclaiming her the first British woman to have undergone reassignment surgery had by this time made her relatively famous. See Cowell, *Roberta Cowell's Story*.

48. Erskine to Benjamin, 10 Nov 1954 and 24 Nov 1954, KILSC-HB, Box 4, Ser. II C. By the time the photo in figure 10 was taken in the studio of Alvin Harris (a friend of Louise Lawrence) in 1954, Angela D. had followed Erskine's example by self-castrating. There is a small collection of photos of Erskine (labeled under her real name) in the Harris-Wheeler Collection, part of the Vern and Bonnie Bullough Collection on Sex and Gender at Special Collections, California State University, Northridge. See Series III: Scrapbooks and Binders, 1949–1954, Box 18, Folder 7. Richard F. Docter describes Harris as a "lingerie fetishist." See, Doctor, *Becoming a Woman*.

49. "Obituary: John 'Bunny' Breckinridge," *SFGate*, November 9, 1996. Accessed August 15, 2024. https://www.sfgate.com/news/article/OBITUARY-John-Bunny-Breckinridge-2959951.php.

50. Erskine to Benjamin, 9 May 1954, KILSC-HB, Box 4, Ser. II C.

51. MacLane's public performances and her search for publicity justify providing her full name. Stryker, "Aleshia Brevard Crenshaw Interviews."

52. MacLane was the friend who begged Erskine to perform surgery on her. Erskine refused and called on Benjamin for support, demonstrating the triangular relationships at play. Benjamin to Erskine, 15 Oct 1953, KILSC-HB, Box 4, Ser. II C.

53. Erskine to Benjamin, 28 Feb 1954, 10 Feb 1954, and 8 Mar 1953, KILSC-HB, Box 4, Ser. II C. Benjamin, rather unethically, tells Erskine that MacLane's case was being handled by Dr. Worden, a psychiatrist also treating Erskine (Benjamin to Erskine, 4 Mar 1954). Erskine's enormous faith that Worden would handle these cases sensitively seems to have been unjustified, since his co-authored publication makes virtually no distinction between psychologically troubled individuals like MacLane and quite rational and stable trans women like Erskine. Worden and Marsh, "Psychological Factors in

Men Seeking Sex Transformation." Benjamin later wrote to Kinsey: "The transvestites who have met him or have read his article are either disappointed, indignant, or very unhappy about it. I understand, of course, that Dr. Worden is not interested in these people except as material for some research. He has made valuable observations, but as a physician he has undoubtedly done more harm than good." Benjamin to Kinsey, 23 May 1955, KA-Corr., Benjamin, Folder 1.

54. Erskine to Benjamin, 3 May 1954, KILSC-HB, Box 4, Ser. II C.

55. Erskine to Benjamin, 7 Mar 1955, KILSC-HB, Box 4, Ser. II C.

56. Roots of Equality et al., *Lavender Los Angeles*, 9. For more general histories of prohibitions against cross-dressing in the United States, see: Peter Boag, *Re-Dressing America's Frontier Past*, and Bullough and Bullough, *Cross Dressing, Sex, and Gender*. Like these two books, Sears focuses on the nineteenth century in *Arresting Dress*.

57. Erskine to Benjamin, 8 Mar 1954, KILSC-HB, Box 4, Ser. II C.

58. For a fascinating discussion of the difficulties of discussing trans erotic desire in this period, see Aleshia Brevard Crenshaw Interviews. For an example of the tensions that raising erotic desire could produce even within circles of medical professionals who viewed themselves as experts on transsexuality and transgender identities in the 1990s, see the descriptions of two conferences provided in Ekins, "Science, Politics and Clinical Intervention, esp. 308–09.

59. Benjamin later described his use of the word "transsexualist" unfortunate. Benjamin, *The Transsexual Phenomenon*, 16.

60. Benjamin, "Transvestism and Transsexualism," 13–14.

61. Benjamin et al., "Transsexualism and Transvestism—A Symposium."

62. Ekins, "Science, Politics and Clinical Intervention," esp. 310.

63. Erskine did not explicitly discuss the absence of a vagina in the letters, but Benjamin was certainly aware of this fact and would have passed the information on to Kinsey. Benjamin to Erskine, 14 Apr 1955; 6 May 1955; and 19 May 1955, KILSC-HB, Box 4, Ser. II C.

64. On the "reification of orgasm" and Kinsey's role in it, see Jagose, *Orgasmology*, 29. Jagose notes that "Kinsey uses [orgasm's] alleged stability in order to quantify sexual practice: unless it ends in orgasm, sexual activity does not count, in the literal statistical sense, as an event." As Kinsey himself put it, there "is no better unit for measuring the incidences and frequencies of sexual activity"; Kinsey et al., *Sexual Behavior in the Human Female*, 46. See also Germon, "Kinsey and the Politics of Bisexual Authenticity." For more on how Kinsey counted and classified orgasms, see Drucker, *The Classification of Sex*, 96–8 and 120.

65. As Griffith has argued, "accounts of his stringently religious father . . . [are] habitually embellished well beyond documentary evidence." Griffith, "The Religious Encounters of Alfred C. Kinsey." She includes the most widely read biographies in this critique: Jones, *Alfred C. Kinsey*, and Gathorne-Hardy, *Sex the Measure of All Things*.

The fact that the Kinseys had trouble consummating their marriage is less controversial, though Jones's explanation that this was due to an "adherent clitoris" has also been challenged. See Jones, *Alfred C. Kinsey*, and Rodriguez, *Female Circumcision and Clitoridectomy in the United States*, 214n91.

66. Benjamin to Kinsey, 5 Sept 1951, KA-Corr., Benjamin, Folder 1.

67. Her memories of Finochio's are quite depressing: "It was great for someone in her late tweens and early 20s, and my God it was a far cry from Tennessee, but I saw enough of it to say, 'What a terrible—doomed, that's how you were in society back then, the drugs, sitting and praying in front of the mirror, crying about getting old—and they were every bit of thirty. You know. God.'" Aleshia Brevard Crenshaw Interviews, 30.

68. Aleshia Brevard Crenshaw Interviews, 31.

69. Aleshia Brevard Crenshaw Interviews, 72–73.

70. There are numerous references to her financial situation in her letters to Benjamin. See, for example, Erskine to Benjamin, 5 Oct 1954, 25 Dec 1954, and 27 Oct 1955, KILSC-HB, Box 4, Ser. II C.

71. KILSC-HB, Box 25-1, Permissions (1964).

72. Erskine to Benjamin, 27 Dec 1955, KILSC-HB, Box 4, Ser. II C.

73. Erskine to Benjamin, 10 Nov 1955, KILSC-HB, Box 4, Ser. II C.

74. Caen, "Pacific Tell and Tell," 25.

75. Hayes, "Old Films, Organ Revived." For the story of the theatre, see Dewey Cagle, "What's New . . . on the Avenue?" Erskine is mentioned on page 16.

76. The words are as written/remembered by Laub in Laub, "The Clair Elgin Story."

77. A search of the rich documentary evidence housed at the Digital Transgender Archive pulls up at least twenty-nine hits on Laub's name, all glowing descriptions of his contributions to surgical techniques while he was at Stanford and his numerous presentations to the yearly symposium of the Harry Benjamin International Gender Dysphoria Association (now called the World Professional Association for Transgender Health). He is praised in trans publications such as *AEGIS News*, *Chrysalis Quarterly*, *Female Mimics International*, *Gender Review* (Canada), *Metamorphosis Magazine* (Canada), *Renaissance News*, *The Transsexual Voice*, *The TV-TS Tapestry*, and *TransSisters: The Journal of Transsexual Feminism*.

78. Laub, "The Clair Elgin Story."

79. Handwritten list of "Occupations of Operated Male Transsexuals," 11 Jan 1965, KILSC-HB, Box 28 Series VI E. To Series VI. G.

80. Laub, "The Clair Elgin Story."

81. Facts about Patton were obtained in recorded personal interviews (2022) and correspondence with Jamison Green, which remain in the author's personal files.

82. In the 1930s, 1940s, and 1950s, the notion of "bearded ladies" and other "freaks of nature" had already been displayed for decades throughout the country

by the traveling Barnum & Bailey Circus and Shows, feeding the peoples' hunger for "a conjunction between scientific investigation and mass entertainment." Adams, *Sideshow USA*, 27.

83. These initials do not correspond with any of the initials offered in Money and Brennan's 1968 report on six of seven cases on file in the psychohormonal research unit of the Johns Hopkins Hospital involving "females who were convinced they should be males and therefore wanted to become as like males as possible." Money and Brennan, *Sexual Dimorphism in the Psychology of Female Transsexuals*, 487.

84. Benjamin, *The Transsexual Phenomenon*, 178.

85. Pauly, "The Current Status of the Change of Sex Operation," 462.

86. As noted in the September 19, 2008, *Los Angeles Times* Obituary for Marilyn Fithian, written by *Los Angeles Times* staff writer, Elaine Woo, in "Influential Sex Therapist and Researcher."

87. See chapter 11 in this volume for more information about the first wave of gender clinics.

88. See chapter 10 in this volume for more information about the Erickson Educational Foundation.

89. From email correspondence between Jude Patton and Jamison Green, April 27, 2022, in the author's possession.

90. Psychologist Paul Walker took over the transsexualism-related work of the Erickson Educational Foundation when it ceased operation in 1975. He used the name Janus Information Facility to continue distributing information about transsexualism. At that time, Walker was still working at the University of Texas, Medical Branch, in Galveston; he later established a private practice in San Francisco, California, taking Janus Information Facility with him. It was here that Lou Sullivan produced and first distributed his pamphlet, "Information for the Female-to-Male Cross-Dresser and Transsexual" and began his correspondence with hundreds of trans men before he started his own support group and newsletter, *Female-to-Male (FTM)*, in 1986.

91. Paul Walker presided.

92. See chapter 10 in this volume.

93. The literature on this subject is now vast and growing. I will simply repeat the citation to two useful overviews: Biess, "History of Emotions," and Scheer, "Are Emotions a Kind of Practice?" I have developed this perspective in other places, including the unpublished conference paper by Timm, "Queering Friendship."

WORKS CITED

Adams, R. *Sideshow U.S.A.: Freaks and the American Cultural Imagination*. Chicago, IL: University of Chicago Press, 2001.

Bakker, Alex, Rainer Herrn, Michael Thomas Taylor, and Annette F. Timm. *Others of My Kind: Transatlantic Transgender Histories*. Alberta, Canada: University of Calgary Press, 2020.

Benjamin, Harry. (1966). *The Transsexual Phenomenon*. New York: Warner Books, 1997.

———. "Introduction." In *Transsexualism and Sex Reassignment*, edited by Richard Green and John Money, 1–10. Baltimore, MD: Johns Hopkins University Press, 1969.

———. "Transvestism and Transsexualism." *International Journal of Sexology* 7, no. 1 (1953): 12–14.

Benjamin, Harry, Emil Arthur Gutheil, Danica Deutsch, and Robert V. Sherwin. "Transsexualism and Transvestism—A Symposium." *American Journal of Psychotherapy* 8, no. 2 (1954): 219–44, 220.

Biess, Frank. "History of Emotions." *German History* 28, no. 1 (March 1, 2010): 67–80.

Boag, Peter. *Re-Dressing America's Frontier Past*. Berkeley: University of California Press, 2011.

Bullough, Vern L., and Bonnie Bullough. *Cross Dressing, Sex, and Gender*. Philadelphia: University of Pennsylvania Press, 1993.

Caen, Herb. "Baghdad-by-the-Bay." *San Francisco Chronicle*, n.d., clipping in K1-HB25.

Caen, Herb. "Pacific Tell and Tell." *San Francisco Chronicle*, November 13, 1972, 25.

Cagle, Dewey. "What's New . . . on the Avenue?" *Theater Organ Bombarde: Journal of the American Theatre Organ Enthusiasts*, April 1968.

Cowell, Roberta. *Roberta Cowell's Story*. New York: British Book Centre, 1954.

Davis, G. *Contesting Intersex: The Dubious Diagnosis*. New York: New York University Press, 2015.

Davis, H. F. *Beyond Trans: Does Gender Matter?* New York: New York University Press, 2017.

Docter, Richard F. *Becoming a Woman: A Biography of Christine Jorgensen*. New York: Routledge, 2007.

Dreger, A. D. *Hermaphrodites and the Medical Invention of Sex*. Cambridge, MA: Harvard University Press, 1998.

Dreger, A. D., ed. *Intersex in the Age of Ethics*. Hagerstown, MD: University Publishing Group, 1999.

Drucker, Donna J. *The Classification of Sex: Alfred Kinsey and the Organization of Knowledge*. Pittsburgh, PA: University of Pittsburgh Press, 2014.

Eder, S. "The Volatility of Sex: Intersexuality, Gender and Clinical Practice in the 1950s." In *Historicising Gender and Sexuality*, edited by Kevin P. Murphy and Jennifer M. Spear, 166–81. Malden, MA: Wiley-Blackwell, 2011.

Ekins, Richard. "Science, Politics and Clinical Intervention: Harry Benjamin, Transsexualism and the Problem of Heteronormativity." *Sexualities* 8, no. 3 (2005): 306–28.

Gathorne-Hardy, Jonathan. *Sex the Measure of All Things: A Life of Alfred C. Kinsey*. Bloomington: Indiana University Press, 2000.

Germon, Jennifer E. "Kinsey and the Politics of Bisexual Authenticity." *Journal of Bisexuality* 8, nos. 3–4 (2008): 243–58.

Griffith, R. M. "The Religious Encounters of Alfred C. Kinsey." *Journal of American History* 95, no. 2 (2008): 349–77.

Hayes, Elinor. "Old Films, Organ Revived." *Oakland Tribune*, July 6, 1969.

Jagose, Annamarie. *Orgasmology*. Durham, NC: Duke University Press, 2013.

Jones, James H. *Alfred C. Kinsey: A Public/Private Life*. New York, NY: Norton, 1997.

Kinsey, Alfred C., Wardell B. Pomeroy, Paul H. Gebhard, Clyde Martin, and John Bancroft. *Sexual Behavior in the Human Female*. Philadelphia, PA: W.B. Saunders, 1953.

Laub, Donald. "The Clair Elgin Story." Accessed August 14, 2024. https://dlaub.wordpress.com/2011/04/11/the-clair-elgin-story/.

Meyerowitz, J. *How Sex Changed: A History of Transsexuality in the United States*. Cambridge: Harvard University Press, 2002.

Money, John, and John G. Brennan. "Sexual Dimorphism in the Psychology of Female Transsexuals." *Journal of Nervous and Mental Disease* 147, no. 5 (1968): 472–86.

Oosterhuis, Harry. *Stepchildren of Nature: Krafft-Ebing, Psychiatry, and the Making of Sexual Identity*. Chicago, IL: University of Chicago Press, 2000.

Pauly, I. B. "The Current Status of the Change of Sex Operation." *Journal of Nervous and Mental Disease* 47 (1968): 460–71.

Reis, E. *Bodies in Doubt: An American History of Intersex*. Baltimore, MD: Johns Hopkins University Press, 2010.

———. "Divergence or Disorder? The Politics of Naming Intersex." *Perspectives in Biology and Medicine* 50, no. 4 (2007): 535–43.

Rodriguez, Sarah B. *Female Circumcision and Clitoridectomy in the United States*. Rochester, NY: University of Rochester Press, 2014.

Roots of Equality, Tom De Simone, Teresa Wang, et al. *Lavender Los Angeles*. Charleston, SC: Arcadia Publishing, 2011.

Rosenbaum, Jack. "Our Man on the Town." *San Francisco Examiner*, March 21, 1970, and March 30, 1972.

San Francisco Examiner. "Sex Operation on Self Fails." August 19, 1953.

Scheer, Monique. "Are Emotions a Kind of Practice (and Is That What Makes Them Have a History)? A Bourdieuian Approach to Understanding Emotion." *History and Theory* 51, no. 2 (2012): 193–220.

Sears, C. *Arresting Dress: Crossdressing, Law, and Fascination in Nineteenth-Century San Francisco*. Durham, NC: Duke University Press, 2014.

Serano, J. *Whipping Girl: A Transsexual Woman on Sexism and the Scapegoating of Femininity*. Emeryville, CA: Seal Press, 2007.

Stryker, Susan. "Don Lucas Interview: Recorded at Lucas's Home in San Francisco." GLBT Historical Society, June 13, 1997. August 2024. http://www.glbthistory.org.

———. "Aleshia Brevard Crenshaw Interviews." GLBT Historical Society, August 2, 1997. Accessed August 2024. http://www.glbthistory.org.

Tagawa, Beth, "When Crossdressing Was Criminal: Book Documents History of Longtime San Francisco Law." *SF State News*, San Francisco State University, February 2015. August 2024. https://news.sfsu.edu/archive/when-cross-dressing-was-criminal-book-documents-history-longtime-san-francisco-law.html.

Timm, Annette F. "Queering Friendship: What Hirschfeld Could Teach Hegel and Arendt." Paper presented at Rethinking Amity: Workshop in Honor of Michael Geyer, University of Chicago, April 2013.

Woo, E. "Influential Sex Therapist and Researcher." *Los Angeles Times*, September 19, 2008. Accessed May 21, 2022. https://www.latimes.com/archives/la-xpm-2008-sep-19-me-fithian19-story.html.

Worden, Frederic G., and James T. Marsh, "Psychological Factors in Men Seeking Sex Transformation: A Preliminary Report." *Journal of the American Medical Association* 157, no. 15 (April 9, 1955): 1292–98.

7.1. PROFILE: LOUISE LAWRENCE (1912–1976): UNSUNG MOTHER OF THE TRANS COMMUNITY

Ms. Bob Davis and Jules Gill-Peterson

Louise Lawrence (1912–1976) was an important figure in the mid-twentieth-century American trans community. Known for socially "going full time" in 1944 to live as a woman, she is mistakenly regarded as one of the first to do so. It would be more accurate to say that she hailed from a more secretive, prewar generation whose desire for anonymity differed from the visibility forced on transsexuals by doctors and media in the 1950s and 1960s. Lawrence enjoyed the support of her hometown San Francisco LGBTQ community and her network of approximately one hundred transgender correspondents. This diverse group of people wrote to one another for comfort and support, to share tips and erotica, and to pursue relationships by letter. Lawrence, in the role of dominatrix, carried on a lively correspondence with several more submissive transvestites.

To successfully live as Louise without medical transition, Lawrence invented ways to present as a woman. She had the support of two other patients of Harry Benjamin: trans couple Barbara Ann Richards and Richard Wilcox. In addition to emotional backing, Richards and Wilcox helped Lawrence with practical aspects of her womanhood, such as how to dress and remove facial hair through hot wax treatments. Hazel, another close friend and a fellow transvestite, referred Lawrence to the Langley Porter Hospital for help from psychiatric professionals to address the conflict that cross-dressing caused in her marriage. To her sorrow, Lawrence's marriage to Montez, her second wife, ended with Lawrence's decision to live full time as a woman.

Having secured a new social security card, Lawrence found a job at the Hilltop Restaurant in Nob Hill. In her unpublished autobiography she described being a waitress as fortunate: "For as time went on the mere fact that I was in front of people so much was a tremendous factor in helping me to gain the security in myself and my ability to live in my role naturally."[1] Later, she worked as a photographer, circulating through crowds of gay men, lesbians, and countless service members. As she put it:

> This was during the Second World War and so the bars were full of soldiers and sailors on leave. . . . This fact was good for business but also left quite a potential for troublemaking especially in the bars after a few drinks. However I was quickly learning how to handle men in general and drunks in particular. . . . By the time this happened I had become well established in the neighborhood and many of the "regulars" knew me . . . (and) knew me as Louise.[2]

In 1958, the US Army dismissed Lawrence's live-in partner Gay Elkins (a cisgender woman) from her job as a civilian nurse under a medical discharge without benefits. At this same time, the US State Department also revoked Lawrence's new passport, citing her use of a false name. Like many other LGBTQ people in this era, Elkins' and Lawrence's lives and relationship became entangled in the Cold War politics that penalized transgressions of gender and sexuality. Later that year, the State Department and US Army eventually resolved both issues in Elkins' and Lawrence's favor. In the 1960s, they lived together and rented out rooms in their San Francisco apartment house. Lawrence served as the manager, attending to the building's maintenance, plumbing, and electrical repairs.

Lawrence did not consider herself transsexual and had no interest in medical transition. When writing to transsexuals, she followed a policy that "not withstanding my personal feeling that the sex operation is not the proper solution to the problem, except, perhaps, in extreme circumstances, I have made it a policy not to intervene in their own personal ideas and solutions."[3] Nonetheless, Lawrence regularly connected medical and social scientific researchers with trans community members who could educate them. At the Langley Porter Hospital, she collaborated with a team of doctors who, having decided there was no possible cure, were interested in learning about transvestism. She carried on a long friendship with Benjamin, helping establish connections between his office and individuals in her network. Benjamin, aware of Lawrence's personal disinterest in medical transition, wrote to her after Christine Jorgenson's much-publicized return to the United States: "The operation we've discussed so often is legal in Holland and could be performed there—naturally only with the proper medical and psychiatric indications. I am trying to make the necessary contact for those who may need it. *Be happy that you don't.*"[4] [Emphasis added.]

Lawrence later formed a working relationship with Alfred Kinsey. After sitting for an interview with him, she recruited many transvestites, female impersonators, cross-dressers, and transsexuals to participate with his research team. After her death, the bulk of her personal archives, primarily information she sent to Kinsey, as well as her unpublished autobiography, were donated to the Kinsey Institute.

We know little about the last fifteen years of Lawrence's life, except that she spent time living in London and touring the transvestite social worlds of

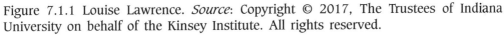

Figure 7.1.1 Louise Lawrence. *Source*: Copyright © 2017, The Trustees of Indiana University on behalf of the Kinsey Institute. All rights reserved.

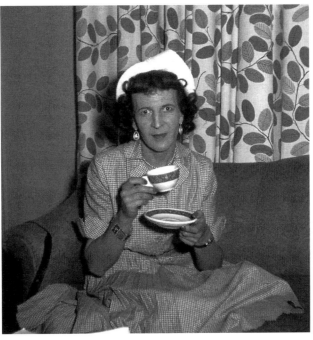

England, France, and Germany. Katherine Cummings, author of *Katherine's Diary: The Story of a Transsexual*, recalls meeting Lawrence in San Francisco in 1968. Cummings wrote that Lawrence, who was then in her mid-fifties, had curly gray hair and was self-possessed and well-spoken. She called Lawrence "a remarkable woman and quite fearless."[5] Lawrence died in 1976.

NOTES

1. Lawrence, Unpublished autobiography, 104.
2. Lawrence, Unpublished autobiography, 112.
3. Lawrence, Unpublished autobiography, 4.
4. Schaefer and Wheeler, "Harry Benjamin's First Ten Cases," 81.
5. Katherine Cummings, personal interview with author, April 18, 2019.

WORKS CITED

Lawrence, Louise. "Lawrence Autobiography 1948–1957." Unpublished manuscript. Box 1, Series A, Folder 3. Louise Lawrence Collection. Kinsey Institute for Research in Sex, Gender, and Reproduction, Bloomington, Indiana.
Schaefer, Leah, and Connie Wheeler. "Harry Benjamin's First Ten Cases (1938–1953): A Clinical Historical Note." *Archives of Sexual Behavior* 24, no. 1 (1995): 73–93.

7.2. PROFILE: VIRGINIA PRINCE (1912–2009)

Dallas Denny

Virginia Prince is an important and controversial figure in transgender history. At a time when trans people lived their lives in isolation and without information, she created a theory of cross-dressing, a nationally distributed magazine, and many support organizations, most of which are still in existence. However, her[1] autocratic style of leadership alienated or drove away many group participants and magazine subscribers, sometimes leading them to form competing organizations—and her exclusionary "no gays, no transsexuals" membership criteria denied many (myself included) admission to the most accessible source for support at the time. Those of us thus ostracized were left isolated and confused.[2]

Born in 1912 in Los Angeles with the name Arnold Lowman, Prince began cross-dressing at the age of twelve and was soon venturing out in public.[3] In 1938 she earned a PhD in chemistry at the University of California San Francisco and later took a position there as a research assistant and lecturer.[4] Around 1941, she attended grand rounds at the Langley Porter Clinic, where early trans activist Louise Lawrence was presented as a study subject. Prince managed to obtain Lawrence's contact information and even visited her home; however, afterward, she was overcome with guilt and shame. This feeling persisted until she visited psychiatrist Karl Bowman, who, on hearing her tell her story, said, "So, what else is new?" He assured her there were others like her and suggested she learn to accept herself. She included his words in every issue of *Transvestia*, a magazine for cross-dressers she edited and published for some twenty years.[5]

Through Lawrence, Prince met, corresponded, and visited with other cross-dressers in the San Francisco area and, eventually, all over the world.[6] In 1952, she and her friends published several issues of a mimeographed digest-sized newsletter that the group called *Transvestia*. It lasted for only a few issues. (In a later iteration in it would be a magazine.) Genny Beemyn notes it was "apparently the first specifically transgender publication in the United States and served as a trial run for wider organizing among crossdressers."[7]

In 1960, Prince relaunched *Transvestia*. Now a magazine, published six times a year, she began with only twenty-five subscribers; by the mid-1960s there were as many as one thousand. *Transvestia* was profusely illustrated and contained articles, letters, editorials, poetry, short fiction, and profiles of cross-dressers. A personals section allowed readers to safely and anonymously contact other readers.[8] These connections slowly grew into supportive trans communities in the United States and around the world. Prince edited the magazine through issue one hundred, which was published in 1979. She contributed to every issue and authored or co-authored articles in professional journals at a time when no other trans person was able to do so.

Prince went on to write several books for her fellow cross-dressers,[9] travel the world to meet with other cross-dressers, and attend trans conferences. In 1961, she founded the social group Hose and Heels Club. Members would arrive in men's garb, carrying two paper bags. One was filled with snacks, the other contained stockings and high heels. At a signal from Prince, attendees would open the bags and don the footwear. At the close of the meeting, members would again change clothing.[10] Prince soon considered forming a new and larger organization with a national and even international focus. She flew to

New York, where she attended a weekend gathering of cross-dressers at the Chevalière d'Eon resort in Hunter, a city in the Catskills. The group enthused about her plans, although some present had reservations about her proposed membership policies. (Harvey Fierstein depicts this first meeting in his play *Casa Valentina*. Based on Michel Hurst and Robert Swope's 2005 photo book portraying mid-twentieth-century cross-dressers, the play opened on Broadway in April 2014 and in London in September 2014.)[11] Virginia told me, in a 1995 oral interview, "I regard that [visit to Casa Susanna] as kind of the fundamental beginning of the whole thing."[12] The resulting organization, Full Personality Expression, eventually evolved into Tri-Ess, the Society for the Second Self.[13]

By age forty or so, Prince was living full time as a woman. She continued to do so and remained engaged in activism until her death in 2009 at age ninety-six.[14]

Figure 7.2.1. Photograph of transgender activist Virginia Prince (1912–2009). *Source*: Courtesy of University of Victoria Libraries, Transgender Archives.

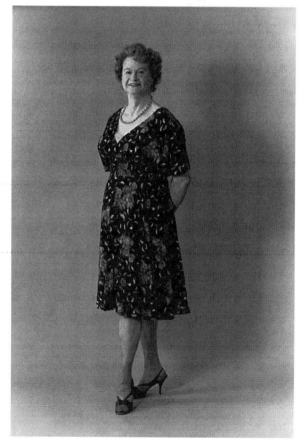

My personal feelings about Prince are mixed. On the one hand, I loathed her for her unnecessary ban on transsexuals and gay cross-dressers in her groups. That policy damaged many of us and held the trans community back. I and many others attempted to persuade her that her championing of heterosexual cross-dressers did not require or justify such discrimination, but she was unmoved. In other ways, I admired Prince. There's a reason for that—in the early 1960s, US Postal Inspectors arrested her for amatory correspondence with another cross-dresser. Wishing to spare her parents the embarrassment of a trial, she pled guilty to a felony. Prosecutors told her they would drop the charges if she would close the Full Personality Expression mailbox and stop publishing *Transvestia*. Most people would have taken that deal, but Virginia refused and was sentenced to prison and placed on probation. She took a big hit for the community, and to an extent that tempers my judgment.[15]

NOTES

1. I use the pronouns "she" and "her" throughout this article. This was Prince's preference.

2. For an account of how Prince's exclusionary policies affected me, see Denny, "First Contact." See also Raynor, *A Year Among the Girls*.

3. Denny, *No Brief Candle*. Over the course of one week in October 1995, Denny recorded interviews with Virginia Prince. A transcript of the interviews in this forthcoming book details Prince's life and activism and is consistent with other sources.

4. Cowan, "Virginia Prince (1912–2009)"; Docter, *From Man to Woman*, 26.

5. In Prince's words: "So I tell him [Karl Bowman] this whole story, and he's sitting there in the swivel chair, and he reaches down and pulls out the lower drawer of his desk, and puts his feet up on the drawer, and swivels around, and pushes back, and puts his hands behind his head, ah, takes a big breath and says, 'So what else is new?'" Denny, *No Brief Candle*.

6. Cowan, "Virginia Prince (1912–2009)."

7. Beemyn, "Transgender History in the United States," 18.

8. Beemyn, "Transgender History in the United States," 18. The Transgender Archive at the University of Victoria has released scans of the entire run of *Transvestia* at https://vault.library.uvic.ca/collections/6576cedf-1282-4089-8351-08f73f4199b4. Accessed December 13, 2020.

9. For instance, in 1967 Prince published the sexist *The Crossdresser and His Wife* in which she encourages readers to rate their spouses on a scale of A through F.

10. Denny, *No Brief Candle*. Prince recounts: "After we had eaten most of the food and just chatted back and forth, I said, 'Okay, time's come. Now take off your

shoes and socks and put on your nylons and your heels.' The theory being that if this guy over here who I had been wondering whether he was an FBI guy has got a pair of heels that will fit him, he's probably like I am."

    11. Manhattan Theatre Club. "Casa Valentina, 2013–2014 Season." For a review, see Brantley, "A Place to Slip into Something Comfortable."

    12. Denny, *No Brief Candle*.

    13. Beemyn, "Transgender History in the United States," 19.

    14. For additional biographical information and more about Prince's activism, see Cowan, "Virginia Prince (1912–2009)"; Docter, *From Man to Woman*; and Ekins and King, "Transgendering."

    15. For a detailed account of this experience, see Prince, "The Life and Times of Virginia" and "How I Became a Convicted Felon."

WORKS CITED

Beemyn, Genny. "Transgender History in the United States." In *Trans Bodies, Trans Selves*, edited by Laura Erickson-Schroth, 1–49. New York: Oxford University Press, 2014.

Brantley, Ben. "A Place to Slip into Something Comfortable: 'Casa Valentina,' a New Play by Harvey Feirstein." *New York Times*, April 23, 2014. Accessed August 5, 2024. https://www.nytimes.com/2014/04/24/theater/casa-valentina-a-new-play-by-harvey-fierstein.html?_r=0.

Cowan, Zagria. "Virginia Prince (1912–2009): A Conflicted Life in Trans Activism." Academia, 2013. Accessed December 13, 2020. https://www.academia.edu/43755193/Virginia_Prince_A_conflicted_life_in_trans_activism.

Denny, Dallas. *No Brief Candle: Virginia Prince, in Her Words and Mine*. Victoria, BC: TransGender Publications. (In press).

———. "First Contact." *Chrysalis Quarterly Online*, August 21, 2013. Accessed October 31, 2020. http://dallasdenny.com/Chrysalis/2013/08/21/first-contact/.

———. "Heteropocrisy: The Myth of the Heterosexual Crossdresser." *Chrysalis Quarterly* 2, no. 4 (Spring 1996): 23–30.

Docter, Richard F. *From Man to Woman: The Transgender Journey of Virginia Prince*. Northridge, CA: Docter Press, 2004.

Ekins, Richard, and Dave King. "Transgendering, Migrating and the Life and Work of Virginia Prince." Paper presented at Gendys 2000, Sixth International Gender Dysphoria Conference, Manchester, England, September 2–3, 2000. Accessed October 31, 2020. http://www.gender.org.uk/conf/2000/king20.htm.

Hurst, Michel, and Robert Swope. *Casa Susanna*. New York: Powerhouse Books, 2005.

Manhattan Theatre Club. "Casa Valentina, 2013–2014 Season." Accessed August 5, 2024. https://www.manhattantheatreclub.com/shows/2013-14-season/casa-valentina/.

Prince, C. V. "166 Men in Dresses." *Sexology* 3 (1962): 520–25.

Prince, Virginia. *The Crossdresser and His Wife*. Los Angeles, CA: Chevalier Publications, 1962.

———. "How I Became a Convicted Felon." *Chrysalis Quarterly* 1, no. 5 (1993): 23–24, 50, 41. Accessed December 13, 2020. http://dallasdenny.com/Writing/wp-content/uploads/2014/01/CQ-23smallpdf.com_.pdf.

———. "The Life and Times of Virginia." *Transvestia*, XVII, no. 100 (1979): 1–120.

Raynor, Darryl. *A Year among the Girls*. New York: Lyle Stuart, 1966.

7.3. PROFILE: A CURBSIDE ENCOUNTER WITH HARRY BENJAMIN (1985–1986)

Sharon Stuart (a.k.a. Thomas Heitz)

Had you been driving along the winding canyon road that passed by Virginia Prince's Hollywood home on a particular July afternoon in 1968, you might have noticed a slender, youthful US Marine Corps captain in uniform engaged in earnest conversation with a tall, round-faced older gentleman. The older man was Harry Benjamin, the world-famous and controversial pioneer of transgender medicine in the United States.[1] I was the US Marine captain, on liberty from Camp Pendleton, where I had been stationed as a judge advocate and court-martial trial prosecutor. Having carried out my official duties earlier that morning, I remained in uniform. Presenting as Tom, I arrived at Prince's house hours late for Benjamin's presentation to a select gathering of the Society for the Second Self (Tri-Ess) chapter members. I parked up the road and walked back to Virginia's front door, ignoring the gentleman perched against one of the parked vehicles smoking a cigarette. Inside, the remains of a buffet luncheon lay scattered about Prince's living room. Tri-Ess members crowded the space, engaged in their business meeting.

Activists Prince and Carol Beecroft founded Tri-Ess, a pioneering organization for male cross-dressers, several years earlier. By 1968, Tri-Ess had become one of a growing number of local, regional, and national organizations for those assigned male at birth who were described as transvestites, transsexuals, cross-dressers, drag queens, and female impersonators. Of all these designations, the word *transsexual*, popularized by Benjamin, was the most well-known.[2]

Virginia directed me outside to meet Benjamin—the man I had just passed on the road.[3] The skies were clear and the temperature mild. He greeted me kindly. There was nowhere to sit, so we leaned against car hoods and bumpers. Later, someone brought lawn chairs. For the next two hours, I had Benjamin's undivided attention.

Our encounter was informal, warm, and reassuring. He asked about my experience in the Marines; my childhood in Kansas City, Missouri; and my thoughts on the Vietnam War. I talked of my childhood—my cross-dressing exploits, my preoccupation with feminine toys, story books, and clothing. He asked about my ethnic history—German on my father's side and Welsh-British on my mother's. He laughed when I told him about my first awakening to the possibility of sex reassignment in 1954, at the age of thirteen, when a sensational story of Christine Jorgensen's transition appeared on the front page of the *Sunday Kansas City Star*. My mother ripped it out of the paper, not realizing that I had already seen it. Benjamin listened, encouraged me, and relieved some of the confusion and tension that I held at the time.

I told him about my marriage of four years (a union now in its sixth decade) and the birth of our first of three daughters. He asked, "Would you divorce your wife and leave your child to live the rest of your life as a woman?" I answered no. We agreed I was not a candidate for sex reassignment surgery. He was adamant and well-known for his refusal (based on legal concerns) to recommend surgery for those who were married.

In 1963, while still in law school in Kansas City, I found early editions of Prince's publication *Transvestia* at a newsstand. Now, a few weeks earlier in 1968, I had met her in person when I was invited to her home for a day and shared a meal in a swanky Hollywood restaurant. In an essay published in *Transvestia*, Virginia proposed the word *trangenderist* to describe those who cross-dressed but did not pursue sex reassignment surgery or those who lived and dressed as women full- or part-time. The word *transgender* derived from this term, and it became the word I preferred.

After years of painful secrecy, fear, and self-doubt, I had suddenly found Prince and Benjamin, two people who possessed (each in their own way) the experience, training, and dedication to help others discover their gender paths. In the subsequent years, I presented alternately as Tom and as Sharon, expressing both parts of myself with equal facility and with time for both genders. I think of myself as *bigendered*,[4] signifying parallel modes of gender expression. I consider the term analogous in meaning and effect to words such as *bilingual*, *biracial*, and *bi-ethnic*.

It was Prince and Benjamin who offered me the validation and knowledge that I required to live with what psychiatric professionals now refer to as *gender dysphoria*. That's another false term. Thanks to those two and that day, I have lived my life with *bigender euphoria*.

NOTES

1. As the first physician in America to publicly provide hormone therapy for sex reassignment, Benjamin had endured sensationalized publicity, attacks from social conservatives, and ridicule from comedians and talk show hosts.
2. Transsexuals were decidedly unwelcome in Prince's groups. Most other groups of the time followed her lead. There were a few transsexual-only groups, but there wasn't much mixing of cross-dressers and transsexuals.
3. The antismoking movement had started in the 1960s, and Prince, a stickler for rules, forbade smoking inside her house.
4. Prince disapproved of the term *bigender*. She said it sounded like "big-ended" and would be confused with bisexual.

7.4. PROFILE: LOUIS G. SULLIVAN (1951–1991): CHANGING THE PARADIGM ABOUT SEX AND GENDER

Jamison Green

Louis Graydon Sullivan, born with a female body in Wisconsin in 1951, was not destined to become a woman. It took a long time for Sullivan to understand and define himself, a journey documented in his meticulous diaries, now housed in the San Francisco Public Library. In these pages, Sullivan detailed his extensive sexual and gender exploration and eventual self-identification as a gay man. He struggled to categorize himself during an era with no words for his particular experience, first identifying as a transvestite considering sex change, retreating to a feminine expression, later returning to a transvestic self-concept, and finally, pursuing medical transition to become a man, all the while sexually attracted to gay men.

In 1975, Sullivan and his boyfriend left Wisconsin and moved to San Francisco, where he immersed himself in the gay and transvestite culture. In 1976, after reaching out to a psychologist at the Center for Special Problems about joining their transsexual support group (all male-to-female), he saw a newspaper article about Steve Dain, a high school teacher who transitioned (and had lost his job for it) in a nearby town. Sullivan realized he was not alone. In 1979, Sullivan met Dain and sought his advice about the mechanics of a physical female-to-male transition. Dain encouraged him not to relinquish his sexual orientation (as the protocols then required) but instead learn to accept and define himself without conforming to physician stereotypes. Sullivan obtained approval to medically transition from Wardell Pomeroy, a psychologist and former collaborator with Alfred Kinsey, at the National Sex Forum. Sullivan started testosterone that fall and underwent chest reconstruction the following summer. That same year, he created a pamphlet—*Information for the Female-to-Male Crossdresser and Transsexual*—that was distributed through the Janus Information Facility, a service run by psychologist Paul Walker, a gay man and founding president of the Harry Benjamin International Gender Dysphoria Association.

Sullivan wanted Don Laub to perform his genital surgery, as he had done for Dain. According to Walker, both Laub and Norman Fisk (the psychiatrist who worked with Laub's sex reassignment program) asserted that "they want to free the world of homosexuality by offering sex change surgery."[1] Walker advised Sullivan not to lie about his sexual orientation, even if it led to a denial for services. Eventually, another surgeon, Michael Brownstein, performed Sullivan's genital reconstruction.

Sullivan believed that the unexplored experiences of gay and bisexual trans men merited attention in the scientific literature. Walker referred Sullivan to Eli Coleman and Walter Bockting, psychologists at the University of Minnesota. Bockting first met with Sullivan in 1987, and thanks to the rich vein of access and information gleaned from Sullivan, Bockting and Coleman subsequently published a number of papers on trans men and sexuality, HIV, and trans resilience.

Sullivan participated in a videotaped interview with psychiatrist Ira Pauly, who then showed the video at the 1989 Harry Benjamin Scientific Symposium in Cleveland.[2] At this conference, Bockting also challenged the theory linking gender identity to sexual orientation advanced by Ray Blanchard and colleagues. Up to that point, most researchers did not believe that gay or bisexual trans men existed.[3] Bockting's reports on Sullivan's experience began to shift scientific understanding regarding sex and gender paradigms. Bockting recalled:

> Lou has inspired many, including me, to continue research to understand the experiences and identity development of transgender men

who are attracted to, and have sex with, other men. In 1991, with funding from the American Foundation for AIDS Research, I developed the first HIV prevention intervention for transgender people and made sure it included both transmasculine and transfeminine individuals; in other words, it was not limited to transgender women. After that, with funding from the Minnesota Department of Health, we broadened this intervention to affirm diversity in gender, sexual orientation, and sexual health within the trans community, again inclusive of trans men who have sex with men. This led to the first NIH [National Institutes of Health]–funded HIV-prevention research grant that included this part of the community (in 2001), and the rest is history.

Since then, many more trans men have come out as gay or bisexual, and they got involved to address their own sexual health and HIV prevention needs. However, I would say even today, the issue remains understudied and neglected. So, while it is now widely accepted that gender identity and sexual orientation are distinct, the issue of transgender men who are living with HIV remains an issue in need of greater visibility. And this is [over 35] years since Lou disclosed that he was diagnosed with AIDS. . . . It was very brave of him.[4]

Motivated by his 1987 AIDS diagnosis, Sullivan had inaugurated the transmasculine support and information group FTM in 1986, and he launched the quarterly *FTM Newsletter* in 1987. He disclosed publicly that he had AIDS in June 1990, and he died March 2, 1991, three months shy of his fortieth birthday. His efforts to build transmasculine community and pride even as he knew he was dying inspired a new generation of trans activism focused on health as well as civil and human rights.

NOTES

1. Sullivan, Martin, and Ozma, *We Both Laughed*, 338.
2. Katz, "AIDS: The FTM Response."
3. Walter Bockting and Jamison Green, personal email communication, October 26, 2020.
4. Bockting and Green, personal email communication.

WORKS CITED

Katz, Nathan. "AIDS: The FTM Response and the Death of Lou Sullivan." *Out History*, September 28, 2013. Accessed June 15, 2021. https://outhistory.org/exhibits/show/man-i-fest/exhibit/aids.

Sullivan, Lou, Ellis Martin, and Zach Ozma. *We Both Laughed in Pleasure: The Selected Diaries of Lou Sullivan.* New York: Nightboat, 2019.

8
TRANS-FOCUSED PSYCHOLOGY AND PSYCHIATRY IN THE UNITED STATES: 1910–1990

Dallas Denny, Jamison Green, and Hansel Arroyo

PART I: THEORIES OF CAUSATION AND ETIOLOGY OF GENDER INCONGRUENCE

The fields of psychiatry and psychology developed in Europe in the 1800s, with distinctively different approaches to mental health, and both fields have evolved significantly through the contributions of practitioners in the United States.[1] Since *disorderly* behavior is often presumed to be indicative of a mental problem, it's not surprising that the expression of gender identities or behaviors that fail to conform to expected patterns of masculinity or femininity, especially when accompanied by an intent to change one's body or prescribed gender identity, have historically been seen as manifestations of mental disorder. While the field of healthcare has largely moved away from this view, some mental health practitioners still cling to old theories, while others strive to assist transgender and gender-diverse (TGD) people in developing resilience and the skills necessary for survival in what can often be a hostile world.

Understanding this history is crucial to grasping the current state of trans peoples' relationship to the present medical and mental health systems in the United States. This chapter provides an overview of the trans-focused theories and theoreticians who established the paradigms that trans people and their mental health professional allies are breaking free of in the twenty-first century.

EARLY PSYCHOLOGICAL MODELS

Freudian psychoanalytic drive theory postulates that the fusion of aggressive and sexual drives plays an important role, and these conflicts are focused on the genitals. Studies that included transgender women theorized that the male–female dualism of destructive and constructive elements, respectively, would influence the individual's desire to become female to be deserving of love and to ameliorate aggressive tendencies.[2] It would explain, for example, that a desire for breasts would supply their unmet oral needs from childhood. Studies that included transgender men described a rejection of the female form and role as a rejection of feelings of "passivity, helplessness, vulnerability, lack of control, and the susceptibility for being dominated."[3] It would similarly explain that a desire for a penis would protect them from their fears of penetration. Freudian castration anxiety theories influenced some to think that transgender people had a preoccupation with their genitals, viewing them as defective, mutilated, missing parts, deformed, split, or rotted—leading to feelings of incompleteness, defectiveness, depression, and overall preoccupation with "concerns of bodily defectiveness and a distorted body image."[4]

Psychoanalysts depicted what was then referred to as transsexualism not as a single or independent diagnostic category but rather an "association with several clinical conditions," adding that it was a "consequence of the inability to develop appropriate gender identity in accordance with anatomy." They considered what is now called gender-affirming treatment, surgery in particular, an intervention that "constitutes a sanctioning of the transsexual's pathological view of reality and cannot resolve the underlying conflict."[5]

Since its inception in psychiatry, the goals of psychoanalysis and psychotherapy have been to understand the individual's psychological nature to provide relief for existing mental disorders. Initially, the mental health field viewed transgender people as stricken with various mental disorders. These views, rooted in psychoanalytic theory, categorized transsexualism as a disorder of "defective object relations, aggression and sexuality, castration anxiety, rebirth fantasies, gender envy, and warding off decompensation,"[6] or as "sociopaths seeking notoriety, masochist homosexuals, or borderline psychotics."[7] Early studies defined transgender people as having "profound disturbance in core gender identity" or even as having a form of psychosis, giving rise to the use of multiple terms including genuine transvestism, metamorphosis sexualis paranoica, psychopathia transsexualis, eonism, sex role inversion, true transsexual or inverted homosexuality, paranoia transsexualis, escape from genital sexuality, psychosexual inversion, and psychosexual hermaphroditism.[8]

Early psychoanalytic models based presumed disturbances on problems with object relations, often a disturbance in the mother-child dyad. The *Role of the Mother* sections of Leslie Lothstein's paper on the psychodynamics and sociodynamics of transsexualism postulated that mothers who actively discouraged effeminate behavior and cross-dressing also encouraged their children's passive dependency by quelling their individuality.[9] Robert J. Stoller, an American professor of psychiatry and researcher at the Gender Identity Clinic at the University of California Los Angeles (UCLA) in the 1960s through the 1980s, presented the most comprehensive theory of transgender identity and behavior as caused, for the most part, by the mother's wishes. These models argued that the disturbance in object-relations lead "to dysregulation of intrapsychic boundaries and an attempt, on the part of the patient, to incorporate an alternate persona."[10]

Theories in object relations described the cause of the so-called disturbance in gender identity as being linked with a childhood replete with losses, deaths, and separations, causing a conspicuous lack of socialization and failure to establish meaningful relationships. In adolescents, this social isolation led to further estrangement. Psychoanalysts understood this isolation to be the reason transgender people sought identification within the gay community but observed that after being unable to adopt a "homosexual orientation the transsexual was soon outcast."[11] Clinicians believed these patterns of social withdrawal and interpersonal isolation led to the "magical idea of attaining satisfying object relations through sex change."[12]

Although there have been many sympathetic psychoanalysts who worked with transgender people, for most of the twentieth century these clinicians focused on "curing" transgender people of a "disease" through a process now known as conversion therapy—now widely recognized as a cause of psychological harm.[13] Tragically, this approach by the psychiatric community led many people to view transgender individuals as mentally ill. Those who did not respond to psychoanalysis were frequently institutionalized and received a variety of aversion therapies.[14]

Early sexologists did not reject psychological etiologies for transgenderism but often focused on the search for a biological justification. Dominant theories included the possible effects of prenatal sex steroids on brain lateralization, sexual orientation, and gender identity.[15] Since sex hormones were discovered only in 1910 and synthesized for mass production only in the 1950s,[16] mid-twentieth-century thinkers on the social aspects and science of sex, gender, and sexuality generally offered simplistic and classical assumptions about human nature and stereotypical beliefs about male and female psyches.[17]

In 1910, Magnus Hirschfeld, a Jewish physician in Germany, pioneered an approach to care for transgender individuals that involved changing bodies to match one's gender identity. Subsequent hormonal and surgical treatment approaches in the mid-twentieth century continued under similar frameworks, rejecting, at least in part, transgenderism as a mental health concern requiring a mental health intervention.

Models in the early twentieth century included the thinking that humans had both female and male characteristics. People manifesting both traits were labeled transvestites. The model, developed or at least popularized by Sigmund Freud, was termed *bisexuality*: "There is no pure masculinity or femininity either in the biological or psychological sense."[18]

Followers of this model believed transfeminine individuals possessed male anatomy and female chromosomes, and transmasculine individuals were the opposite. Such thinking legitimized medical and surgical intervention and placed transgender individuals in the same space as those who were intersex. This bisexuality theory received publicity when US citizen Christine Jorgensen underwent gender-affirming surgery in Denmark in 1952.[19] Christian Hamburger, Jorgensen's endocrinologist, psychiatrist George Stürup, and surgeon Erling Dahl-Iversen postulated in the *Journal of the American Medical Association* that Jorgensen was a "genuine transvestite."[20] In other words, she was thought to have characteristics of both men (her body) and women (her personality, gender expression, and psyche). Since her mind could not be changed, she required feminine hormones and reconstructive surgery to harmonize her body and mind.

In the 1950s, John Money and the team at Johns Hopkins Hospital introduced the concept of gender, differentiating it from sex, and by studying hermaphrodites, they theorized the role of child development on gender. They concluded that the most reliable 'prognosticator' of a person's gender role was the sex of assignment (that is, the declaration of sex made at birth by the birthing attendant, physician, or midwife, based on the appearance of the infant's genitalia as male or female), not biologic categories of chromosomal sex, gonadal sex, hormonal sex, internal reproductive structure, or morphology of external genitalia."[21]

In the 1990s, a model referred to as gender transposition postulated that prenatal hormonal neurotransmitter levels and postnatal social programming influenced gender identity. This model suggested links among steroid hormones, brain structure, and sexual behavior in nonhuman animals[22] and stated that at critical gestational points, hormone-induced structural brain differentiation occurred. Advances in brain imaging, hormonal analysis, and genetic studies in the twenty-first century may yield more nuanced understanding of human variations and gender identity and expression,[23] yet we still have a long way to go to understand the complex and diverse interplay between psyche and soma.

EARLY SOCIAL MODELS

Early social theories described gender incongruence as not only a psychological disorder but also a social phenomenon. The interaction between the transgender person's behaviors (for example, gender role and expression) brought them into contact with their social environment. The outcome of this interaction varied drastically with racial, regional, cultural, and socio-educational differences and perceived attractiveness or the ability to pass as cisgender. At the time, and with the help of the social phenomenon of Jorgensen, shifts in public opinion fostered the formation of a transgender subculture, which opened opportunities to study its dynamics.

Theories based on this interface between individual and society, or intersocial realm, led to the concept of the *stigmatized homosexual*. The stigmatized homosexual model postulated that a homosexual individual who could not tolerate the explicit and implicit stigma, social sanctions, and punishments of being a homosexual in society would relinquish their "choice" and adopt a transgender role.[24] The theory argued that this reaction would not only reduce the individual's tensions and cognitive dissonance but also render them more socially acceptable. Sociological theories about transgender people stressed the importance of role status and the *progression of roles,* defined by Levine, Shaiova, and Mihailovic as a "transformation from an extremely ambivalent, confused gender role during childhood and primary school years, to one involving homosexuality in post-adolescence, to that of a drag queen (experimental cross-dressing) to that of a self-declared, permanently cross-dressed transsexual."[25]

The radical behavioral model introduced by psychologist B. F. Skinner[26] took the position that complex human behavior was for the most part the product of environmental reinforcement. Skinner's model did not imply that all infants were a tabula rasa—blank slate—or that behavior was unaffected by biological underpinnings but was, rather, a component of it. Models based on radical behaviorism proposed that gender identity was a social construct imposed on the sex recorded at birth. Feminists extrapolated on the belief that societal roles influenced humans in "becoming" either men or women while developing feminist standpoint theory, a conviction also explored by philosophers such as Michel Foucault and Jacques Lacan. Most recently, philosopher Judith Butler popularized this by stating that gender identity is performance, that is, people "do" gender, and the "script" of gender performance is transmitted through generations based on cultural norms.[27] Because of the harm caused by those who claim a trans person's declared gender is not real, Butler later clarified this position with respect to trans people, noting that this interpretation of social construction is "a false, misleading, and oppressive use of the theory" and "one should be free to determine the course of one's gendered life."[28]

Despite early treatment paradigms for transgender people, throughout the remainder of the twentieth century the prevailing model for gender identity was one championed by John Money and Joan and John Hampson.[29] This team developed a theory of psychosexual neutrality: gender identity in humans is not dependent on genetics or hormonal state or internal or external genitalia but is primarily psychological, developing only as a child ages in a sort of imprinting process, and so could be channeled in infants and young children.[30] According to Money's model, gender identity was not ingrained, a view that meshed well with efforts of the era to undo a long history of attributing sex roles in society to sex-based brain differences.[31]

Money and his team believed that gender identity was based heavily on environmental factors. Permutations in environmental influences, like child-rearing techniques or one's passive response to visible anatomy, determined gender identity. In either instance, the idea that gender identity was malleable normalized surgery on intersex individuals who, they believed, should be directed to accept the gender identity that matched the anatomy a surgeon preferred or felt was the easiest surgery to perform.[32] It followed that, if gender identity was malleable, then treatment approaches for transgender people would also include efforts to change it. Bodies of study focused on the success of various methods of externally manipulating gender identity with attention to, among other elements, age of treatment.[33]

CURRENT PSYCHOLOGICAL AND SOCIAL MODELS

Paradigm shifts occurred as our understanding evolved in both the psychological and social sciences. The framework shifted away from the view that transgender people were mentally ill or a product of their environmental upbringing; the framework also shifted away from a binary (man, woman) perspective to a view of gender as existing on a spectrum. In the realm of transgender medical interventions, the framework has shifted from a sex-change model to an individualized-care model, based on a person's embodiment goals.[34] This shift emphasizes a healthy model of gender variability, acknowledging that psychopathology discovered in gender-diverse people was often the result of the social stigma, harassment, and violence most TGD people experience; this trauma can leave lifelong psychological scars.

Modern models consider the biological bedrock that influences the psychology and behavior of individuals. These models center on prenatal testosterone levels and their influence on brain development and behavior, including its effects on sex-typical childhood behaviors[35] during play. Traditional models assumed that sex-typical behavior, childhood play, and toy choices were acquired behaviors that were learned socially and involved a process of cognitive development, which led to sex-related behaviors. A wide range of studies—including those that look at genetic variations, maternal treatment with hormones, and physiological hormonal variability—have demonstrated that prenatal testosterone influences sex-typical behavior, playmate, and activity preferences in infants.[36] Female infants with a virilizing form of congenital adrenal hyperplasia, a genetic disorder that results in exposure to high levels of prenatal androgens, show increases in what is labeled male-typical behavior (for instance, physical aggression) and a reduction in what is commonly labeled female-typical behaviors (for example, empathy).[37]

Early hormonal environment also may play a role in the emergence of psychiatric disorders, which differ in frequency between sexes. Examples include autism spectrum disorder, obsessive compulsive disorder, and Tourette syndrome,[38] which are more common in males. In particular, the incidence of autism spectrum disorder has been reported to be higher (7.8%) in transgender individuals than in cisgender individuals.[39] Such models contribute to the idea that prenatal hormones have an effect on the development of sex-related variation and human behavior.

Modern psychological and social thought continues to move away from pathologizing transgender people. A major turning point occurred in 2019, when the World Health Organization removed "gender identity disorder" as a category of mental illnesses in the *International Classification of Diseases Revision 11* (*ICD-11*), which became effective worldwide January 1, 2022.[40] Under the chapter on sexual health, new language emerged—"gender incongruence"—thus no longer labeling transgender people as mentally ill. However, under the current medical system in the United States, if a person needs help to pay for treatment (such as through health insurance), there must be a diagnosis that justifies the treatment. The US system has not yet implemented the changes in ICD-11. In September 2021, The US Department of Health and Human Services issued a twenty-five-page letter labeled "Updated Recommendations for Immediate Action on ICD-11."[41] Until this transition is complete across all our medical systems, trans people in the United States remain stuck with the *Diagnostic and Statistical Manual of Mental Disorders Fifth Edition, Text Revision* (*DSM-5-TR*) diagnosis of gender dysphoria as the entryway to trans-affirming healthcare covered by third-party payors (private or public insurance plans).

PART II: THEORY-DRIVEN PRACTICE

In the 1960s, the original diagnostic categories like transvestite and eonist, which originated in Europe with early sexologists, expanded to include new diagnostic labels—for instance, transsexual—to describe those who wished to modify their bodies and gender roles. Because most mental health professionals viewed gender identity and presentations that varied from binary norms as, simultaneously, a symptom of mental illness and as a diagnostic category in its own right, their reaction was often one of rejection toward gender-affirming palliative therapies.

After Jorgensen's sex reassignment came to the attention of psychoanalysts through the news and the publication of Hamburger, Stürup, and Dahl-Iversen's 1953 article in the *Journal of the American Medical Association*,[42] notable scholars in the field declared Jorgensen psychotic[43] and gender-affirming treatment "collusion with delusion"[44] and "collaboration with psychosis."[45] Psychiatrists Charles Socarides[46] and Paul McHugh[47] perpetually attacked gender-affirmative interventions, with the goal of ending affirming practices; McHugh continues these assaults to this day.[48] In 1979, psychiatrist Thomas Szasz expressed sympathy with feminist Janice Raymond's attacks on gender-affirming treatment.[49] Medical schools consistently exposed psychiatrists-in-training to these sorts of views. As an example, internist Charles Ihlenfeld, who was extraordinarily sympathetic toward his transgender patients under the tutelage of Harry Benjamin, later retrained as a psychiatrist, temporarily shifting his attitude toward gender-affirming treatment: "Whatever surgery did, it did not fulfill a basic yearning for something that is difficult to define. This goes along with the idea that we are trying to treat superficially something that is much deeper."[50]

Attempts to find the causes of gender-variant behavior went hand in hand with attempts to eradicate it. Notwithstanding their ineffectiveness, every technique in the medical armamentarium has been used in attempts to change the sexual orientations and gender identities of often unwilling subjects; these include psychoanalysis, psychotherapy, religious counseling, hypnosis, exorcism,[51] psychoactive drugs, electroconvulsive and insulin shock, estrogen therapy for transmasculine people and testosterone injections for transfeminine people, psychodrama, abreaction, desensitization, referrals to prostitutes, aversive electrical and chemical interventions, commitment to mental institutions, imprisonment, and lobotomy.[52] None were effective.

Attempts to cure gender-variant people were excessive and inappropriate. Some cures were claimed as successes, or at least initially seemed to have worked. In 1974, psychiatrist Robert Bak reported the psychoanalytic cure of a cross-dresser. However, at the time of Bak's publication, his patient, now known as Renée Richards, had overcome her internal conflict and was scheduled for vaginoplasty with surgeon Georges Burou in Casablanca.[53] More commonly, clinicians practiced draconian methods to cure problems that weren't problems at all. Nowhere is this more evident than in the attempts of British and American behaviorists to eliminate cross-dressing and feminine identification in males:

> In the first published account of aversion therapy with a crossdresser, Lavin, et al. (1961) kept a 22-year-old married man awake for days with amphetamines, giving him frequent injections of apomorphine to make him violently sick to his stomach while he was forced to look at slides of himself in a crossdressed state. Treatment did not stop until the subject became confused and his vital signs became abnormal. Barker, et al. (1963) required a heterosexual crossdresser who sought treatment for his transvestism to dress and undress 400 times in six days. He was given electric shock to his feet (or, after it had become conditioned to become an aversive stimulus, a buzzer sounded) to signal him to undress. . . . We must remember that this

extremely aversive treatment was given for behaviors which were essentially harmless and which could have been dealt with in any number of less aversive ways.[54]

These treatments led in some instances to catastrophe. In a paper published in 1963, researcher A. J. Cooper reported a month-long hospitalization for a patient who developed cardiac problems after being given amphetamines, kept awake for a week, and given drugs to make him nauseous.[55] At least one patient died as the result of such stress.[56] Transgender activist Denny wrote: "If you have a bit of imagination—a word, I know, I should not use at a meeting of behavior analysts—you can see this man, this crossdresser, wild-eyed and perspiring from the amphetamines, smelling of vomit, going into cardiac distress. It's a scene straight out of Stanley Kubrick's *A Clockwork Orange*—but let me remind you that the protagonist in the film brutalized and killed people. Cooper's patient merely sometimes wore women's clothing."[57] Despite these treatments to "cure" people who were not harming themselves or others, the clinicians apparently never questioned whether what they were doing was justified, or for that matter, whether nonaversive methods should have been tried first.[58] Aversion therapy persisted in the United States through the 1990s. Less harmful but certainly indeed coercive conversion therapy is still practiced in the United States—in states where it's still legal.[59]

The lack of success of "curative" treatment methods eventually opened the door to gender-affirming treatment. Benjamin cited the inability of these techniques to change the desires, identities, and gender presentations of subjects and used this as a launching point for his argument that, due to their collective ineffectiveness, the most humane approach (in extreme cases, he was quick to point out) was to empower patients to live as they pleased.[60]

Health professionals, from sexologist Hirschfeld in 1920s Germany to surgeons Elmer Belt in Los Angeles and Burou in Casablanca to endocrinologist Hamburger and his team in Denmark, had long endeavored to provide gender-affirming treatment to TGD people. The gender identity clinics that sprang up in the 1960s provided collaborative and organized multidisciplinary treatment environments, generated hundreds of journal articles, and produced more than a few books about transsexualism.[61] The personnel at the clinics were sympathetic toward TGD people, but they accepted only a minority of applicants. Until their closure in 1979, they operated entirely under a medical model that presumed transsexualism was a mental illness, one that usually coexisted with other mental illnesses. This bias colored the literature and theories of causation, as well as the associated research questions, of what was then called gender dysphoria.

The clinics were not universally unkind to their TGD clients,[62] but they were quick to deny treatment to most applicants. Much of their intellectual output was designed to differentiate those deemed worthy of treatment from those who were not. In 1965, psychiatrist Ira Pauly divided those seeking surgery into genuine transsexuals and pseudotranssexuals, with the latter seeking hormones and surgery to "rationalize their homosexuality."[63] In a pair of articles published in 1974, psychiatrists Ethyl Person and psychoanalyst Lionel Ovesey also divided transfeminine transsexuals into two types: primary and secondary, based on age and sexual orientation.[64] Despite the fact that the originators of these clinical categories found them inadequate,[65] clinicians widely embraced them. These categories continue to hold sway in some circles today, although some in the field have called for an end to such nonsense.[66]

In the 1980s, sexologist Ray Blanchard proposed modification of Person and Ovesey's typology to homosexual and non-homosexual.[67] In 1989, he coined the diagnosis *autogynephilia*, which he described as a paraphilia, to wit, "a male's propensity to be sexually aroused by the thought of himself as a female."[68] Sexologist and anesthesiologist Anne Lawrence and psychologist J. Michael Bailey[69] are proponents of this controversial concept, which took a major step back in time and re-pathologized transfeminine transgender people. While some transfeminine people saw themselves in the diagnosis, others did not. The diagnosis was especially onerous, as first it postulated a special status that applied only to "secondary" transsexuals and, second, created a "have you stopped beating your wife" scenario in which any late-transitioning trans woman who denied sexual arousal via cross-dressing was deemed either self-deluding or lying.

Another unfortunate concept was the sexist mother-blame theory of psychiatrist Stoller.[70] Stoller was a prolific writer who produced three books and many articles on transsexualism. Based on case studies of three feminine young boys and extrapolating from Freud's psychoanalytic theories and ethologist Konrad Lorenz' discovery of imprinting in nonhuman animals,[71] Stoller "argued the primary cause of transsexualism was faulty imprinting of appropriate gender (sex-role stereotypes)," caused by emotionally empty[72] bisexual[73] mothers,[74] sometimes aided by absent, uninvolved fathers.[75]

> It appears that transsexualism, starting in early childhood, may occur when a bisexual woman marries a passive man. . . . The father can

cope with his marriage and family only by being absent, at least during the infancy and childhood of his son; his wife survives by letting him be absent and by comforting herself in her life-long depression as well as in her personal anguish by taking her infant son back in upon her body as a continuing comfort . . . so that he feels himself to be a female despite the evidence of his senses that he is anatomically a male.[76]

Stoller and other clinicians embraced Person and Ovesey's primary/secondary duality; however, the category they assigned to transsexuals was largely based on the age at which they came out, their ability to pass, attractiveness, and sexual orientation and was not, as postulated, a matter of "types." The case of a transfeminine woman Stoller and Harold Garfinkel called "Agnes" in print perfectly illustrated the problems with this methodology. In 1958, at age nineteen, Agnes became one of Stoller's patients and the subject of a study by sociologist Harold Garfinkel. Stoller and Garfinkel discussed the details of Agnes' case in a chapter in the latter's edited 1967 text *Studies in Ethnomethodology.*[77] Garfinkel's interactions with Agnes, which consisted of recorded interviews, "is widely believed to be, in sociologist Kristen Schilt's words, 'the first sociological case study of a transitioning person. . . .' It may also be the first American case study of a transgender person in transition."[78]

Stoller and Garfinkel considered Agnes to be intersex, as that was what she had told them. Upon reaching puberty, she said, her body had begun to spontaneously feminize. They believed her, even after extensive tests failed to confirm her claims: "Agnes was wholly unlike any other intersexed patient that the doctors had encountered in their own observations or in the medical literature. The doctors pondered, publicly and privately, what this represented, and they used her case study in scholarly presentations and publications. Three medical doctors joined Stoller in authoring 'Pubertal Feminization in a Genetic Male.' "[79] They hypothesized that Agnes had "a diffuse lesion of the testis" which had produced the estrogen which had, in turn, produced her breasts.[80] The source of Agnes' "natural" femininity turned out to be her mother's estrogen tablets, which she had been taking since age twelve.[81] "After having kept it from me for eight years, with the greatest casualness, in mid-sentence, and without giving the slightest warning it was coming, she revealed that she had never had a biological defect that had feminized her but that she has been taking estrogens since age 12."[82]

To his credit, Stoller was forthcoming about having believed Agnes' claims of spontaneous feminization: "Stoller presented his findings on Agnes in 1963 at the International Psychoanalytic Congress in Stockholm and also published them in scholarly journals."[83] (Compare this to Money's disgraceful behavior in the case of David Reimer[84] and George Rekers' in the case of Kirk Andrew Murphy.[85]) Agnes's revelation was, without doubt, a professional blow to Stoller; he was forced to recant the findings he had presented, years before, on her case, and the discovery was doubtless a factor in a disappointed Stoller writing in 1982, "After 30 years . . . both the treatments and the patients (of both sexes) have been, at most, near misses."[86] In one tongue-in-cheek sentence, Stoller informs the reader of his opinion not only that transsexual women are not "really" women but also that after decades of investigation, his theory of causation had not borne fruit. Stoller's reaction, too, reveals him to be something of a sore loser, upset, as was Garfinkel, that Agnes had manipulated the treatment paradigm to meet her needs.[87]

Joanne Meyerowitz noted the conflicting motivations of those seeking treatment and those who provided (or did not provide) treatment: "In short, the patients mistrusted the doctors, and the doctors mistrusted the patients."[88] Unfortunately, rather than acknowledging the complex dynamics involved in treatment under the medical model of the clinics, clinicians blamed transsexuals, considering them unreliable and manipulative.[89]

Many TGD people and clinicians revile psychiatrist and lawyer Richard Green for his clinical psychiatric research with children (the Sissy Boy study, described below). It was indeed abhorrent. Nevertheless, Green made many contributions toward gender-affirming treatment and gay rights. In the 1960s, he wrote hormone and surgery letters while working in Benjamin's New York office. He played a major role in the creation of the first gender clinic in the United States at Johns Hopkins University; worked at the Hopkins and UCLA gender clinics early in his career and later at the clinic at Charing Cross Hospital in London; documented hostile attitudes of American physicians toward transsexuals; played an active role in the push to remove homosexuality from the American Psychiatric Association's *DSM*; took a very early position (1974) in support of same-sex marriage; was a founding member of the Harry Benjamin International Gender Dysphoria Association (HBIGDA); was one of the eight people who created the original HBIGDA *Standards of Care*; and served as president of HBIGDA from 1997 to 1999. He was the primary editor of the first book about gender-affirming care[90] and wrote five other books and many research articles. He wrote the first journal articles supporting transsexual people as parents, the earliest of which, 1978's "Sexual Identity of 37 Children Raised by Homosexual or Transsexual Parents" was, for years, the only citable article that attorneys could use to help trans parents in divorce proceedings retain custody or even visitation with their minor children.[91] He was the founding editor of the prestigious peer-reviewed journal *Archives of Sexual Behavior* and he served as editor for thirty years. He was a member of the committees of psychiatrists who produced the *DSM-III* and *DSM-IV*, served as a professor at four universities, and retrained late in his career as a lawyer and worked tirelessly on behalf of TGD people and gender-affirming care.[92]

Green began working with feminine boys while in medical school at Johns Hopkins in the late 1950s. He and Money published two papers in 1961 that described characteristics among the boys they studied and offered recommendations for managing these "psychic hermaphrodites" to enable them to lead a stable and productive life.[93] These recommendations, based on Lorenz' discovery of imprinting in geese, did not specifically mention coercive methods but were decidedly geared toward encouraging feminine boys to become more "boyish."

After medical school, Green trained as a psychiatrist at UCLA, where he met Stoller, "the only other psychiatric researcher in the US focused on gender identity."[94] At the university's gender clinic, he was soon treating transsexual patients. While working with Stoller, Green initiated what he (insensitively) called the Sissy Boy study.[95] He identified a cohort of 150 young boys whom he believed to be pre-transsexual and followed them into adulthood; selection criteria were based on reports by many of the adult transsexual women that Stoller and Green had studied who told the researchers that as young boys they had been extravagantly feminine. To Green's surprise, most of the boys tracked in the study came to identify in adulthood as gay men. Ninety-eight percent desisted from cross-dressing and feminine identities[96]—an astonishing and entirely unexpected finding.

The study was unfortunately muddled, because during therapy sessions the parents of Green's subjects were told to encourage masculine behavior and discourage feminine displays, and the boys were urged to play with stereotypical boys' toys and repeat statements affirming boyhood and manhood.[97] These interventions were in and of themselves coercive and no doubt viewed by most of the boys as aversive.[98] We will never know what might have transpired had the subjects received affirmative care or at least not been discouraged in their feminine mannerisms and modes of dress—or maybe we do, for studies of feminine boys that do not attempt to instill masculine behavior and identities also show their subjects typically grow up to become gay men.[99] Green himself pointed out that only one boy in his control group was transsexual as an adult.[100] Green's Sissy Boy and similar studies eventually came under attack by former patients, mental health patients, and LGBTQ advocates.[101]

Meyerowitz described Green as distancing himself from conversion therapies,[102] and indeed, we found no mention of the Sissy Boy study in his autobiography.[103] He criticized psychologist and Southern Baptist minister George A. Rekers, his successor at UCLA, for his use of aversion therapy. Nevertheless, Green seemed to maintain the position throughout his life as outlined in his 1961 article with Money that a homosexual outcome is less painful than a transsexual one.[104] Rekers and Kenneth Zucker held similar opinions.[105]

Rekers was a cofounder, in 1983, of the faith-based anti-GLBTQ Family Research Council, of which the Southern Poverty Law Center says "[FRC] bills itself as 'the leading voice for the family in our nation's halls of power,' but its real specialty is defaming LGBTQ people."[106] His views on homosexuality were negative in the extreme, and he promulgated them by, among other things, testifying as a paid expert in court.[107] In 1974, Rekers coauthored an article with Norwegian psychologist Ivar Lovaas in which the feminine behavior of a five-year-old boy, whom they referred to as "Kraig," was targeted for extinction with operant conditioning techniques.[108] The home component of "Kraig's" treatment included physical punishment—namely, spanking by his father and getting red "punishment" tokens for behavior the researchers considered "feminine," for instance, playing with dolls.[109] Rekers and Lovaas considered their treatment a success, concluding that "he was indistinguishable from any other boy in terms of gender-related behaviors" and "the boy's sex-typed behaviors have become normalized."[110]

"Kraig's" real name was Kirk Andrew Murphy.[111] After his mother saw Green on television talking about feminine traits in boys, she took her son to UCLA for evaluation. Rekers, then a graduate student, was chosen to work with "Kraig."[112] In a tragic mirroring of the case of Reimer,[113] Kirk Murphy committed suicide on December 21, 2003. "Murphy became increasingly miserable and filled with self-hatred. He grew up to be gay—but, unable to accept his sexuality, he committed suicide at age 38."[114] His family believes his death was a direct result of Rekers' and Lovaas' interventions.[115] During treatment, and even afterward, the situation at home was, according to Murphy's family, grim:

> The punishment Kirk's father dealt out consisted of beatings with a belt—sometimes so harsh that the boy was left with welts 'up and down his back and on his buttocks,' according to Kaytee [Kirk's mother].[116]

> 'I took some of the red chips and I put them on my side,' a tearful Mark [Kirk's brother] told CNN, going on to describe what it was like to monitor the stacked chips as they accumulated over the course of the week.[117]

Rekers repeatedly lauded "Kraig's" treatment as a success story and continued to do so after Murphy committed suicide. Kirk "had the prestige of appearing in 17 of Rekers' articles as evidence of a successful outcome."[118] To be blunt, Rekers knew about the ultimate failure of "Kraig's" treatment and, like Money in the case of Reimer, ignored and denied the evidence. He continued to do so in writing until at least 2009.[119]

Reker's 1974 paper with Lovaas launched a "three-decade career as a leading national expert in trying to prevent children from becoming gay."[120] That career came to an effective end in 2010, when *Miami New Times* broke the story of Rekers' two-week-long European vacation in the company of a gay male escort he had hired on the "pornographic gay escort" website rentboy.com.[121] As he had in the case of Kirk Murphy, Rekers denied the evidence, claiming the relationship was not sexual and that his companion was along merely to carry luggage, but ensuing politicization of the incident in the 2020 Florida governor's race catapulted Rekers into the national spotlight.[122]

Despite the obvious presence of transgender men in their caseloads and, eventually, in the clinical literature, clinicians developed and clung to notions that they were an order of magnitude less common than transgender women, were psychologically and behaviorally more "normal" than transgender women,[123] and were sexually interested exclusively in women; consequently, they were largely ignored or overlooked in the literature. When transgender men were mentioned in the literature, they were typically stereotyped as John Wayne wannabes. When psychiatrist Lothstein finally published a book about transgender men in 1983, he employed defamatory and insulting language, misgendered and dead-named individuals, and placed quotation marks around their names, pronouns, and body parts.[124] Fourteen years later, sociologist Aaron Devor published the next research-driven text about transmasculine people—this one affirming and definitive.[125]

Things began to change—slowly. In 1985, the Stanford Gender Dysphoria Program rejected Louis Graydon Sullivan as a patient because he identified as a gay man, spurring him to embark on a campaign to convince psychiatrists and psychologists that TGD men could identify and live successfully as gay men. Almost as if to prove his point, Sullivan passed away tragically in 1991 from complications of AIDS. Shortly before his death, he wrote in his diary: "They told me at the gender clinic that I could not live as a gay man, but it looks like I will die as one."[126] One week before his death, Sullivan asked Jamison Green, one of the editors of this volume (no relation to Richard Green), to keep San Francisco's FTM support group's newsletter, *FTM*, alive;[127] Jamison agreed, and managed the group as well until August 1999.[128] From its tenuous start,[129] networks of trans men of every sexual orientation found one another and gained support. Gradually, as it became clear that their numbers were on par with assigned-male-at-birth individuals and that many transmasculine people, like Sullivan, identified as gay men, the attitudes of clinicians began to change.

A clinician who stood out in his interest in transmasculine people was psychiatrist Pauly. Pauly collaborated with Benjamin in the early 1960s and was quick to acknowledge female-to-male transsexuals in the medical literature and suggest they were present in significant numbers.[130] Green and Money's 1969 edited text *Transsexualism and Sex Reassignment* includes chapters about adult transmasculine and transfeminine people, both by Pauly.[131] In 1974, he wrote that the widely held belief by clinicians of low incidence of transsexualism in female-bodied people was inaccurate and suggested the ratio of TGD men to TGD women might approach 1:1.[132] He was prescient. Pauly was exceptional also in his understanding that many of the frustrations clinicians experienced in dealing with TGD people were artifacts of the treatment model and suggested that clinicians were as much a cause of conflict in treatment as their patients.

The medical model did not endure. Its demise was hastened by the skullduggery of McHugh and Jon Meyer, who succeeded in closing the gender clinics. Thanks to the cogent analysis of patient-doctor interactions by psychologist Suzanne Kessler and sociologist Wendy McKenna and further analysis by anthropologist Anne Bolin,[133] a new, healthy person model arose within fledgling trans communities and soon spread to treatment communities.[134] Those clinging to mental illness models of gender variance are few today and are viewed as troglodytes by adherents of the new model. Many therapists, psychiatrists, psychologists, and researchers these days are themselves trans.

Patient-caregiver relations are much improved. We should not forget those courageous few who risked their careers and the respect of their peers by daring to provide gender-affirming care to trans people; nor should we forget those who used their positions of authority to deny us the treatment we needed.[135]

The widespread adoption of the healthy transgender model marked a paradigm shift.[136] Clinicians and TGD people came to view questions posited under the medical model as unproductive and irrelevant, and clinicians shifted their attention away from theories based on the mental illness model to begin offering gender-affirming medical care. This movement began with clinicians in the 1970s and 1980s who observed that TGD clients weren't struggling *en masse* with pathology but rather the stress associated with the rejection, stigmatization, and hostility they experienced due to their minority status as transgender.[137] And by the end of the 1990s, TGD scholars and trainees in medicine, psychiatry, psychology, sociology, and social work were publishing research papers and entering practice and contributing to and broadening the collective knowledge base.

A few of the prescient cisgender mental health professionals who led the way were sexologist and psychotherapist Leah C. Schaefer, who had been an associate of Benjamin in New York City; Scheafer's collaborator and frequent co-author, psychologist Christine Wheeler; and social services innovator, psychologist, and educator Barbara Warren. In the Chicago area, Scheafer's niece, forensic psychologist Randi Ettner, authored several books advocating compassionate care for transsexual people, beginning with *Confessions of a Gender Defender* and *Gender Loving Care*. In the latter book, Ettner postulated that the paradigm shift began with "revolutionary technological advances" enabling surgeons to do better and more sophisticated genital reconstruction, more and better psychosocial research demonstrating the biological roots of gender diversity and outcomes data, and better information dissemination via the Internet.[138] These developments were crucial and so was the increasing visibility and self-advocacy of TGD people.

In the mid-1970s to 1980s, San Francisco psychologist Paul Walker and psychotherapist Lin Fraser recognized the veracity of transgender people's identities and set about to help them live their best lives. Transgender counselor Gianna Israel, one of the first openly trans women to present herself as a gender specialist and privately provide counseling, collaborated with cisgender psychiatrist Donald E. Tarver II, who worked in public health and private practice, to deliver medical, mental health, and social services to the gender diverse population in San Francisco. Together, they created one of the first comprehensive guides to educate general audiences; transgender people; and medical, mental health, and community-based organizations about the TGD community's needs and concerns. Their book *Transgender Care* strove to depathologize TGD people and inspire healthcare professionals to treat them with respect. They informed TGD people what they should expect from a responsive and knowledgeable healthcare provider, and how to recognize when they were being shortchanged or gaslighted.

In 1992, the Tom Waddell Clinic, a part of San Francisco's Department of Public Health and a leader in HIV care, opened its clinic for evening appointments on Transgender Tuesdays to provide hormonal care and general primary healthcare for uninsured, often unhoused transgender residents of the city. Psychiatrist Dan Karasic advocated for the civil rights and ethical treatment of TGD people in diverse settings, from universities to the streets, courtrooms, and prisons. Karasic also worked within the American Psychiatric Association to reform diagnostic terminology and criteria.[139] In 2004, social worker Arlene Istar Lev published her extensive and pathbreaking book *Transgender Emergence: Therapeutic Guidelines for Working With Gender-Variant People and Their Families*, a resource for the burgeoning cohort of healthcare professionals eager to learn about TGD people.

Countless other professionals across the country developed compassion for and the ability to listen to TGD people; TGD individuals rose up, entered the helping professions, and carried out research and interventions to make the world safe for themselves and others like them. Their efforts led to a worldwide effort to reform the rigid, conformist, and punitive attitudes that birthed psychology and psychiatry. As the twenty-first century dawned, inclusive workplaces bloomed, legislators enacted laws and regulations to ensure nondiscrimination, and healthcare education expanded to include training on gender identity. As we strive to learn more about the human condition, we embrace the rich experience of TGD people whose shared stories educate, enlighten, and inspire the clinicians who serve them.

NOTES

1. For summaries of the history of these two approaches to mental health, see Kendra Cherry's "The Origins of Psychology."

2. Lothstein, "Psychodynamics and Sociodynamics," 226.
3. Lothstein, "Psychodynamics and Sociodynamics," 227.
4. Lothstein, "Psychodynamics and Sociodynamics," 226.
5. Socarides, "The Desire for Sexual Transformation," 125.
6. Lothstein, "Psychodynamics and Sociodynamics," 214.
7. Belli, "Transsexual Surgery: A New Tort?" 2144.
8. Lothstein, "Psychodynamics and Sociodynamics," 214.
9. Lothstein, "Psychodynamics and Sociodynamics," 218–25.
10. Ettner, Monstrey, and Coleman, *Principles of Transgender Medicine and Surgery*, 4–5.
11. Lothstein, "Psychodynamics and Sociodynamics," 226.
12. Lothstein, "Psychodynamics and Sociodynamics," 226.
13. Yarbrough, *Transgender Mental Health*.
14. Shtasel, "Behavioral Treatment of Transsexualism," 362–67.
15. Gooren, "The Endocrinology of Transsexualism," 3–14.
16. Money, *The Adam Principle*, 119.
17. Money, *The Adam Principle*, 246–61.
18. Freud, *Three Contributions to the Theory of Sex*, 79.
19. See chapter 6 of this volume.
20. Hamburger, Stürup, and Dahl-Iversen, "Transvestism," 396.
21. Slagstad, "The Political Nature of Sex," 1072; Money, Hampson, and Hampson, "Hermaphroditism," 284–300; Money, Hampson, and Hampson, "An Examination of Some Basic Sexual Concepts," 301–19. See chapter 8.1. Profile: Joseph Lobdell.
22. Dörner et al., "Gene- and Environment-Dependent Neuroendocrine Etiogenesis of Homosexuality and Transsexualism," 141–50.
23. Rosenthal, "Challenges in the Care of Transgender and Gender-Diverse Youth," 581–91.
24. Lothstein, "Psychodynamics and Sociodynamics," 226.
25. Levine, Shaiova, and Mihailovic. "Male to Female: The Role Transformation of Transsexuals," 175.
26. Skinner, *The Behavior of Organisms*.
27. Butler, "Performative Acts and Gender Constitution."
28. Williams, "Gender Performance: The TransAdvocate Interviews Judith Butler."
29. See chapter 14 in this volume.
30. Money, Hampson, and Hampson, "Imprinting and the Establishment of Gender Role," 293; Diamond, "A Critical Evaluation of the Ontogeny."
31. See Diamond, "A Critical Evaluation of the Ontogeny." In 1965, anatomist and psychologist Milton Diamond published a devastating critique of this theory.
32. Dreger, *Intersex in the Age of Ethics*, 12.
33. Meyerowitz, *How Sex Changed*, 98–129.

34. Coleman et al., "Standards of Care for the Health," 167–71.
35. Hines, "Sex-Related Variation in Human Behavior," 448–56.
36. Hines, "Sex-Related Variation in Human Behavior."
37. Hines, "Sex-Related Variation in Human Behavior."
38. Hines, "Sex-Related Variation in Human Behavior."
39. Ettner, Monstrey, and Coleman, *Principles of Transgender Medicine*, 2nd ed., 105–06.
40. World Health Organization. *International Classification of Diseases 11th Revision*.
41. National Committee on Vital and Health Statistics. "Updated Recommendations for Immediate Action on ICD-11."
42. Hamburger, Stürup, and Dahl-Iversen, "Transvestism."
43. Wiedeman, "Letter to the Editor," 1167.
44. Wiedeman, "Letter to the Editor," 1167.
45. Meerloo, "Letter to the Editor," 263–64.
46. Socarides, "The Desire for Sexual Transformation." "Charles Socarides was the standard bearer for psychoanalysts relentlessly arguing that homosexuals [and transsexuals] were mentally ill." See Green, *Gay Rights/Trans Rights*, 33.
47. Ogas, "Spare Parts," 12–15.
48. McHugh, "Psychiatric Misadventures," 497–510; McHugh, "Surgical Sex," 34–38.
49. Szasz, "Male and Female Created He Them."
50. This quote, which appeared in a 1976 interview of Ihlenfeld by D. Greene in *The National Observer*, is cited by Zagria Cowan on her Gender Variance Who's Who website. See also Oppenheim, Garrett, "Ihlenfeld Cautions on Hormones."
51. Barlow, Abel, and Blanchard, "Gender Identity Change in a Transsexual," 387–95.
52. Schechter, *Surgical Management of the Transgender Patient*; Smith, Bartlett, and King, "Treatments of Homosexuality in Britain," 427.
53. See Richards and Ames, *Second Serve*, for the first part of her story, and Richards, *No Way Renée*, for her later views.
54. Denny, "Behavioral Treatment in Gender Dysphoria," 54–56.
55. Cooper, "A Case of Fetishism and Impotence Treated by Behaviour Therapy," 649–52.
56. Smith, Bartlett, and King, "Treatments of Homosexuality in Britain," 427.
57. Denny, "Behavioral Treatment in Gender Dysphoria," 75.
58. Denny, "Behavioral Treatment in Gender Dysphoria," 54–56. For a recent and extensive discussion of this unethical, needless, and dangerous treatment, see Reay, *Trans America*, 161–68.
59. Wikipedia, "Kenneth Zucker," https://en.wikipedia.org/wiki/Kenneth_Zucker. As of July 2022, conversion therapy is banned in twenty states and the District of

Columbia, according to the Movement Advancement Project, Conversion "Therapy" Laws. Practitioners in the United States include George A. Rekers and Gene Abel, and in Canada, Kenneth Zucker, at what was then the Clarke Institute of Psychiatry in Toronto. According to Wikipedia, Zucker "has treated about 500 preadolescent gender-variant children to have them accept the gender identity they were assigned at birth."

60. Benjamin, "The Transsexual Phenomenon," in its entirety.

61. See chapter 11 in this volume.

62. Although certainly some staff members were insensitive and even cruel.

63. Meyerowitz, *How Sex Changed*, 174; Pauly, "Male Psychosexual Inversion," 172–81.

64. Person and Ovesey, "The Transsexual Syndrome in Males: I," 4–20, and Person and Ovesey, "The Transsexual Syndrome in Males: II," 174–93. For definition and discussion, see "A Proliferation of Gender Clinics" section in chapter 11 of this book.

65. Reay, *Trans America*, 137.

66. Jurysta and Hladki. "Primary and Secondary Transsexualism, Really?" 5590–91.

67. Blanchard, "Typology of Male-to-female Transsexualism," 247–61.

68. Lawrence, "Autogynephilia," 135.

69. Lawrence, "Autogynephilia"; Bailey, *The Man Who Would be Queen*.

70. See Herdt, "Robert J. Stoller in the Clinic and the Village." At the same time, Stoller also believed masculinity and femininity were controlled by an innate biological force.

71. Lorenz, "Der Kumpan in der Umwelt des Vogels," 289–413; Hess, "Imprinting in Animals," 81–90.

72. Stoller, *Sex and Gender*, 113.

73. Stoller, *Sex and Gender*, 114.

74. Dr. Em, "Sexist History at the Heart of the 'Science' on Transsexualism"; Stoller, *Sex and Gender*.

75. See Pollak, *The Creation of Doctor B*. Psychiatrist Leo Kanner and psychologist Bruno Bettelheim considered emotionally distant mothers to be the primary cause of autism and Asperger syndrome. For decades, this theory induced guilt in parents of individuals on the autism spectrum. It was, of course, not true. Bettelheim, who popularized Kanner's theory and introduced the term *refrigerator mother*, was eventually revealed to be a fraud. Almost everything about him, including his medical credentials, was a lie.

76. Stoller, "Parental Influences in Male Transsexualism," 155.

77. Stoller and Garfinkel, "Passing and the Managed Achievement of Sex Status," 116–85.

78. Goldberg, "Reframing Agnes." Goldberg does not provide a citation for Schilt's words but presumably they are from the film *Framing Agnes*, directed by Joynt.

79. Schwabe et al., "Pubertal Feminization in a Genetic Male," 762–75.

80. Meyerowitz, *How Sex Changed*, 160.

81. Meyerowitz, *How Sex Changed*, 161.
82. Garfinkel, "Appendix to Chapter 5," 285–88.
83. Meyerowitz, *How Sex Changed*, 160.
84. See chapter 14 in this volume.
85. In this chapter, below.
86. Stoller, " 'Near Miss': Sex Change Treatment and its Evaluation," 283. Stoller became skeptical about the trans surgeries. In 1975, "[H]e wondered about the long-term benefits to patients, and he criticized his colleagues for their gung-ho attitude toward surgery." Meyerowitz, *How Sex Changed*, 267.
87. Goldberg, "Reframing Agnes."
88. Meyerowitz, *How Sex Changed*, 162.
89. Meyerowitz, *How Sex Changed*, 161. It would not be clinicians but rather three nonclinicians who would eventually examine the medical model and discover its shortcomings. See Kessler and McKenna, *Gender: An Ethnomethodological Approach*, and Bolin, *In Search of Eve*.
90. Green and Money, *Transsexualism and Sex Reassignment*.
91. Green, "Sexual Identity of 37 Children Raised by Homosexual or Transsexual Parents," 692–97; Green, "Transsexuals' Children," (1998); Green, "Parental Alienation Syndrome," 9–13.
92. Green, *Gay Rights/ Trans Rights*.
93. Green and Money, "Incongruous Gender Role." See also Green and Money. "Effeminacy in Pre-Pubertal Boys," 286–91.
94. Green, *Gay Rights/Trans Rights*, 25.
95. Green, *The Sissy Boy Syndrome*.
96. Brody, "Boyhood Effeminacy and Later Homosexuality"; Green, *The Sissy Boy Syndrome*; Singh, Bradley, and Zucker, "A Follow-up Study of Boys with Gender Identity Disorder"; Weinrich, "Transsexuals, Homosexuals, and Sissy Boys."
97. Green and Stoller, with Lawrence E. Newman, provided the rationale for this approach in a 1972 paper in *Archives of Gender Psychiatry*.
98. Some subjects were seemingly ashamed of their feminine mannerisms and wanted to become more masculine—or at least said so. In the repressive environment of Green's study, the boys were hardly free to say what they really wanted or how they really felt.
99. Weinrich, "Transsexuals, Homosexuals, and Sissy Boys," 322–35; Singh, Bradley, and Zucker, "A Follow-up Study of Boys With Gender Identity Disorder."
100. Green, *The Sissy Boy Syndrome*, 261.
101. Goulding, "UCLA Study Tried to Change Children's Gender Identity"; Meyerowitz, *How Sex Changed*, 265.
102. Meyerowitz, *How Sex Changed*, 265–66.
103. Green, *Gay Rights/Trans Rights*.
104. Ashley, "Homophobia, Conversion Therapy," 361–83.

105. Zucker, "Treatment of Gender Identity Disorders in Children," 27–45.
106. Southern Poverty Law Center, "Family Research Council."
107. Rothaus, "Antigay Witness Costly."
108. Rekers and Ivar. "Behavioral Treatment," 173–90.
109. Rekers and Lovaas, "Behavioral Treatment," 180, 185–86.
110. Rekers and Lovaas, "Behavioral Treatment," 173.
111. Ashley, "Homophobia, Conversion Therapy," 373; Bronstein and Joseph, "Therapy to Change."
112. Bronstein and Joseph, "Therapy to Change"; Burroway, "What You Didn't See on CNN's 'The Sissy Boy Experiment.'"
113. See chapter 14 in this volume.
114. Szalavitz, "The 'Sissy Boy' Experiment."
115. Bronstein and Joseph, "Therapy to Change"; Melloy, "Did "Cure" for "Feminine Boy" Lead to Suicide"; Szalavitz, "The 'Sissy Boy' Experiment."
116. Melloy, "Did "Cure" for "Feminine Boy" Lead to Suicide."
117. Melloy, "Did "Cure" for "Feminine Boy" Lead to Suicide."
118. Pyne, "The Governance of Gender Non-Conforming Children," 86.
119. Bronstein and Joseph, "Therapy to Change"; Szalavitz, "The 'Sissy Boy' Experiment."
120. Bronstein and Joseph, "Therapy to Change."
121. Bullock and Thorp, "Christian Right Leader"; Bullock and Thorp, "How George Alan Rekers and His Rent Boy got Busted by *New Times*"; Bullock and Thorp, "Reporters Find Tragic Story amid Embarrassing Scandal."
122. In a bizarre counterpoint to previous efforts to expunge boys' femininity, in the current day gender-affirming treatment of TGD children is under attack and has been outlawed in some states. See chapters 12 and 18.2 in this volume.
123. Reay, "*Trans America*," 77.
124. Lothstein, *Female-to-Male Transsexualism*.
125. Devor, *FTM: Female-to-Male Transsexuals in Society*.
126. Sullivan, *We Both Laughed in Pleasure*, 371.
127. Sullivan, *We Both Laughed in Pleasure*, 419.
128. Jamison Green, personal communication to Dallas Denny, October 27, 2022.
129. Sullivan's 1990 book *Information for the Female-to-Male Cross-Dresser and Transsexual* was also transformative for many trans men. It was originally self-published as a pamphlet in 1980, with a second edition in 1985, and a third edition in 1990.
130. Pauly, "Male Psychosexual Inversion," cited by Reay, *Trans America*, 68.
131. Pauly, "Adult Manifestations of Male Transsexualism," 37–58; Pauly, "Adult Manifestations of Female Transsexualism," 59–87.
132. Pauly, "Female Transsexualism: I," 487–507.
133. Kessler and McKenna, *Gender*; Bolin, *In Search of Eve*.

134. Denny, "Transgender Communities in the United States," 171–91.

135. An excellent study of the cultural norms and lack of clinical experience and research contributing to uncertainty in the field is stef m. shuster's *Trans Medicine*.

136. Ettner, "*Gender Loving Care*," xiii–xiv.

137. McLemore, "A Minority Stress Perspective."

138. Ettner, "*Gender Loving Care*," xiii–xiv.

139. For an overview of the issues in diagnoses, see Karasic and Drescher, *Sexual and Gender Diagnoses*.

WORKS CITED

Ashley, Florence. "Homophobia, Conversion Therapy, and Care Models for Trans Youth: Defending the Gender-Affirmative Approach." *Journal of LGBT Youth* 17, no. 4 (2020): 361–83.

Bailey, Michael. *The Man Who Would Be Queen*. Washington, DC: Joseph Henry Press, 2003.

Bak, Robert C., and Walter A. Stewart. "Fetishism, Transvestism, and Voyeurism: A Psychoanalytic Approach." In *American Handbook of Psychiatry*, 2nd ed., Vol. 2, edited by S. Arieti and E. Brady, 352–63. New York: Basic Books, 1974.

Barlow, David H., Gene G. Abel, and Edward B. Blanchard. "Gender Identity Change in a Transsexual: An Exorcism." *Archives of Sexual Behavior* 6, no. 5 (September 1977): 387–95.

Belli, Melvin M. "Transsexual Surgery: A New Tort?" *Journal of the American Medical Association* 239, no. 20 (1978):2143–48.

Benjamin, Harry. *The Transsexual Phenomenon: A Scientific Report on Transsexualism and Sex Conversion in the Human Male and Female*. Ace Publications, 1966.

Blanchard, Ray. "The Concept of Autogynephilia and the Typology of Male Gender Dysphoria." *Journal of Nervous and Mental Disease* 177, no. 10 (1989): 616–23.

———. "Typology of Male-to-Female Transsexualism." *Archives of Sexual Behavior* 14, no. 3 (1985): 247–61.

Bolin, Anne. *In Search of Eve: Transsexual Rites of Passage*. South Hadley, MA: Bergin & Garvey, 1988.

Brody, Jane E. "Boyhood Effeminacy and Later Homosexuality." *New York Times*, C1, December 16, 1986. Accessed July 12, 2022. https://www.nytimes.com/1986/12/16/science/boyhood-effeminancy-and-later-homosexuality.html.

Bronstein, Scott, and Jessi Joseph. "Therapy to Change 'Feminine' Boy Created a Troubled Man, Family Says." *CNN*, June 10, 2011. Accessed August 12, 2022. http://www.cnn.com/2011/US/06/07/sissy.boy.experiment/index.html.

Bullock, Penn, and Brandon K. Thorp. "Christian Right Leader George Rekers Takes Vacation with 'Rent Boy.'" *Miami New Times*, May 6, 2011. Accessed August 15, 2022. https://www.miaminewtimes.com/news/christian-right-leader-george-rekers-takes-vacation-with-rent-boy-6377933.

———. "How George Alan Rekers and his Rent Boy Got Busted by *New Times*." *Miami New Times*, May 13, 2011. Accessed August 15, 2022. https://www.miaminewtimes.com/news/how-george-alan-rekers-and-his-rent-boy-got-busted-by-new-times-6366835.

———. "Reporters Find Tragic Story Amid Embarrassing Scandal." *CNN*, June 10, 2011. Accessed August 15, 2022. http://www.cnn.com/2011/US/06/08/rekers.sissy.boy.experiment/index.html.

Burroway, Jim. "What You Didn't See on CNN's 'The Sissy Boy Experiment.'" *Box Turtle Bulletin*, June 8, 2011. Accessed August 15, 2022. http://www.boxturtlebulletin.com/2011/06/08/33993.

Butler, Judith. "Performative Acts and Gender Constitution: An Essay in Phenomenology and Feminist Theory." *Theatre Journal* 40, no. 4 (1988): 519–31. https://doi.org/10.2307/3207893.

Cherry, Kendra. "The Origins of Psychology: From Philosophical Beginnings to the Modern Day." Verywellmind, 2020. Accessed July 9, 2022. https://www.verywellmind.com/a-brief-history-of-psychology-through-the-years-2795245.

Coleman, Eli, Walter Bockting, Marsha Botzer, et al. "Standards of Care for the Health of Transsexual, Transgender, and Gender-Nonconforming People, Version 7." *International Journal of Transgenderism* 13, no. 4 (2012): 165–232.

Cooper, A. J. "A Case of Fetishism and Impotence Treated by Behaviour Therapy." *British Journal of Psychiatry* 109, no. 462 (1963): 649–52.

Denny, Dallas. "Behavioral Treatment in Gender Dysphoria: A Review of the Literature and a Call for Reform." *TV-TS Tapestry Journal* 69 (Fall 1994): 54–56. Accessed August 8, 2024. http://dallasdenny.com/Writing/2011/10/25/behavioral-treatment-of-gender-dysphoria/.

———. "Changing Models of Transsexualism." *Journal of Gay & Lesbian Psychotherapy* 8, no. 1 (2004): 25–40.

———. "The Paradigm Shift is Here!" *AEGIS News*, 4 (1995): 1. Accessed August 17, 2022. http://dallasdenny.com/Writing/2013/04/29/the-paradigm-shift-is-here-1995/.

———. "Transgender Communities in the United States in the Late Twentieth Century." In *Transgender Rights*, edited by P. Currah, R. M. Juang, and S. P. Minter, 171–91. Minneapolis: University of Minnesota Press, 2006. Accessed August 8, 2024. http://dallasdenny.com/Writing/2014/03/01/transgender-communities-in-the-united-states-in-the-late-twentieth-century-2006/.

Devor, Holly. *"FTM: Female-to-Male Transsexuals in Society."* Bloomington: Indiana University Press, 1997.

Diamond, Milton. "A Critical Evaluation of the Ontogeny of Human Sexual Behavior." *Quarterly Review of Biology*, 40, no. 2 (June 1965): 147–75.

Dörner, Günter, Ingrid Poppe, F. Stahl, J. Kölzsch, and R. Uebelhack. "Gene- and Environment-Dependent Neuroendocrine Etiogenesis of Homosexuality and Transsexualism." *Experimental and Clinical Endocrinology* 89, no. 2 (1981): 141–50. https://doi.org/ 10.1055/s-0029-1211110.

Dr. Em. "Sexist History at the Heart of the 'Science' on Transsexualism, Part II: Robert Stoller, True Trans." Uncommon Grounds Media: Material Humanism, 2020. Accessed July 10, 2022. https://uncommongroundmedia.com/robert-stoller-true-trans/.

Dreger, Alice Domurat. *Intersex in the Age of Ethics*. Hagerstown, MD: University Publishing Group, 1999.

Ettner, Randi. *Confessions of a Gender Defender*. Evanston, IL: Chicago Spectrum Press, 1996.

———. *Gender Loving Care: A Guide to Counseling Gender Variant Clients*. New York: W. W. Norton, 1999.

Ettner, Randi, Stan Monstrey, and A. Evan Eyler. *Principles of Transgender Medicine and Surgery*. New York: Haworth Press, 2007.

Ettner, Randi, Stan Monstrey, and Eli Coleman. *Principles of Transgender Medicine and Surgery*. 2nd ed. New York: Routledge, 2016.

Freud, Sigmund. *Three Contributions to the Theory of Sex*. 2nd ed. New York: Nervous and Mental Disease, 1920.

Garfinkel, Harold. "Appendix to Chapter 5." In *Studies in Ethnomethodology*, edited by Harold Garfinkel, 285–88. New York: Prentice-Hall, 1967.

Goldberg, R. L. "Reframing Agnes." *Paris Review*, April 26, 2019. Accessed July 10, 2022. https://www.theparisreview.org/blog/2019/04/26/reframing-agnes/.

Gooren, Louis. "The Endocrinology of Transsexualism: A Review and Commentary." *Psychoneuroendocrinology* 15, no. 1 (1990): 3–14. https://doi.org/10.1016/0306-4530(90)90041-7.

Goulding, Susan Christian. "UCLA Study Tried to Change Children's Gender Identity Starting in the 1960s, Say Two Educators." *Orange County Register*, November 18, 2019. Accessed July 13, 2022. https://www.ocregister.com/2019/11/18/2-subjects-discuss-trauma-as-kids-involved-in-uclas-now-defunct-gender-identity-study/.

Greene, D. "A Doctor Tells Why He'll No Longer Treat Transsexuals." *National Observer*, October 16, 1976, 14. As cited in Zagria Cowan's A Gender Variance Who's Who website. Accessed July 9, 2022. https://zagria.blogspot.com/2013/11/charles-l-ihlenfeld-1937-sexologist.html#.YskenHbMJD9.

Green, Richard. *Gay Rights/ Trans Rights: A Psychiatrist/Lawyer's 50-Year Battle*. Self-published, Richard Green, 2018.

———. "Parental Alienation Syndrome and the Transsexual Parent." *International Journal of Transsexualism* 9, no. 1 (2006): 9–13.

———. "Robert Stoller's *Sex and Gender:* 40 Years On." *Archives of Sexual Behavior* 39 (2010): 1456–65.

———. "Sexual Identity of 37 Children Raised by Homosexual or Transsexual Parents." *American Journal of Psychiatry* 135, no. 6 (1978): 692–97.

———. *The Sissy Boy Syndrome: The Development of Homosexuality.* New Haven, CT: Yale University Press, 1987.

———. "Transsexuals' Children." *International Journal of Transgenderism* 2, no. 4 (1998). Accessed December 16, 2022. https://www.acthe.fr/upload/1445876170-green-r-1998-transsexuals-s-children.pdf.

Green, Richard, and John Money. "Incongruous Gender Role: Nongenital Manifestations in Pre-Pubertal Boys. *Journal of Nervous and Mental Disease* 131, no. 2 (1960): 160–68.

———. "Effeminacy in Prepubertal Boys: Summary of Eleven Cases and Recommendations for Case Management." *Pediatrics* 28 (1961): 286–91.

———, eds. *Transsexualism and Sex Reassignment.* Baltimore, MD: Johns Hopkins University Press, 1969.

Green, Richard, Lawrence E. Newman, and Robert Stoller. "Treatment of Boyhood 'Transsexualism': An Interim Report of Four Years' Experience." *Archives of General Psychiatry* 26, no. 3 (1972): 213–17.

Hamburger, Christian, George K. Stürup, and Erling Dahl-Iversen. "Transvestism: Hormonal, Psychiatric, and Surgical Treatment." *Journal of the American Medical Association* 152, no. 5 (May 30, 1953): 391–96. https://doi: 10.1001/jama.1953.03690050015006.

Herdt, Gilbert. "Robert J. Stoller in the Clinic and the Village." *Psychoanalysis and History* 22, no. 1 (2020): 15–34.

Hess, Eckhard. "Imprinting in Animals." *Scientific American* 198, no. 3 (1958): 81–90.

Hines, Melissa. "Sex-Related Variation in Human Behavior and the Brain." *Trends in Cognitive Sciences* 14, no. 10 (2010): 448–56. https://doi.org/10.1016/j.tics.2010.07.005.

Israel, Gianna E., and Donald E. Tarver II. *Transgender Care: Recommended Guidelines, Practical information & Personal Accounts.* Philadelphia, PA: Temple University Press, 1997.

Joynt, Chase, dir. *Framing Agnes.* 2022. Accessed July 13, 2022. https://www.framingagnes.com/.

Jurysta, Fabrice, and Gaëlle Hladki. "Primary and Secondary Transsexualism, Really?" *European Psychiatry* 33 (March 2016): 5590–91. Accessed July 10, 2022. https://www.sciencedirect.com/science/article/abs/pii/S0924933816022045.

Karasic, D., and J. Drescher. *Sexual and Gender Diagnoses of the Diagnostic and Statistical Manual (DSM): A Reevaluation.* Binghamton, NY: Haworth Press, 2005.

Kessler, Suzanne J, and Wendy McKenna. *Gender: An Ethnomethodological Approach.* New York: John Wiley & Sons, 1978.

Kuhn, Thomas S. *The Structure of Scientific Revolutions.* Chicago, IL: University of Chicago, 1962.

Lawrence, Anne A. "Autogynephilia: An Unappreciated Paraphilia." *Advances in Psychosomatic Medicine* 31 (October 10, 2011): 135–48.

Lev, Arlene Istar. *Transgender Emergence: Therapeutic Guidelines for Working with Gender-Variant People and Their Families.* New York: Haworth Clinical Practice Press, 2004.

Levine, Edward M., Charles H. Shaiova, and Miodrag Mihailovic. "Male to Female: The Role Transformation of Transsexuals." *Archives of Sexual Behavior* 4, no. 2 (1975): 173–85. https://doi.org/10.1007/BF01541081.

Lorenz, Konrad. "Der Kumpan in der Umwelt des Vogels. Der Artgenosse als auslösendes Moment sozialer Verhaltensweisen (The Companion in the Bird's Environment. The Conspecific as a Triggering Moment of Social Behavior)." *Journal für Ornithologie* 83, no. 137–215 (1935): 289–413.

Lothstein, Leslie M. "Psychodynamics and Sociodynamics of Gender-Dysphoric States." *American Journal of Psychotherapy* 33, no. 2 (1979): 214–38.

Lothstein, Leslie Martin. *Female-to-Male Transsexualism: Historical, Clinical, and Theoretical Issues.* Boston, MA: Routledge & Kegan Paul, 1983.

McHugh, Paul R. "Psychiatric Misadventures." *American Scholar* 61, no. 4 (1992): 497–510.

———. "Surgical Sex." *First Things: The Journal of Religion, Culture, and Public Life* 147 (November 2004): 34–38.

McLemore, K. A. "A Minority Stress Perspective on Transgender Individuals' Experiences with Misgendering." *Stigma and Health* 3, no. 1 (2018): 53–64. https://doi.org/10.1037/sah0000070.

Meerloo, Joost A. M. "Letter to the Editor: Change of Sex and Collaboration with the Psychosis." *American Journal of Psychiatry* 124, no. 2 (1967): 263–64.

Melloy, Kilian. "Did 'Cure' for 'Feminine Boy' Lead to Suicide of 38-Year-Old Man?" EdgeMediaNetwork, June 7, 2011. Accessed December 16, 2022. https://www.edgemedianetwork.com/story/120616.

Meyerowitz, Joanne. *How Sex Changed: A History of Transsexuality in the United States.* Cambridge, MA: Harvard University Press, 2002.

Money, John. *The Adam Principle: Genes, Genitals, Hormones, and Gender: Selected Readings in Sexology.* Buffalo, NY: Prometheus Books, 1993.

Money, John, John L. Hampson, and Joan G. Hampson. "An Examination of Some Basic Sexual Concepts: The Evidence of Human Hermaphroditism." *Bulletin of the Johns Hopkins Hospital* 97 (1955): 301–19.

———. "Hermaphroditism: Recommendations Concerning Assignment of Sex, Change of Sex, and Psychologic Management." *Bulletin of the Johns Hopkins Hospital* 97 (1955): 284–300.

---. "Imprinting and the Establishment of Gender Role." *Obstetrical and Gynecological Survey* 13, no. 2 (April 1958): 293–294.

Movement Advancement Project. "Conversion 'Therapy' Laws." Accessed July 9, 2022. https://www.lgbtmap.org/equality-maps/conversion_therapy.

National Committee on Vital and Health Statistics. "Updated Recommendations for Immediate Action on *ICD-11*." September 10, 2021. Accessed December 16, 2022. https://ncvhs.hhs.gov/wp-content/uploads/2021/09/NCVHS-ICD-11-recommendations-for-HHS-Sept-10-2021-Final-508.pdf.

Ogas, Ogi. "Spare Parts: New Information Reignites a Controversy Surrounding the Hopkins Gender Identity Clinic." *City Paper* (Baltimore), March 9, 1994, 10, 12–15.

Oppenheim, Garrett. "Ihlenfeld Cautions on Hormones." *Transition* 8 (February 1979). Pages unnumbered.

Pauly, Ira B. "Adult Manifestations of Female Transsexualism." In *Transsexualism and Sex Reassignment*, edited by Richard Green and John Money, 59–87. Baltimore, MD: Johns Hopkins University Press, 1969.

---. "Adult Manifestations of Male Transsexualism." In *Transsexualism and Sex Reassignment*, edited by Richard Green and John Money, 37–58. Baltimore, MD: Johns Hopkins University Press, 1969.

---. Female Transsexualism: I." *Archives of Sexual Behavior* 3, no. 6 (1974): 487–507.

---. "Male Psychosexual Inversion: Transsexualism. A Review of 100 Cases." *Archives of General Psychiatry* 13, no. 2 (1965): 172–81.

Person, Ethyl, and Lionel Ovesey. "The Transsexual Syndrome in Males: I. Primary Transsexualism." *American Journal of Psychotherapy* 28 (1974): 4–20.

---. "The Transsexual Syndrome in Males: II. Secondary Transsexualism." *American Journal of Psychotherapy* 28 (1974): 174–93.

Pollak, Richard. *The Creation of Doctor B.: A Biography of Bruno Bettelheim*. New York: Simon & Schuster, 1997.

Pyne, Jake. "The Governance of Gender Non-Conforming Children: A Dangerous Enclosure." *Annual Review of Critical Psychology* 11 (January 2014): 79–96.

Raymond, Janice G. *The Transsexual Empire: The Making of a She-Male*. London: Women's Press, 1979.

Reay, Barry. *Trans America: A Counter-History*. Medford, MA: Polity Press, 2020.

Rekers, George A., and Lovaas O. Ivar. "Behavioral Treatment of Deviant Sex-Role Behaviors in a Male Child." *Journal of Applied Behavior Analysis* 7, no. 2 (Summer 1974): 173–90.

Richards, Renée. *No Way, Renée: The Second Half of My Notorious Life*. New York: Simon & Schuster, 2007.

Richards, Renée, and John Ames. *Second Serve: The Renée Richards Story*. New York: Stein & Day, 1983.

Rosenthal, Stephen M. "Challenges in the Care of Transgender and Gender-Diverse Youth: An Endocrinologist's View." *National Review of Endocrinology* 17, no. 10 (October 2021): 581–91. doi: 10.1038/s41574-021-00535-9.

Rothaus, Steve. "Antigay Witness Costly." *Tampa Bay Times*, May 12, 2010. Accessed August 12, 2022. https://www.tampabay.com/archive/2010/05/12/antigay-witness-costly/.

Schechter, Loren S. *Surgical Management of the Transgender Patient.* Amsterdam: Elsevier, 2016.

Schwabe, Arthur D., David H. Solomon, Robert Stoller, and Jason P. Burnham. "Pubertal Feminization in a Genetic Male with Testicular Atrophy and Normal Urinary Gonadotropin." *Journal of Clinical Endocrinology and Metabolism* 22 (August 1962): 834–45.

Shtasel, T. F. "Behavioral Treatment of Transsexualism: A Case Report." *Journal of Sex & Marital Therapy* 5, no. 4 (1979): 362–67. https://doi.org/10.1080/00926237908407080.

shuster, stef m. *Trans Medicine: The Emergence and Practice of Treating Gender.* New York: New York University Press, 2021.

Singh, Devita, Susan J. Bradley, and Kenneth J. Zucker. "A Follow-up Study of Boys with Gender Identity Disorder." *Frontiers in Psychiatry*, 12 (March 29, 2021): pages unnumbered. https://doi.org/10.3389/fpsyt.2021.632784.

Skinner, Burrhus F. *The Behavior of Organisms.* New York: Appleton-Century-Crofts, 1938.

Slagstad, Ketil. "The Political Nature of Sex—Transgender in the History of Medicine." *New England Journal of Medicine* 384, no. 11 (2021): 1070–74. https://doi.org/10.1056/NEJMms2029814.

Smith, Glenn, Annie Bartlett, and Michael King. "Treatments of Homosexuality in Britain Since the 1950s—and Oral History: The Experience of Patients." *British Medical Journal* 32, no. 8 (February 21, 2004): 427.

Socarides, Charles W. "The Desire for Sexual Transformation: A Psychiatric Evaluation of Transsexualism." *American Journal of Psychiatry* 125, no. 10 (1969): 1419–25. https://doi.org/10.1176/ajp.125.10.1419.

Southern Poverty Law Center. "Family Research Council." Accessed August 12, 2022. https://www.splcenter.org/fighting-hate/extremist-files/group/family-research-council.

Stoller, Robert J. "'Near Miss': Sex Change Treatment and its Evaluation." In *Eating, Sleeping and Sexuality*, edited by M. R. Zales, 258–83. New York: Brunner/Mazel, 1982.

———. "Parental Influences in Male Transsexualism." In *Transsexualism and Sex Reassignment*, edited by Richard Green and John Money, 153–69. Baltimore, MD: Johns Hopkins University Press, 1969.

———. *Sex and Gender: On the Development of Masculinity and Femininity*. London: Hogarth Press, 1968.

Stoller, Robert, and Harold Garfinkel. "Passing and the Managed Achievement of Sex Status in an 'Intersexed' Person." In *Studies in Ethnomethodology*, edited by Harold Garfinkel, 116–85. New York: Prentice-Hall, 1967.

Sullivan, Lou. *Information for the Female-to-Male Cross-Dresser and Transsexual*. Seattle, WA: Ingersoll Gender Center, 1990.

———. *We Both Laughed in Pleasure: The Selected Diaries of Lou Sullivan, 1961–1991*, edited by Ellis Martin and Zach Ozma. New York: Nightboat Books, 2019.

Szalavitz, Maia. "The 'Sissy Boy' Experiment: Why Gender-Related Cases Call for Scientists' Humility." *Time*, June 8, 2011. Accessed July 12, 2022. https://healthland.time.com/2011/06/08/the-sissy-boy-experiment-why-gender-related-cases-call-for-scientists-humility/.

Szasz, Thomas. "Male and Female Created He Them." *New York Times*, section BR, 3, June 10, 1979. Accessed July 9, 2022. https://www.nytimes.com/1979/06/10/archives/male-and-female-created-he-them-transexual.html.

Waltz, Mitzi M. "Mothers and Autism: The Evolution of a Discourse of Blame." *American Medical Association Journal of Ethics* 17, no. 4 (April 2015): 353–58. Accessed July 10, 2022. https://journalofethics.ama-assn.org/article/mothers-and-autism-evolution-discourse-blame/2015-04.

Weinrich, James D. "Transsexuals, Homosexuals, and Sissy Boys: On the Mathematics of Follow-up Studies." *Journal of Sex Research* 21, no. 3 (August 1985): 322–35.

Wiedeman, George H. "Letter to the Editor." *Journal of the American Medical Association* 152, no. 12 (1953): 1167.

Williams, Cristan. "Gender Performance: The TransAdvocate Interviews Judith Butler." *TransAdvocate*, n.d. Accessed December 15, 2021. https://www.transadvocate.com/gender-performance-the-transadvocate-interviews-judith-butler_n_13652.htm.

Yarbrough, E. *Transgender Mental Health*. 1st ed. Washington, DC: American Psychiatric Association, 2018.

World Health Organization. *International Classification of Diseases 11th Revision*. 2019. Accessed December 15, 2021. https://icd.who.int/en.

Zucker, Kenneth. "Treatment of Gender Identity Disorders in Children." In *Clinical Management of Gender Identity Disorders in Children and Adults*, edited by Ray Blanchard and Betty W. Steiner, 27–45. Washington, DC: American Psychiatric Association, 1990.

8.1. PROFILE: JOSEPH ISRAEL LOBDELL (1829–1912)

Bambi Lobdell

Joseph Lobdell,[1] née Lucy Ann Lobdell, was born 1829 in Westerloo, New York.[2] As a young child, he wandered the woods so often his mother had to bell him to keep track of his whereabouts.[3] At the age of ten, after voicing a desire for an education, he was given the task of managing livestock to earn money to pay for tuition. To protect the livestock from predators, he taught himself how to shoot, eventually earning a reputation as a superior marksman in adulthood, and the nickname The Female Hunter of Delaware County.[4]

In 1852, he moved with his family to Long Eddy, New York, where he taught at the small village's first school. His family compelled him to marry George Slater.[5] Lobdell shocked the community by disobeying Slater, wearing men's clothes, doing men's work, cutting his hair short, disagreeing with ministers, and openly advocating for women's rights.[6] In October 1855, after Slater abandoned his family, Lucy reclaimed the name Lobdell, secured his newborn infant with his parents, and, wearing men's clothing, left the area.[7]

In October 1855, Joseph Israel Lobdell entered Bethany, Pennsylvania, and established a singing school. He was welcomed by the townspeople and was known as "a general favorite among the girls."[8] He wooed one woman but the day before their wedding, word got out that Lobdell "was not a man but a woman," and an all-male tar-and-feather crew chased him out of town.[9]

In the spring of 1856, Lobdell traveled to Minnesota, ending up in Manannah as La-Roi Lobdell.[10] As a multiskilled hard worker, he bunked with other men and was considered "offensive to none . . . and a 'hale fellow well met.'"[11] In 1858, "by accident, 'Satan, with the aid of original sin,' exposed Lobdell's sex," and Lobdell was arrested and tried for his gender performance: "One Lobdell, being a woman, falsely impersonates a man."[12] However, the judge found Lobdell competent and dismissed the case, and Lobdell was freed.[13] Rejected by the general populace and without work, he returned to Long Eddy, penniless, and still presenting as male.

Lobdell's hard luck persisted. In 1860 he signed himself into the County Poor House in Delhi, New York.[14] In 1861, Marie Perry arrived, and shortly thereafter, the two left the poorhouse. They were married by a member of the clergy and returned to Perry's hometown of Whitman, Massachusetts.[15] They lived on Perry's father's estate, where Lobdell was described as a "hard-working, industrious citizen and exemplary family man."[16] Eventually, Perry's family suspected "'Joe' was not all that he pretended to be" and had him arrested and jailed for months.[17] After Perry successfully pleaded for Lobdell's release, they left the area. This was the third time Lobdell had first been accepted into a community and then rejected and expelled, so the wilderness might have seemed safer than civilization. From 1864 to 1878, the couple wandered the woods near the New York–Pennsylvania border.[18] Lobdell built rough cabins, hunted and trapped, and traded game and pelts for supplies.[19]

During this time, local newspapers noted every time Lobdell and Perry came into any town. They described Perry as pretty, but the masculine Lobdell as a "raving maniac," a "strange creature, haggard and insane, wandering the countryside like a beast."[20] People of this time felt gender roles and presentation were dictated by biology, so Lobdell's gender nonconformity was viewed as so deviant and disorderly that it was assumed to be a sign of insanity. Articles reported his periodic arrests for vagrancy and highlighted Lobdell's gender variance by referring to him as "the man-woman" and "it."[21] They noted Lobdell and Perry's marriage as a relationship that was curious but constant, referring to them as "the female hunter and her wife, Marie."[22] Newspapers in larger cities, such as *The New York Times* and *The Boston Globe*, were kinder, and Lobdell's life story was reported as the exciting adventure of a superior marksman.[23]

In 1880, Lobdell was committed to the Willard Insane Asylum at Ovid, New York.[24] Lunacy testimonials claimed as proof of insanity that Lobdell wore men's clothes, claimed to be a man, and considered Marie his wife. P. M. Wise, the attending physician at Willard Asylum, published "Case of Sexual Perversion," the first medical case study in the United States to describe a person who would today be understood as transgender.[25]

Wise diagnosed Lobdell with "a rare form of mental disease" and focused on Lobdell's masculine presentation and behaviors and his "perverted" sexual proclivities.[26] Wise presents Lobdell's account of intimacy in his married life but seems skeptical about whether he and Perry had sex: "From this statement, it *appears* that she made frequent *attempts* at sexual intercourse with her companion and *believed* them successful; that she *believed* herself to possess virility and the coaptation of a male; that she had not experienced connubial content with her husband but with her late companion nuptial satisfaction was complete."[27] Scholars point to Wise's use of the term *lesbian*, the first use of this word in the medical literature, but Wise used the word as an adjective, not as a noun to define an identity:[28] "An incident occurred in 1876 to interrupt the quiet monotony of this Lesbian love."[29] Wise concluded that Lobdell's case was a "clinical curiosity," establishing the precedent for US academic publications to conflate gender diversity with mental illness.[30]

Lobdell died in the Binghamton Insane Asylum in 1912.[31]

Figure 8.1.1. A young Lobdell. *Source*: Wikimedia Commons. Public domain.

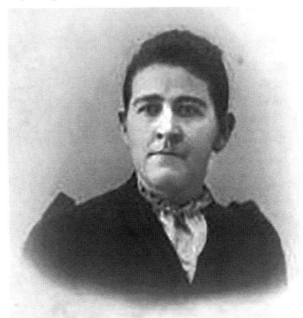

NOTES

1. Bambi Lobdell is second cousin, four times removed, to Joseph Lobdell.
2. Lobdell, *Narrative of Lucy Ann Lobdell*, 3.
3. Lobdell, *Narrative of Lucy Ann Lobdell*, 4.
4. Lobdell, *Narrative of Lucy Ann Lobdell*, 30.
5. Wise and Willard, "Case of Sexual Perversion," 88. Lobdell, *Narrative of Lucy Ann Lobdell*, 13. While Lobdell presents marriage to Slater as something desired, Wise reports that "it was after the earnest solicitation of her parents and friends that she consented to marry, in her twentieth year, a man for whom, she has repeatedly stated, she had no affection and from whom she never derived a moment's pleasure, although she endeavored to be a good wife."
6. Lobdell, *Narrative of Lucy Ann Lobdell*, 1–47.
7. Lobdell, *Narrative of Lucy Ann Lobdell*, 41–47.
8. *Evening Gazette*. "The Man-Woman," 1.
9. *Evening Gazette*. "The Man-Woman," 1.
10. Smith, *A Random Historical Sketch of Meeker County*, 103.
11. Smith, *A Random Historical Sketch of Meeker County*, 105.

12. Smith, *A Random Historical Sketch of Meeker County*, 105.
13. Smith, *A Random Historical Sketch of Meeker County*, 106.
14. *New York Times*, "Extraordinary Narrative," 5.
15. *Omaha Daily Boo*, "Defied Father for Lover," 6.
16. *Omaha Daily Boo*, "Defied Father for Lover," 6.
17. *National*, "Marie's Joe"; *Boston Globe*, "Wife of a Woman," 11.
18. Kiernan, "Psychological Aspects of the Sexual Appetite," 203.
19. *Wayne Citizen*, "Death of the 'Hunter of Long Eddy.'"
20. *Stamford Mirror*, "The Female Hunter of Long Eddy," 2; *Port Jervis Evening Gazette*, "The Man-Woman, Lucy Ann Lobdell in Town."
21. *Wayne Citizen*, "The Maniac Man-Woman"; *Port Jervis Evening Gazette*, "The Man-Woman, Lucy Ann Lobdell in Town"; *Honesdale Citizen*, "Sidebar About Lobdell Leaving Jail With Marie."
22. *Warren Ledger*, "A Queer Married Couple," 1; *Evening Gazette*, "Romantic Lunatics"; *Wayne County Citizen*, "Lucy Ann Lobdell."
23. *Boston Globe*, "Wife of a Woman," 11.
24. Delaware County Clerk's Office, "In the Mattter of Lucy Ann Slater, A Supposed Lunatic."
25. Wise and Willard, "Case of Sexual Perversion," 87.
26. Wise and Willard, "Case of Sexual Perversion," 90.
27. Wise and Willard, "Case of Sexual Perversion," 90.
28. Wise and Willard, "Case of Sexual Perversion," 88.
29. The first term used as an identity for homosexuals was *invert*, as sexologists believed same-sex desire was created by having the wrong soul or brain inside the body. Believing that women did not experience sexual desire, sexologists first focused on nonnormative sexual activities of men. The earliest scientific explanation for homosexuality claimed that homosexual men had the brains or souls of women in their bodies, which influenced their form of desire. In the 1860s, Karl Heinrich Ulrichs presented his theory about same-sex attraction in men, stating he knew firsthand the symptoms and the problems as he, himself, suffered from the condition. He claimed that one man out of five hundred had this condition and he called these men "urnings," female souls trapped in male bodies, suffering from a hereditary, congenital condition that was not perverse or immoral, but rather physiological. In 1864, he published *Vindex* (Book 1 in the collection *The Riddle of Man-Manly Love*, which, in 1994, introduced Ulrichs's work to English-speaking readers). Ulrichs sought to vindicate the rights of gay men and described urnings as "mental hermaphrodites." This condition was presented as distinctly male since Ulrichs, like all sexologists, presumed that women were naturally and passively heterosexual. In 1869, Karl Westphal published his theory of sexual inversion, describing effeminate male and masculine female same-sex attraction in *Archive for Psychiatry and Nervous Disorders*. See also

"Sexual Inversion in Women" by Havelock Ellis in which he presents his four types of female inverts, based mostly on gender presentation.

30. Wise and Willard, "Case of Sexual Perversion," 91.

31. Bureau of Vital Statistics, "Death Certificate Lucy Ann Slater."

WORKS CITED

Boston Globe. "Wife of a Woman." November 21, 1890, 11.

Bureau of Vital Statistics. "Death Certificate Lucy Ann Slater." City of Binghamton, NY, May 28, 1912.

Delaware County Clerk's Office. "In the Matter of Lucy Ann Slater, A Supposed Lunatic." Delhi, New York, May 31, 1880. Testimony of Sidney Lobdell, John Lobdell, Harry Welsh and William Main.

Ellis, Havelock. "Sexual Inversion in Women." *Alienist and Neurologist: A Quarterly Journal of Scientific, Clinical and Forensic Psychiatry and Neurology* 16 (1895): 141–58.

Evening Gazette. "Romantic Lunatics." September 21, 1876.

Evening Gazette. "The Man-Woman. Lucy Ann Lobdell, the Female Huntress of Wayne." August 10, 1896, 1.

Honesdale Citizen. "Sidebar about Lobdell Leaving Jail with Marie." September 21, 1876.

Kiernan, James G. "Psychological Aspects of the Sexual Appetite." *Alienist and Neurologist* 12 (1891): 203.

Lobdell, Bambi. *A Strange Sort of Being. The Transgender Life of Lucy Ann/Joseph Israel Lobdell 1829–1912.* Jefferson, NC: McFarland, 2011.

Lobdell, Lucy Ann. *Narrative of Lucy Ann Lobdell, the Female Hunter of Delawaree and Sullivan Counties.* New York: Self-published, 1855.

National. "Marie's Joe." December 13, 1890, 3.

New York Times. "Death of a Modern Diana: The Female Hunter of Long Eddy—the Strange History of Lucy Slater—Her Career as a Huntress, a Pauper, A Minister, and a Vagrant—Dressed in Men's Clothing She Wins a Girl's Love." October 2, 1879, 2.

New York Times. "Extraordinary Narrative." August 25, 1871, 5.

Omaha Daily Boo. "Defied Father for Lover." December 22, 1890, 6.

Port Jervis Evening Gazette. "The Man-Woman, Lucy Ann Lobdell in Town." n.d.

Smith, A. C. *A Random Historical Sketch of Meeker County, Minnesota: From Its First Settlement to July 4th, 1876.* Llitschfield, MN: Belfoy & Joubert. 1877. Accessed October 18, 2022. https://archive.org/details/randomhistorical00smit/page/n13/mode/2up?ref=ol&view=theater.

Stamford Mirror. "The Female Hunter of Long Eddy: A Raving Maniac." November 14, 1871, 2.

Ulrichs, Karl Heinrich. *The Riddle of Man-Manly Love. 1864–1879*. Translated by Michael Lombrdi-Nash. Amherst, NY: Prometheus Books, 1994.

Warren Ledger. "A Queer Married Couple." Novemnber 15, 1883, 1.

Wayne Citizen. "Death of the 'Hunter of Long Eddy." October 16, 1879.

———. "The Maniac Man-Woman." November 2, 1871.

Wayne County Citizen. "Lucy Ann Lobdell." November 9, 1871.

Westphal, Karl. *Contrary Sexual Instinct: Symptom of a Neuropathic (Psychopathic) Condition*. Translated by M. Lombardi-Nash. Jacksonville, FL: Urania Manuscripts, 2006. Original work published in *Archive for Psychiatry and Nervous Disorders* 2 (1869): 73–108.

Wise, P. M., and N. Y. Willard. "Case of Sexual Perversion from Alienist and Neurologist." *Alienist and Neurologist* 4, no. 1 (1983): 87–91. Accessed December 12, 2020. https://search.proquest.com/openview/a840246cdc94b904f753056d8fa5398c/1?pq-origsite=gscholar&cbl=51134.

8.2. PROFILE: DAVID O. CAULDWELL (1897–1959)

Carolyn Wolf-Gould

In 1946, Dr. David O. Cauldwell, an army contract surgeon and neuropsychiatrist for the US War Department, left patient care to become the editor of the question-and-answer section of a trendy, quasi-scientific magazine called *Sexology*.[1] From 1947 to 1956, he published extensively about transsexuality, transvestism, and hermaphroditism, breaking taboos and creating a critical but more liberal climate for discussion of these topics. Cauldwell asked and answered the questions: What is this phenomenon? Why are people like this? How do we treat people like this? Although he had no formal training in sexology, Cauldwell touted himself as an expert by dint of his communication with thousands of transgender people who peppered him with questions. He published pamphlets, case reports, and essays in a rambling, opinionated style. His prolificacy and medical degree rendered him the public authoritative voice on transsexualism for the decade. He credited himself with coining the term *transsexual*, although others attribute this definition to Magnus Hirschfeld or Harry Benjamin.[2]

In 1949, Cauldwell published *Psychopathia Transexualis*, setting the cultural standard for viewing transsexuality as weird, offensive, mentally unhealthy, and the result of a "poor hereditary background and a highly unfavorable childhood environment."[3] He described the case of Earl, a person assigned female at birth, who identified as male. When Earl first visited Cauldwell's home, Cauldwell found him an "inoffensive guest" who dressed as a male in the house and a female outside, admitted to a crush on a girl, and appeared "more puzzled than determined to live as a male."[4] After some time, Cauldwell received a frantic telegram and second visit from Earl, who arrived disheveled and broke after sleeping on park benches and having been in police custody. Earl, now desperate, explained his plan for transition to an astonished Cauldwell, who felt his proposal was "impossible" and that a surgically constructed penis "is of no material use on a female and has no more sexual feeling than a fingernail."[5]

Earl's protracted visit wore on his host. Eventually, Cauldwell contacted Earl's family who reported that Earl wormed money from his relatives, preferring to "live parasitically,"[6] and harbored death wishes against them. Cauldwell described Earl's psychopathic practices: "seduction, parasitism, violation of the social codes in numerous ways, frequently kleptomania and actual thievery, pathological lying, and other criminal and unsocial tendencies."[7] He based the development of this psychopathic state on an underlying mental illness. "When an individual fails to mature according to his (or her) proper biological and sexological status, such an individual is psychologically (mentally) deficient. The psychological condition is in reality the disease."[8]

Cauldwell spoke out against surgeons who mutilated healthy breasts or castrated people. In his publication, "Sex Transmutation—Can One's Sex Be Changed?" he asserted that the removal of healthy gonadal tissue was "an act which either borders on criminality or is criminal" and that surgery never affects a true change in sex.[9] He disparaged the transgender and gender-diverse (TGD) people who wrote asking him where to find surgeons. "The psyche is already ill and sanity is seriously involved when an individual develops a compulsion to be rid of his natural organs. . . . Mutilating surgery cannot preserve such a psyche and it cannot restore sanity to the insane."[10]

Despite his beliefs about surgery, Cauldwell left behind a mixed legacy. He published long letters from TGD people, acknowledging their experience, if not with the affirmation they craved. He normalized the phenomenon, noting that "transsexuality is far more prevalent than it is suspected of being."[11] While many conflated transsexuals and homosexuals, Cauldwell stated that "trans-sexuals are individuals of one sex and apparently psychologically of the opposite. Trans-sexuals include heterosexuals, homosexuals, bisexuals, and others. A large element of transvestites have trans-sexual leanings."[12] Through his publications, American people heard the voices of transgender people firsthand. Most importantly, TGD people found descriptions that mirrored their own experiences, a tantalizing glimpse of a wider community.

Upon Cauldwell's death, controversial activist Virginia Prince[13] eulogized Cauldwell as a friend to transvestites—someone who answered their letters and emphasized that their activities "were not dangerous, criminal, or immoral."[14] She forgave him his doubts, because "he, at last, did much to explain and take the sting out of the problem for the benefit of non-TV's who might read sexology. . . . In recent years he took positions in regard to sex-conversion surgery, that the writer thought were unfair but he was entitled to his opinions."[15]

NOTES

1. Elkins and King, "Pioneers of Transgendering," 2.
2. Elkins and King, "Pioneers of Transgendering," 1.
3. Cauldwell, "Psychopathia Transexualis," 1.
4. Cauldwell, "Psychopathia Transexualis," 2.
5. Cauldwell, "Psychopathia Transexualis," 3.
6. Cauldwell, "Psychopathia Transexualis," 4.
7. Cauldwell, "Psychopathia Transexualis," 5.
8. Cauldwell, "Psychopathia Transexualis," 1.
9. Cauldwell, "Sex Transmutation," 22.
10. Cauldwell, "Questions and Answers," 7.
11. Cauldwell, "Questions and Answers," 32.
12. Cauldwell, "Questions and Answers," 1.
13. See profile of Virginia Prince in chapter 7.2 of this volume. Prince also harbored doubts about the value of surgical transitions.
14. Prince, "In Memorium." 45.
15. Prince, "In Memorium." 45.

WORKS CITED

Cauldwell, David O. "Questions and Answers on the Sex Life and Sexual Problems of Trans-Sexuals: Trans-Sexuals are Individuals of One Sex and Apparently Psychologically of the Opposite Sex. Trans-Sexuals Include Heterosexuals, Homosexuals,

Bisexuals and Others." *International Journal of Transgenderism* 5, no. 2 (2001): 1–33. Reprinted from 1950.

———. "Psychopathia Transexualis." *International Journal of Transgenderism* 5, no. 2 (2001): 1–6. Reprinted from 1949.

———. "Sex Transmutation—Can One's Sex Be Changed? There's But a Thin Genetic Line Between the Sexes, but the Would-Be Transmutee Battles Forces More Stubborn than the Genes." *International Journal of Transgenderism* 5, no. 2 (2001): 1–31. Reprinted from 1951.

Ekins, Richard, and David King. "Pioneers of Transgendering: The Popular Sexology of David O. Cauldwell." *International Journal of Transgenderism* 5, no. 2 (2001): 1–8.

Prince, Virginia. "In Memoriam." *Transvestia* 1, no. 1 (1960): 45. Accessed August 8, 2024. https://vault.library.uvic.ca/concern/generic_works/47c6e7a5-d411-4cc8-9f4e-1210a9e84302?locale=en

8.3. THE RELIGIOUS RESPONSE TO MEDICAL INTERVENTIONS

Carolyn Wolf-Gould

In the middle of the twentieth century, many transgender people began to fear or report harm from their faith communities due to their wish to pursue medical interventions. Simultaneously, religious organizations, their leaders, and congregants reacted to the visibility of transgender healthcare, grappling with how new medical practices could be reconciled with existing religious texts and tenets. Many transgender people left their places of worship and found—or created—spiritual homes that affirmed the medical and surgical procedures that brought them spiritual and/or bodily peace. Others struggled to conform to entrenched religious expectations.

In 1978, as part of its public educational mission, the Erickson Educational Foundation published a pamphlet entitled *Transsexualism Religious Aspects*, offering statements from clergy of various faiths on gender-affirming surgical procedures.[1] Each of these statements urged compassion for transsexual people. Many endorsed medical interventions, although the preface stated that individual views did not necessarily reflect that of the contributors' faith organization. Clergy from Baptist, Catholic, Christian Science, nondenominational, Episcopal, Jewish, Lutheran, and Presbyterian faiths reflected on a central question: Are these medical interventions a sin against God? Many referenced the healing ministry of Christ, who restored health and wholeness to those who suffered from physical or emotional distress. A Baptist minister compared the transformation of a transsexual he worked with to being born again and urged the responsible provision of surgery, when needed. A Christian Science pastor fell short of endorsing medical interventions, recommending instead absolute love and affirmative prayer. A Rabbi explained that Biblical law prohibits castration and related acts. Furthermore, as the sexual status of one postsurgery remained undefined, surgery violated Jewish law, as it pertains to one's obligations in marital, personal, and ritual matters. He recommended avoiding surgery unless the condition was a threat to one's life or health, at which point Jewish law offered acceptance.

Many religious bodies offer specific guidelines around medical transitions. Most mainstream Protestant religions affirm gender-diverse people and their right to surgical transitions. The Bible and Christian history contain figures who defied gender role expectations, including Deborah, Queen Esther, and Joan of Arc. The Protestant beliefs from *Of Justification by Faith*[2] offer reassurance that the acceptance of Christ ensures salvation. Nonetheless, gender-affirming surgeries create theological problems for many faiths and sects whose leaders believe it (1) threatens God's sovereignty by challenging the ordained gender binary; (2) invokes controversy about the relationship between body and soul; (3) defiles the body, which was created by an omniscient God in God's image; and (4) encourages nonheteronormative and nonprocreative sexuality.[3]

Christian traditions outside the Protestant mainstream are less accepting. Jehovah's Witnesses refuse to baptize someone after gender surgery (seen as mutilation of the body) and equate biologic sex with gender identity.[4] The Latter-day Saints (Mormons) have no official policy regarding transgender individuals but will not baptize someone considering surgery.[5] Those who have already undergone surgery may be baptized, pending approval from the governing body of the church. Seventh-day Adventists assert that incongruence between the body and soul is a sin and expect members to live in their sex assigned at birth.[6] Evangelical and Catholic churches have historically opposed same-sex relationships and gender transitions, stating they violate divine personhood manifest through sexuality. The Catholic tradition rejects genital surgery on the basis of Directive 53,[7] which prohibits sterilization unless the procedure will cure or alleviate severe pathology and no simpler procedure is available. No Pope has ever publicly addressed the issue of gender-affirming surgery, though surgeon Donald Laub requested papal guidance in 1968 and received permission from Pope Paul VI to operate on trans people under the doctrine of the whole.[8]

Rabbis interpret Jewish law and the Talmud to render a range of liberal to conservative opinions on gender surgery.[9] Scholars recognize that while Judaism's legal tradition assumes a gender binary, people do not always fit into this binary package, and discourse regarding intersex individuals and the influence of genetics and hormones led to debate on treatments for gender incongruence. Discussion revolves around two central questions: Is surgery permitted under Jewish law, and is someone who has undergone gender-affirming surgery considered to have changed gender with respect to religion's norms?

Muslim scholars debate the acceptance of surgeries based on Islamic theology, with most holding the opinion that these procedures were sinful and prohibited (haram).[10] Others offer more liberal interpretations, including Ayatollah Khomeini who, after being moved by the story of a transgender woman, issued a fatwa on the permissibility of gender surgery in Islam. However, to be gay in Iran is a sin punishable by death; gay individuals continue to face intense pressure to transition for safety.[11]

Buddhist spirituality, as interpreted by Western world traditions, remains neutral on issues related to gender identity, instead providing spaces for people to learn and practice, although some teachings encourage letting go of gender identity on the path to releasing the illusion of selfhood.[12] Others argue that to be present in Buddhist practice, one must be present and comfortable in the body and that medical treatments assist with this process. My Buddhist teachers assure me that these seemingly conflicting truths can be comfortably held in the palm of one hand.[13]

NOTES

1. Erickson Educationall Foundation, *Transsexualism Religious Aspects*.
2. Calvin, "Of Justification by Faith," 1–40.
3. Sharzer et al., "Religious Attitudes Toward Gender-Confirming Surgery," 227–28.
4. jw.support, "Watchtower View of Transgenderism."
5. Human Rights Campaign, "Stances of Faiths on LGBTQ Issues"; Sharzer et al. "Religious Attitudes Toward Gender-Confirming Surgery," 228–29.
6. Seventh-day Adventist Church, "Statement on Transgenderism."
7. US Conference of Catholic Bishops, *Ethical and Religious Directives*, 19.
8. Laub, *Second Lives, Second Chances*, 73–74.
9. Sharzer et al., "Religious Attitudes Toward Gender-Confirming Surgery," 234–36.
10. Sharzer et al., "Religious Attitudes Toward Gender-Confirming Surgery," 237–38.
11. Hamedani, "The Gay People Pushed to Change Their Gender."

12. Sharzer et al., "Religious Attitudes Toward Gender-Confirming Surgery," 241.
13. Personal conversation with Corday Selden, Michael Selden, and Mark Imbrie, June 24, 2021.

WORKS CITED

Calvin, John. *Justification by Faith*, edited by Nate Pickowicz and translated by John Allen. Petersborough, Ontario, Canada: H&E Publishing, 2018.

Erickson Educational Foundation. *Transsexualism Religious Aspects*. 1978. Accessed May 7, 2021. https://archive.org/details/transsexualismrethirnoau/mode/2up.

Laub, Donald. *Second Lives, Second Chances*. Toronto, Ontario: ECW Press, 2019.

Hamedani, Ali. "The Gay People Pushed to Change Their Gender." *BBC News*. November 5, 2014. Accessed June 13, 2021. https://www.bbc.com/news/magazine-29832690.

Human Rights Campaign. "Stances of Faiths on LGBTQ Issues: Church of Jesus Christ of Latter-day Saints (Mormons)." Human Rights Campaign Resources. Accessed May 7, 2021. https://www.hrc.org/resources/stances-of-faiths-on-lgbt-issues-church-of-jesus-christ-of-latter-day-saint.

jw.support. "Watchtower View of Transgenderism." 2019–2021. Accessed May 7, 2021. https://jw.support/watchtower-view-of-transgenderism/.

Seventh-day Adventist Church. "Statement on Transgenderism." *Official Statements*. April 12, 2017. Accessed May 7, 2021. https://www.adventist.org/official-statements/statement-on-transgenderism/.

Sharzer, Leonard, David Jones, Mehrdad Alipour, and Kelsey Jacob Pacha. "Religious Attitudes Toward Gender-Confirming Surgery." In *Gender Confirmation Surgery*, by Loren Schecter, 237–57. Switzerland: Springer Nature Switzerland AG, 2020.

US Conference of Catholic Bishops. *Ethical and Religious Directives for Catholic Health Care Services*. 6th ed. Washington DC: US Conference of Catholic Bishops, June 2018. Accessed May 7, 2021. https://www.usccb.org/about/doctrine/ethical-and-religious-directives/upload/ethical-religious-directives-catholic-health-service-sixth-edition-2016-06.pdf.

9

THE COSTS OF MEDICALIZATION

Kyan Lynch, Carolyn Wolf-Gould, Dallas Denny, and Jennifer Lee

INTRODUCTION: A CAUTIONARY TALE OF MEDICALIZATION

On May 11, 1982, *New York Times* journalist Lawrence K. Altman depicted a strange new illness in his article "New Homosexual Disorder Worries Health Officials."[1] This sickness, one characterized by unexplained immune system collapse, was what researchers were beginning to refer to as AIDS, for acquired immunodeficiency disease, or GRID for gay-related immunodeficiency.[2] Though acknowledging that some heterosexual men and women, including those who use injection drugs, had also been affected by the outbreak, Altman predominantly used the term *GRID* throughout the article.[3]

When describing a matter of public health, language shapes the rapidity and extent of governmental response, educational programming, policy decisions, access to funding, and public opinion.[4] In the case of HIV/AIDS, the term *GRID*—along with its various degrading euphemisms, including gay plague, gay cancer, and WOGS, or the Wrath of God Syndrome[5]—has been partly responsible for over forty years of stigmatization and the subsequent loss of countless lives.[6] Far more insidious than simple name calling, the significance of these terms lies in the explicit connection drawn between the gay lifestyle, the theoretical homosexual body, and disease. Conflating being gay with being diseased can be correctly described as pathologization, or the process through which an experience or identity is constructed as an illness, problem, or abnormality. To pathologize homosexuality is to view the sexual orientation as a pathway to suffering.

As biomedical researchers studied HIV and its mechanisms of disease, members of the public and certain physicians creatively applied preexisting bias to try to make sense of the crisis. In addition to demonizing promiscuity more generally, theories that emphasized the relative permeability of the "fragile anus" over the "rugged vagina" were particularly popular.[7] This discourse is certainly pathologizing. It can also be described using a similar, though not perfectly synonymous, term: *medicalizing*. Medicalization is frequently characterized as "a process by which nonmedical problems become defined and treated as medical problems, usually in terms of illness and disorders."[8] In the above example, desiring and having receptive anal sex is conceptualized as some sort of anatomical malpractice. One implication is that gay men do not have the requisite expertise to understand their own bodies. Rather, medical professionals must be relied on to define and distinguish normal/healthy sex from abnormal/unhealthy sex and, in doing so, control the problem. These two steps, defining a problem in medical terms and placing the problem under the control of medical professionals, are critical in the medicalization process.[9]

The medicalization of gay sex during the HIV/AIDS crisis was particularly galling for the activists and allies who had already fought medicalization and won. Roughly one decade prior, thanks to persistent advocacy, homosexuality was removed from the *Diagnostic and Statistics Manual* (*DSM*). Consider the following quote attributed to activist Michael Lynch: "Like helpless mice we have peremptorily, almost inexplicably, relinquished the one power we so long fought for . . . the power to determine our own identity. And to whom have we relinquished it? The very authority we wrested it from in a struggle that occupied us for more than a hundred years: the medical profession."[10] This quote illustrates the painful paradox that gay activists faced in the early 1980s: to survive, they needed the help of the medical establishment, but needing the medical establishment meant succumbing to medicalization. The data did not lie; gay men acquired and died from HIV/AIDS at far higher rates than any other demographic. Ending the epidemic would necessarily require medical intervention, expertise, and leadership.

As it turned out, the upper echelons of the medical establishment largely abdicated, leaving a vacuum that people living with AIDS, gay rights activists, and their allies (particularly lesbian veterans of the women's rights movement) were determined to fill.[11] Highlighting research articles, staging protests, and demanding access to treatment options, groups such as AIDS Coalition to Unleash Power (ACTUP), Gay Men's Health Crisis, and the National Association of People with AIDS rejected the traditionally meek role of "patient" in favor of an active role in their own salvation.[12] Some argue that, by joining with and catalyzing the medical profession in response to the HIV/AIDS epidemic, these pioneering activists successfully staved off the remedicalization of homosexuality.[13] Others argue that targeted recommendations for more recent advances in biomedical HIV prophylaxis indicate that the medicalization of gay sex continues.[14] Regardless, the gay activists of the 1980s and 1990s undoubtedly changed the dynamic between the medical establishment and the gay community by refusing to be relegated back to the margins.

HISTORICAL ECHOES

Medical professionals initially struggled to differentiate homosexuality and transgenderism. Given this, one might expect that the members of the LGBTQIA+ population would have faced medicalization together. On the contrary, just as homosexuality was working its way out of the *DSM*[15]—thanks, in large part, to gender transgressing advocates and activists[16]—the first mentions of gender variance were being entered into this so-called psychiatrist's bible.[17] Though hardly the first time that gender-transgressive people were regarded as abnormal by medical professionals, the introduction of transvestism (1968) and later transsexualism (1980) into the *DSM* marked a new level of awareness and medicalization of transgender and gender-diverse (TGD) people. Formally a part of the psychiatric pantheon of disease, performing and/or desiring to perform a nonnormative gender became codified as a medical problem therefore deserving of medical treatment and within the scope of medical professionals.

In our modern medical system, in which all healthcare is documented, administered, and paid for using diagnostic codes, a formal diagnosis is, in essence, a ticket to ride. Much of this book is dedicated to telling the story of how that ride was built, replete with examples of the various medical breakthroughs and surgical advances that have made gender-affirming medical care satisfying for some and lifesaving for others.

As ever, the ride is not free. There are costs to medicalization. For many TGD people, affirming medical care arrived too late, was too limited, or too far out of reach. For others, the very physicians who claimed they could help were the ones who caused the most pain. There are costs for seeking care and costs for being denied it; there are costs for meeting medical requirements for care and costs for existing outside them. Perhaps the highest cost is the one Lynch feared at the onset of the AIDS epidemic: relinquishing the power to determine our own identity.

A STORY OF MEDICALIZATION IN FIVE PARTS

In this chapter, we present five short, self-contained pieces, each documenting a different cost of medicalization. Though potentially unanswerable, these stories raise critical, haunting questions: Is the ride worth the cost? Can medicalization and liberation coexist? Is medicalization inherently inequitable? What does it mean to do no harm? Can anyone claim to be an expert on someone else's body?

We begin with the story of Pauli Murray, a trailblazer and revolutionary upon whose shoulders we all stand. In her own field of law, Murray's work was ahead of its time. Though she had no formal medical training, her clinical reasoning was prescient. Searching for a way to understand her own attractions and gender identity, Murray sought guidance from medical professionals; she found the answers lacking, as have so many others before and since. Now, with the benefit of hindsight, we see that the medical establishment was not yet even asking the right questions.

PROFILE: PAULI MURRAY (1910–1985), BY CAROLYN WOLF-GOULD

Pauli Murray, born in 1910 and named Anna Pauline, was an influential African American lawyer, activist, writer, community organizer, and eventually, an Episcopal priest.[18]

Her maternal grandmother, Cornelia, born into slavery, was the child of a woman who had been raped by her owner's son—a heritage that left Murray with skin lighter than her African American classmates and darker than the family who raised her.[19] She fought insistently for civil rights, women's rights, and the end of *Jane Crow*, a term she coined to describe the intersectional discrimination she faced in her own life. She worked largely behind the scenes and, despite her remarkable accomplishments—including her pivotal role in the landmark cases Brown v. Board of Education and Reed v. Reed—is largely unknown. While she toiled in support of human rights, she struggled internally with her own gender identity and sexual orientation, striving to define herself in an era that lacked the necessary language and resources.

Murray claimed the most significant fact of her childhood was that she was an orphan.[20] Her mother died suddenly when Murray was three years old. Her father, unable to manage a house with six children, sent her to live with her Aunt Pauline Fitzgerald in North Carolina.[21] Three years later, her father was committed to the Crownsville State Hospital for the Negro Insane, where he was clubbed to death with a baseball bat by a white guard.[22]

A precocious child, Murray stood out as an avid reader and excellent student. She preferred masculine clothing and chores and adopted the name Paul (later Pauli) for herself as a teen. She was teased at her all-Black school for her light color, intellect, and left handedness, Murray never truly fit in. As she attempted to access educational and extracurricular activities, she repeatedly encountered and resisted the systems of Jim Crow that restricted the lives of African Americans. She graduated from high school at fifteen, the first in her class. She was editor-in-chief of the school paper, president of the literary society, and played the forward position on the basketball team.[23] After graduation she rejected the opportunity to attend the North Carolina College for Negroes. She applied to Columbia University and soon learned her life was constrained not only by race but also by gender. Columbia didn't accept women.

She eventually attended Hunter College but left school after the Wall Street crash of 1929, when she lost the jobs that supported her education.[24] After five years of odd jobs and poverty, she applied to a graduate program in sociology at the University of North Carolina, a school that refused to admit African Americans. Murray unsuccessfully challenged this rule, pointing out that members of her slave-owning family had attended the school and even served on the board.[25] Murray repeatedly faced denials of admittance to schools of higher education, first because of race and, later, because of her gender. When her application to Harvard Law School was denied based on gender, she wrote, "Gentlemen, I would gladly change my sex to meet your requirements, but since the way to such change has not been revealed to me, I have no recourse but to appeal to you to change your minds on this subject. Are you to tell me that one is as difficult as the other?"[26]

Although Murray's autobiography chronicles much of her life's journey, she omitted any description of her personal struggle to understand her own sexual orientation and gender identity and her decades-long attempt to medically transition.[27] Archival material unearthed by her biographer revealed Murray's agonized exploration around her attraction to women and identification as a male.[28] To understand herself, she researched sexual deviance and latched onto the work of Havelock Ellis, who coined the term *pseudo-hermaphrodite* to describe those whose gender identity was incongruent with their assigned sex at birth. She believed her attraction to women affirmed her masculine identity and suspected she harbored male genitalia inside her abdomen.[29] At times she identified as a mixed-gender person. "Maybe two got fused into one with parts of each sex . . . male head and brain (?), female-ish body, mixed emotional characteristics." More often, she identified as "a girl who should have been a boy."[30] Murray suffered from a series of mental breakdowns related to her dysphoria and for years tried unsuccessfully to find doctors who would experiment on her with masculine hormones—but at this time, the care she sought didn't exist.[31] The documentary *My Name is Pauli Murray* chronicles the despair she felt as she reached out to clinicians, asking for care that didn't exist at the time.[32]

Murray served as a powerful activist, but much of her work took place out of the limelight. In 1940, years before Rosa Parks, Murray refused to move to the broken seats at the back of a bus when ordered to do so by the driver and landed in jail. She met Eleanor Roosevelt while advocating for a sharecropper who had been sentenced to death for shooting his white landowner in self-defense. Roosevelt and Murray developed a long and joyful friendship. She was the first African American to attain a Doctor of Jurisprudence degree from Yale University. When asked by the women's division of the Methodist Church to develop a pamphlet on segregation laws in the United States, she wrote a book with 746 pages, *States' Laws on Race and Color*, in which she described the extent and insanity of segregation. Supreme Court Justice Thurgood Marshall referred to it as the bible for Brown v. Board of Education.[33] Marshall's team employed Murray's reasoning to argue and win this defining legislation. Justice Ruth Bader Ginsberg credited Murray with the legal strategy she employed to persuade the Supreme Court to bar sex discrimination in the absence of an equal rights amendment, by applying the Fourteenth Amendment's equal protection clause to gender.[34] In Reed v. Reed, Ginsburg's first brief to the Supreme Court, Ginsburg listed Murray as well as her ACLU colleague Dorothy Kenyon, although neither directly participated in its writing. "We're standing on their shoulders," said Ginsburg. "We're saying the same things they said, but now at last society is ready to listen."[35]

In the 1960s, Murray plunged into both the civil rights and women's rights movements, organizing and advocating for numerous causes. In 1965,

Figure 9.1 Pauli Murray, 2007. *Source*: Carolina Digital Library and Archives, UNC University Library.

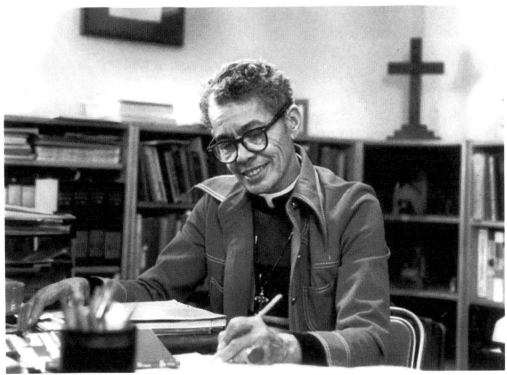

after suggesting a women's march on Washington, Betty Friedan contacted her, and soon after, during a women's rights conference, Murray, Friedan, and a group of like-minded women launched the National Organization for Women.

Later in life, Murray grew disillusioned with the ways "the civil-rights movement was sidelining women [and the] women's movement was sidelining minorities and poor people."[36] After the death of her life partner Irene Barlow, she entered New York's General Theological Seminary to become an Episcopal priest, despite the fact that the Episcopal church refused to ordain women.[37] This ban was lifted in 1977, shortly after she received her degree.[38] She died in 1985 and, in 2012, was sainted in the Episcopal Church as an exemplary member of its "communion of saints" for being a source of inspiration and for her "advocacy of the universal cause of freedom and as the first African American female priest ordained by the Episcopal Church."[39]

In a 1976 interview, Murray reflected on her activism. "In not a single one of these little campaigns was I victorious. In other words, in each case,

I personally failed, but I have lived to see the thesis upon which I was operating vindicated. And what I very often say is that I've lived to see my lost causes found."[40] A poet, Murray left us with "Dark Testament," a poem about the broken places and dreams of African American people that, paradoxically, inspired her to hope.

> Hope is a crushed stalk
> Between clenched fingers
> Hope is a bird's wing
> Broken by a stone . . .
> Hope is a song in a weary throat.
> Give me a song of hope
> And a world where I can sing it.[41]

∾

As evident from this brief biography, Murray's life was lived in the intersections, in the complicated interplay of race, gender, and class, in the gap between "how it has always been" and "how it could be." She was, in every way, a visionary. Having performed her own research, Murray saw the potential benefits of testosterone therapy; however, despite her repeated efforts for gendering-affirming care, her physicians clung to the cisheteronormative party line, offering only estrogen supplementation or psychiatric hospitalizations. Just as she was turned away by white supremacist and patriarchal institutions of higher learning, so too, was she pathologized by a medical establishment—also riddled with racism and misogyny[42]—that was keener to uphold socially accepted gender roles than to explore the true nature of gender.

Murray's story illustrates several substantial costs to medicalization. First, being defined by a medical framework reduces the fullness of gender diversity to that which fits within the medical imagination at any given sociocultural moment. Second, within the medical context, seeking treatment automatically implies that there is a problem. Within the Western medical model, forged from the advances in natural sciences that revolutionized the profession in the nineteenth century,[43] there has historically been a dividing line between bodily and/or organic ailments and mental illness.[44] Organic diseases can be observed, imaged, managed, and excised. Mental ailments, in contrast, have been considered to be more mysterious in origin and have been variously described as biological disorders, collections of undesirable behaviors, and personal flaws, depending on the time and theoretical orientation of the clinician.[45] Since Murray's physicians could not find an organic cause to her distress, they relegated her concerns to the realm of the psychiatric. This assumption produced two harmful sequelae. Finding no organic error or imbalance underpinning her distress, her clinicians refused to use organic treatments to mitigate her distress. In addition, labeled mentally unwell, Murray's visionary insights were written off as unreliable (a tactic that would be used again by the psychiatric establishment to discredit LGBT activists arguing to remove homosexuality from the *DSM*[46]).

Finally, Murray suffered because the romanticized notion of Western medical empiricism was never based on objective truth. Rather, the scientific empiricism, logical positivism, and their current-day successor, evidence-based medicine, touted by the Western medical establishment can be more accurately described by what Chanda Prescod-Weinstein terms *white empiricism*.[47] According to Prescod-Weinstein, white empiricism is "the phenomenon through which only white people (particularly white men) are read as having a fundamental capacity for objectivity."[48] White empiricism involves "a denial of a knower's competence based on ascribed identity" and a "willingness to ignore empirical data."[49] When combined, the emphasis on evidence as fact in Western medicine provides a predicate for eliminating "culture, contexts, and the subjects of knowledge production from consideration, a move that permits the use of evidence as a political instrument where power interests can be obscured by seemingly neutral technical resolve."[50] In other words, what the medical community deemed to be true for Murray cannot and should not be accepted as the truth without turning a critical eye. Simultaneously, the unchallenged medicalization of the transgender experience uplifts the medical profession as the arbiters of gender truth, inarguably (albeit silently) informed by centuries of racism, misogyny, homophobia, and transphobia.

Murray was ahead of her time, but it would be naive to assume that, had she simply lived in a more modern era, she would have received the care she deserved. The US medical system was not born out of a desire to care for all Americans equitably, nor can it claim to do so today.[51] In the following piece, Dallas Denny tells the shameful story of how the medical system failed a transgender man in need of care.

PROFILE: LACK OF ACCESS TO MEDICAL TREATMENT AND HOW IT AFFECTED ROBERT EADS (1945–1999), BY DALLAS DENNY

> I wish I could understand why they did what they did, why they had to feel that way, and I know in a way they've contributed to my dying here. But I can't hate them. I don't hate them. I feel sorry for them. . . . I guess what makes me most sad is they probably felt like they did the right thing.
>
> —Statement by Robert Eads in Kate Davis's film *Southern Comfort*[52]

Throughout the 1990s I operated the American Educational Gender Information Service, an Atlanta-based national nonprofit 501(c)(3) corporation. One of my primary functions as director was to provide referrals for medical and psychological care for trans people. I soon amassed a worldwide database of surgeons, endocrinologists, electrologists, therapists, and other professionals. Between 1990 and 1999 I provided thousands of referrals in person and by phone, fax, US mail, and (after 1993) email.[53]

Robert Eads was a trans man in his mid-forties when I met him in 1991 at the first Southern Comfort, a transgender conference based in Atlanta. At that time, he lived in Florida, but in 1996, he relocated to rural Toccoa, Georgia, one hundred miles northeast of Atlanta. He was a polite and well-liked man. Every time I saw him, he was dressed in black or wearing his plaid jacket. He walked with a cane due to a back injury.[54]

Eads phoned me around the time of his move to Georgia and asked for a referral to a gynecologist. I gave him the names of three who worked with trans people. One was the go-to source for Atlanta-area trans men. I had consulted the second for follow-up to my vaginoplasty, and he expressed a willingness to treat other transgender people. The third had recently performed a hysterectomy on a trans man of my acquaintance. I told Eads I had more names in case the referrals I made didn't work out. He and I didn't speak again about this matter, and I assumed he had obtained treatment.

In fact, Eads had not been treated. More than twenty gynecologists and a number of hospitals refused to see him—including the three doctors to whom I had referred him.[55] At a time when prompt medical action might have saved his life, Eads and his friend Debbie, who made phone calls on his behalf, were unable to find a physician willing to provide treatment. Excuses ranged from "I'm not taking new patients" to worries about the reaction of female patients to Eads's presence in the waiting room.[56]

We don't know if immediate surgery would have saved Eads's life, as according to his friend Maxwell Anderson, Eads ignored his symptoms for years, but certainly, it might have. Just as certainly, without appropriate and timely medical treatment, he had no chance of surviving. Anderson wrote, "in the end, it was Robert himself who did the most damage by ignoring the signs his own body had been showing him for years. There are doctors out there who will treat us. The key is persistence, and honesty."[57]

Through the efforts of filmmaker Kate Davis, the world soon knew about Eads and his health difficulties. Davis's 2002 documentary film *Southern Comfort* followed him, his lover, Lola Cola, and his friends and family through the last year of his life.[58] Eads was determined to live long enough to give a farewell speech at the 1998 Southern Comfort Conference, and he did.[59] He died on January 17, 1999, from metastatic ovarian cancer, at age fifty-three.[60]

Trans people, their allies, and audiences the world over were shocked and outraged that Eads was refused treatment by physicians who had the ability to save his life. So was I. And so should you be.

Robert Eads deserved treatment for ovarian cancer. He deserved dignity, respect, and compassion from his healthcare providers. He deserved so much more than he was given. Ultimately, Eads carried two official diagnoses according to the medical establishment: ovarian cancer and gender identity disorder (according to the *DSM-IV*, the active edition at his time of death[61]). His would-be physicians' biases toward one prevented them from treating the other, and Eads paid the ultimate price.

Unfortunately, anti-trans violence and discrimination have been features of US society since its founding.[62] Given this reality, while not all transgender individuals desire to pass as cisgender, many have found that it is the safest way to survive.[63] Additionally, transgender people—particularly Black, brown, indigenous, and immigrant transgender people—have been systematically shut out of traditional means of employment and have therefore been more likely to pursue sex work as a source of income.[64] This confluence of circumstances has created strong incentives for transgender people to pursue body modifications to achieve a physique that society deems to be in line with their gender.[65]

The American medical system offers medical and procedural ways to achieve cisnormative results. However, the medical system is built to serve some and not others. TGD individuals are routinely blocked from accessing affirming medical interventions for body modification due to inability to pay and/or insurance companies denying coverage for "cosmetic" procedures,[66] as well as discrimination based on immigration status,[67] nonbinary identity,[68] racial and/or ethnic identity,[69] participation in sex work,[70] age,[71] carceral status,[72] and other societal markers of marginalization. Additionally, surgical body modification procedures were developed to achieve aesthetics in line with Eurocentric beauty standards,[73] requiring would-be patients to acquiesce to their surgeon's racialized conception of masculine and feminine features. In the absence of affirming, accessible, and culturally responsive care, a vacuum forms, one that both well-intentioned and nefarious players have rushed to fill.

THE PROBLEM WITH SILICONE INJECTIONS, BY DALLAS DENNY

Since the mid-1940s men and women have enhanced their body contours with injections of liquid silicone—sometimes in minute quantities and often in quantities measured in liters.[74] Silicone has been and continues to be directly injected in small and large quantities into almost every part of the human body by physicians and lay "practitioners." Because the cost for injections is hundreds of dollars as opposed to thousands for cosmetic surgery to achieve the same purpose and because silicone can be administered serially, further reducing the economic burden, sex workers, women of color, women of low socioeconomic status, and especially trans women have been and continue to be willing and often enthusiastic participants, in spite of efforts to educate them about the dangers of silicone injected in large quantities by unlicensed and untrained practitioners in nonmedical settings.[75]

THE SILICONE STORY

Silicon is the fourteenth element. In the periodic table of elements, it is placed below carbon and above germanium. Silicones are colorless oil- and rubber-like polymers and have a variety of industrial, medical, and household uses.

In post–World War II Japan, US Army quartermasters discovered drums of silicone transformer-insulating fluid had gone missing from the docks at

Figure 9.2. American Educational Gender Information Services advisory on silicone, *Chrysalis Quarterly*, Summer, 1991. Graphic by Margaux Ayn Schaefer. *Source*: Dallas Denny; public domain.

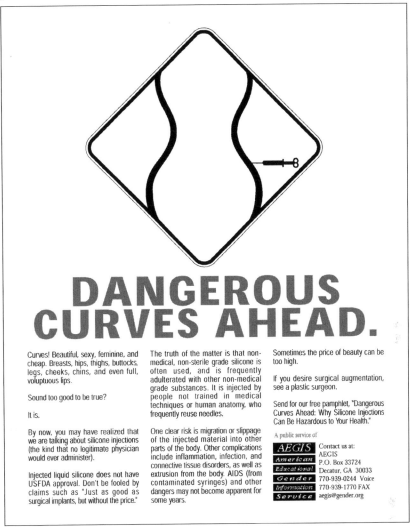

Yokohama Harbor. Upon investigation, authorities discovered the pilfered silicone was being injected into the breasts of local prostitutes to enhance their body contours and westernize their faces.[76] It was a safer (but certainly not safe!) alternative to the paraffin injections that were popular in Japan at the time. The practice soon spread to the United States, where silicone injections became popular, especially with socialites, sex workers, women of color, and transgender women.[77]

Since those post–World War II days, silicone oil has been used around the world to change the shape of the human body. It is directly injected into almost every part of the body by physicians and lay people and is sometimes self-injected. In men and women, it is used to remove wrinkles; disguise acne and other skin imperfections; enlarge lips, thighs, breasts, calves, and buttocks; modify jawlines; and create the appearance of high cheekbones. Trans women use silicone to disguise heavy brow ridges and Adam's apples. In men, it is used to increase the size of the scrotum or penis and mimic athletic musculature. Silicone is also used as filler in breast, gluteal, cheek, jaw, and other implants.[78] Quantities injected vary from one or two milliliters in the face to three or four liters in thighs, breasts, hips, and buttocks and up to fifteen liters overall.[79] Untrained lay people often use industrial-quality silicone[80] and sometimes adulterate or replace silicone with paraffin, vegetable or mineral oil, or lanolin.[81] The results are often horrific.

For many years physicians were open to and some even specialized in injection of silicone in large quantities, but most ceased when the Federal Food and Drug Administration (FDA) classified injected silicone as a drug in 1964. In 1991, the FDA went further, forbidding the injection of liquid silicone for aesthetic purposes. Today the FDA allows some physicians to inject tiny quantities into the face, but they risk censure or loss of license if they don't comply with guidelines. However, lay practitioners continue to inject silicone in large quantities, often at pumping parties in private homes or the back rooms of beauty salons.

PROBLEMS WITH SILICONE INJECTIONS

Medical emergencies and deaths caused by silicone can occur within hours of injection or years or decades later when the silicone migrates to noninjected parts of the body. When globules of silicone block blood vessels, stroke and tissue death follows.[82] When silicone migrates to the lungs, the result is sometimes fatal respiratory distress. In 2005, Schmid and colleagues reported the development of silicone embolism syndrome with fatal outcome in six of thirty-three hospitalized illegally injected individuals.[83] Risk is directly related to the amount of silicone injected but can develop even after the injection of minute quantities in the face. The buttocks seem to pose the most extreme risks.[84]

Gravity is an inexorable force. Over years, gravity may cause silicone to migrate downward, leading to severe disfigurement.[85] This can result in tissue death of body parts and require amputation. Migration can also cause death due to respiratory distress or stroke.

MEDICAL AND LEGAL RESPONSE TO SILICONE

By the 1960s, articles in medical journals were reporting negative effects, medical emergencies, and deaths related directly to the injection of silicone, and today the problem is well documented.[86] Legal authorities, however, initially did not seem to have silicone on their radar. This changed in 1992, after a transgender woman named Sophia Pastel died after traveling from Norfolk, Virginia, to Atlanta to receive massive quantities of silicone in her buttocks. Dr. Mark Kononen at the Georgia State Medical Examiner's Office took an interest in the case and went to the trans community for answers.[87] Fred Kennedy Glenn was soon arrested and convicted for causing Pastel's death. As a result of this case, authorities have prosecuted similar cases, usually to great effect.

∽

In the case of silicone injections, it is critical to recognize the context in which lay practitioners operating within transgender communities offer the service. Turned away from legal and formalized transition-related care, TGD people desperately pursue options to relieve gender dysphoria, make themselves more desirable sexually, achieve intracultural status, and/or approach a sense of safety.[88] Though dangerous, nonlicensed injection providers and TGD individuals who self-inject[89] do so because the use of fillers and other nonsurgical injections works to improve self-body image and self-esteem in transgender individuals.[90] In other words, the practice exists because members of the community found a way to achieve a desired outcome when the medical profession failed to help.

Similarly, among ACT UP's most successful methods of HIV/AIDS activism was the development and deployment of knowledge within its ranks.[91] Partnering with pharmacologist Iris Long, activists Peter Staley and Mark Harrington became lay experts in promising pharmacotherapies and the many convoluted drug approval pathways, ultimately scoring multiple significant victories in the fight against the epidemic.[92] Roughly a decade earlier, Dallas Denny deployed the same strategy when faced with medical obstinacy. Rather than pay a cost she deemed too high, Dallas Denny used the hard-earned knowledge that she had accrued and took matters into her own hands.

PROFILE: NOT SCREWED UP ENOUGH, BY DALLAS DENNY

In 1979, I went to the gender clinic at Vanderbilt University, requesting sex reassignment. There, I paid the not inconsequential fee of three hundred dollars and poured out my heart to a number of interviewers. After I finished intake interviews and a battery of psychological tests, Dr. Embree McKee told me the clinic would not be offering me gender reassignment therapy. I asked where I could go for a second opinion. "San Francisco," said the doctor. "That's the only other place." San Francisco was more than 2,300 miles away from Nashville.

And why could I not receive treatment here and now? McKee explained: (1) I had been successfully married for five years; (2) I was not sexually attracted to males; (3) I had two college degrees; and (4) I had a professional position as a protective services worker. Clearly, I was not dysfunctional enough to qualify for treatment. I was devastated. After a formal evaluation, a team of experts had concluded I was not transsexual. What the hell, then, was I? And why did I so desperately want to be a woman?

I straightaway took myself across the quad to Vanderbilt's first-rate medical library. There, for months, I researched, photocopied, and read anything and everything in the stacks about transsexuals and transsexualism. I found Harry Benjamin's 1966 *The Transsexual Phenomenon,* Richard Green and John Money's 1969 *Transsexualism and Sex Reassignment* (both of which were helpful), several volumes by psychiatrist Robert Stoller (which weren't), and hundreds of articles in psychiatric, urological, surgical, and general medical journals.

Every word of research confirmed what the Vanderbilt clinic had just told me. Transsexuals were poorly adjusted in every possible way. We were impulsive, narcissistic, manipulative, and histrionic. We acted out sexually. We had poor work histories and frequently had run-ins with the police and court systems. We had highly stereotyped notions of maleness and femaleness. We often had comorbid psychiatric disorders.[93] The term *comorbid*, of course, falsely presumed that transsexualism was itself a mental disorder. According to the experts, transsexuals were everything I was not.

And yet I knew I was transsexual. I would later come to understand that this self-perpetuating literature reflected the cultural biases of the time far more than it did the transsexual clients it libeled. In the short term, though, that research and so-called knowledge served only to devastate me further. And so, after I had exhausted every other option, I made what I considered then—and remain certain of today—was a rational and measured life-changing decision. I forged a prescription for diethylstilbestrol,[94] a form of estrogen, and in so doing, became the person I am today. As soon as I was able to find a legal source for estrogen, I visited a therapist, obtained a hormone letter, and stopped writing my own prescriptions—had I not taken the initiative, I would be living in a quite different body today.

There are medical risks associated with the administration of human sex hormones and their analogs, and it's essential to monitor blood chemistry. The opportunity today to work in concert with a medical professional is a privilege I and many others were not afforded.[95] It has become far easier to find a compassionate helping professional who will set a dosage and write a prescription and monitor your health. I urge those seeking hormones to follow my later example, and not my earlier one.

༄

Despite displaying some of the medical system's worst qualities, Denny's story has a happy ending. Following in the footsteps of countless gender rebels before her, and foreshadowing successful advocacy yet to come, Denny refused to believe the "experts" and instead forged her own path forward. Rather than accepting the stereotypical, absurd, and demeaning caricature that the medical establishment upheld as the transsexual standard, she reclaimed her right—and power—to determine her own identity.

In our fifth and final piece, we will explore a remarkable example of self-determination, resistance, and resilience in the face of medical abuse and abandonment.

HOUSE BALLROOM CULTURE, BY JENNIFER LEE

I am a member of the House and Ballroom Community (HBC), a culture that evolved from the drag shows and pageants of the 1920s Harlem Renaissance. In 1977, Crystal Labeija, a trans woman of color, founded the House of Labeija—historically credited as the first house established within the ballroom community—in response to the discrimination and gender-based violence queer people of color (QPOC) experienced in the drag circuits.[96] The HBC culture emerged as kinship groups formed these houses, a family-like community structure. The HBC subculture includes family units, with housing, parents (senior members who act as mothers and fathers and provide safe housing, mentorship, and support), and children (young people who have usually been rejected by families, spiritual homes, or the larger society).[97] House members live in their truth and compete against other houses in the joyful and celebratory performance art known as "balls" or ballroom.[98]

The HBC community defies hegemony, with no boundaries around gender and sexuality. Marlon Bailey, a HBC member and highly regarded scholar, described the system in his 1980s Detroit community, which was comprised of QPOCs who endorsed a six-part gender system for "walking the ball"; participants represented "butch queens (biological males who have sex with men), femme queens (male-to-female transgender individuals), butch queens up in drags (biological men who have sex with men and sometimes cross-dress but do not live as women), butches (masculinity in a person born female, whether identifying as lesbian or trans man), women (biological females who are feminine women regardless of sexual orientation) and men (heterosexual men who live as men.)."[99] Categories such as these evolve over time, as HBC members develop more nuanced and fluid understandings of gender and sexual expansiveness and liberation. The HBC is often the only community that affirms QPOC identities and existence with love, respect—represented by cash prizes, trophies, and ballroom status recognition during competition—and care.

Cultural labor refers to our performance work and the work of creating these life-affirming communities that enhance our health and wellness within systems that typically fail QPOC.[100] Notably, the increased burden of HIV on QPOC also inspired the HBC to organize health services to foster liberation from the intersectional, systemic oppressions that have led to healthcare inequities in our community. The labor of the HBC community to turn HIV/AIDS prevention from a culture of risk into a culture of support has been called an *intravention*, meaning that the "HIVAIDS prevention activities are conducted and sustained through practices and processes within at-risk communities themselves"[101] rather than individual-focused interventions, generally based on research that lacks cultural analyses.[102] We have overhauled HIV care centers by insisting that their systems offer affirming, transition-related care, including cultural responsiveness training for staff, trauma-informed care, and clinician education regarding implicit bias and healthcare inequities.

The community protects itself through such intraventions, and by embodying a culture of intraventions, we are self-sustaining and constantly evolving to respond to new emerging issues (for example, COVID-19, the rise in trans violence and murders).[103] Our communities of caring serve as alternate social spheres and sites of refuge—places for enjoyment and personal connection.[104] We decolonize our own minds by giving voice to our shared history of racial and cultural oppression and speaking against our stigmatization as dangerous, dysfunctional, and vectors of disease.[105] In sum, we challenge the dominant, normative logic of health interventions by maintaining collective forms of intravention and care.

HBC members who work for or with AIDS services or community-based organizations share educational information; disseminate safer-sex kits; and connect individuals to medical and mental healthcare, insurance navigators, and support services. To further health justice, there are homegrown, grassroots spaces created by HBC members to facilitate access to these service providers and community organizing (for example, #HouseLivesMatter, Destination Tomorrow, Prince Janae's House, Life 4 All, Ballroom We Care, and Keeping Ballroom Community Alive Network). Our kinship structure encourages involved members to share resources, as well as parents to take an active role, to offer "daily parental guidance to Ballroom kids on issues such as intimate/romantic relationships, sex, gender and sexual identities, health, gender-affirming care, and body presentation."[106] Unconditional sibling love also provides daily support for us to thrive through shared lived experience.

The QPOC of ballroom are at the forefront of changing the culture of health, with intraventions and kinship models showing what it means to provide holistic trans-affirming care. Our revolutionary acts showcase our intelligence, political savvy, and social connections. With our strength, we foster wellness and remarkable resilience within our community.[107]

The HBC is an inspiring response to the medicalization paradox. Rather than relying on a system built to discriminate, HBC founders created a system designed to be nurturing, resourceful, and self-sustaining. The community-led intraventions, championed by HBC, offer an alternative blueprint through which the TGD and medical communities can truly partner, share expertise, and center biopsychosocial wellness.

I find hope in their example. A medical doctor myself, I believe that medicine has a role to play in supporting gender transition. I work within the medical system, and I am a beneficiary of medical and surgical transition-related care. Ultimately, though, buying into a system built on the entrenched belief that nonnormative gender identities are indicative of pathology, rather than naturally occurring phenomena, comes at a steep personal and collective cost. Western medical systems were built to treat disease, not nurture difference.

Just as transgender people (and particularly trans people of color) were integral in the fight to remove homosexuality from the *DSM* in 1973, transgender activists and allies, including my illustrious coeditors, have fought to curtail medical overreach, minimize gatekeeping, and center transgender voices in the medical conversation.[108] The publication of the World Professional Association for Transgender Health *Standards of Care* is a rebellion against traditional medicalization, as it is a means through which transgender individuals are emboldened to set the terms.

As of this writing, it is indisputable that the transgender experience is defined in medical terms, understood within a medical framework, and addressed through medical treatment. The costs of this medicalization are high and inequitably distributed. However, the example of the HBC, the advocacy of transgender individuals and groups, and the increasing numbers of transgender medical professionals[109] indicate that significant changes in the medical professional-transgender patient dynamic are ahead. In this modern era of transgender medicine, we refuse to be relegated to the margins of our own medical care.

NOTES

1. Altman, "New Homosexual Disorder Worries Health Officials," C1–C6.
2. Altman, "New Homosexual Disorder Worries Health Officials," C1.
3. Altman, "New Homosexual Disorder Worries Health Officials," C1–C6.
4. Michie, "A Few Words About AIDS," 328.
5. Royse and Birge, "Homophobia and Attitudes," 867.
6. Quinn, "Forty Years of AIDS," 3.
7. Treichler, "AIDS, Homophobia and Biomedical Discourse," 267.
8. Conrad, Mackie, and Mehrotra, "Estimating the Costs of Medicalization," 1943.
9. Torres, "Medicalizing to Demedicalize," 161.
10. Lynch, "Living with Kaposi's," 40.
11. Martos, Wilson, and Meyer. "Lesbian, Gay, Bisexual, and Transgender (LGBT) Health," 5.
12. Wright, "Only Your Calamity," 1794.
13. Conrad and Angell, "Homosexuality and Remedicalization," 36.

14. Wolfgang and Portinari, "The PrEP Recommendation," 275.
15. Drescher, "Out of DSM," 565.
16. James, "Queer People of Color Led the LGBTQ Charge"
17. Drescher, "Queer Diagnoses," 441–42.
18. If Murray had lived in another decade, she might have identified as transgender and preferred different pronouns. But she lived in a gender-binary culture, and her struggle to find words to describe her experience over time was a defining life theme. Changing her pronouns to ones that might better reflect her gender identity today feels presumptuous, given that she referred to herself with feminine pronouns and kept her gender exploration private; Rosenberg, *Jane Crow*, xvii. With respect for her complex lived experience and time in history, I use feminine pronouns in this piece. I similarly bow to Simmons-Thorne and the Pauli Murray Center for History and Social Justice for alternative approaches to the use of pronouns for Murray and other historical figures, when personal choice was unknown. See Simmons-Thorne, "Pauli Murrray and the Pronominal Problem."
19. Rosenberg, *Jane Crow*, 3.
20. Rosenberg, *Jane Crow*, 16.
21. Rosenberg, *Jane Crow*, 16.
22. Rosenberg, *Jane Crow*, 27–28.
23. Schulz, "The Many Lives of Pauli Murray."
24. Schulz, "The Many Lives of Pauli Murray."
25. Schulz, "The Many Lives of Pauli Murray."
26. Rosenberg, *Jane Crow*, 138–39.
27. Murray, *Song in a Weary Throat: Memoir of an American Pilgramage*; Rosenberg, *Jane Crow The Life of Pauli Murray*, 6.
28. Rosenberg, *Jane Crow*, 2–3.
29. Schulz, "The Many Lives of Pauli Murray."
30. Schulz, "The Many Lives of Pauli Murray."
31. Rosenberg, *Jane Crow*, 2–3.
32. Cohen and West, *My Name is Pauli Murray.*
33. Schulz, "The Many Lives of Pauli Murray."
34. White, "The Dynamic Woman Who Shaped Ruth Bader Ginsburg."
35. White, "The Dynamic Woman Who Shaped Ruth Bader Ginsburg."
36. Schulz, "The Many Lives of Pauli Murray."
37. Schulz, "The Many Lives of Pauli Murray."
38. Schulz, "The Many Lives of Pauli Murray."
39. *Duke Today*, "Pauli Murray Named to Episcopal Sainthood."
40. McNeil, Interview with Pauli Murray, 1976.
41. Murray, "Dark Testament."
42. Byrd and Clayton, "Race, Medicine, and Health Care in the United States," 115.

43. Starr, "Professionalization and Public Health," S28; Makari, "On the Shifting Boundaries of Medicine," 206–07.

44. Zachar and Kendler, "Psychiatric Disorders," 560.

45. Lafrance and McKenzie-Mohr, "The DSM and Its Lure of Legitimacy," 126.

46. Uyeda, "How LGBTQ+ Activists Got 'Homosexuality.'"

47. Prescod-Weinstein, "Making Black Women Scientists Under White Empiricism," 421.

48. Prescod-Weinstein, "Making Black Women Scientists Under White Empiricism," 426.

49. Prescod-Weinstein, "Making Black Women Scientists Under White Empiricism," 426.

50. Goldenberg, "On Evidence and Evidence-Based Medicine," 2622.

51. Ortega and Roby, "Ending Structural Racism in the US Health Care System," 613.

52. This quote is also used by Ravishankar, "The Story of Robert Eads."

53. Denny, "The Impact of Emerging Technologies on One Transgender Organization."

54. Anderson, "Remembering Robert."

55. I have often wondered what went sideways with the referrals I made—especially the ob-gyn who had performed a hysterectomy on another trans man only a few months earlier.

56. McIntosh, "Teaching Transgender Issues Through Documentary and Southern Comfort."

57. Anderson, "Remembering Robert," 50.

58. Davis, *Southern Comfort*.

59. It was an extraordinary emotional moment and Eads gave a wonderful speech.

60. Eads wasn't the only subject in Davis's film to experience cavalier treatment at the hands of medical professionals. At 00:10:25 and 1:06:00 segments, Cas and Stephanie Piotrowski describe how complications from Cas's top surgery went untreated because his surgeon went on leave immediately after he "stopped cutting." In the 00:10:25 segment, Cas says wryly, "All these young guys coming up ask 'What questions should I ask?' I say you'd better find out about when he's taking his vacation."

After Ead's death, Lola Cola founded the Robert Eads Health Partnership Program (later Project) for trans men. For many years, there was a Robert Eads Health Care Day for trans men during the Southern Comfort Conference. Attendees were given access to every sort of medical service in a supportive setting. After the Southern Comfort Conference moved to Fort Lauderdale in 2015, the project remained in Atlanta. It was hosted in Atlanta at Transgender Health & Education Alliance's Peach State Conference in 2015 and 2016 and was thereafter maintained by Dr. Alan Perry until the advent of Paradise Conference in Atlanta in October 2021. Blake Alford, personal communications, 2019, 2021; see also Reiser, "Transgender Conference Moves to South Florida," and Walker, "THEA Peach State Conference Returns."

61. Bradley et al., "Interim Report of the *DSM-IV* Subcommittee on Gender Identity Disorders," 340.

62. Stryker, "A Hundred-Plus Years of Transgender History," 46.

63. Bockting et al., "Stigma, Mental Health, and Resilience in an Online Sample of the US Transgender Population," 943.

64. Winter et al., "Transgender People: Health at the Margins of Society," 394.

65. Wilson et al., "The Use and Correlates of Illicit Silicone or 'Fillers,'" 1717; Padilla et al., "Trans-Migrations: Border-Crossing and the Politics of Body Modification Among Puerto Rican Transgender Women," 269; Sergi and Wilson. "Filler Use Among Trans Women," 88.

66. Dubov and Fraenkel, "Facial Feminization Surgery," 4.

67. Gonzalez et al., "'A Center for Trans Women Where They Help You,'" 61.

68. Scandurra et al., "Health of Non-Binary and Genderqueer People," 4.

69. Smart et al., "Transgender Women of Color in the US South," 172.

70. Radix and Goldstein, "Issues in the Care and Treatment of Transwomen Sex Workers," 393–94.

71. Porter et al., "Providing Competent and Affirming Services," 368; Witten, "Health and Well-Being of Transgender Elders," 27; Abreu et al., "Impact of Gender-Affirming Care Bans," 2.

72. McCauly et al., "Exploring Healthcare Experiences," 35.

73. Plemons, "Gender, Ethnicity, and Transgender Embodiment," 5; Gonsalves, "Gender Identity," 1022.

74. Kulick, *Travesti*, 5.

75. See Denny, "Dangerous Curves," for a graphic description of the long-term effects of silicone injection.

76. Chasan, "The History of Injectable Silicone Fluids."

77. Chasan, "The History of injectable Silicone Fluids."

78. Silicone sometimes leaks from implants. This motivated the FDA to call a moratorium on the use of silicone as filler. The ban lasted fourteen years before being lifted in 2006. See Associated Press, 2006.

79. Kulick, *Travesti*, 5.

80. Usually caulk from home improvement stores.

81. "Auto-Shop Silicone Used for Injection"; see also Denny, "Dangerous Curves."

82. FDA News Release, "FDA Warns Against Use."

83. Schmid et al., "Silicone Embolism Syndrome."

84. Roth, "Risks of Unlicensed Silicone Buttocks Injections."

85. Denny, "Cheekbones from Hell."

86. Chaplin, "Loss of Both Breasts."

87. Denny, "Cheekbones from Hell."
88. Padilla et al., "Trans-Migrations," 269; Tucker and Love, "Realness," 160–61.
89. Hines, Laury, and Habermann. "They Just Don't Get Me," e82.
90. Kelly et al., "Psychosocial Differences," 5.
91. Aizenman, "How to Demand a Medical Breakthrough."
92. Volberding, "How to Survive a Plague," 1298–99.
93. Stone, "Psychiatric Screening."
94. I picked diethylstilbestrol over other estrogens as a result of my review of the literature. When, years later, the dangers of the drug became known, I switched to Premarin. Luckily, I have suffered no unwanted side effects related to my use of diethylstilbestrol.
95. . . . and yet all is not well. It can still be difficult to obtain hormones, and people of color and of low socioeconomic status can have a particularly difficult time.
96. Lawrence, "History of Drag Balls," 4.
97. Bailey, "Performance as Intravention," 260, 267.
98. Arnold and Bailey, "Constructing Home and Family," 3; Bailey, "Performance as Intravention," 254.
99. Bailey, "Performance as Intravention," 5; Bailey, "Gender/Racial Realness," 260.
100. Bailey, "Performance as Intravention," 257.
101. Friedman et al., "Urging Others to Be Healthy," 250; Bailey, "Performance as Intravention," 259.
102. Bailey, "Performance as Intravention," 257.
103. Bailey, "Performance as Intravention," 266.
104. Arnold and Bailey, "Constructing Home and Family," 3.
105. Friedman et al., "Urging Others to be Healthy," 259; Bailey, "Performance as Intravention," 259.
106. Bailey, "Performance as Intravention," 267.
107. Lee, "The House We Built."
108. Stryker, "Transgender Activism."
109. Kvach, Weinand, and O'Connell, "Experiences of Transgender and Nonbinary Physicians," 201.

WORKS CITED

Abreu, Roberto L., Jules P. Sostre, Kirsten A. Gonzalez, Gabriel M. Lockett, Em Matsuno, and Della V. Mosley. "Impact of Gender-Affirming Care Bans on Transgender and Gender Diverse Youth: Parental Figures' Perspective." *Journal of Family Psychology* 36, no. 5 (2022): 643–52.

Aizenman, Nurith, "How to Demand a Medical Breakthrough: Lessons from the AIDS Fight." *NPR*, February 9, 2019. Accessed August 15, 2022. https://

www.npr.org/sections/health-shots/2019/02/09/689924838/how-to-demand-a-medical-breakthrough-lessons-from-the-aids-fight.

Altman, Lawrence K. "New Homosexual Disorder Worries Health Officials." *New York Times*, May 11, 1982, C1–6.

Anderson, Maxwell. "Remembering Robert." *Transgender Tapestry Journal* 103 (2003): 46–50. Accessed October 26, 2021. https://archive.org/details/transgendertapes1032unse/page/50/mode/2up.

Arnold, E. A., and M. M. Bailey. "Constructing Home and Family: How the Ballroom Community Supports African American GLBTQ Youth in the Face of HIV/AIDS." *Journal of Gay and Lesbian Social Services* 21, no. 2–3 (2009): 171–88.

Associated Press. "FDA Lifts Ban on Silicone Breast Implants." *Fox News*, November 18, 2006. Accessed February 3, 2021. https://www.foxnews.com/story/fda-lifts-ban-on-silicone-breast-implants.

Associated Press. "Man Charged in Silicone Injection Death." *Gainesville (GA) Sun*, February 13, 1993.

"Auto-Shop Silicone Used for Injection." *Oakland (CA) Tribune*, February 18, 1993, A8.

Bailey, Marion. "Gender/Racial Realness: Theorizing the Gender System in Ballroom Culture." *Feminist Studies* 37, no. 2 (2011): 365–86.

———. "Performance as Intravention: Ballroom Culture and the Politics of HIV/AIDS in Detroit." *Souls* 11, no. 3 (2009): 253–74.

Bockting, Walter O., Michael H. Miner, Rebecca E. Swinburne Romine, Autumn Hamilton, and Eli Coleman. "Stigma, Mental Health, and Resilience in an Online Sample of the US Transgender Population." *American Journal of Public Health* 103, no. 5 (2013): 943–51.

Bradley, Susan J., Ray Blanchard, Susan Coates, et al. "Interim Report of the *DSM-IV* Subcommittee on Gender Identity Disorders." *Archives of Sexual Behavior* 20, no. 4 (1991): 333–43.

Byrd, W. Michael, and Linda A. Clayton. "Race, Medicine, and Health Care in the United States: A Historical Survey." *Journal of the National Medical Association* 93, no. 3 Suppl (2001): 11S.

Chaplin, C. H. "Loss of Both Breasts from Injections of Silicone (with Additive)." *Plastic and Reconstructive Surgery* 44, no. 5 (1969): 447–50.

Chasan, Paul E. "The History of Injectable Silicone Fluids for Soft Tissue Augmentation." n.d. Accessed February 2, 2021. https://www.drchasan.com/blog/published-articles/history-injectable-silicone-fluids-soft-tissue-augmentation.

Chauncy, George. *Gay New York: Gender, Urban Cullture, and the Making of the Male Gay World 1980–1940*. New York: Basic Books, 1994.

Cohen, Julie, and Betsy West, Directors. *My Name Is Pauli Murray*. Storyville Films. 2021. 91 min. https://www.imdb.com/title/tt11092594/.

Conrad, Peter, and Alison Angell. "Homosexuality and Remedicalization." *Society* 41, no. 5 (2004): 32–39.

Conrad, Peter, Thomas Mackie, and Ateev Mehrotra. "Estimating the Costs of Medicalization." *Social Science & Medicine* 70, no. 12 (2010): 1943–47.

Davis, Kate, Dir. *Southern Comfort*. Q-Ball Productions. 2002. Accessed October 26, 2021. https://www.imdb.com/title/tt0276515/.

Denny, Dallas. "Cheekbones from Hell, or Injected Silicone: Bad News." *TV-TS Tapestry* 61 (1992): 46–48.

———. "Dangerous Curves: Injectable Silicone Can Lead to Disfigurement and Death." Workshop presented at Trans Lives Conference, Farmington, CT, April 26, 2014.

———. "The Impact of Emerging Technologies on One Transgender Organization." Dallas Denny: Body of Work. 2001. Accessed October 26, 2021. http://dallasdenny.com/Writing/2013/08/22/the-impact-of-emerging-technologies-on-one-transgender-organizationthe-impact-of-emerging-technologies-on-one-transgender-organization the-impact-of-emerging-technologies-on-one-transgender-organizatio/.

Diagnostic and Statistical Manual of Mental Disorders: DSM-IV. Washington, DC: American Psychiatric Association, 1994.

Drescher, Jack. "Out of DSM: Depathologizing Homosexuality." *Behavioral Sciences* 5, no. 4 (2015): 565–75.

———. "Queer Diagnoses: Parallels and Contrasts in the History of Homosexuality, Gender Variance, and the *Diagnostic and Statistical Manual*." *Archives of Sexual Behavior* 39, no. 2 (2010): 427–60.

Dubov, Alex, and Liana Fraenkel. "Facial Feminization Surgery: The Ethics of Gatekeeping in Transgender Health." *American Journal of Bioethics* 18, no. 12 (2018): 3–9.

Duke Today Staff. "Pauli Murray Named to Episcopal Sainthood." July 14, 2012. Accessed June 14, 2021. https://today.duke.edu/2012/07/saintmurray.

Federal Food and Drug Administration News Release. "FDA Warns Against Use of Injectable Silicone for Body Contouring and Enhancement." November 13, 2017. Accessed October 16, 2022. https://www.fda.gov/news-events/press-announcements/fda-warns-about-illegal-use-injectable-silicone-body-contouring-and-associated-health-risks

Friedman, Samuel, Carey Maslow, Melissa Bolyard, Milagros Sandoval, Pedro Mateau-Gelabert, and Alan Neaigus. "Urging Others to Be Healthy: 'Intravention' by Injection Drug Users as a Community Prevention Goal." *AIDS Education and Prevention* 16, no. 3 (2004): 250–63.

Garber, E. A. "A Spectacle in Color: The Lesbian and Gay Subcullture of Jazz Age Harlem." In *Hidden From History: Reclaiming the Gay and Lesbian Past*, eds. Martin Duberman, Martha Vicinus, and George Chauncey, 318–31. New York: New American Library, 1989.

Goldenberg, Maya J. "On Evidence and Evidence-Based Medicine: Lessons from the Philosophy of Science." *Social Science & Medicine* 62, no. 11 (2006): 2622.

Gonsalves, Tara. "Gender Identity, the Sexed Body, and the Medical Making of Transgender." *Gender & Society* 34, no. 6 (2020): 1005–33.

Gonzalez, Kirsten A., Roberto L. Abreu, Cristalís Capielo Rosario, Jasmine M. Koech, Gabriel M. Lockett, and Louis Lindley. "'A Center for Trans Women Where They Help You': Resource Needs of the Immigrant Latinx Transgender Community." *International Journal of Transgender Health* 23, no. 1–2 (2022): 60–78.

Hines, Dana D., Esther R. Laury, and Barbara Habermann. "They Just Don't Get Me: A Qualitative Analysis of Transgender Women's Health Care Experiences and Clinician Interactions." *Journal of the Association of Nurses in AIDS Care* 30, no. 5 (2019): e82.

James, Scott. "Queer People of Color Led the LGBTQ Charge, but Were Denied the Rewards." *New York Times*, June 22, 2019.

Kelly, Patrick J., Anne S. Frankel, Paul D'Avanzo, Katie Suppes, Adrian Shanker, and David B. Sarwer. "Psychosocial Differences between Transgender Individuals With and Without History of Nonsurgical Facial Injectables." *Aesthetic Surgery Journal Open Forum* 3, no. 1 (2021): ojaa050.

Kulick, Don. *Travesti: Sex, Gender, and Culture Among Brazilian Transgendered Prostitutes.* Chicago, IL: University of Chicago Press, 1998.

Kvach, Elizabeth J., Jamie Weinand, and Ryan O'Connell. "Experiences of Transgender and Nonbinary Physicians During Medical Residency Program Application." *Journal of Graduate Medical Education* 13, no. 2 (2021): 201–05.

Lafrance, Michelle N., and Suzanne McKenzie-Mohr. "The DSM and Its Lure of Legitimacy." *Feminism & Psychology* 23, no. 1 (2013): 126.

Lawrence, Tim. *'Listen and You Will Hear All the Houses that Walked Here Before': A History of Drag Balls, Houses, and the Culture of Voguing.* July 16, 2013. Accessed August 19, 2024. https://www.timlawrence.info/articles2/2013/7/16/listen-and-you-will-hear-all-the-houses-that-walked-there-before-a-history-of-drag-balls-houses-and-the-culture-of-voguing.

Lee, Jennifer. "The House We Built in Challenging the Status Quo: House and Ballroom Community Leadership and Health Justice." PhD diss., CUNY School of Public Health, 2020. https://academicworks.cuny.edu/sph_etds/47/.

Lynch, Michael. "Living with Kaposi's." *Body Politic* 88 (November 1982): 31–37.

Makari, George. "On the Shifting Boundaries of Medicine." *Lancet* 373, no. 9659 (2009): 206–07.

Martos, Alexander J., Patrick A. Wilson, and Ilan H. Meyer. "Lesbian, Gay, Bisexual, and Transgender (LGBT) Health Services in the United States: Origins, Evolution, and Contemporary Landscape." *PloS One* 12, no. 7 (2017): e0180544.

McCauley, Erin, Kristen Eckstrand, Bethlehem Desta, Ben Bouvier, Brad Brockmann, and Lauren Brinkley-Rubinstein. "Exploring Healthcare Experiences for Incarcerated Individuals Who Identify as Transgender in a Southern Jail." *Transgender Health* 3, no. 1 (2018): 35.

McIntosh, Heather. "Teaching Transgender Issues Through Documentary and Southern Comfort." *MP: An Online Feminist Journal* 3, no. 4 (2012): 75–76. Accessed October

26, 2021. http://academinist.org/wp-content/uploads/2010/06/MP0304_05Teaching+Southern+Comforts.pdf.

McNeil, Genna Rae. Interview with Pauli Murray, February 13, 1976. Interview G0044. Southern Oral History Program Collection (#4007). Accessed September 28, 2022. https://docsouth.unc.edu/sohp/html_use/G-0044.html.

Michie, Helena. "A Few Words About AIDS." *American Literary History* 2, no. 2 (1990): 328–38.

Murray, Pauli. "Dark Testament," Verse 8. In *Dark Testament and Other Poems*. 2018. Accessed October 17, 2022. https://travelingasafamily.tumblr.com/post/165548861414/dark-testament-verse-8-by-pauli-murray.

———. *Song in a Weary Throat: Memoir of an American Pilgramage*. New York, NY: Liverlight, 2018.

Ortega, Alexander N., and Dylan H. Roby. "Ending Structural Racism in the US Health Care System to Eliminate Health Care Inequities." *JAMA* 326, no. 7 (2021): 613–15.

Padilla, Mark B., Sheilla Rodríguez-Madera, Nelson Varas-Díaz, and Alixida Ramos-Pibernus. "Trans-Migrations: Border-Crossing and the Politics of Body Modification Among Puerto Rican Transgender Women." *International Journal of Sexual Health* 28, no. 4 (2016): 261–77.

Pauli Murray Center for History and Social Justice, "Pronouns, Gender, & Pauli Murray." n.d. Accessed October 11, 2023. https://www.paulimurraycenter.com/pronouns-pauli-murray.

Plemons, Eric. "Gender, Ethnicity, and Transgender Embodiment: Interrogating Classification in Facial Feminization Surgery." *Body & Society* 25, no. 1 (2019): 3–28.

Porter, Kristen E., Mark Brennan-Ing, Sand C. Chang, et al. "Providing Competent and Affirming Services for Transgender and Gender Nonconforming Older Adults." *Clinical Gerontologist* 39, no. 5 (2016): 366–88.

Prescod-Weinstein, Chanda. "Making Black Women Scientists under White Empiricism: The Racialization of Epistemology in Physics." *Signs: Journal of Women in Culture and Society* 45, no. 2 (2020): 421–47.

Quinn, Thomas C. "Forty Years of AIDS: A Retrospective and the Way Forward." *Journal of Clinical Investigation* 131, no. 18 (2021): e154196.

Radix, Asa, and Zil Goldstein, "Issues in the Care and Treatment of Transwomen Sex Workers." In *Transgender Sex Work and Society*, edited by Larry Nuttbrock, 394–94. New York: Harrington Park Press.

Ravishankar, Mathura. "The Story about Robert Eads." *Journal of Global Health*, January 18, 2013. Accessed August 21, 2020. https://archive.is/20130914005716/http://www.ghjournal.org/jgh-online/the-story-about-robert-eads/#selection-393.2-393.286.

Reiser, Emon. "Transgender Conference Moves to South Florida." *Southern Florida Business Journal*, September 17, 2014. Accessed October 26, 2021. https://www.bizjournals.com/southflorida/news/2014/09/17/transgender-conference-moves-to-fort-lauderdale.html.

Rosenberg, Rosalind. *Jane Crow: The Life of Pauli Murray*. New York: Oxford University Press, 2017.

Roth, Jeffrey. "Risks of Unlicensed Silicone Buttocks Injections." Las Vegas Plastic Surgery. n.d. Accessed February 2, 2021. https://www.jjrothmd.com/blog/risks-of-unlicensed-silicone-buttocks-injections/.

Royse, David, and Barbara Birge. "Homophobia and Attitudes Towards AIDS Patients Among Medical, Nursing, and Paramedical Students." *Psychological Reports* 61, no. 3 (1987): 867–70.

Scandurra, Cristiano, Fabrizio Mezza, Nelson Mauro Maldonato, et al. "Health of Non-Binary and Genderqueer People: A Systematic Review." *Frontiers in Psychology* 10 (2019): 1453.

Scarce, Michael. "Harbinger of Plague: A Bad Case of Gay Bowel Syndrome." *Journal of Homosexuality* 34, no. 2 (1997): 1–35.

Schulz, Kathryn. "The Many Lives of Pauli Murray." *The New Yorker*, April 10, 2017. Accessed January 20, 2021. https://www.newyorker.com/magazine/2017/04/17/the-many-lives-of-pauli-murray.

Schmid, Andreas, Assaf Tzur, Lidiya Leshko, and Bruce P. Krieger. "Silicone Embolism Syndrome: A Case Report, Review of the Literature, and Comparison with Fat Embolism Syndrome." *Chest* 127, no. 6 (2005): 2276–81.

Sergi, Francesco D., and Erin C. Wilson. "Filler Use Among Trans Women: Correlates of Feminizing Subcutaneous Injections and Their Health Consequences." *Transgender Health* 6, no. 2 (2021): 82–90.

Simmons-Thorne, Naomi. "Pauli Murray and the Pronominal Problem: A De-Essentialist Trans Historiography." *Activist History Review*, May 30, 2019. Accessed August 19, 2024. https://activisthistory.com/2019/05/30/pauli-murray-and-the-pronominal-problem-a-de-essentialist-trans-historiography/.

Smart, Benjamin D., Lilli Mann-Jackson, Jorge Alonzo, et al. "Transgender Women of Color in the US South: A Qualitative Study of Social Determinants of Health and Healthcare Perspectives." *International Journal of Transgender Health* 23, no. 1–2 (2022): 164–77.

Starr, P. "Professionalization and Public Health: Historical Legacies, Continuing Dilemmas." *Journal of Public Health Management and Practice* 15, no. 6 (2009), S28.

Stone, C. B. "Psychiatric Screening for Transsexual Surgery." *Psychosomatics* 18, no. 1 (1977): 25–27.

Stryker, Susan. "A Hundred-Plus Years of Transgender History." In *Transgender History: The Roots of Today's Revolution*. 2nd ed. New York: Seal Press, 2017: 46.

———. "Transgender Activism." *GLBTQ: An Encyclopedia of Gay Lesbian Bisexual Transgender and Queer Culture*. 2004. Accessed August 19, 2024. http://www.glbtq.com/social-sciences/transgender_activism.

Treichler, P. A. AIDS, Homophobia and Biomedical Discourse: An Epidemic of Signification. *Cultural Studies* 1, no. 3 (1987): 263–05.

Tucker, Ricky, and Gia Love. "Realness." In *And the Category Is*. Boston, MA: Beacon Press, 2022: 160–61.

Uyeda, Ray Levy. "How LGBTQ+ Activists Got 'Homosexuality' out of the DSM." *JSTOR Daily*, May 26, 2021. Accessed August 19, 2024. https://daily.jstor.org/how-lgbtq-activists-got-homosexuality-out-of-the-dsm/.

Volberding, Paul A. "How to Survive a Plague: The Next Great HIV/AIDS History." *JAMA* 317, no. 13 (2017): 1298–99.

Walker, Dionne. "THEA Peach State Conference Returns to Atlanta for Second Year." *Georgia Voice*, October 31, 2016. Accessed October 26, 2021. https://thegavoice.com/news/georgia/thea-peach-state-conference-returns-atlanta-second-year/.

White, Meghan. "The Dynamic Woman Who Shaped Ruth Bader Ginsburg." National Trust for Historic Preservation. October 6, 2015. Accessed June 14, 2021. https://savingplaces.org/stories/how-pauli-murray-helped-shape-notorious-rbg#.YMeS3TZKjPY.

Wilder, C. S. *In The Company of Black Men: The African Influence on African American Culture in New York City*. New York: New York University Press, 2001.

Wilson, Erin, Jenna Rapues, Harry Jin, and Henry Fisher Raymond. "The Use and Correlates of Illicit Silicone or 'Fillers' in a Population-Based Sample of Transwomen, San Francisco, 2013." *Journal of Sexual Medicine* 11, no. 7 (2014): 1717–24.

Winter, Sam, Milton Diamond, Jamison Green, et al. "Transgender People: Health at the Margins of Society." *Lancet* 388, no. 10042 (2016): 390–400.

Witten, Tarynn M. "Health and Well-Being of Transgender Elders." *Annual Review of Gerontology and Geriatrics* 37, no. 1 (2017): 27–41.

Wolfgang, Simone, and Denise Portinari. "The PrEP Recommendation: The Inscribed Disease in a Healthy Body." *Social Medicine* 12, no. 3 (2020): 272–79.

Wollina, Uwe. "Silicone Injections." *Journal of Cutaneous and Aesthetic Surgery* 5, no. 3 (2012): 197.

Wright, Joe. "Only Your Calamity: The Beginnings of Activism by and for People with AIDS." *American Journal of Public Health* 103, no. 10 (2013): 1788–98.

Zachar, Peter, and Kenneth S. Kendler. "Psychiatric Disorders: A Conceptual Taxonomy." *American Journal of Psychiatry* 164, no. 4 (2007): 557–65.

Section III

ENCOUNTERS WITH THE MAINSTREAM

Section III of this volume describes the emergence of the interdisciplinary field of transgender healthcare and its early struggle to attain legitimacy within US mainstream medical practice. In chapter 10, sociologist and sexologist Aaron Devor reveals the story of Reed Erickson, a wealthy trans man who established the Erickson Educational Foundation, an organization that promoted and legitimized transgender healthcare from 1964 to 1976. In chapter 11, Dallas Denny chronicles the opening of the Johns Hopkins clinic in 1966 and the subsequent proliferations of US gender clinics, a period that ended in 1979 with the rapid closure of these facilities after a scathing critique by psychiatrist Paul McHugh. Denny writes from the largely unpublished perspective of a desperate community whose hopes for good care were often dashed by interactions with these clinics. In chapter 12, Carolyn Wolf-Gould discusses the various human and civil rights organizations that formed in the 1960s and fought for the rights of people of color communities, women, LGB people, and eventually transgender and gender-diverse (TGD) people. In chapter 13, Jamison Green describes the evolution of professional guidelines in transgender healthcare, with discussion on the evolution of insurance coverage and legal intersections.

In chapter 14, Carolyn Wolf-Gould and endocrinologist Joshua Safer explain past and current theories on the biological underpinnings of gender identity. This is followed by two short commentaries: the first, a profile on Eugen Steinach and his work to effect sex changes in rodents and identify sex hormones, a story that exposes the glitches and triumphs of research around the etiology of sexual and gender diversity; the second illustrates how "born this way" etiologic theories meant to normalize the TGD experience may exist as a double-edged sword.

In chapter 15 clinician researcher George Brown and Carolyn Wolf-Gould describe Brown's career as one of the first researchers to employ big data to study and document the health problems and disparities of American TGD people. This chapter is followed by a commentary on the troubled history of ethical research violations in the field of TGD research and the new standards that guide contemporary research efforts. A second commentary explores the troubled relationship between TGD people with the Department of Defense and how the Veterans Health Administration has begun to address discrimination by developing increasingly inclusive policies.

Trans pioneers profiled in section III include Marsha P. Johnson and Sylvia Rivera, who championed the plight of TGD communities of color, creating support structures for sex workers, street youth, and others living in poverty—setting the stage for contemporary medical programs that target HIV and gender healthcare for these populations today. We describe the lives and work of Denny and Green, co-editors of this volume, as early and ongoing trans activists, writers, and community organizers.

10

LEGITIMIZING TRANS

Reed Erickson (1917–1992) and the
Erickson Educational Foundation

Aaron Devor

In the 1960s, average Americans and American medical practitioners knew next to nothing about the existence or experiences of trans people.[1] Those few who possessed some awareness generally presumed that trans people suffered from a mental disorder and that their "delusions" should neither be encouraged nor tolerated.[2] It was in this milieu that Reed Erickson established the Erickson Educational Foundation, an organization that profoundly transformed public and medical opinions about trans people.[3]

WHO WAS REED ERICKSON?

Erickson was born on October 13, 1917, in El Paso, Texas.[4] By February 1928, the Erickson family, then including a younger sister, had moved to Philadelphia.[5] Following high school, Erickson enrolled at Temple University in Philadelphia, taking, and doing poorly in, a secretarial course.[6] In 1938, Erickson's mother Ruth died,[7] and in 1940 Erickson's father remarried and moved his family and lead recycling business, Schuylkill Metals, to Baton Rouge, Louisiana.[8]

Erickson worked at Schuylkill Metals and then enrolled at Louisiana State University, becoming, in 1945, the first woman graduate in the mechanical engineering program.[9] Erickson moved back to Philadelphia but found it impossible to get work as a woman engineer.[10] While there, Erickson became involved with a left-leaning, racially integrated, largely homosexual group[11] and deepened a love affair with a politically radical, white Jewish woman, Anne (pseudonym), who remained a strong progressive influence on him for decades.[12] In 1953, Erickson settled in Baton Rouge, where he again worked for the family business[13] until taking it over upon Robert Erickson's death in 1962.[14]

In the mid-1950s, Erickson began to gradually transform from living as a butch lesbian to increasingly presenting as a man. At first, Erickson wore masculine clothing at a time when very few women did so,[15] and after becoming a patient of Harry Benjamin in October 1963 at age forty-six, he further masculinized with hormone therapy under Benjamin's care.[16] In November 1963, Erickson legally changed his name,[17] and in May 1965, he had his sex changed on his birth certificate.[18]

Figure 10.1. Reed Erickson and Aileen Ashton. *Source*: Courtesy of the author.

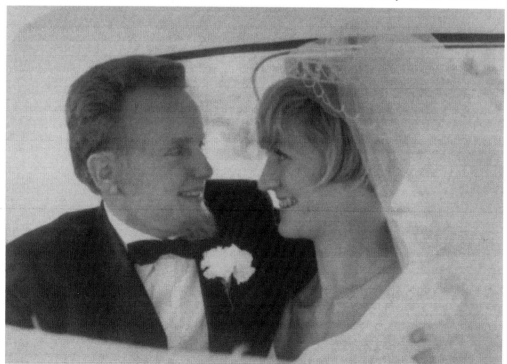

In 1964, in a New York City bar, Erickson met the woman who was to become the mother of his children. Aileen Ashton, a former Paris can-can dancer and gentleman's escort, was originally from New Zealand.[19] They married among family and friends in a church wedding in March 1966 in Christchurch, New Zealand.[20] In September 1968, Ashton gave birth to their daughter,[21] conceived via an anonymous donor insemination performed by a New York City physician and arranged by Johns Hopkins psychologist John Money.[22] In May 1972, they adopted their son immediately upon his birth in Baton Rouge.[23]

In 1972, Erickson moved his family to Mazatlán, Mexico,[24] where they lived in a large and ornate custom-built home called the Love Joy Palace. By August 1974, he and Ashton divorced,[25] with Erickson claiming he had paid her a settlement of twenty million dollars.[26] Erickson met his second wife, Evangelina Trujillo Armendarez, when he visited the tourist bureau where she worked and where he had gone looking for a translator for the book *A Course in Miracles*.[27] They married in Baton Rouge, Louisiana, in January 1977[28] and again in May 1977, in Mazatlán.[29] They eventually became estranged due to Erickson's increasingly debilitating use of legal and illegal drugs, but they were still officially married until his death.[30]

People who knew Erickson frequently described him as an astute businessman. Upon inheriting control of the family business, he grew Schuylkill Metals from an already successful enterprise to a sophisticated operation that he sold to Arrow Electronics in 1969 for more than five million dollars.[31] By the 1970s, he had parlayed his personal fortune into thirty to forty million dollars through canny real estate deals, some of which involved the discovery of, and income from, oil deposits.[32] Individuals close to him at this time recalled his income as varying between one hundred thousand dollars and five hundred thousand dollars monthly for many years.[33]

Later in his life, after many successful and productive years as a businessman and philanthropist, Erickson became enamored of a wide range of New Age and spiritual pursuits. Initially in search of higher consciousness, he and his friend John Lilly explored the use of ketamine as a possible path to enlightenment.[34] Later, Erickson may have also used the drug to self-medicate for a self-diagnosed cancer.[35] Sadly, Erickson's drug use grew beyond his control, sorely degraded his once very sharp mind, and left him with only a tenuous and intermittent grasp on reality. He died a much diminished man in a humble hotel room in Mazatlán in January 1992.[36]

INTRODUCING THE ERICKSON EDUCATIONAL FOUNDATION

Erickson decided to put some of his enormous wealth to work in the service of others by creating a nonprofit foundation, the Erickson Educational Foundation (EEF), incorporated in the state of Louisiana on June 26, 1964.[37] Although the Foundation did occasionally request donations,[38] Erickson funded the EEF himself. Similarly, while the EEF boasted an advisory board that included such well-known individuals as Reverend Ted McIlvenna,[39] Money, Evelyn Hooker,[40] and Anke Ehrhardt,[41] the members of this board contributed little to the vision or operations of the EEF beyond the prestige and legitimacy provided by their names on EEF materials.[42]

The EEF's published aims were "to provide assistance and support in areas where human potential was limited by adverse physical, mental, or social conditions or where the scope of research was too new, controversial, or imaginative to receive more traditionally oriented support."[43] Erickson described the EEF as "primarily a medical research foundation" whose purpose was "to underwrite or initiate essential but unusual medical type research projects"[44] by providing seed money to initiatives likely to be able to develop independently.[45] Specifically, "Too long neglected by the scientific and helping professions, the problem of gender dysphoria (transsexualism) became a focal point for Foundation endeavors."[46] The EEF actively worked on issues concerning transsexualism from 1964 to 1976.[47]

The EEF was always a small organization with a big budget and a huge social impact. Erickson stood at the head, making all fundamental decisions and micromanaging most of the everyday operations.[48] Over the years of trans-focused activities, the EEF maintained offices in Baton Rouge and New York City. One full-time staff person ran each office, supervising a staff bookkeeper and part-time clerks. Erickson largely remained in the background while staff handled most telephone or postal inquiries through the Baton Rouge offices. Zelda Suplee, long-time EEF executive director and trusted advisor to Erickson, managed publicity from the New York office.[49]

The EEF focused on three areas: supporting homophile rights organizations, primarily ONE Inc.;[50] advancing the cause of trans social acceptance; and exploring New Age lifestyles and personal growth. The first two were inherently intertwined during a time when sexual and gender minorities were considered so alike that activists, medical practitioners, members of the public, and even those minorities themselves made few meaningful distinctions between them. ONE Inc. began in 1952 as a monthly magazine dedicated to homosexual issues and later expanded to include an educational arm, the ONE Institute for Homophile Studies.[51] Erickson looked to build and make use of ONE Inc.'s infrastructure as a vehicle for communicating and building support for his view that trans people were legitimately deserving of medical treatment and that, with proper gender affirmation, could productively integrate into society. The EEF's third area of activity, New Age projects, was unrelated to the development of trans medicine in the United States.

The EEF's financial support of ONE Inc. began in 1964 after Erickson replied to an appeal for donors sent to ONE's mailing list. He phoned with an invitation for an officer of ONE to visit with him in Baton Rouge, all expenses paid. One of the founders of ONE, Dorr Legg, went to Baton Rouge to learn more despite some incredulity among ONE staff, with Legg summarizing their impression as: "This is just a Southern queen who wants a date for the weekend and was willing to send an airplane ticket."[52] Under Erickson's guidance, ONE established a nonprofit organization, the Institute for the Study of Human Resources (more commonly known as ISHR, pronounced: ISH-er), to receive charitable donations.[53] Thus began a funding relationship that ended in the 1990s with protracted court battles over the Milbank Estate, a piece of property in Los Angeles worth more than two million dollars. During the intervening years, the EEF channeled upwards of two hundred thousand dollars to ONE through ISHR. That support, and the proceeds from the sale of ONE's court-ordered portion of the disputed Milbank Estate, contributed to the survival of ONE[54] and its eventual growth into today's ONE National Gay & Lesbian Archives at the University of Southern California Libraries, the largest repository of lesbian, gay, bisexual, transgender, and queer materials in the world.[55]

After a decade of work promoting public and professional support for medical treatment and social acceptance for trans people (described in more detail below), Erickson's focus turned away from trans issues and toward New Age spiritual and personal development projects.[56] Two such projects supported by the EEF stand out because of their continued influence. In the first, the EEF funded the first edition of the quasi-religious spiritual guide *A Course in Miracles* (1976),[57] a series of three books " 'scribed' by Dr. Helen Schucman through a process of inner dictation that she identified as coming from Jesus." *A Course in Miracles* has been translated into twenty-seven languages with millions of copies sold worldwide.[58] The EEF also provided financial support to Erickson's close friend, John Lilly, for his groundbreaking research demonstrating the now accepted fact that dolphins engage in intraspecies communications.[59]

THE EEF'S WORK FOR TRANS PEOPLE

In the mid-1960s, when Erickson founded the Erickson Educational Foundation, the public—including medical personnel—knew little about transsexualism. Those physicians who knew anything at all about trans people usually endorsed the prevailing opinion that transsexualism was a delusional mental illness, closely related to homosexuality, and best treated by psychiatrists. Few approved of hormonal or surgical treatment, and those who did risked being viewed as quacks by the public and their peers.[60] The few doctors who supported affirming medical treatment for transsexual people "respected one another as liberal pioneers in a conservative profession"[61] and saw themselves as pursuing justice for a misunderstood minority.

Erickson used his foundation to lead and support those who he believed could shift public opinions and policies about trans rights and healthcare. At the same time, the EEF offered direct services to individual trans people and supported groups that offered such services. The central goal of Erickson and the EEF was to establish transsexuality as a bona fide medical condition, which, when properly treated, could support trans people to become productive and respectable contributors to mainstream heteronormative middle-class society, no different from other middle-class members of their affirmed gender.[62] As noted in the EEF-produced film, *I Am Not This Body*, "The Erickson Educational Foundation . . . is endeavoring to encourage research and medical and professional cooperation and better public understanding of a problem endured by many individuals through no fault of their own. The transsexual is seeking the opportunity to function as a complete person, fulfilling his or her potential as a worthy member of society."[63] The EEF's activities took a three-pronged approach to building acceptance for trans people: (1) providing advice and referrals for trans individuals to sympathetic professionals or peer support and advocacy groups, (2) offering public advocacy and education about the needs and strengths of trans people, and (3) supporting research and professional development among people whose work might bring them into contact with trans people.

APPROACH 1: ADVICE AND REFERRALS

The EEF staff in the Baton Rouge office answered letters and some phone calls from trans people asking for advice and referrals, while executive director Suplee, who also did most of the EEF's public education and outreach, answered most phone inquiries from the New York office. Suplee served as the face of the EEF and is remembered as one who provided sympathetic and kindly personal advice to trans people who visited the New York office. One trans woman remembered Suplee's advice as lifesaving at a time when suicide seemed to be her best option. After swallowing a bottle of sleeping pills, she called the office to "say good-bye to a woman there who had given me some literature." Suplee asked the police to trace the call and send an ambulance. The woman later remembered, "I was alone, and if not for that sweet woman on the other end of the phone line at the Erickson Educational Foundation . . . I would not be here."[64]

Sarah Santana, who ran the Baton Rouge office between 1971 and 1975, recalled that they typically received twenty to forty letters a week, and maintained ongoing correspondence with approximately 150 people. She estimated that she devoted sixty percent of her workweek to correspondence with trans people who wrote asking for information about medical and legal steps required for transition. The EEF kept state-by-state, up-to-date information about laws, policies, and practices concerning identification documents, as well as a comprehensive nationwide referral list of supportive professionals. Santana recalled that the EEF reply letters consisted of a set of standard paragraphs addressing common questions strung together with more personalized content. If requested, these letters included contact information for two or three physicians as geographically close to the letter writer as possible.[65] By late 1971, the EEF's list of sympathetic physicians willing to take referrals of trans patients had grown to 250 names.[66] One Canadian trans woman remembered the value of these services in a letter to the EEF:

> I am writing . . . to express my deepest appreciation, for the help you gave me freely, in . . . my hours and years of need in the late sixties and early seventies . . . maybe we can meet someday, and I'll give you a warm embrace for being that angel in the night who saved my life from so many thousand miles away . . . and I'll sing your praises all the way to heaven's door, along with Zelda's, and beyond.[67]

During this period, many US locales had laws that required people to wear at least three items of clothing that matched their legal sex. In some states, it was impossible to get one's sex legally changed, while in all others it was a difficult and costly process. As a result, the vast majority of trans people risked arrest for considerable periods of time. To reduce the likelihood of arrest for cross-dressing, the EEF issued identification cards which stated: "The undersigned is required to live in the gender of his/her choice for six months or more as a pre-requisite to sex-reassignment surgery." The Foundation suggested that card carriers also hold a corroborating doctor's note.[68] At least one recipient of an EEF identification card considered it so meaningful that she kept it for more than fifty years.[69]

The EEF also funded other organizations that supported individual trans people. For example, in response to a 1967 request from Dr. Robert W. Deisher, the EEF provided ongoing funding of approximately $250 per month for more than ten years[70] to the Seattle Counseling Service, which, until forced to close in 2022, proudly proclaimed itself to be "the oldest LGBTQ-focused community mental health agency in the world."[71] In San Francisco, an EEF grant of approximately $200 per month went to the National Transsexual Counseling Unit from 1969 to 1974 to pay the costs of rent, a salary for a counselor, typewriters, and a copy machine.[72] The work of the National Transsexual Counseling Unit, according to the EEF, included "counseling individuals and educating the public on transsexualism through street and studio radio programs, TV interviews, and arranging meetings with civic, administrative, social and other agency personnel, in an effort to improve the personal, social and economic condition of [trans] people."[73] One of the founders of the National Transsexual Counseling Unit, Suzan Cooke, described it this way:

> The roots of our organization were in . . . the Compton's Cafeteria Riots . . . the main mission of our organization was to help ourselves and our peers get through the process of changing sex. . . . We taught them how to get ID, who to see to get hormones. . . . We found people . . . who would let them crash at their place until they could get a place of their own. We told people how to dress and act when they saw a doctor. We didn't give people a script. We told them to tell the truth to the doctors. That the doctors were willing to help. . . . We helped people connect with sensitive people in both the welfare and employment offices. We had lawyers and friendly bail bonds offices we could refer people to. Mostly, though, we listened and offered our own experiences. Shared what we knew and learned from what others had to offer.[74]

APPROACH 2: PUBLIC EDUCATION AND ADVOCACY

Between 1964 and 1975, the EEF functioned as the strongest public voice advocating for the acceptance of trans people. During this period, a great deal of what appeared in public media and a large proportion of public lectures on the topic of transsexualism can be directly or indirectly traced to the auspices of the EEF. These resources included the organization's newsletters, advice pamphlets, and educational films; newspaper and magazine articles; radio and television discussions; reference works; and speakers at a wide range of public gatherings. The EEF set out to literally define what *trans* meant in the public mind, as demonstrated in 1969 when Benjamin and Money drafted definitions of the terms *transsexual, transsexualism, transvestite,* and *transvestism*. The EEF sent their definitions "to 105 medical and lay dictionaries and encyclopaedias to update incorrect or obsolete definitions and to be included in revised editions where hitherto omitted."[75]

The *EEF Newsletter* was published several times a year, starting with the spring 1968 edition and continuing until summer 1976, with one final publication in Spring 1983. Suplee wrote the newsletters under Erickson's supervision.[76] Newsletters had the EEF logo across the top of the page, ran four to eight pages of two-column text, double-sided, on thick, letter-sized, colored paper—designed to impress. The newsletters brought together a wide range of information on trans issues and research and on other topics of interest to the EEF. In an era when most trans people felt alone in the world, and when even professionals found it difficult to access sources of information, the *EEF Newsletter* served as a uniquely valuable resource.

The contents included a mixture of news items and reports on the activities of people of interest to, or associated with, the EEF. In the beginning, Erickson clipped many of the news items himself.[77] Later, the EEF hired a clipping service to cut and compile articles into large scrapbooks.[78] The EEF distributed its newsletter free of charge to approximately one thousand subscribers, as well as to others whom Erickson thought would benefit.[79] In 1975, the *EEF Newsletter* claimed a mailing list of twenty thousand.[80] A 1983 mailing list included all public libraries in the United States, all vendors and business associates, the address books of Erickson and the EEF, all EEF grant recipients, and individual subscribers in thirty-three US states.[81]

The EEF's pamphlet series functioned as another major informational source during this era. The pamphlets were 5 × 8 inches, written in plain language, printed with colorful card stock covers on good quality paper, and

Figure 10.2. *EEF Newsletter*. *Source*: Courtesy of the author.

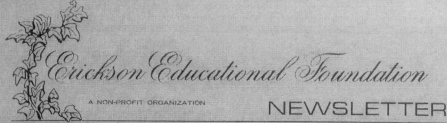

THE NEW FOUNDATION STYLE

"... There has developed in this country a degree of public blandness which does us no credit. Neither in business, nor in the professions, nor in government, is there enough encouragement to independent activities by young men. The 'organization man' is not merely a slick phrase. He is a growing menace to us ... Foundations ought to stand against this kind of thing. They should begin by encouraging both variety and energy of expression in their own staffs. They should put a premium in diversity in their grant-making and be ready to give a hand to the unorthodox ... They should contribute in as many ways as they properly can to honest public discussion of issues which are controversial."

McGeorge Bundy, Director of the Ford Foundation
FORTUNE, April 1968

AVANT GARDE IN CONCEPT

The Erickson Educational Foundation is proud to have anticipated Mr. Bundy's counsel. In 1964, this Foundation was established by Reed Erickson to assist where human potential was limited by physical, mental or social conditions, or where scope of research was too new, controversial or imaginative to encourage traditionally oriented support.

Reflecting this concept is the newest member of our Advisory Board, Rev. Ted McIlvenna, director of the Glide Foundation Urban Center, Glide Methodist Church, San Francisco, and founder of the rapidly expanding Council on Religion and the Homophile.

SEX AND GENDER ROLE RESEARCH — Psychosexual Research

Although millions of Americans have serious gender identity problems, little top level research was being done. EEF initiated and supported the Harry Benjamin Foundation in order to assist pioneer Harry Benjamin, M.D., endocrinologist, and his associates in their work with transsexual and transvestite patients.

Lecturing before medical groups at leading universities and hospitals through the country and in many articles, Dr. Benjamin stressed the vital need of enlightenment among allied as well as the medical disciplines.

The Transsexual Phenomenon by Dr. Benjamin (Julian Press, 1966) was the first scientific report on 15 years study of hundreds of patients and on the sex conversion operation then not yet performed in the United States.

"A CHANGING OF SEX BY SURGERY BEGUN AT JOHNS HOPKINS"

This N.Y. Times headline Nov. 21, 1966, was one of many that startled the American public. The Gender Identity Clinic at this major medical center had quietly started its work with transsexuals and the related cases of the Hermaphrodite and the Klinefelder syndrome. EEF helped support the committee, cooperating with John Money, Ph.D., Associate Professor of Medical Psychology and Pediatrics, as well as the surgical team at Johns Hopkins.

The first patients were referred through the Harry Benjamin Foundation after thorough testing, treatment and counseling indicated the operation was the only solution to the unendurable condition of sex variance. Thousands of poignant letters followed the news of hope for the alienated person who felt imprisoned in the wrong external sex role (body), spotlighting the need for further research and treatment facilities throughout the country.

Clinical psychologist John G. Brennan, formerly of Wellington, New Zealand, is currently at Johns Hopkins working on the psychology of transsexualism, under EEF grant, collecting and evaluating research data at the Gender Identity Clinic.

It is gratifying to know that several other large medical centers have now initiated the study of transsexualism and the performance of the conversion operation.

NEW YORK ACADEMY OF SCIENCES MEETING

In January, 1967, in the Division of Psychology, the following papers were presented and later published in the February 1967 issue of the Academy's Transactions:

The Transsexual Phenomenon by Harry Benjamin
The Endocrine Status of the Transsexual Patient by Herbert S. Kupperman
A Report of the Sexual Histories of Twenty-Five Transsexuals by Wardell B. Pomeroy
Vernal Aptitude in Eonism and Prepubertal Effeminacy by John Money and Ralph Epstein
Psychological Testing of Transsexuals: A Brief Report of the Results from the Wechsler Adult Intelligence Scale, the Thematic Apperception Test, and the House-Tree-Person Test by Ruth Rae Doorbar
Transsexual Gynecological Aspects by Leo Wollman
The Transsexual Patient: A Problem in Self-Perception by Henry Guze

were sixteen to forty pages long. The Brooklyn-based technical writer Harriet Slavitz researched and wrote the pamphlets, which Erickson then scrutinized for accuracy and to ensure that they always maintained a positive tone.[82] The EEF distributed their pamphlets free of charge in conjunction with EEF public events and on request through the postal system with an optional postage and handling fee of twenty-five cents each[83] or one dollar for a set.[84]

The series consisted of nine titles, three of which were updated and reissued in second editions and three of which were available only to professionals: *Some Legal Aspects of Transexualism* (1970); *Legal Aspects of Transexualism and Information on Administrative Procedures* (1971 and 1973); *Information for the Family of the Transexual and Children with Gender Identity Disturbances* (1971); *Religious Aspects of Transexualism* (1972 and 1978); *Counseling the Transexual: Five Conversations with Professionals in Transexual Therapy* (1973) (for professionals only); *An Outline of the Medical Management of the Transexual* (1973) (for professionals only); *Information on Transexualism for Law Enforcement Officers* (1974) (for professionals only); *Guidelines for Transexuals* (1974 and 1976); and *Transsexualism: Information for the Family* (1977).[85]

Together, these pamphlets covered a wide swath of useful information for trans people and other interested parties. Easy to understand, practical, and comprehensive information on the topics covered was unavailable from any other source at the time—and remained unrivaled for many years to come. Trans people and professionals alike found them invaluable, attested to by the fact that they often held on to them for decades. Researcher Suzanne Kessler only parted with her copies when she donated her collection of *EEF Newsletters* and pamphlets to the University of Victoria Transgender Archives in 2017, and trans woman Brandy Herbert kept her copies until 2020, when she offered them to the Transgender Archives. Organizations as diverse as the American Medical Association, American Association of Sex Educators and Counselors, and the National Conference of Christians and Jews endorsed the pamphlets in their publications.[86]

The EEF campaign to educate the public also focused on the production and distribution of films and other media. For example, the Fall 1970 *EEF Newsletter* announced the completion of the twenty-eight-minute first-of-its-kind educational cinéma vérité film *I Am Not This Body*, sponsored by the EEF, filmed in their New York offices, and produced by Sunrise Films. Structured as a conversation, the film presented media-personality Pamela Lincoln, who was seeking to learn about transsexualism; Lynn Raskin, a preoperative

Figure 10.3. EEF pamphlet. *Source*: Courtesy of the author.

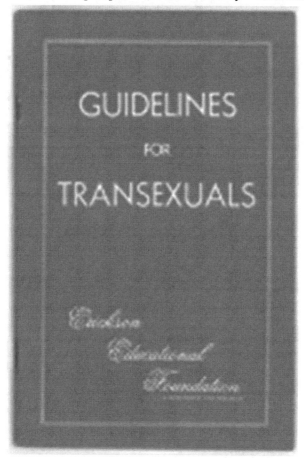

trans woman;[87] Deborah Hartin, a postoperative trans woman; Leo Wollman, a physician colleague of Harry Benjamin; and Suplee, EEF's executive director.[88] Over the next year alone, the EEF showed the film to physicians, psychiatrists, psychologists, social workers, civil servants, police, and lawyers at the First Miami Gender Identity Symposium; during grand rounds at the Department of Obstetrics and Gynecology of the College of Medicine in Syracuse, New York; to a large audience of faculty and medical students at the University of Florida Medical School; to a symposium on Benjamin's book *The Transsexual Phenomenon* at Fairleigh Dickinson University; to eight hundred attendees at the National Council on Family Relations annual meetings in Estes Park, Colorado; and to paramedics and a sex-education class for teachers and professionals at the State University of New York at Stony Brook.[89] The EEF rented the film to interested parties for thirty-five dollars.[90]

In keeping with the EEF philosophy that public education would improve the situation of trans people and inspire more physicians to respectfully provide appropriate medical treatment, EEF newsletters reported on recent books and films, newspaper and magazine articles, scholarly articles, and radio and television shows that advanced a positive view of trans people. The Summer 1976 *EEF Newsletter* exemplifies this practice. The contents included a report on a new book, *Transvestites and Transsexuals: Mixed Views,* by EEF grant recipient Deborah H. Feinbloom[91] and an eighteen-minute documentary film *I'm Something Else.*[92] This issue provided quick précises of newspaper articles from across North America, including items that appeared in publications from New York, Newark, Philadelphia, New Orleans, Denver, Milwaukee, Savanah, San Jose, and Norfolk in the United States and from Calgary and Toronto in Canada.[93] The newsletter made special note of a letter to the popular newspaper advice columnist, Dear Abby. A concerned mother asked Abby, "Shouldn't it [transsexualism] be kept a secret?" to which Abby replied, "Hold up your head. You have nothing to be ashamed of."[94] This issue similarly approvingly quoted a *Newsweek* article as saying that transsexuals are "neither psychopath nor deviate."[95] It also noted a thirteen-page illustrated article in the *Boston Phoenix Report* entitled "Transexuality"[96] as "the longest news feature article we have seen on the subject." The same Summer 1976 issue also briefly mentioned four television shows on transsexualism that aired in New York City; a four-part television series on transsexualism shown in Columbus, Ohio; a two-part radio program on transsexualism presented on a Hollywood radio station; and a radio show on transsexualism in New York City.[97]

The EEF placed a program of speaking engagements before a wide variety of audiences high on its agenda. The favored format consisted of an EEF staff person (most often Suplee) accompanied by an authoritative professional who interviewed one or more trans people, who were specifically chosen for the task because their gender presentation was virtually indistinguishable from cisgender, white, middle-class, "respectable" heteronormativity. The goal of these talks was to demonstrate that trans people who received their desired medical treatment could leave behind their "deviance" and become fully integrated productive members of "normal," white, middle-class society.[98] For example, in the 1970s, Kessler and McKenna, authors of the classic *Gender: An Ethnomethodological Approach,*[99] regularly engaged a group from the EEF to educate their college classes. McKenna recalled of the trans representatives that "every single one was attractive, credible, articulate and somebody who was able to get the students to sympathize with them, with their story. They were people it was impossible to see as any other gender than they presented themselves."[100]

The EEF newsletters proudly reported that their audiences included lawyers, criminologists, and prison personnel; general practitioners, psychiatrists, gynecologists, endocrinologists, and clinical counselors; business leaders; social workers; religious leaders; and other interested members of the public. The EEF speakers presented to groups of all sizes, often in formal settings, such as professional association meetings, university lecture halls, or hospital grand rounds. The Fall 1970 *EEF Newsletter* boasted: "It is impossible to report in detail the increasing number of significant lectures being delivered before professional groups by specialists in the transsexual field. However, [the] outstanding mileage record is held by Dr. Leo Wollman, whose various speaking engagement trips have ranged from Istanbul, Milan, Nairobi, Mainz, Barcelona, Malaga, and Costa Del Brava to domestic meetings, and Dr. John Money, who has covered the area 'down under.'"[101]

APPROACH 3: SUPPORT FOR RESEARCH AND PROFESSIONAL DEVELOPMENT

The EEF also offered financial support for research projects, provided opportunities for researchers to collaborate, and assisted in bringing attention to research findings. The EEF worked toward these goals by implementing and funding a granting program that supported most of the early US researchers active in the field of trans health. The EEF also brought researchers together in small seminars, facilitating scholarly and professional connections through these workshops, and by mentioning their new publications in the *EEF Newsletter*. On a larger scale, the EEF sponsored the first international symposia on trans topics, which generated the formation of the Harry Benjamin International Gender Dysphoria Association, later known as the World Professional Association for Transgender Health.[102]

The first researcher supported by Erickson's EEF was Erickson's physician, Benjamin. Erickson provided Benjamin with a three-year research grant (January 1965 to December 1967) of $18,000 per year (the median annual income in the United States in 1965 was $6,900[103]) in support of the Harry Benjamin

Foundation "to investigate the nature, causes and treatment of . . . transsexualism." The researchers associated with the Harry Benjamin Foundation met monthly at Benjamin's offices at 44 East 67th Street in New York City. They compared outcomes for three groups of patients: one group who was tested before and one year after undergoing "conversion operations"; another group who was examined before starting hormone treatments and again six months into treatment; and a third group who was one-year postoperative for whom "their mental and emotional status and their usefulness to society in their new role of the opposite sex [was] to be evaluated."[104]

This small research group included Benjamin, psychometrist Ruth Rae Doorbar, psychiatrist Richard Green, psychologist Henry Guze, hormone researcher Herbert Kupperman, sexologist Money, Kinsey co-interviewer Wardell Pomeroy, and gynecologist and hypnotherapist Leo Wollman—several of whom went on to become major influences in sex research. Erickson attended most meetings, and there were other occasional attendees.[105]

The EEF's support of these meetings greatly impacted the field of trans medicine, including the founding of the first gender identity clinic in the United States at Johns Hopkins University in Baltimore, Maryland. The Harry Benjamin Foundation, the EEF, and Money (also a member of the EEF advisory board) spearheaded the endeavor. A November 21, 1966, press release specifically cited Money's encouragement as a motivating factor in launching this clinic. The statement then went on to say: "Many [patients] have been referrals from the Harry Benjamin Foundation of New York. . . . The Benjamin Foundation was endowed by the Erickson Educational Foundation, which is also the sole source of research support for the Hopkins endeavor."[106] The EEF provided more than twenty-thousand dollars as start-up funding for the first two years of the clinic's operations.[107]

Another product of EEF-sponsored research meetings and funding was the second book on the subject of transsexualism: *Transsexualism and Sex Reassignment*.[108] Edited by Green and Money and published by Johns Hopkins University Press in 1969, it contained a foreword by Erickson; an introduction and chapters by Benjamin; chapters by Harry Benjamin Foundation attendees Green, Money, Guze, Pomeroy, Doorbar, and Wollman; and chapters by EEF grantee Ira Pauly and by Christine Jorgensen's physician, Christian Hamburger.[109]

The EEF also conducted a grants program that provided seed money to support much of the early research about trans people. Many of those so supported—and the work they produced—became influential in shaping the course of trans medicine in the United States. Money, perhaps one of the most (in)famous,[110] published approximately two thousand articles, books, chapters, refereed journal articles, and reviews; Money also received sixty-five honors, awards, and degrees.[111] The EEF provided a research grant to Ehrhardt for her doctoral and postdoctoral research under the tutelage of Money. The EEF funded Money and Ehrhardt to write the book *Man & Woman, Boy & Girl* (1972).[112] Ehrhardt subsequently authored more than two hundred publications in the field of sex research.[113]

Other influential grantees went on to lead new medical and research centers serving trans people, thereby further extending the accessibility of gender-affirming care. Psychologist Paul Walker, who also started out working under Money at the Johns Hopkins clinic, eventually became the director of the Gender Clinic of the University of Texas Medical Branch in Galveston, Texas, and later, the director of the Janus Information Facility, the successor organization to EEF.[114] June Reinisch, an EEF grantee for her doctoral research,[115] later became the director of the Kinsey Institute for Research in Sex, Gender, and Reproduction in Bloomington, Indiana, and published more than one hundred scientific papers.[116]

Vern Bullough, another notable EEF grantee, received fifteen thousand dollars per year for six years (1970–1976), which resulted in four books out of his lifetime oeuvre of nearly fifty books and more than one hundred articles.[117] Other EEF grant recipients included John Brennan, Harold Christenson, C. J. Dewhurst, Norman Fisk, Stanley Krippner, Donald Laub, Elizabeth McCauley, Marie Mehl, Jon K. Meyer, Ira Pauly, Richard Pillard, Richard Sabatino, and Ira Yolem.[118] The EEF tax returns for 1969–1970 listed almost $74,000 in grants to various projects, while the 1971–1972 return itemized $98,000 in grants and 1972–1973 claimed $85,000.[119] In these three years alone, the sum total of the EEF's research grants ($257,000) amounted to roughly the equivalent of $1,824,408 in 2022.[120]

In addition to supporting researchers, the EEF—intending to build networks and encourage further growth in the field of trans research—put considerable effort into organizing, promoting, and funding symposia to facilitate the exchange of ideas and the cementing of research relationships. In addition to the Harry Benjamin Foundation research group, the EEF organized, and EEF grantees participated in, a myriad of smaller meetings, seminars, and symposia in diverse locations. The EEF also made a point to encourage attendance at, and report about, programs organized by others.

The year 1972 was notable for the sheer number of such professional symposia. According to reports in the *EEF Newsletter*, EEF grantees or employees presented on more than fifty occasions at professional meetings including the Society for the Scientific Study of Sex,[121] the American Association of Sex Educators and Counselors, the Southern Correctional Institute, the American Humanistic Psychology Association,[122] the American College of Surgeons,[123] the American Psychiatric Association,[124] the First International Symposium on Sex Education,[125] the Southeastern Society of Plastic and Reconstructive Surgeons,[126] the Yale University Medical Centre,[127] Lincoln Hospital Lutheran Medical Center,[128] and St. Vincent's Hospital in New York.[129] The University of Nebraska Medical School,[130] Purdue University,[131] Adelphi College, Hunter College, Queens Community College, and William Paterson College[132] also offered academic venues for EEF speakers in 1972.

While the EEF was based in the United States, its influence stretched across the Atlantic into Europe and Israel and across the Pacific to Japan, Australia, and New Zealand. As EEF grantees and representatives traveled to other countries to confer with their colleagues and present their work, Erickson envisioned still larger gatherings as opportunities to strengthen and speed the growth and dissemination of knowledge that would advance understanding, proper medical treatment, and social acceptance of trans people. To that end, the EEF sponsored the three first-ever international conferences concerned with trans people, out of which grew the Harry Benjamin International Gender Dysphoria Association (HBIGDA), now known as the World Professional Association for Transgender Health (WPATH).

The First International Symposium, Gender Identity: Aims, Functions, and Clinical Problems of a Gender Identity Unit, took place at the Piccadilly Hotel in London, England, over the weekend of July 25–27, 1969. Co-sponsored by the EEF (with the work of Suplee) and the Albany Trust of London (with the organizational assistance of Doreen Cordell of the Albany Trust) and chaired by Professor C. J. Dewhurst of Queen Charlotte Hospital of London, the event hosted at least fifty attendees.[133] The ten speakers hailed from England and the United States and included Member of Parliament David Kerr, John Money, Richard Green, Zelda Suplee, Manchester attorney David Green, and representatives from several London Hospitals. Ironically, conference organizers only allowed the media to attend a briefing after the event, even though the symposium program proclaimed: "The international cooperation of scientists, researchers, teachers and social workers, as well as the active assistance of socially concerned citizens and the use of every medium of communication, are needed to make the public aware of the scope of this problem, and of the need to reduce the social waste and human misery associated with it."[134]

The Second International Symposium on Gender Identity took place at the Marienlyst Hotel in Elsinore, Denmark, September 12–14, 1971. This occasion featured thirty speakers from the United States, Canada, England, Denmark, Sweden, the Netherlands, and Japan, including George Stürup and Paul Fogh-Anderson, who were among Jorgensen's doctors. The organizers divided presentations into sessions on the Psychological, Hormonal and Surgical Management of Transsexualism; Sociological and Legal Aspects of Transsexualism; and Possible Etiological Factors in Transsexualism.[135] A message from Benjamin at the opening set a tone for the symposium:

> I trust that in the lectures to follow, attention will be paid to possible organic causes for the development of the transexual disorder and not only to the frequently overemphasized psychological ones. If the latter were the only cause, why then is psychotherapy not more helpful than it actually is . . . we should not forget the patient. He or she will have to be relieved of suffering no matter what the cause. . . . Valuable lives have been salvaged and miserable ineffectual men have become reasonably well adjusted women, and vice versa. In this way, not only an individual, but also society has been served.[136]

The final EEF symposium, the Third International Symposium on Gender Identity, organized by Suplee and Ehrhardt,[137] took place at the Hotel Libertas in Dubrovnik, Yugoslavia, September 8–10, 1973. The conference featured nineteen presentations to a gathering of approximately thirty people from the United States, Canada, Denmark, Sweden, the United Kingdom, the Netherlands, and Japan. Money chaired the meeting, and speakers included several EEF grantees: Bullough on "Transsexualism in the Past," Pauly on "A Body Image Scale for Evaluating Transsexuals," Wollman on "The Female Transsexual,"[138] Laub on "Rehabilitation Program for Gender Dysphoria Syndrome by Surgical Sex Change," and Ehrhardt on "Exposure to Pre-Natal Androgens-Sex Differences in Behavior."[139]

Two years later, February 28–March 2, 1975, Suplee assisted EEF grantee Laub at Stanford University to organize the fourth symposium in this series. In honor of Benjamin's ninetieth birthday, they named the conference the Harry

Benjamin Fourth International Symposium on Gender Identity,[140] but despite this aspirational title, the only contributor to the published proceedings from outside the United States was Roy MacKenzie from the Faculty of Medicine at the University of Calgary in Canada.[141] While conferences for professionals devoted to improving understanding and treatment of trans people continued in subsequent years, after 1975, the EEF, true to its stated funding policy of only providing seed money, no longer took leadership in making them happen.

THE ENDING AND LEGACY OF THE EEF

By late 1976, Erickson's interests had shifted to a stronger focus on New Age spirituality. On November 1, 1976, the EEF's New York office closed with a plan to concentrate all operations at the Moreland Avenue office in Baton Rouge.[142] Not long after, the "EEF granted permission for the public information distribution and research to be taken over at the Gender Clinic of the University of Texas Medical Branch in Galveston, Texas, and the Janus Information Facility was established by Walker, Gender Clinic director . . . and Suplee, former EEF director."[143] With that move, the EEF ceased to be an organization centrally focused on trans advocacy and support.

The closing of the EEF precipitated a huge gap in resources, as evidenced by responses from trans and research communities. Heino F.L. Meyer-Bahlburg of the State University of New York at Buffalo's Office of Psychoendocrinology sent a representative letter that read:

> I am shocked that the EEF will suddenly cease to exist. The EEF has been a most important clearinghouse for information and often a first ray of hope for countless unhappy people. In addition, the foundation and, in particular, you personally has [sic] brought us together and kept us in contact with each other. Thus, for all involved, this will be a hard felt loss. I want to thank you for all your past efforts, and I sincerely hope that there will be some way to have the functions of the EEF live on with some other means.[144]

Indeed, some of the pamphlets produced by the EEF and some of the referrals work done by the EEF lived on through the work of the Janus Information Facility, which subsequently passed the torch to Jude Patton and Joanna Clark, who operated an organization known as J2CP.[145] By 1991, Clark (then known as Sister Mary Elizabeth) turned over this work started by the EEF to Denny of the American Educational Gender Information Service until it too closed in 2000.[146]

The EEF announced the closing of its New York offices and the need to step away from trans activities just before the Fifth International Gender Dysphoria Symposium, February 10–13, 1977, hosted by the Eastern Virginia Medical School in Norfolk, Virginia. The introductory text in the program for the symposium included these words: "Just prior to the meeting we have learned that the Erickson Educational Foundation, which we all consider a vital force in the area of transsexualism, will cease to exist. This impartial educational agency has been of inestimable value to the field. The conference planning committee will schedule a business meeting in lieu of one of the discussion periods to discuss the expected effect of this event on the field and to brainstorm about the implications of this."[147] Before the symposium was over, attendees decided to launch the HBIGDA, chose the founding committee, and conceived of the first HBIGDA *Standards of Care*.[148] Of the EEF's many legacies, HBIGDA, which later changed its name to WPATH, has become the world's largest professional association serving trans communities worldwide. With more than thirty-six hundred individual members from fifty-six countries, it is best known for the publication of its authoritative *Standards of Care* and its Global Education Institute.

By 1977, when the EEF stopped doing trans work, many more trans people knew there were others like them and had some idea about how and where to obtain medical treatment and other kinds of supports. Gender clinics existed throughout North America where previously none had existed, and doctors were more equipped to offer gender-affirming care. Researchers and medical providers shared data among themselves and published their findings. The new networks between trans people and with and between the professionals who served them were growing, and sometimes even flourished. The EEF's influence extended beyond trans communities and those with whom they worked. Thanks to the EEF's educational campaigns, tens, if not hundreds of thousands of people, had received some basic education about the lives of trans people.

In its twelve years of active trans-focused work, the EEF served as a catalyst and accelerant in transforming the social and scientific landscape for trans people in mid-twentieth-century America, so much so that it would be difficult to overestimate the impact of the EEF in advancing the legitimization of trans existence in the eyes of the US public and professionals. Erickson used the EEF as a vehicle to promote the idea that being trans was a valid medical condition that, when properly treated, could allow trans people to become fully productive and contributing members of society, virtually indistinguishable from their cisgender peers. The door that this work opened initially most benefited white, middle-class individuals who could pass for cisgender, that is, those trans people most likely to be acceptable to mid-twentieth-century Americans in positions of power and authority. The accomplishment of these essential first steps, laid a foundation on which much has since been built, to the continuing benefit of subsequent generations of increasingly diverse trans people.

NOTES

1. During the period under discussion, the only words used to describe trans people were *transsexual* and *transvestite*. I have chosen to use the more modern word *trans* as a general term to include both.

2. Meyerowitz, *How Sex Changed.*

3. This chapter would not have been possible without the contributions of many. My thanks go to the people who provided interviews, to my colleague Pam Duncan, and research assistants Nicholas Matte, Josephine MacIntosh, Theresa Vladicka, Kimi Dominic, and Jen Kostuchuck. Special thanks to my wife, Lynn Greenhough, for her ongoing wise counsel and patience. Funding was provided at various points by the Social Sciences and Humanities Research Council of Canada and the University of Victoria.

4. Birth certificate for Reed Erickson, October 13, 1917, File No. 3919, Texas State Board of Health, Bureau of Vital Statistics; Maris Harry, April 13, 1999.

5. Ada Bello, in discussion with the author, June 22, 1997.

6. Report issued by the US Federal Bureau of Investigation in response to FOIPA request no. 415686/190-HQ-1243634. May 26, 1998. File no. 100-26128 p. 2, private collection of Aaron Devor.

7. "Start of Reinsberg Family Tree: AR 11491 Sys # 000200186." Available from Leo Baeck Institute, Center for Jewish History, 15 W. 16th St. New York, NY, 10011. lbaeck@lbi.cjh.org.

8. Judy Wollowitz, in discussion with the author, June 5, 1997.

9. Letter from Edward McLaughlin Dean of Engineering LSU, July 21, 1997, private collection of Aaron Devor.

10. Wollowitz, in discussion with the author, June 30, 1997.

11. Wollowitz, in discussion with the author, June 5, 1997; Ben Kimmelman, in discussion with the author, December 15, 1997.

12. Bello, in discussion with the author, June 22, 1997; Anonymous 1, in discussion with the author, July 12, 1997.

13. Anonymous 1, in discussion with the author, July 12, 1997.

14. Sarah Santana, in discussion with the author, June 8, 1994.

15. Bello, in discussion with the author, June 22, 1997.

16. Benjamin, Medical records files, private collection of Aaron Devor.

17. Birth certificate for Reed Erickson, October 13, 1917. Texas State Department of Health, Bureau of Vital Statistics. https://dshs.texas.gov/vs/birth/.

18. Birth certificate for Reed Erickson, October 13, 1917.

19. Monica Erickson, in discussion with the author, June 3, 1996.

20. Wedding invitation addressed to Harry Benjamin, private collection of Aaron Devor.

21. Birth announcement, private collection of Aaron Devor.

22. James W. Lorio, in discussion with the author, July 23, 1997.

23. Rosalie Cangelosi, in discussion with the author, July 26, 1997.

24. Monica Erickson, email message to author, October 21, 2003.

25. Copy of divorce decree in the private collection of Aaron Devor.

26. Donald Laub, in discussion with the author, September 12, 1997.

27. ACIM, "Reed Erickson Funded First Edition of ACIM"; Hector Marin, in discussion with the author, September 14, 2018.

28. Helen Kleinstiver, in discussion with the author, July 28, 1997.

29. Marin, in discussion with the author, September 14, 2018.

30. Marin, in discussion with the author, September 14, 2018.

31. Frank Coates, in discussion with the author, July 22, 1997.

32. Laub, in discussion with the author, September 12, 1997; Coates, in discussion with the author, July 22, 1997; Erickson, in discussion with the author, June 03, 1996.

33. Erickson, in discussion with the author, June 3, 1996; Kleinstiver, in discussion with the author, July 28, 1997.

34. "Proposal for Support of a Scientific Program by John Lilly, M.D." (n.d., estimated to be from Fall 1982), private collection of Aaron Devor; "Summary of Results with Ketamine Research by John C. Lilly, M.D." (November 23, 1982), private collection of Aaron Devor; "Proposal for the Training of Professionals in the Enhancement of Intelligence and Humour with the Use of Isolation, Solitude and Confinement in 2-Person Sessions using Tanks and Ketamine HCL" (December 5, 1982), private collection of Aaron Devor.

35. Erickson, in discussion with the author, June 3, 1996.

36. Death certificate for Reed Erickson, Folio 43594, issued April 24, 1997, by Civil Registrar, Mazatlán, Sinaloa, Mexico, private collection of Aaron Devor.

37. Erickson Educational Foundation Articles of incorporation, 1964, private collection of Aaron Devor.

38. Erickson Educational Foundation, *A Tax-Exempt Non-Profit Organization*.
39. Erickson Educational Foundation, "Avant Garde in Concept," 1.
40. Erickson Educational Foundation, "Welcome, Dr. Evelyn Hooker," 3.
41. Erickson Educational Foundation, "Welcome Aboard," 2.
42. Coates, in discussion with the author, July 22, 1997.
43. Erickson Educational Foundation brochure, n.d., private collection of Aaron Devor.
44. Erickson Educational Foundation, *A Tax-Exempt Non-Profit Organization*.
45. Erickson Educational Foundation, "Fruition—Then and Now," 4.
46. Erickson Educational Foundation brochure, n.d., private collection of Aaron Devor.
47. Reed Erickson, letter to Paul Walker, April 15, 1982, private collection of Aaron Devor.
48. Kleinstiver, in discussion with the author, July 25, 1997.
49. Leonore Tiefer, in discussion with the author, July 24, 1997; Santana, in discussion with the author, December 11, 1997; McKenna and Kessler, in discussion with the author, December 28, 1997.
50. Devor and Matte, "ONE Inc. and Reed Erickson."
51. White, *Pre-Gay L.A.*
52. Dorr Legg, in discussion with Bullough, December 15, 1993, private collection of Aaron Devor.
53. Legg, in discussion with Bullough, December 15, 1993, private collection of Aaron Devor,
54. Devor and Matte, "ONE Inc. and Reed Erickson."
55. ONE National Gay & Lesbian Archives at the USC Libraries, "ONE Archives at the USC Libraries."
56. Erickson Educational Foundation, "Foundation Future," 1.
57. ACIM, "Reed Erickson Published First Edition of ACIM."
58. ACIM, "A Course in Miracles."
59. Erickson Educational Foundation, "Human/Dolphin Communication," 3.
60. Meyerowitz, *How Sex Changed*, 122.
61. Meyerowitz, *How Sex Changed*, 213.
62. Nicholas Matte, "Historicizing Liberal Amcrican Transnormativities."
63. Erickson Educational Foundation, "I Am Not This Body," 2.
64. Confidential email message from D. L. to author, June 4, 2004, private collection of Aaron Devor.
65. Santana, in discussion with the author, December 11, 1997.
66. Erickson Educational Foundation, "Progress," 2.
67. Rev Linda T O'Connell, D. D., letter to Erickson Educational Foundation, February 12, 1981, private collection of Aaron Devor.

68. Erickson Educational Foundation, "Identification Card for Cross-Dressing," 3.

69. Email message from Brandy Herbert to the author, May 5, 2021, private collection of Aaron Devor.

70. Dr. Robert W. Deisher, letter to Erickson Educational Foundation, February 10, 1977, private collection of Aaron Devor; Erickson Educational Foundation Ledger of cheques written 1971–1975, private collection of Aaron Devor.

71. Capitol Hill Seattle Blog, "The 'Oldest LBGTQ-Focused.'"

72. Cooke, "Suzan Cooke Interview"; Erickson Educational Foundation Ledger of cheques written 1971–1975, private collection of Aaron Devor.

73. Erickson Educational Foundation, "On the Lighter Side," 4.

74. Cooke, "The Transsexual Counseling Service."

75. Erickson Educational Foundation, *Erickson Educational Foundation Newsletter* 1, no. 2 (1969), 1.

76. Santana, in discussion with the author, December 11, 1997.

77. Erickson, letter to Dwight Billings, September 19, 1983, private collection of Aaron Devor.

78. These scrapbooks were delivered by the author to the University of Victoria Transgender Archives in 2017. AR417 Reed Erickson fonds, accession 2017-034. Special Collections and University Archives, Transgender Archives Collection, University of Victoria 2017-34.01 to 2017-034.08.

79. Suplee, "Harvey Plaks Investigative Interview."

80. Erickson Educational Foundation, "Now Read This," 1.

81. Erickson Educational Foundation, *Subject: Mailing List for EEF Newsletter*, March 4, 1983, private collection of Aaron Devor.

82. Santana, in discussion with the author, December 11, 1997.

83. Erickson Educational Foundation, "New EFF Pamphlet," 3.

84. Erickson Educational Foundation, "Pamphlets Available," 3.

85. Wilchins, "Riki Anne Wilchins (1952–)." *Transsexual* has been spelled with either one *s* or two before becoming established in the now-accepted double *s* form. One of the earliest published papers on the topic was Cauldwell, "Psychopathia Transexualis." Benjamin's *The Transsexual Phenomenon* spelled it as is now most commonly done, after which time it became the standard spelling. However, in 1994, Riki Anne Wilchins and Denise Norris started the activist organization The Transexual Menace—spelled with one *s*.

86. Erickson Educational Foundation, "Pamphlet Publicity," 2.

87. In this period, all transsexual-identified people were presumed to be desirous of a medical transition that culminated in genital surgery. *Preoperative* and *postoperative* were standard terms referencing whether or not a person had undergone genital surgery. Trans people were not considered to be fully transitioned until they were postoperative.

88. Erickson Educational Foundation, "I Am Not This Body," 2.

89. Erickson Educational Foundation, "Miami Marches On" and "Grand Rounds in Gainesville," 1–2; Erickson Educational Foundation, "New Jersey Next," 1; Erickson Educational Foundation, "Family Action Conference," 1; Erickson Educational Foundation, "An EEF First at SUNY," 2.

90. Erickson Educational Foundation, "College Class Presentations," 3.

91. Erickson Educational Foundation, "Valuable New Book," 5.

92. Erickson Educational Foundation, "Audio-Visual Aids," 2.

93. Erickson Educational Foundation, "In the News," 4.

94. Erickson Educational Foundation, "Queries in the Press," 5.

95. Erickson Educational Foundation, "Magazine Material," 4.

96. Erickson Educational Foundation, "The Boston Phoenix Report," 5.

97. Erickson Educational Foundation, "On the Air," 3.

98. Matte, "Historicizing Liberal American Transnormativities."

99. Kessler and McKenna, *Gender: An Ethnomethodological Approach*.

100. Kessler and McKenna, in discussion with the author, December 28, 1997.

101. Erickson Educational Foundation, "Platform Notes," 3.

102. Devor, "International Symposia."

103. US Census Bureau, "Current Population Reports."

104. Benjamin, letter to Miss Frances Kahn, December 03, 1966, private collection of Aaron Devor.

105. Minutes of Harry Benjamin Foundation meetings, January 30, 1965, to September 29, 1967, private collection of Aaron Devor.

106. The Johns Hopkins University and Johns Hopkins Hospital Office of Institutional Public Relations (November 21, 1966) Press Release. "Statement on the Establishment of a Clinic for Transsexuals at the Johns Hopkins Medical Institutions," private collection of Aaron Devor.

107. Erickson Educational Foundation, Board meeting minutes, October 4, 1965,

108. The first being Benjamin's pioneering 1966 book, *The Transsexual Phenomenon*.

109. Green and Money, *Transsexualism and Sex Reassignment*.

110. Near the end of a long and very influential career, Money was exposed as having suppressed vital information related to what came to be known as the John/Joan case. See Colapinto, *As Nature Made Him*.

111. Wikipedia, "John Money."

112. Money and Ehrhardt, *Man & Woman*; Ehrhardt, in discussion with the author, July 24, 1997.

113. Ehrhardt, "Anke A Ehrhardt."

114. Erickson Educational Foundation, "Janus Information Facility," 5; "Now In San Francisco," 1; and "Information Pleases," 1.

115. Erickson Educational Foundation, "Fruition—Then and Now," 4.
116. Indiana University, "June Reinisch."
117. Williams, "Vern Bullough, Ph.D. In Memoriam."
118. Erickson Educational Foundation, *Erickson Educational Foundation Newsletter* (1968–1983).
119. Erickson Educational Foundation, Income Tax Forms 990-AR June 1, 1969, to May 31, 1970; June 1, 1971, to May 31, 1972; June 1, 1972, to May 31, 1973, private collection of Aaron Devor.
120. CPI Inflation Calculator, "US Inflation Calculator: 1635–2021," Department of Labor data. Accessed July 22, 2020. https://www.in2013dollars.com/us/inflation/1971.
121. Erickson Educational Foundation, "New York Symposium on TS," 1.
122. Erickson Educational Foundation, "On the Agenda," 2.
123. Erickson Educational Foundation, "Surgeons Hear Hoopes," 3.
124. Erickson Educational Foundation, "Educating the Sex Educators," 3.
125. Erickson Educational Foundation, "In Tel Aviv," 2.
126. Erickson Educational Foundation, "In Jacksonville," 4.
127. Erickson Educational Foundation, "In New Haven," 2.
128. Erickson Educational Foundation, "On the Agenda," 4.
129. Erickson Educational Foundation, "In Manhattan," 2.
130. Erickson Educational Foundation, "News from Nebraska," 2.
131. Erickson Educational Foundation, "In Indiana," 2.
132. Erickson Educational Foundation, "College Class Presentations," 3.
133. Antony Grey, in discussion with the author, August 23, 1999.
134. First International Symposium on Gender Identity, program brochure (1969) and Transcript of Proceedings, private collection of Aaron Devor.
135. Second International Symposium on Gender Identity program (1971), private collection of Aaron Devor.
136. Erickson Educational Foundation, *Erickson Educational Foundation Newsletter* 4, no. 4 (1971), 1.
137. Ehrhardt, in discussion with the author, July 24, 1997.
138. At this time, professionals referred to transsexual people in terms of their sex assigned at birth. Thus, a person called a "female transsexual" then would now be known as a transmasculine person or a trans man.
139. Third International Symposium on Gender Identity program (1973), private collection of Aaron Devor.
140. Suplee, letter to Reed Erickson, April 21, 1975, private collection of Aaron Devor.
141. Green and Laub, "The Fourth International Conference on Gender Identity. Selected Proceedings."
142. Suplee, letter to "Dear Friend," September 30, 1976, private collection of Aaron Devor.

143. Erickson Educational Foundation, "Janus Information Facility," 5.

144. Meyer-Bahlburg, letter to Erickson Educational Foundation, February 1, 1977, private collection of Aaron Devor.

145. The organization was named J2CP to reflect the first and last names of its founders: Joanna Clark and Jude Patton.

146. Denny, email message to author, July 27, 1999.

147. Fifth International Gender Dysphoria Symposium program (1977), private collection of Aaron Devor.

148. Please refer to chapter 13 in this volume for further details about HBIGDA and WPATH.

WORKS CITED

ACIM Foundation for Inner Peace. "A Course in Miracles." Accessed August 18, 2024. https://acim.org/acim/en.

ACIM Foundation for Inner Peace. "Reed Erickson Funded First Edition of ACIM. Forty Years of Publishing a Course in Miracles." May 11, 2016. Accessed August 17, 2024. https://acim.org/reed-erickson-funded-first-edition-of-acim/.

Benjamin, Harry. *The Transsexual Phenomenon*. New York: Julian Press, 1966.

Capitol Hill Seattle Blog. "The 'Oldest LGBTQ-Focused Community Mental Health Agency in the World' Is About to Close Its Doors in Seattle—UPDATE." March 2, 2022. Accessed August 18, 2024. https://www.capitolhillseattle.com/2022/03/the-oldest-lgbtq-focused-community-mental-health-agency-in-the-world-is-about-to-close-its-doors-in-seattle/#:~:text=After%20more%20than%2050%20years,%2C%E2%80%9D%20the%20SCS%20announcement%20reads.

Cauldwell, D. O. "Psychopathia Transexualis." *Sexology* 16 (1949): 274–80.

Colapinto, John. *As Nature Made Him: The Boy Who Was Raised as a Girl*. New York: HarperCollins, 2000.

Cooke, Suzan. "Suzan Cooke Interview." Interview by Susan Stryker. GLBT Historical Society, January 10, 1998. Accessed August 18, 2024. https://revolution.berkeley.edu/assets/Suzy-Cooke-Interview-full.pdf.

———. "The Transsexual Counseling-Service and the National Transsexual Counseling Unit's Purpose." August 29, 2012. Accessed August 18, 2024. Archived content from the Women Born Transsexual website. https://web.archive.org/web/20230520001800/https://womenborntranssexual.com/2012/08/29/the-transsexual-counseling-service-and-national-transsexual-counseling-units-purpose/.

Devor, Aaron. "International Symposia." WPATH World Professional Association for Transgender Health, 2013. Accessed August 18, 2024. https://www.wpath.org/about/history/international-symposia.

Devor, Aaron H., and Nicholas Matte. "ONE Inc. and Reed Erickson: The Uneasy Collaboration of Gay and Trans Activism, 1964–2003." *GLQ: A Journal of Gay and Lesbian Studies* 10, no. 2 (2004): 179–209.

Ehrhardt, Anke A. "Anke A Ehrhardt, PhD." HIV Center for Clinical and Behavioral Studies. Accessed August 18, 2024. https://www.hivcenternyc.org/anke-ehrhardt-phd.

Erickson Educational Foundation. *A Tax-Exempt Non-Profit Organization*, 1966. Private collection of Aaron Devor.

———. "An EEF First at SUNY." *Erickson Educational Foundation Newsletter* 4, no. 4 (1971). Private collection of Aaron Devor.

———. "Audio-Visual Aids." *Erickson Educational Foundation Newsletter* 9, no. 1 (1976). Private collection of Aaron Devor.

———. "Avant Garde in Concept." *Erickson Educational Foundation Newsletter* 1, no. 1 (1968). Private collection of Aaron Devor.

———. "*The Boston Phoenix Report*." *Erickson Educational Foundation Newsletter* 9, no. 1 (1976). Private collection of Aaron Devor.

———. "College Class Presentations." *Erickson Educational Foundation Newsletter* 5, no. 2 (1972). Private collection of Aaron Devor.

———. "Educating the Sex Educators." *Erickson Educational Foundation Newsletter* 5, no. 2 (1972). Private collection of Aaron Devor.

———. "Family Action Conference." *Erickson Educational Foundation Newsletter* 4, no. 3 (1971). Private collection of Aaron Devor.

———. "Foundation Future." *Erickson Educational Foundation Newsletter* 7, no. 1 (1974). Private collection of Aaron Devor.

———. "Fruition—Then and Now." *Erickson Educational Foundation Newsletter* 10, no. 1 (1983). Private collection of Aaron Devor.

———. "Human/Dolphin Communication." *Erickson Educational Foundation Newsletter* 10, no. 1 (1983). Private collection of Aaron Devor.

———. " 'I am Not this Body.' " *Erickson Educational Foundation Newsletter* 3, no. 2 (1970). Private collection of Aaron Devor.

———. "In Indiana." *Erickson Educational Foundation Newsletter* 5, no. 2 (1972). Private collection of Aaron Devor.

———. "In Jacksonville." *Erickson Educational Foundation Newsletter* 5, no. 3 (1972). Private collection of Aaron Devor.

———. "In Manhattan." *Erickson Educational Foundation Newsletter* 5, no. 3 (1972). Private collection of Aaron Devor.

———. "In New Haven." *Erickson Educational Foundation Newsletter* 5, no. 2 (1972). Private collection of Aaron Devor.

———. "In the News." *Erickson Educational Foundation Newsletter* 9, no. 1 (1976). Private collection of Aaron Devor.

———. "In Tel Aviv." *Erickson Educational Foundation Newsletter* 5, no. 3 (1972). Private collection of Aaron Devor.

———. "Information Pleases." *Erickson Educational Foundation Newsletter* 2, no. 2 (1969). Private collection of Aaron Devor.

———. "Janus Information Facility." *Erickson Educational Foundation Newsletter* 10, no. 1 (1983). Private collection of Aaron Devor.

———. "Miami Marches On." *Erickson Educational Foundation Newsletter* 4, no. 1 (1971). Private collection of Aaron Devor.

———. "New EEF Pamphlet." *Erickson Educational Foundation Newsletter* 6, no. 1 (1973). Private collection of Aaron Devor.

———. "New Jersey Next." *Erickson Educational Foundation Newsletter* 4, no. 2 (1971). Private collection of Aaron Devor.

———. "New York Symposium on TS." *Erickson Educational Foundation Newsletter* 5, no. 1 (1972). Private collection of Aaron Devor.

———. "News from Nebraska. *Erickson Educational Foundation Newsletter* 5, no. 5 (1971). Private collection of Aaron Devor.

———. "Now In San Francisco." *Erickson Educational Foundation Newsletter* 10, no. 1 (1983). Private collection of Aaron Devor.

———. "Now Read This." *Erickson Educational Foundation Newsletter* 8, no. 1 (1975). Private collection of Aaron Devor.

———. "On the Agenda." *Erickson Educational Foundation Newsletter* 5, no. 1 (1972). Private collection of Aaron Devor.

———. "On the Air." *Erickson Educational Foundation Newsletter* 9, no. 1 (1976). Private collection of Aaron Devor.

———. "On the Lighter Side." *Erickson Educational Foundation Newsletter* 4, no. 1 (1971). Private collection of Aaron Devor.

———. "Pamphlet Publicity." *Erickson Educational Foundation Newsletter* 7, no. 1 (1974). Private collection of Aaron Devor.

———. "Platform Notes." *Erickson Educational Foundation Newsletter* 3, no. 2 (1970). Private collection of Aaron Devor.

———. "Progress." *Erickson Educational Foundation Newsletter* 4, no. 3 (1971). Private collection of Aaron Devor.

———. "Progress in New York City." *Erickson Educational Foundation Newsletter* 5, no. 2 (1972). Private collection of Aaron Devor.

———. "Queries in the Press." *Erickson Educational Foundation Newsletter* 9, no. 1 (1976). Private collection of Aaron Devor.

———. "Quoting Dr. Benjamin." *Erickson Educational Foundation Newsletter* 4, no. 4 (1971), private collection of Aaron Devor.

———. "Surgeons Hear Hoopes." *Erickson Educational Foundation Newsletter* 5, no. 1 (1972). Private collection of Aaron Devor.

———. "Valuable New Book." *Erickson Educational Foundation Newsletter* 9, no. 1 (1976). Private collection of Aaron Devor.

———. "Welcome Aboard." *Erickson Educational Foundation Newsletter* 5, no. 1 (1972). Private collection of Aaron Devor.

———. "Welcome, Dr. Evelyn Hooker." *Erickson Educational Foundation Newsletter* 4, no. 1 (1971). Private collection of Aaron Devor.

Green, Richard, and Donald R. Laub Sr. "The Fourth International Conference on Gender Identity. Selected Proceedings." *Archives of Sexual Behavior* 7, no. 4 (1978): 244–48.

Green, Richard, and John Money, eds. *Transsexualism and Sex Reassignment*. Baltimore, MD: Johns Hopkins University Press, 1969.

Indiana University. "June Reinisch." Indiana University Honors and Awards. Accessed August 18, 2024. https://honorsandawards.iu.edu/awards/honoree/9006.html.

Inflation Calculator. "One Hundred Dollars in 1971 Is Worth $670.85 Today." Accessed July 22, 2020. https://www.in2013dollars.com/us/inflation/1971.

Kessler, Suzanne, and Wendy Mckenna. *Gender: An Ethnomethodological Approach*. Chicago, IL: University of Chicago Press. 1978.

Matte, Nicholas. "Historicizing Liberal American Transnormativities: Medicine, Media, Activism, 1960–1990." PhD diss., University of Toronto, 2014.

"Median Family Income Up About 5 Percent in 1965 (Advance Data for Families and Unrelated Individuals from March 1966 Sample Survey)." US Census Bureau, Series P-60, No. 49. August 10, 1966. Accessed August 18, 2024. https://www.census.gov/library/publications/1966/demo/p60-049.html.

Meyerowitz, Joanne J. *How Sex Changed: A History of Transsexuality in the United States*. Cambridge: Harvard University Press, 2004.

Money, John, and Anke Ehrhardt. *Man & Woman, Boy & Girl*. Baltimore, MD: Johns Hopkins University Press, 1972.

ONE National Gay & Lesbian Archives at the USC Libraries. Accessed August 18, 2024. https://one.usc.edu/.

Suplee, Zelda. "Harvey Plaks Investigative Interview." Interview by Harvey Plaks. *Reed Erickson Collection*. Transgender Archives, University of Victoria, July 29, 1988.

White, C. Todd. *Pre-Gay L.A.: A Social History of the Movement for Homosexual Rights*. Chicago, IL: University of Chicago Press, 2009.

Wikipedia. "John Money." Last modified July 23, 2021. Accessed August 18, 2024. https://en.wikipedia.org/wiki/John_Money.

Wilchins, Riki Anne. "Riki Anne Wilchins (1952–) Computing, Activist." A Gender Variance Who's Who. March 27, 2014. Accessed August 18, 2024. https://zagria.blogspot.com/2014/03/riki-anne-wilchins-1952-computing.html#.YQBlmERKjIV.

Williams, Walter L. "Vern Bullough, Ph.D. In Memoriam." *Journal of Homosexuality* 54, no. 4 (2008): 341–44.

11

BLINDED BY THE BINARY
A Critique of the Mid-Twentieth Century Gender Clinics

Dallas Denny

In November 1966, the prestigious Johns Hopkins University announced it would be opening a clinic to provide transition-related medical care for transsexuals[1]—including what is today called gender affirmation surgery. Within a few years, more than forty such university-affiliated facilities would open in the United States and Canada. The clinics, which were experimental by design, provided therapy, hormones, breast augmentation, genital and other surgeries, and social services to the few applicants who were accepted; most were interviewed and then rejected. Treatment was predicated on the assumption that transsexuals were mentally ill, and medical providers at most of the clinics subjected patients to extraordinary and often bizarre gender-stereotypical requirements regarding their dress, appearance, names, marital status, and sometimes sexual behavior. In some cases, patients were required to participate in clinical studies and make themselves available for follow-up. Noncompliance in the smallest measure or failure to meet the clinicians' expectations about gender identity, dress, or body type typically resulted in dismissal from the programs.[2]

Most practitioners at the clinics, and, for that matter, most of the patients, were blinded by the gender binary. They, like most other Americans of the day, were simply unable to see it or see beyond it. In the 1960s and 1970s, the terms *sex* and *gender* were used interchangeably and most people—and this included both clinicians and applicants at the clinics—gave little or no thought to the possibility of a middle ground between the two traditional sexes: stereotypically male or stereotypically female.[3] They saw only the binary.[4] Treatment consisted of an all-or-nothing migration from one gender to the other, and the gender clinics were the authoritative issuers of the passports to care. The minority of applicants who were accepted for sex reassignment were required to take hormones, cross-live, and undergo genital reconstruction. After this treatment, they were counseled to drop their transsexual and gay friends, hide their pasts, and disappear into society, "cured" of their non-cisgender nonheteronormative "ailments." The professional literature produced by the clinics reflected this binary thinking and was often contemptuous and condescending toward the transsexual people who came to them for help.

Most of these clinics abruptly closed when, in 1979, Johns Hopkins psychiatrists Paul McHugh and Jon Meyer conspired to publish a severely methodologically flawed cherry-picked post hoc report on surgical outcomes that concluded there was no objective advantage in terms of social rehabilitation to genital reassignment surgery in male-to-female transsexuals—and such was Hopkins' prestige that most of the clinics that had risen in its wake closed in the months that followed. A few were reorganized as for-profit centers. An exception was the University of Minnesota, where the Program in Human Sexuality (now the Eli Coleman Institute for Gender and Sexual Health) took on responsibility for treating transsexual clients when the existing clinic closed.[5]

Before their closure, the gender clinics of the 1960s and 1970s offered a legal, institutional pathway for those who sought sex reassignment. The model was far from perfect, serving too few and relying on cisgender, heteronormative evaluations to determine patient eligibility, yet their establishment and the select compassionate doctors and researchers who worked in them marked a critical step toward gender-affirming care for transsexuals.

Long before the advent of the university-based gender clinics, the first gender-affirming medical treatments in the Western world came about due to compassion for gender-variant people on the part of specific clinicians. This is not to say money didn't change hands—certainly it did—but in each case the primary motivation, in my estimation, was to provide care and relief to suffering people. These pioneering physicians and sexologists put themselves at considerable risk of censure from their peers by the very act of helping. Most physicians of the day would have let a transsexual die by suicide before agreeing to treat them.[6]

In 1919, Magnus Hirschfeld's Institut für Sexualwissenschaft in Berlin opened its doors to anyone with questions about their sexuality or gender identity, and people from all over the world visited and sometimes worked there.[7] In 1940s England, pioneering plastic surgeon Sir Harold Gillies agreed to construct a phallus for an unhappy and desperate Michael Dillon.[8] In the 1960s, in the middle of his long life and career, German-born US endocrinologist Harry Benjamin agreed to see a transsexual referred by the Kinsey Institute and soon had a waiting room full of similar patients.[9] When news of Christine Jorgenson's sex reassignment in Denmark made headlines worldwide in 1951, she and her medical team were deluged with letters from people asking for the same procedures.[10] From the mid-1950s on, Elmer Belt in Los Angeles, Georges Burou in Casablanca, and others around the world performed gender-affirming surgery on transsexual women.[11]

Pioneers like Jorgenson who sought gender-affirming treatment were the social architects of their own gender transitions.[12] In those times, a change of sex, as it was then called, was not a familiar concept, and before 1952 there were no visible and widely known role models in the United States for those who would soon come to be called transsexuals. Most individuals had no language and no one to guide them as they sought to obtain medical treatment to support their visions of their bodies, their identities, and their lives. Those who came after Jorgenson followed her famous case history as a beacon. They, too, sought medical assistance in a time of limited access to information, and most attained help from medical personnel only through persistence, creativity, and hard work.[13]

THE FORMATION OF THE GENDER IDENTITY CLINIC AT JOHNS HOPKINS MEDICAL SCHOOL

In 1957, Richard Green was a first-year medical student at Johns Hopkins. Because he had written a paper on hermaphroditism, he was referred to psychologist and sexologist John Money. Money took Green to meet the family of a patient he called a "psychic hermaphrodite," and, as Green noted in his memoir, "That launched my career."[14]

Five years later, Money introduced Green to Benjamin. Benjamin invited Green to sit in on his interactions with his transsexual patients; Green accepted and was soon writing letters of support for what we today call gender-affirming surgeries.[15] At Benjamin's office, he met an assortment of professionals with a shared interest in transsexualism, including psychologist Henry Guze, gynecologist and hypnotherapist Leo Wollman, Kinsey co-interviewer Wardell Pomeroy, hormone researcher Herbert Kupperman, attorney Robert Sherwin, and psychometrist Ruth Rae Doorbar. Most members of this informal group contributed to Green and Money's 1969 edited text *Transsexualism and Sex Reassignment* and were likely members of the Harry Benjamin Foundation and supported financially by the Erickson Educational Foundation.[16]

Green's and Money's interests in intersexuality had grown to include transsexualism. At Hopkins, Money queried endocrinologist Claude Migeon, gynecologist Howard Jones Jr., and plastic surgeons John Hoopes and Milton Edgerton about their willingness to treat adults who wanted to change their sex[17] and received an enthusiastic response. At the December 10, 1965, meeting of the Benjamin Foundation, Green announced that Johns Hopkins was forming a committee to consider experimental transsexual surgery; the Erickson Educational Foundation would underwrite some of the expense.[18] One year later, Hopkins announced the opening of the first US gender clinic via a press release sent to the *New York Times*.[19]

A PROLIFERATION OF GENDER CLINICS

Johns Hopkins, a private research university founded in 1876, was, and remains, one of the world's most prestigious centers for higher education. In its 2020 annual ranking of institutions of higher education, the long-running weekly magazine *Times Higher Education* ranked Hopkins number twelve overall in a field of nearly fourteen thousand schools and, in 2016, number twenty-four for prestige.[20] Such was the reputation of Hopkins that other universities now felt empowered and perhaps even expected to announce gender programs of their own.[21] Within a few years, more than forty university-affiliated gender clinics opened across the United States and in Canada. They were located at, among other places, the University of Virginia in Charlottesville; Toronto, Ontario; the University of Minnesota; Stanford University in California; Emory University in Atlanta; and Duke University in North Carolina.[22]

The principals and staff of the Hopkins clinic came from a variety of disciplines, and their motivations varied. Personnel included gynecologists, urologists, surgeons, endocrinologists, psychiatrists, psychologists, social workers, nurses, electrologists, orderlies, administrators, office staff, and the occasional sexologist. Aside from the sexologists, few had experience or training in sex or gender, primarily because those subjects were then rarely taught, written about, or practiced. Some, like Money, participated because they saw the treatment of transsexuals as an adjunct to their primary interests. Some, like Green, saw it as a way to advance their careers or expand their professional turf. Some saw it as a test of their abilities and an opportunity to learn new skills. All wanted to help unhappy and often desperate people: "Among those willing to investigate the sex-reassignment procedure as a method of therapy for a specific psychopathology were surgeons for whom this represented a unique experience and challenge to perfect techniques heretofore restricted to the treatment of congenital malformations, and traditionally the province of the urologist and gynecologist, rather than the plastic surgeon."[23]

Some of the personnel at the clinics were, without a doubt, themselves trans. If so, they kept it secret. In the voluminous literature generated by the gender clinics, I've been unable to find a single journal article or medical textbook I can identify as authored or co-authored by an out trans clinician. In his 2018 memoir, Green wrote about coming across a stash of dresses at the home of a noted and unmarried British psychiatrist.[24] A book chapter written in 1990 used the birth name of a gender clinic staff member who later transitioned. There were perhaps others, but to the best of my knowledge no trans-identified staffers seem to have published during this time. It would be a decade or more after the opening of the clinic at Hopkins before trans people were able to work openly in the helping professions, and more than two decades before their professional publications on trans issues would begin to see print by academic publishers.[25]

Whatever their professional aspirations or personal identities and despite the shortcomings of the clinics, clinicians at the gender clinics intended to do good in the world by trying to understand the motivations of transsexual people and alleviating their suffering.[26] Some clinic staff members worked for free, or almost so, as funding for the clinics was generally shaky and sometimes nonexistent.[27] Funding was a challenge, as their work was considered experimental: their purpose was to use the scientific method to study transsexualism and transsexuals themselves.[28]

Consequently, the mission to advance medical knowledge of transsexualism often trumped altruism. Helping transsexuals with their transitions was at best an ancillary goal. The centers marked their success and ensured grants would continue primarily by the numbers of professional presentations, books, book chapters, and articles published in refereed journals, and not necessarily by the number of people they helped. Their patients suffered from this emphasis on research over care—and they suffered also because of the clinics' strict admission criteria and guidelines for the minority who were accepted for treatment. Most clinics offered hormones and surgery to surprisingly few patients, as clinicians typically viewed sex reassignment as a last-ditch effort to save those with whom other therapies and interventions had failed."[29]

The clinics operated under the then almost universal assumption that transsexualism was a form of mental illness that impaired psychological function and resulted in profound unhappiness and social dysfunction. It would be best to cure transsexuals of their "delusions,"[30] but since they were strangely resistant to every form of medical and psychiatric treatment,[31] caring physicians could at least help those most profoundly affected by providing them with palliative care that would render them less unhappy and better able to contribute to society.[32] This effort to enable transsexual people to conform to social stereotypes of the day through medical technology constitutes what is known as the medical model of transsexualism. Unfortunately, clinicians counseled these lucky few to divest themselves of any friends and memorabilia from their past lives and to go proudly forth to live in society, masquerading as cisgender and hiding their transsexualism from anyone they might meet. Many transsexuals followed this advice, often to their psychological detriment.[33]

Benjamin solidified this argument in his groundbreaking 1966 book *The Transsexual Phenomenon*. He advanced the idea of a syndrome marked by great anguish and distress in people who wished to be members of their non-natal sex.[34] Certainly, he must have seen great emotionality in his patients. Even today, many transgender people deny or wrestle privately with their gender identity and ask for help only at the point of anguish and despair; this was more extreme in the 1960s, when information and support or even a friendly ear were almost impossible to find. People in highly emotional states present an entirely different clinical picture than those at ease with themselves, and on initial presentation, many of the patients at the clinics were in a state of desperation.

Benjamin argued that those with the syndrome could not be dissuaded from their wishes, but for those most profoundly affected, their psychic pain could be alleviated by medical treatment, namely, hormones and genital surgery. The psychiatric condition would not be cured, but individuals with the syndrome could be rendered happier and more at ease in their bodies. I cannot know Benjamin's private opinion, but certainly his was the only approach he could have taken at that time in his attempts to convince his peers to provide compassionate treatment for transsexuals.

In their edited 1969 text *Transsexualism and Sex Reassignment*, Green and Money advanced an interdisciplinary treatment protocol based on Benjamin's model. Patients would be treated in a special clinic by a group of personnel representing a variety of disciplines, including surgery, endocrinology, psychology, electrology, cosmetology, religion, and law. In this controlled setting, applicants could be evaluated and studied and thereby stimulate research articles that would lead to increased understanding of transsexualism.

With their restrictive experimental approach and centering around the medical model of transsexualism, the clinics rigorously screened applicants and turned most away. Reasons for rejection were many, varied from clinic to clinic, and included the following:

The applicant was

- a cross-dresser and not transsexual;
- "actually" a gay man or lesbian;
- married;
- a parent;
- heterosexual in the gender assigned at birth;
- psychotic or mentally unstable;
- unable to afford the clinic's fees;
- too young or too old;
- physically impaired;
- unable or unwilling to pay the clinic's fees;
- a criminal;
- a sex worker;
- economically successful (that is, employed in a high-paying position).

The applicant was considered

- unlikely to pass successfully in the target gender;
- not considered sexually attractive in their target gender;

- unlikely or unwilling to be available for follow-up;

- likely to be noncompliant with lifestyle requirements;

- a malingerer or publicity seeker;

- likely to be litigious;

- unwilling or unable to make lifestyle adjustments (change of career, mode of personal presentation, cessation of contact with friend and loved ones, or even sexual behavior).

The applicant failed to

- be hyperfeminine or hypermasculine in appearance and manner when cross-dressed;

- report a history of playing with toys and wearing clothing of the nonbirth gender from an early age;

- report cross-dressing from an early age;

- demonstrate an unwavering lifelong commitment to sex reassignment.

The list was highly subjective and seemingly endless.[35] An applicant's ability to pass in cisgender heteronormative society remained a core objective of clinicians who provided treatment.

Clinicians' fixation on the binary often dictated who received care. In their 1978 ethnographic study, Suzanne Kessler and Wendy McKenna recounted conversations on the subject of judging applicants: One clinician "said that he was more convinced of the femaleness of the male-to-female transsexual if she was particularly beautiful and was capable of evoking in him those feelings that beautiful women generally do. Another clinician told us that he uses his own sexual interest as a criterion for deciding whether a transsexual is really the gender she/he claims."[36]

After evaluation, transfeminine applicants to the clinics were generally assigned to one of two diagnostic categories described by Ethyl Person and Lionel Ovesey in 1974: primary transsexual or secondary transsexual.[37] Those relegated to the primary category were typically young, feminine in appearance and behavior, and sexually interested in men. Many were active in and had found a home in lesbian and gay communities. Most had come out as gay or transsexual early on, and some had been cast out of their homes by their parents. Because their appearance often was not gender-normative and because many were marginalized by intersectional issues like race and homelessness, finding and keeping employment was difficult or impossible; consequently, they had little money to pay the fees the clinics demanded, even for initial evaluation.

Those considered secondary transsexuals tended to be older, better educated, and well-established as husbands, fathers, and workers, most in what was then considered male-centric or even male-only positions. Many had histories in the military. Most were sexually interested only in women. They tended to be masculine in appearance and unable, in the eyes of the clinicians, to pass convincingly as female.

Not surprisingly, "primary transsexuals" were more likely to be considered for feminizing treatment than "secondary transsexuals." The reason for this seems obvious: in the eyes of the clinicians, they were, as a group, considered more likely to live normative lives as women than those whose bodies had masculinized under the influence of decades of testosterone. "Secondary transsexuals" were more likely to be considered "just" cross-dressers and were turned away in large numbers.[38]

Paradoxically, even though they were more likely to be offered counseling and eventual hormonal and surgical treatment, primary transsexuals were often unable to pay the required fees. Equally paradoxically, secondary transsexuals, most of whom could manage the fees and afford feminizing medical treatment, were usually not offered treatment.

In retrospect, it seems likely there were never two categories of transfeminine transsexuals. In my opinion, the differences in appearance, demeanor, and lifestyle observed by the clinic's clinicians weren't so much due to personality differences or clinical "types" as it was to the age at which applicants walked through the doors. Younger applicants, who were viewed by clinicians as naturally feminine as a class, were viewed as acceptable candidates. Similarly, those who were unable or unwilling or couldn't figure out how to live authentically or who had simply lacked the courage to act found themselves locked into typical male career, matrimonial, and parenthood tracks as their bodies continued to masculinize. When they presented in middle or late adulthood with adult male bodies, they seemed to the clinicians to be poor candidates. The real and perhaps only difference between primary transsexuals and secondary transsexuals seen by the clinics was an age difference of twenty, thirty, or forty years.

Researchers and clinicians viewed transsexual men, first, as rare, and second, as presenting a clinical picture that varied little from applicant to applicant. They believed them to be universally sexually attracted to women. In spite of evidence showing this was not the case, including Lou Sullivan's death from AIDS-related complications in 1991,[39] this belief persisted into the 1990s. In a chapter in my 1998 edited textbook *Current Concepts in Transgender Identity,* psychiatrist Ira Pauly, who knew Sullivan, self-referentially wrote:

> Pauly had reported in 1974 that all female-to-male transsexuals were homosexual. These biological females who were unable to accept their sex of birth and assignment, and who developed a male gender identity, all wished to pursue a relationship with a nonhomosexual woman. Pierce et al. (1981) confirmed this observation that the wives and/or girlfriends of a group of female-to-male transsexuals whom she studied were all heterosexual women with no homosexual experience. Both partners to this social and sexual liaison considered themselves to be heterosexual, normal, or straight. This finding was generally accepted and continued to be the case even as late as 1987 when Blanchard et al. reported that "typologies exist in male-to-female transsexuals, but not in female-to-male transsexuals."[40]

Pauly, influenced by Sullivan, realized transsexual men were not all alike, but for other clinicians, change was slow to come.

> Both transsexual men and transsexual women realized that chances of acceptance at the gender clinics were higher if they presented histories that conformed to the expectations of the clinicians at the clinics. Allucquére Rosanne "Sandy" Stone has written eloquently about this. In his memoir *Becoming a Visible Man,* Jamison Green noted that some transsexuals assumed the clinicians were right: we *were* all alike. "As long as we were kept separate from each other, many of us felt that fitting the psychological model was the only way to get access to medical treatment. In 1999, I heard a physician declare, 'All *my* FTMs want tattoos,' as if this proved 'his' FTMs were typical men, or that FTMs who didn't want tattoos were somehow less authentic than 'his' FTMs. An additional consequence of this monolithic analysis is that we ourselves labor under the mistaken assumption that we are all alike."[41]

A LIBELOUS LITERATURE

The staff considered applicants to the clinics patients rather than clients. This established a medical dynamic that profoundly defamed and disempowered the transsexuals who applied for and attended the clinics, not only in terms of who would get treatment and who wouldn't, but also in the very language of the research articles the clinics generated and published. This literature, written almost exclusively by clinicians affiliated with one or another of the gender clinics, often employed hostile and pejorative language and self-fulfilling research designs. Staff decided who was and who wasn't transsexual and admitted or rejected applicants accordingly; the medical literature they subsequently generated validated the staff's ideas of who was a true transsexual and thus deserving of treatment; who was to be rejected as a gay man or woman or a cross-dresser; and who was simply, in the estimation of the authors, confused or seeking attention. The clinicians then employed this literature to admit or reject future applicants, establishing a self-fulfilling set of definitions and criteria for treatment that served to perpetuate their own biases.[42]

The literature propagated the cisnormative, heteronormative, and sexist views of the researchers, beliefs based on the binary vision of sex and gender that then dominated American culture. The clinicians expected to produce attractive, passable, sexually alluring postoperative women and the occasional masculine heterosexual man[43] who would dress in appropriate hyperfeminine and hypermasculine clothing and go out into the world, if not cured, then at least prepared to lead "normal" lives as heterosexuals in their new genders. The staff considered those who might fall short of these standards unsuitable candidates for gender reassignment. They advised those who weren't laser-focused on hormones and genital surgery, those who didn't subscribe to John Wayne/Marilyn Monroe stereotypes of masculinity and femininity, those who were still figuring themselves out, and those who did not want to cross the binary gender divide immediately and forever to go elsewhere.[44]

Books and journal articles from this period reflect this discriminatory thinking in a variety of ways. First, the literature of the day was filled with slurs, accusations, and name-calling; I have called it "a collection of papers by clinicians explaining to other clinicians how to deal with such troublesome people."[45] In later analysis, I explicitly condemned the research generated by these clinics, noting:

Much of the supposedly objective literature is characterized by moral pronouncements, outrageous attacks on the nature and appearance of transsexual people, and the use of nomenclature and pronouns which are offensive (deliberately, in some cases) to transsexual people. This is but the visible tip, however, of what lies under the surface of a literature which presumes transsexuals are what the medical community has always supposed them to be: manipulative, dishonest, maladjusted, sexual stereotypes. It is a literature which gives permission to its authors to write whatever they wish about transsexuals, with no fear of censure.[46]

Occasionally, authors unabashedly stated their moral distaste for sex reassignment. For example, Donald Laub and Norman Fisk opened an article in the journal *Plastic and Reconstructive Surgery* in 1974 with the sentence "To change an individual's God-given anatomic sex is a repugnant concept." This statement, astonishing in a medical journal, went unremarked until 1991, when I pointed it out in *Chrysalis*, a journal I then edited.[47]

There were cheap shots and name-calling. Long after the closure of the gender clinics in 1979 and 1980, Betty Steiner's distaste for transsexuals surfaced like a Freudian slip in an otherwise nonjudgmental descriptive passage about treating transsexuals: "The realistic assessment of gender-dysphoric patients must take into account that there are some individuals who could never pass as members of the opposite sex, regardless of how skillfully they are dressed and made up. A six-foot-five, 300-pound trucker will never pass as a woman, but will always look like 'a guy in drag.'"[48] Steiner's statement might be objectively true, but it was cruel, irrelevant, and needless. More subtle was psychoanalyst Robert Stoller, who frequently voiced his concerns about sex reassignment. In 1982 he wrote, of transsexuals and sex reassignment, "After 30 years . . . both the treatments and the patients (of both sexes) have been, at most, near misses." In this tongue-in-cheek sentence, Stoller informs the reader of his opinion that transsexuals are not, after medical treatment, real men and women.[49]

Snide remarks like Stoller's, above, were uncommon, but present nonetheless. Witness Money and Clay Primrose's sly put-down of transsexuals who took the initiative to learn about what was going on with them: "Transsexuals . . . are distinguishable from females at large by their lack of special attraction to the helpless newborn and their imagery in coital fantasies. It is possible, though, that transsexuals will change their conception of the female stereotype to include these features after reading this article, since they are often influenced by reading about their condition."[50] Money and Primrose's remark illustrates a phenomenon described by sociologist Irving Goffman: when an individual is stigmatized, whatever he or she does is interpreted and interpretable as problematic in light of the stigma.[51] Thus, when transsexuals endeavored to learn more about their situation—something that would be considered admirable in expectant mothers or grandfathers with cancer—their resourcefulness was viewed as emblematic of their condition. Clinicians characterized transsexuals as unreliable and manipulative.[52]

The literature was filled with pronominal misgendering, peppered with unnecessary quotation marks around names, body parts, and pronouns, and rife with terms like *male transsexual* (for trans women) and *female transsexual* (for trans men) designed to tell the reader what gender transsexuals "really" were.[53] These practices had the demeaning effect of stripping transsexuals of their own agency and self-determination: "It has long been considered appropriate for others to make decisions about which pronoun to use with transsexuals, regardless of the self-perception of the transsexuals themselves, but it is decidedly not okay to do so with nontranssexuals. Quite simply, when it comes to transsexualism, the usual rules of propriety do not apply, and no one seems to notice that they have been set aside, even in the hallowed pages of medical and psychological journals."[54]

Despite its many problems, the literature from this period did advance understanding of transsexuals and transsexualism, especially with descriptions of the surgical and other medical techniques used for treatment. However, for every article that helped, another contributed little or added to the accumulating pile of papers that systematically maligned and stigmatized transsexuals.[55]

THE CARROT AND THE STICK: TREATMENT AND MISTREATMENT AT THE GENDER CLINICS

The gender clinics provided treatment transsexuals desperately wanted—primarily, acknowledgment of their condition, hormones, surgery, and social support. But clinic clinicians, fearful of being called to task by the medical community for being too liberal with hormones and surgery and under financial constraints as well, rationed those commodities, offering them only to a minority of clients. The staff, following the treatment suggestions from Benjamin's *The Transsexual Phenomenon* and Green and Money's *Transsexualism and Sex Reassignment,* served as gatekeepers, and keep the gates they did. In its thirteen years of existence, the Gender Identity Clinic at Johns Hopkins performed gender-affirmation surgery on only thirty patients.[56] This averages to fewer than three per year.

The application procedures at the clinics were time-consuming, expensive, and onerous, and getting approved for feminizing or masculinizing treatment even more so. In the Winter 1991/1992 issue of the journal *Chrysalis Quarterly,* I reprinted the restrictive admission requirements of the gender clinic at Case Western Reserve University in Ohio. The description of the twenty-one-step process filled the better part of two pages of the magazine.[57]

The process to meet requirements for hormone therapy at Case Western included participation in a battery of psychological tests; multiple interviews with social workers (including a four-hour interview devoted to spouses, family members, and friends); assignment to and interviews with a primary and secondary clinician; repeated and lengthy case reviews by the entire clinical team; a commitment to long-term psychotherapy; and finally, after all criteria were met, a referral to an internist or endocrinologist to discuss hormone therapy.[58] The clinic guidelines required further extensive evaluation and testing prior to gender-affirming surgery.

Requirements to stay in a program could be as strenuous as criteria for admission. Transsexuals had no choice but to follow the rules, no matter how unnecessary or distasteful. Demands could include, and sometimes did, being required to change one's job (and indeed, sometimes one's occupation); construct falsified personal histories as a member of the target gender; divest oneself of friends and possessions that did not "match" the target gender, have sexual experiences with members of the same or biologically other sex; or divorce a beloved long-term spouse. One transsexual woman told me that as part of the screening process for admission she was required to sit naked in a chair in front of fully clothed staff.

Failure to comply with even the most bizarre request could and frequently did result in ejection from a program. In my 1991 *Chrysalis* article I included histories of a transsexual woman who was required to change her birth name, even though her first and middle names worked well as a woman's name; another woman who was told to experiment with homosexuality, even though she was clear with staff that she was exclusively attracted to women; and another who was required to give up her high-paying job as an aircraft technician to go back to school and retrain as a nurse.

The following quotations are from the first few transsexual women I interviewed.

CQ: Didn't you have a name that worked in both genders?

Amy: Yes. My first name was Lonnie—I had started to spell it Loni—and my second name worked, too. But the clinic told me I had to change it.

CQ: Wasn't it just a suggestion?

Amy: No, they told me I had to change it or forget about the program.[59]

Jenna: I was working as an aircraft maintenance technician. I really liked it. My psychiatrist told me that I had to quit. I think he did so on advice from the gender clinic. He said it wasn't a very feminine thing to do. I said, "I'm not into flower arranging or basket weaving!" He made me quit, and I entered a continuing education program.

Despite his insistence that I would turn out to be lesbian, I didn't. My work now is exciting, but you know—I really liked working as an aircraft technician.[60]

Several interviewees described a lack of promised follow-through by the clinics for hormonal therapy and genital reassignment surgery.

Carla: I had done everything right, and they weren't being forthcoming with what I needed. It took three years to get a letter for hormones. Three years after going into real-life test, they still hadn't approved my surgery. They kept saying that I would get it soon, but "soon" never came.[61]

In the literature, several researchers characterized these demands as requests—a fallacy, given the reality on the ground at the clinics.[62] In one case, I documented that to receive treatment, transsexuals were required to participate in the clinic's research program.[63]

Anthropologist Anne Bolin perfectly described the imbalance of power: "Inherent to the *Standards of Care* and in the policy relations of caretaker to client is an inequity in power relations such that the recommendation for surgery is completely dependent on the caretaker's evaluation. This results in a situation in which the psychological evaluation may be, and often is, wielded like a club over the head of the transsexual who so desperately wants that surgery."[64] As one of the interviewees in my 1991 *Chrysalis* article told me about her clinician, "He banged his fist on the table. 'We're not here to negotiate! You've heard our terms. Take them or leave them.' "[65]

The following excerpt is from a remarkable article in the August 1980 issue of *The Gateway,* the newsletter of the Golden Gate Girls/Guys support group. The unnamed author of the article characterized the speaker as shockingly unprofessional. I have redacted the speaker's name. "[The speaker] gave three criteria by which a person is diagnosed a 'transsexual': (1) the inner feeling of being from the other sex; (2) a past history of activities usually associated with the other sex; and (3) a heterosexual orientation post-operatively. This last point raised much dissent in the group, and [she] curtly explained that her Program made this distinction and that those who disagreed with it were more than welcome to take their business elsewhere."[66]

An attitude of arrogance was not uncommon at the clinics. The clinicians viewed themselves as the experts, and who the hell were transsexuals to second-guess their methods? It was a theme in my personal experience and the experiences of the interviewees in my *Chrysalis* article and others I have interviewed since and was, I believe, widespread throughout the clinic system. This hubris and other abusive treatment were directly attributable to the power dynamics inherent in the medical model. Unfortunately, few clinicians questioned or understood the power they held over their patients and ignored or were blissfully unaware of critiques of practices at the clinics called into questions by Kessler and McKenna and, later, Bolin.

Dissent was not an option for those who sought treatment at the gender clinics. As the anonymized speaker described above makes clear, gender clinics were resistant to pushback and sometimes expelled those who complained or questioned them or their theories. In the above excerpt, the author's characterization of the speaker underscores her absence of care for transsexuals, not only as patients, but also as people. "[The speaker] proved to be a master at cold stares and one-sentence 'answers.' It was impossible to pry a concerned or empathetic word from her."[67] While the clinics did manage to provide medical services and social support that allowed a handful of clients to alter their bodies and successfully transition gender roles, many applicants faced mistreatment, and most outright rejection.

The clinicians were also blind to the intersectional barriers to care faced by trans people of color and/or those whose backgrounds differed from that of the clinic employees. Most staff members were white, educated, able-bodied, and middle/upper class and, like most of America at that time, oblivious to how microaggressions, institutionalized racism, classism, ableism, and sexism permeated the medical culture.

Of course, the clinics and clinicians got many things right. The hormonal, surgical, and general medical care they gave to those lucky enough to be admitted to their programs were in general excellent, and the personnel were licensed and professional. The clinics cooperated with one another, and the resulting collegial atmosphere stimulated research. At a time when little was known about gender dysphoria, their books, journal articles, and papers read at professional conferences advanced the medical and psychological knowledge of transsexuals and transsexualism, introduced new surgical techniques and hormonal regimens, and examined dynamics of doctor-patient interactions in the clinics and the problems that resulted.

THE CLOSURE OF THE GENDER CLINICS

The late 1970s marked a dramatic shift in transsexual healthcare and sociocultural knowledge about transsexuals. In 1976, the Erickson Educational Foundation ceased funding gender-affirming programs and research. In 1978, Kessler and McKenna took the first objective look at the medical model of treatment prevalent at the gender clinics in the United States.[68] In 1979, the Harry Benjamin International Gender Dysphoria Association was formed and published the initial version of its *Standards of Care*;[69] 1979 also marked the publication of Janice Raymond's polemic *The Transsexual Empire* and the rapid domino-like closure of gender clinics across the United States. It was also the year I first sought treatment.

McHugh, the newly appointed chair of the psychiatry department at Johns Hopkins, engineered the closing of the Hopkins clinic and boasted of it in a 1992 article in the magazine *American Scholar*. He expanded on this in 2004 in an online article:

> Until 1975, when I became psychiatrist-in-chief at Johns Hopkins Hospital, I could usually keep my own counsel on these matters. But once I was given authority over all the practices in the psychiatry

department I realized that if I were passive I would be tacitly co-opted in encouraging sex-change surgery in the very department that had originally proposed and still defended it. I decided to challenge what I considered to be a misdirection of psychiatry and to demand more information both before and after their operations.[70]

Once ensconced as the head of the psychiatry department at Hopkins, McHugh did as he had promised: he set about engineering the closure of the university's gender identity clinic. He understood little about transsexualism and misunderstood much,[71] but he was clever enough to approach Meyer, the disaffected former head of the gender identity clinic at Hopkins and convince him to contrive and submit for publication a study that purported to show "no objective advantage in terms of social rehabilitation" for genital reassignment surgery in male-to-female transsexuals. Written by Meyer and his secretary Donna Reter, the article, "Sex Reassignment: Follow-Up" appeared in 1979 in the journal *Archives of General Psychiatry*.[72]

Just about everyone involved in the treatment of transsexuals smelled a rat, and its name was McHugh. The study was methodologically flawed, appeared to have been constructed from data gathered post hoc in support of the article's thesis, and was timed to appear when Money, the principal proponent of the gender clinic at Hopkins, was out of the country. The study's findings were at odds with other, better-engineered follow-up studies. At an October 1, 1979, press conference to which the popular press was invited and academics were not, Meyer promoted the study and announced the closure of the clinic at Johns Hopkins.[73]

When Money found out about McHugh's hijinks, he was thunderstruck: "'No one at the Gender Identity Clinic was informed about the press conference,'" Money asserted. "It was done behind everyone's back. I was on my way to Prague for a professional convention when the press conference was announced."[74] Researcher Ogi Ogas neatly summarized the dramatic effect of the press conference: "Thus, after 13 years of highly acclaimed research, counseling, and surgery, SRS [sex reassignment surgery] was terminated at a press conference held without the consent of the clinic itself and based upon a single study that the majority of gender professionals regard as questionable."[75]

As Ogas predicted, reviewers immediately characterized the study as misleading or fraudulent,[76] but McHugh and Meyer managed to get stories planted in practically every newspaper and popular news magazine in the world, on the three major US television networks, and on innumerable local television and radio stations. Such was the prestige of Johns Hopkins that, now that it had closed its gender clinic and withdrawn its support of sex reassignment therapies, within months most of the other university-affiliated gender clinics closed their doors; the remaining few became for-profit businesses. For more than a decade, any mention of gender-affirming care for transsexualism would resurrect Meyer and Reter: "But the Hopkins study . . ."

THE HAPPY AFTERMATH

McHugh's efforts to eradicate transsexual surgery ultimately failed. Certainly, he succeeded in closing the gender clinics, but in their place a free enterprise network of helping professionals sprang up in the United States. Before long the free market to which transsexuals had turned before the opening of the gender clinics found a new life. Practitioners like Harry Benjamin and Wollman in New York,[77] Ira Dushoff in Florida, and Stanley Biber in Colorado had provided services throughout the heyday of the gender clinics and continued after their closure—and new practitioners appeared. Transsexuals could again freely choose providers from lists of electrologists, therapists, endocrinologists, surgeons, and support groups. Trans community publications like Phoebe Smith's remarkable *Transsexual Voice* and the International Foundation for Gender Education's *TV-TS Tapestry Journal* included lists of helping professionals that grew throughout the 1980s and early 1990s, and Erickson Educational Foundation successor organizations like the Janus Information Facility, Joanna Clark and Jude Patton's J2CP, FTM International, and the American Educational Gender Information Service compiled lists of caregivers and successively provided referrals until the end of the twentieth century. By that time, of course, a world of information was available instantly on the internet. In this thriving marketplace, it was easier to find sympathetic and helpful service providers, and that's just what transsexuals, including me, did.

In May 1994, I wrote a letter to McHugh in which I chastised him for presuming to attack transsexuals without bothering to learn anything about them—and then I told him his efforts to eliminate transition-related treatment for transsexuals had backfired:

> I'm sure you'll be pleased to know that despite the immediate effect of causing other clinics to close, the closing of the gender clinic at Johns Hopkins caused the rise of a consumer-centered movement

which has made hormonal and surgical treatment available to any American who desires it [and can afford it]. There is now a vast network of support groups and private practitioners which provide the transsexual individual with information and support. You actually did transsexual people a favor by moving to Hopkins and working to close the clinic there.[78]

Not surprisingly, McHugh did not reply.

AFTERWORD

Although I was later licensed as a psychological examiner by the state of Tennessee and was myself a clinician for many years, my involvement with the early gender clinics was limited to my own experience as an applicant rather than as an employee. At the time I sought treatment, I knew next to nothing about transsexualism, for my life had been an informational desert in that regard. I, like almost all other Americans, didn't understand or even know about the distinction between sex and gender. But while I might not have known much, I understood that, despite what I had been told at Vanderbilt University's gender clinic, I was transsexual, and after reading the psychological and medical literature on transsexualism, I was certain something improper and disturbing was underway at the gender clinics.

I'd like to say for a final time that for the most part the staff at the clinics were as blinded by the binary as I was. Being in the business of sex reassignment did not necessarily provide insight. Unfortunately, staff were also blind to the power differential, or perhaps simply didn't care, or in some cases, perhaps both.[79] And so the literature didn't question the medical model of transsexualism or even discuss it at length, except in theoretical articles. Consequently, the researchers and clinicians were blind to their bias and deaf to analyses of the medical model when they began to show up.[80]

Raymond's 1979 screed *The Transsexual Empire,* a critique of transsexualism and an attack on transsexuals, was fraudulent. It posed as a work of science and was considered such by many, but it was merely a diatribe translated into print. Her "research subjects" did not seem to exist; the methodology section of her doctoral dissertation fails to mention them.[81] Her "data," in the form of quotations, came not from her apparently nonexistent subjects, but primarily from a satirical letter written by transsexual Angela Douglas and printed in the August-September 1977 issue of the lesbian journal *Sister*.[82]

In a 1982 critique in the journal *Social Problems*, Dwight Billings and Thomas Urban, like Raymond, criticized transsexuals for adherence to the gender binary, but as I have said, it was Kessler and McKenna and later Bolin who looked at the beliefs about sex and gender and the power dynamics in play at the gender clinics.[83] Their books made the shortcomings and short-sightedness of the clinics manifest and set the stage for gender revolution. Unfortunately, these works appeared too late to affect the trajectory of the gender clinics—and when Kessler, McKenna, and Bolin were published, they didn't seem to be on the reading lists of those who had worked at the gender clinics anyway. Aside from the snow-blind review of Bolin's *In Search of Eve* by Charles Mate-Kole, her work and that of Kessler and McKenna seems to have gone unnoticed and unremarked by clinicians.[84]

In this century we are seeing the rise of a new generation of gender clinics that are not rooted in heteronormativity and the gender binary, nor do their clients generally call themselves transsexual[85]—and they do not ration gender-affirming care. Hopkins itself once again has a center for transgender health and is performing gender-affirming surgeries.[86] So does Vanderbilt University, where, in the late 1970s, I was denied care.[87]

Most of these clinics operate on the model that ultimately replaced the medical model of transsexual: gender affirmation. They provide hormones and surgery and applicants are not accepted or rejected based on personal appearance, gender identity or presentation, sexual orientation, race, income level, marital status, or focus on hormones or surgery. I'm certain these clinics aren't perfect, but I'm convinced they're an order of magnitude more respectful toward and less disempowering of their transgender clients than the clinics of the 1960s and 1970s. See our discussion of this new wave of gender clinics in chapter 16 of this volume.

POSTSCRIPT: THE NATURE OF SCIENCE

My intent in this chapter has not been to malign the many compassionate and empathetic clinicians who worked hard on behalf of their transsexual patients but to excoriate a highly flawed treatment model that prevented thousands of transsexuals from getting help at the gender clinics of the 1960s and 1970s.

I have named some of the most egregious offenders at the gender clinics to make my points, but I have no wish to call out the staff of the clinics as a whole. Most, as I have said repeatedly in this chapter, had the best of intentions and did their utmost on behalf of their transsexual clients. They were, however, hampered by the then lack of differentiation between sex and gender, by a general lack of information about gender dysphoria, and by a medical model that viewed transsexuals as seriously mentally ill. They were blinded by the binary, as, at that time, so was I. But most were also blinded by the medical model. Few questioned it, and most were so enmeshed in the model that they were unable to see it—to the point that when the model came under criticism, it was sociologists and anthropologists and transsexuals, and not the clinicians who worked with transsexuals under the model, who challenged it.

Scientific theories rise and eventually fall under the weight of accumulated data; thus, we move forward—slowly and often painfully, but inexorably. The mental illness model of transsexualism still, of course, has its holdouts, but they seem increasingly out of touch and curmudgeonly.[88] Scientific revolutions don't happen overnight and, I suppose, can never be considered to be completed. After all, six hundred years after Nicolaus Copernicus' proposal that the earth revolves around the sun, not everyone believes it. I'm talking about you, flat Earthers.

Snow-blindness in science is unfortunately common. When you are in a consensual reality, it can be difficult to see or even imagine anything beyond what is apparent. In the case of the early gender clinics, I see parallels between the medical model of transsexualism and other scientific models and the people working within them. One of my favorite books is Stephen Jay Gould's *The Mismeasure of Man*.[89] Gould took a retrospective look at the mental measurement movement in the United States, and what he found was both illuminating and disturbing—a body of research that was based on erroneous scientific assumptions about human intelligence and the fascistic eugenics movement, and was fueled by unconscious bias, experiments that ultimately did nothing to improve the body of knowledge, and in one case, intentional scientific fraud. In looking at photos in a 1912 book by psychometrist Henry H. Goddard,[90] Gould realized that an unknown someone, and perhaps Goddard himself, had crudely retouched photos of members of the "Kallikaks," a family of supposedly feeble-minded and demented individuals who resided in the Pine Barrens of New Jersey. The eyes and mouths of the subjects had been strangely retouched with ink, giving them an otherworldly appearance that made it easy to believe the suppositions about them. Just as Laub and Fisk's 1974 "repugnant concept" remark was ignored and probably subconsciously overlooked for seventeen years, in the more than one-half century since the publication of Goddard's book, no one before Gould had remarked on or apparently even noticed the retouching of the Kallikak photos.

The intent of most mental measurers was pure, but those involved were blind to the idea that their view of human intelligence was harmful and inaccurate. This is exactly what happened with the staff at the early gender clinics.[91]

Science progresses by fits and starts, and its practitioners and adherents are often resistant to new ideas. Science is, however, driven by data and is as objective as human beings are able to get about the universe that surrounds us. The data eventually prevail. False theories topple under the weight of accumulated data, and new and generally more accurate models take their place. But old models have their adherents, and many resist or ridicule new models and ideas and sometimes question or disbelieve data. It can take decades or even centuries for old models to be replaced with new. Meanwhile, much harm can be done. In the case of mental measurement, millions of human beings were viewed as genetically inferior and incapable of functioning in a normal fashion, often on the basis of immigration status or country of origin; tens of thousands were involuntarily hospitalized, some for life, and hundreds were involuntarily sterilized. The loss of human potential was profound.

Data that contradict current models are often initially disregarded, and those who generate such data can find themselves criticized, ridiculed, and marginalized for daring to suggest or promote or run experiments that interrogate current models. Human beings, scientists and medical personnel included, are as likely as anyone to be consciously unaware of the system under which they operate and to resist change. We are all susceptible to and often mirror the attitudes of our families, friends, co-workers, and society, and we adhere to what we have learned through formal education and personal experience. Staff of the gender clinics were limited by the language and mores of the time, the idea that transsexualism was a mental illness, and the focus of the clinics in which they valued research over helping others. I cannot find it in my heart to blame the workers[92] for the way I and others were treated, but I can and do find fault with the system and the model under which gender clinics worked and lament the damage they caused to transsexuals. I'm just glad a new and less disempowering model is in place.

NOTES

1. I use the terms *transsexual* and *transsexualism* in their historical context. The term *transgender* and other associated identities didn't come into fashion until the early mid-1990s.

2. My thanks to Aaron Devor for his feedback on this chapter, Leah Squires, for her exceptional editing skills, and my fellow editors Carolyn Wolf-Gould and Jamison Green for their careful and insightful edits.

3. In a series of papers published in the early 1950s, John Money and John and Joan Hampson argued that sex was multivariate and not a unitary phenomenon. Their work formed the basis for the eventually dissociation of sex and gender in scientific thought and popular culture. See the Early Social Models in chapter 8 of this volume.

4. There were exceptions, of course. Coeditor of this volume Jamison Green has pointed out that early on, gay men and especially lesbians made significant inroads on this binary paradigm. Femme/Butch roles, for example, antagonized the gender binary. Transgender men, many of whom had been active in lesbian circles, were naturally on the front lines as society began to differentiate sex and gender. Clearly, transgender people as well as cisgender researchers were interrogating the gender binary.

5. The Program in Human Sexuality did not offer genital surgery. Unlike the Hopkins-style binary approach to gender identity and presentation, the Program in Human Sexuality was open to alternatives. I have always believed this ahead-of-its-time attitude was largely due to the influence of Coleman, who joined the program in 1978.

6. Nine of ten physicians in the United States, in fact. See Green, Stoller, and MacAndrew, "Attitudes Toward Sex;" Green, "Physician Emotionalism." See also Green, *Gay Rights, Trans Rights*, 124–25, 131–33.

7. Mancini, *Magnus Hirschfeld*; Meyerowitz, *How Sex Changed*, 19–20. See also chapter 3 in this volume.

8. Hodgkinson, *Michael Nee Laura*, 76. See chapter 4 in this volume.

9. Green, *Gay Rights, Trans Rights*, 116. See chapter 6 in this volume.

10. Hamburger, "The Desire for Change of Sex." See chapter 6 in this volume.

11. Meyerowitz, *How Sex Changed*, 46–48. See chapter 4 in this volume. See Burou, "Male-to-Female Transformation," for a discussion, with illustrations, of his pioneering work. See chapters 2–4 in this volume for discussions of the European origins of medical treatment of transgender people in the United States. See also chapter 5 in this volume for a discussion of gender variance in Indigenous peoples in what would become the United States.

12. Denny, "Black Telephones, White Refrigerators."

13. For instance, in her 1979 autobiography, Phoebe Smith documents the extraordinary lengths she went to in order to obtain medical treatment. Smith wrote hundreds of letters to federal and Georgia officials, pleading her case, to little effect.

14. Green, *Gay Rights, Trans Rights*, 24. Green became a psychiatrist and, later, a lawyer and was primary editor of the groundbreaking 1969 book *Transsexualism and Sex Reassignment*, which advanced a multidisciplinary model for treating transsexuals. For many years, he was the editor of the journal *Archives of Sexual Behavior*. He was also the author of the 1987 book *The Sissy Boy Syndrome: The Development of Homosexuality*, which describes an unfortunate and abusive long-term study in which feminine-identified boys were deprived of girls' clothing and toys and encouraged to be more masculine.

15. Green, *Gay Rights, Trans Rights*, 119–20.

16. Green, *Gay Rights, Trans Rights*, 121–22. See chapter 10 in this volume.

17. The new name for this was *sex reassignment*.

18. Green, *Gay Rights, Trans Rights*, 126. Green's statement is confirmed by a press release from the Erickson Foundation. For more about Erickson's remarkable work and personal history, see chapter 10 in this volume.

19. Green, *Gay Rights, Trans Rights*, 125–26. See Buckley, "A Changing of Sex by Surgery"; Hastings, "Inauguration of a Research Project."

20. Times Higher Education, "World University Rankings 2020"; Smith, "The 24 Most Prestigious Universities."

21. Aaron Devor, personal communication, 2020. If Hopkins could open a clinic without suffering censure or legal repercussions, then perhaps it would be safe for other universities to do the same.

22. Researcher Sky Syzygy and I recently combined the lists of gender centers we had been collecting.

23. Money and Schwartz, "Public Opinion and Social Issues in Transsexualism," 255.

24. Green, *Gay Rights, Trans Rights*, 154.

25. So long as we were telling our personal stories, we could get published. When we were so presumptuous as to write about the social or treatment aspects of transsexualism or cross-dressing, no academic or medical publisher was interested. We had a lot to say, but with the exceptions of Louise Lawrence, Virginia Prince, and perhaps a few others, we were limited to magazines and self-help books marketed to others in the trans community. I have written and presented about this exclusion (Denny, "All We Were Allowed to Write"). Allucquére Rosanne (Sandy) Stone's 1991 book chapter "The Empire Strikes Back" is considered by many to be the opening shot for trans studies. Here, for arguably the first time, a trans woman was talking about transsexualism in an academic textbook. By 1994, books by a variety of out trans writers were being published by mainstream presses (for instance, Bornstein, *Gender Outlaw*, and Rothblatt, *The Apartheid of Sex*). My 1998 book *Gender Dysphoria: A Guide to Research* was, I believe, the first book-length text about transsexualism by an out trans person to be published by an academic press.

26. cf. Edgerton, "The Role of Surgery."
27. Fritz and Mulkey, "The Rise and Fall of Gender Clinics."
28. Witkin, "Hopkins Hospital."
29. Meyerowitz, *How Sex Changed*, 208–255; Denny, "The Politics of Diagnosis," 12.
30. See Meerloo, "Change of Sex and Collaboration with the Psychosis."
31. cf. Bak and Stewart, "Fetishism, Transvestism, and Voyeurism." The "cured" patient in this paper was in actuality Richard Raskind, later known as Renée Richards.
32. Haynes, "The World Health Organization Will Stop Classifying Transgender People." The World Health Organization dropped transsexualism as a mental disorder only in 2019.
33. Presbyterian minister and licensed family and marital therapist Erin Swenson told me in 1997 that when her story appeared in Atlanta newspapers, she was contacted by an elderly transsexual woman who was living in a high-rise care facility on a fixed income. At the woman's request, Swenson agreed to meet her for lunch. As they ate, the woman told Swenson that upon the advice of the Emory University gender clinic, she had cut herself off from those she had known before and during her transition and forged a new life, telling no one about her past. Swenson was the first person the woman had spoken to about her transsexualism since the 1970s, and was likely the last.
34. This argument was based on Benjamin's interactions with his transsexual patients. He was extraordinarily empathetic and sympathetic toward them.
35. Most, or at least some, clinics offered rejected applicants therapy to help them function in their birth genders. How do I know? Because that's what I was offered when I was refused treatment at the gender clinic at Nashville's Vanderbilt University.
36. Bolin, *In Search of Eve*, 107, quoting Kessler and McKenna, *Gender*, 118.
37. Person and Ovesey, "The Transsexual Syndrome in Males: I" and "The Transsexual Syndrome in Males: II." See "Part II: Theory-Driven Practice" in chapter 8 of this volume.
38. Person and Ovesey's primary/secondary approach to transmasculine clinic applicants was extended to transmasculine people but never got much traction. Roback and Lothstein, "The Female Mid-life Sex Change Applicant."
39. Lou Sullivan, who was assigned female at birth and came to identify as a gay man, was instrumental in changing the of opinion of clinicians about what was then called female transsexualism. In 1989, Pauly interviewed Sullivan on camera. See Rohrer, "Lou Sullivan: Battling Gender Specialists," and chapter 7.4 in this volume.
40. Pauly, "Gender Identity and Sexual Orientation."
41. Green, *Becoming a Visible Man*, 44.
42. The literature was a snake that ate its own tail. I wonder how many thousands of transsexuals left the clinics despondent, their hoped-for transitions derailed by this runaway feedback loop.

43. The supposed rarity of transsexual men was another self-perpetuating myth that made its way into the scientific literature.

44. Today, the flaws in this sort of thinking are glaringly apparent, but they were not so much so in the 1960s and 1970s. I reiterate: most Americans of the day, gay men and women and transsexuals included, subscribed to the same heteronormative binary philosophies as the clinicians. There was no available way for the clinicians to categorize or think about their patients.

45. Denny, "Letter to the Editor."

46. Denny, "You Make me Sick!"

47. Denny, "Quotations from the Literature," 6. Having read Laub's autobiography, I'm certain this wasn't his personal view. Perhaps it was Fisk's. What is relevant is that it appeared in a supposedly objective medical journal.

48. Steiner, "Intake Assessment of Gender Dysphoric Patients," 102.

49. Stoller, "Near Miss."

50. Money and Primrose, "Sexual Dimorphism and Dissociation," 472.

51. Goffman, *Asylums*; Goffman, *Stigma*. Rosenhan, "On Being Sane in Insane Places," 33: "Once a person is designated abnormal, all of his other behaviors and characteristics are colored by that label. Indeed, that label is so powerful that many of the [nonmentally ill accomplices masquerading as mental patients'] normal behaviors were overlooked entirely or profoundly misinterpreted."

52. This primary tension between transsexuals and the clinics have been thoroughly addressed in the literature. Kessler and McKenna, *Gender*, and Bolin, *In Search of Eve*, offered early critiques. With the exception of possible critiques in the many transgender publications of the day, the first printed analyses by those personally affected by this appeared in the early 1990s. Denny, "The Politics of Diagnosis"; Stone, "The Empire Strikes Back," and criticisms continue today; cf. Shuster, *Trans Medicine*.

53. After attending the 1997 International Gender Symposium of the Harry Benjamin International Dysphoria Association and seeing instance after instance of this sort of language displayed on slides, Jamison Green (a co-editor of this volume) and I took action. We prepared a survey and distributed it throughout the then still forming transgender community and replicated it ten years later. Not surprisingly, respondents were not in favor of the language used by clinicians. See Green, Denny, and Cromwell, ""What Do You Want Us to Call You?"

54. Denny, "Not Screwed Up Enough." Psychologist Leslie Lothstein was the worst in this regard. Throughout his 1983 book on female-to-male transsexuals, he consistently used hostile and demeaning language to refer to his patients.

55. My favorite example of this is a 1982 article by Donald Milliken entitled "Homicidal Transsexuals: Three Cases." Milliken admits going out of his way to dig up three instances, and even then, one of his subjects was unsuccessful in committing murder. The absurdity of this paper becomes clear when the target population is

randomly changed to "Homicidal Dentists: Three Cases," or "Homicidal Ballet Dancers: Three Cases En Pointe."

56. . . . although Megan Day's "How One of America's Best Medical Schools," notes that the Hopkins Clinic did consult and provide training for more than one thousand surgeries performed elsewhere, "training doctors along the way."

57. Lothstein, *Female-to-Male Transsexualism*, 87–91; Denny, "The Politics of Diagnosis," 10–11.

58. Lothstein, *Female-to-Male Transsexualism*, 87–91.

59. Excerpted from Denny, "The Politics of Diagnosis," 15–16.

60. Excerpted from Denny, "The Politics of Diagnosis," 16.

61. Excerpted from Denny, "The Politics of Diagnosis," 14.

62. cf. Clemmensen, "The 'Real-life Test' for Surgical Candidates."

63. Cooper, "Hormone Treatment." I wrote the author to ask him about this, and he replied that participation in the research program was not in fact mandatory, which begs the question: Why did he document in print that it was?

64. Bolin, *In Search of Eve*, 51.

65. Denny, "The Politics of Diagnosis," 15.

66. Reproduced in Denny, "The Politics of Diagnosis," 3.

67. Reproduced in Denny, "The Politics of Diagnosis," 3.

68. Kessler and McKenna, *Gender*.

69. See chapter 13 in this volume on Harry Benjamin International Gender Dysphoria Association and World Professional Association for Transgender Health.

70. McHugh, "Surgical Sex."

71. How little did McHugh know? In 1994, a trans psychiatrist sent me recent personal correspondence from McHugh in which he expressed utter incredulity at the idea that a male-to-female transsexual could be sexually attracted to women. This document now resides in the Labadie Collection at the University of Michigan in Ann Arbor.

72. Meyer was also in the anti sex reassignment camp. Reter, who as department secretary apparently had no training in mental health, was presumably along for the ride; see Ogas, "Spare Parts," for an excellent recounting of the McHugh and Meyer shenanigans. Incidentally, the operated Johns Hopkins subjects of the study reported improvement following surgery, and not one expressed regret.

73. Such a press conference to announce the publication of a paper in a psychiatric journal was highly unusual. See Ogas, "Spare Parts;" Denny, "The Campaigns Against Transsexuals, Part 1;" and Siotos et al., "Origins of Gender Affirmation Surgery."

74. Ogas, "Spare Parts."

75. Ogas, "Spare Parts."

76. A number of early trans community publications, including the *Journal of Male Feminism*, *The Gateway*, and the *Erickson Educational Foundation Newsletter*

had immediate negative reactions. Reviews in professional journals were also negative. See, for instance, Fleming, Steinman, and Bocknek, "Methodological Problems in Assessing Sex-Reassignment Surgery"; Oppenheim, "The Holes in Meyer's Study" and "Meyer's Study Draws Fire from Leading Authorities."

77. Benjamin also practiced in San Francisco.

78. Denny, "Letter to Paul McHugh."

79. I frequently observed both behaviors among coworkers in my professional positions at a psychiatric hospital, as a child protective services worker, and in a variety of developmental centers.

80. Mate-Kole, "Review of A. Bolin."

81. Raymond's *The Transsexual Empire* is based on the dissertation. In its entirety, *Empire* reads like a QAnon conspiracy theory. Despite it having been taken seriously in feminist and other circles, it should be discounted as an empirical or even rational work.

82. Activist Kay Brown was present when Douglas wrote the letter and attested on the internet that it was satirical in its entirety. She advised Douglas not to submit it. The letter was immediately republished in *Dyke: A Quarterly* 1, no. 5 (1977).

83. In 1978 and 1988, respectively.

84. Mate-Kole, "Review of A. Bolin." Mate-Kole wrongly concluded that Bolin's book was of greater relevance to students of anthropology and sociology than to the many people who should have been reading and taking note of it: clinicians.

85. . . . although some clients doubtless do so identify. The term *transsexual* is now considered archaic by many, as it has been largely superseded by the more recent and more general term *transgender*. It nonetheless remains an identity. Despite the popularity of transgender, not everyone who is gender diverse identifies as such. I happen to claim both transsexual and transgender identities. Many people who might have called themselves transsexual thirty years ago now identify as transgender, but many transsexual people continue to dislike and disavow the latter term because, among other possible reasons, it is not descriptive of their experience.

86. Siotos et al., "Origins of Gender Affirmation Surgery."

87. Why was I denied gender-affirming treatment at Vanderbilt? Because I had two college degrees; because I had a position with the state of Tennessee as a child protective services worker; because I was not sexually interested in men and had been married for six years, I was deemed too functional. Obviously, I was functional in the male role, and somehow that translated into disqualification for gender-affirming therapy. Denny, "Not Screwed Up Enough." See also chapter 9 in this volume.

88. Unfortunately, a new breed of critics has taken up the gauntlet. They seem to be driven by outrage by the very existence of transgender people who somehow, by being on the planet, assault their religious, political, and cultural beliefs. Also unfortunately, due to misinformation and disinformation (and in the case of Great

Britain's *The Cass Review*, I believe, outright scientific fraud), they are getting a lot of traction.

89. Gould, *The Mismeasure of Man*.
90. Goddard, *The Kallikak Family*.
91. The history of mental measurement and its eventual replacement by newer and better models of intelligence and the rise and fall of the medical model of transsexualism are illustrations of what Thomas Kuhn wrote about in his 1968 classic work the *The Structure of Scientific Revolutions*.
92. Other than the few who were purposefully cruel, sadistic, or uncaring.

WORKS CITED

Bak, Robert C., and Walter A. Stewart. "Fetishism, Transvestism, and Voyeurism: A Psychoanalytic Approach." In *American Handbook of Psychiatry*, edited by S. Arieti and E. Brady 2nd ed., 352–63. New York: Basic Books, 1974.

Benjamin, Harry. *The Transsexual Phenomenon*. New York: Julian Press, 1966.

Billings, Dwight B., and Thomas Urban. "The Socio-Medical Construction of Transsexualism: An Interpretation and Critique." *Social Problems* 29 (1982): 266–82.

Blanchard, Ray, Leonard H. Clemmensen, and Betty W. Steiner. Heterosexual and homosexual gender dysphoria. *Archives of Sexual Behavior* 16, no. 2 (1987): 139–52.

Bolin, Anne. *In Search of Eve: Transsexual Rites of Passage*. South Hadley, MA: Bergin & Garvey, 1988.

Bornstein, Kate. *Gender Outlaw: On Men, Women, and the Rest of Us*. New York: Routledge, 1994.

Brown, Kay. "Angela Keyes Douglas." TransHistory, 1998. Accessed July 25, 2020. https://web.archive.org/web/20050305102212fw_/http://www.transhistory.org/history/TH_Angela_Douglas.html.

Buckley, Thomas. "A Changing of Sex by Surgery Begun at Johns Hopkins: Johns Hopkins Becomes First U.S. Hospital to Undertake Program of Sex Change through Surgery." *New York Times*, November 21, 1966, 1. Accessed August 4, 2020. https://ai.eecs.umich.edu/people/conway/TS/TimesArticle.html.

Burou, Georges. "Male-to-Female Transformation." In *Proceedings of the Second Interdisciplinary Symposium on Gender Dysphoria Syndrome*, edited by Donald Laub and P. Gandy, 188–94. Palo Alto, CA: Stanford University Medical Center, 1973. Accessed July 2, 2020. http://ai.eecs.umich.edu/people/conway/TS/Burou/Burou.html.

Cass, Hillary. *The Cass Report: Independent Review of Gender Identity Services for Children and Young People*. 2004. Accessed August 11, 2024. https://cass.independent-review.uk/home/publications/final-report/.

Clemmensen, L. H. "The 'Real-Life Test' for Surgical Candidates." In *Clinical Management of Gender Identity Disorders in Children and Adults*, edited by R. Blanchard and B. W. Steiner, 119–35. Washington, DC: American Psychiatric Press, 1990.

Cooper, M. A. "Hormone Treatment Clinic for Transsexuals." *Hawaii Medical Journal* 43, no. 5 (1984): 142, 144, 146, 149.

Cussins, Jessica. "Sweden Repeals Forced Sterilization for Transgender People." *Psychology Today*, January 25, 2013. Accessed July 27, 2020. https://www.psychologytoday.com/us/blog/genetic-crossroads/201301/sweden-repeals-forced-sterilization-transgender-people.

Day, Megan. "How One of America's Best Medical Schools Started a Secret Transgender Surgery Clinic." *Timeline*, November 15, 2016.

Denny, Dallas. "All We Were Allowed to Write: Transsexual Autobiographies in the Late XXth and early XXIst Centuries." Workshop presented at Fantasia Fair, Provincetown, MA, October 22, 2014. Accessed July 13, 2020.

———. "Are Transsexuals as Reliable as Other People?" *Insight* 6, no. 1 (1990): 5–6.

———. "Black Telephones, White Refrigerators: Rethinking Christine Jorgensen." In *Current Concepts in Transgender Identity*, edited by Dallas Denny, 35–44. New York: Garland Publishing, 1998. Accessed August 11, 2024. http://dallasdenny.com/Writing/2014/02/16/black-telephones-white-refrigerators-rethinking-christine-jorgensen-1998/.

———. "The Campaigns Against Transsexuals: Part I: The Conspiracy at Johns Hopkins University." Presentation at Southern Comfort Conference, Atlanta, GA, September 5, 2013. Accessed July 25, 2020. http://dallasdenny.com/Writing/2014/03/06/the-campaign-against-transsexuals-part-i-2013/.

———, ed. *Current Concepts in Transgender Identity*. New York: Garland Publishing, 1998.

———. *Gender Dysphoria: A Guide to Research*. 1st ed. New York: Garland Publishing, 1994.

———. "Letter to the Editor: Response to Charles Mate-Kole's Review of Ann Bolin's. *In Search of Eve: Transsexual Rites of Passage.*" *Archives of Sexual Behavior* 22, no. 2 (1993): 167–69.

———. "Letter to Paul McHugh." May 20, 1994. Accessed July 25, 2020. http://dallasdenny.com/Writing/2011/11/01/letter-to-paul-mchugh-1984/.

———. "Not Screwed up Enough: Managing Trans Identity Then and Now." Keynote at Trans Awareness Week, University of Missouri at Columbia, MO, November 13, 2013. Accessed July 9, 2020. http://dallasdenny.com/Writing/2014/03/13/im-not-screwed-up-enough-2013/.

———. "The Politics of Diagnosis and a Diagnosis of Politics: The University-Affiliated Gender Clinics, and How They Failed to Meet the Need of Transsexual People." *Chrysalis Quarterly* 1, no. 3 (Winter 1991–1992): 9–20. Accessed July 8, 2020.

http://dallasdenny.com/Writing/2013/10/05/the-politics-of-diagnosis-and-a-diagnosis-of-politics-1991/. Reprinted in *Transgender Tapestry* 1, no. 98 (Summer 2002): 17–27.

———. "Quotations from the Literature." *Chrysalis Quarterly* 1, no. 1 (Spring 1991): 6. Accessed July 22, 2020. http://dallasdenny.com/Writing/wp-content/uploads/2013/12/Chrysalis-V.-1-No.-1-aa10.pdf.

———. "Writing Ourselves." *TransSisters: Journal of Transsexual Feminism* 8 (Spring 1995): 38–39. Reprinted in *Proceedings of Third International Conference on Transgender Law and Employment Policy*, edited by Phyllis Frye, P. Houston. TX: International Conference on Transgender Law & Employment Policy, 1994. Accessed July 13, 2020. http://dallasdenny.com/Writing/2011/10/05/writing-ourselves/.

———. "You Make Me Sick!: A Critique of the Psychological and Medical Literature of Transsexualism." Paper presentation at Trans-Progressing Symposium, Fantasia Fair, Provincetown, MA, October 17–24, 2004. Accessed July 9, 2020. http://dallasdenny.com/Writing/2013/08/24/you-make-me-sick-2004/.

Douglas, Angela. "Letter to the Editor." *Sister*. August–September 1997.

Downing, Lisa, Iain Morland, and Nikki Sullivan. "Pervert or Sexual Libertarian: Meet John Money, 'The Father of F***ology.'" *Salon*, 2015. Accessed July 3, 2020. https://www.salon.com/2015/01/04/pervert_or_sexual_libertarian_meet_john_money_the_father_of_fology/. Excerpted from Downing, Lisa, Iain Moreland, and Nikki Sullivan. *Fuckology: Critical Essays on John Money's Diagnostic Concepts*. Chicago, IL: University of Chicago Press, 2014.

Edgerton, Milton T. "The Role of Surgery in the Treatment of Transsexualism." *Annals of Plastic Surgery* 13, no. 6 (1984): 473–81.

Ehrhardt, Anke. *John Money: A Tribute on the Occasion of his 70th Birthday*, xi–xvi. New York: Haworth Press, 1991.

Fleming, Michael, Steinman Carol, and Gene Bocknek. "Methodological Problems in Assessing Sex-Reassignment Surgery: A reply to Meyer and Reter." *Archives of Sexual Behavior* 9, no. 5 (October 1980): 451–56.

Fritz, Melanie, and Nat Mulkey. "The Rise and Fall of Gender Clinics in the 1960s and 1970s." Bulletin of the American College of Surgeons, April 1, 2021. Accessed August 22, 2021. https://bulletin.facs.org/2021/04/the-rise-and-fall-of-gender-identity-clinics-in-the-1960s-and-1970s/.

Goddard, Henry H. *The Kallikak Family: A Study in the Heredity of Feeble Mindedness*. New York: MacMillan, 1912.

Goffman, Erving. *Asylums: Essays on the Social Situation of Mental Patients and Other Inmates*. New York: Doubleday, 1961.

———. *Stigma: Notes on the Management of Spoiled Identity*. Englewood Cliffs, NJ: Prentice-Hall, 1963.

Gould, Stephen Jay. *The Mismeasure of Man*. New York: W. W. Norton, 1981.

Green, Jamison. *Becoming a Visible Man.* 2nd ed. Nashville, TN: Vanderbilt University Press, 2020.
Green, Jamison, Dallas Denny, and Jason Cromwell. "What Do You Want Us to Call You? Respectful Language." *Transgender Studies Quarterly* 5, no. 1 (2018): 100–10.
Green, Richard, Robert J. Stoller, and C. MacAndrew. "Attitudes Toward Sex Transformation Procedures." *Archives of General Psychiatry* 15 (1966): 178–82.
Green, Richard. *Gay Rights, Trans Rights: A Psychiatrist/lawyer's 50-year Battle.* Printed by the author, 2018.
———. "Physician Emotionalism in the Treatment of the Transsexual." *Transactions of the New York Academy of Sciences* 29, no. 4 (1967): 440–43.
———. *The Sissy Boy Syndrome: The Development of Homosexuality.* New Haven, CT: Yale University Press, 1987.
Green, Richard, and John Money, eds. *Transsexualism and Sex Reassignment.* Baltimore, MD: Johns Hopkins University Press, 1969.
Green, Richard, Robert J. Stoller, and Craig MacAndrew. "Attitudes Toward Sex Transformation Procedures." *Archives of General Psychiatry* 15 (1966): 178–82.
Hamburger, Christian. "The Desire for Change of Sex as Shown by Personal Letters from 465 Men and Women." *Acta Endocrinologica* 14, no. 4 (1953): 361–75.
Hastings, Donald W. "Inauguration of a Research Project on Transsexualism in a University Medical System." In *Transsexualism and Sex Reassignment*, R. Green and J. Money, eds., 243–52. Baltimore, MD: Johns Hopkins University Press, 1969.
Haynes, Suyin. "The World Health Organization Will Stop Classifying Transgender People as Having a 'Mental Disorder.'" *Time*, May 28, 2019. Accessed July 17, 2020. https://time.com/5596845/world-health-organization-transgender-identity/.
Hodgkinson, Liz. *Michael Nee Laura.* London: Columbus Books, 1989.
"Infighting Rages at Hopkins." *The Gateway* 2, no. 6 (December 1979): 9–10. Accessed July 25, 2020. https://www.digitaltransgenderarchive.net/files/4x51hj12b.
International Alliance for Male Feminism. "That Infamous Meyer-Reter Report." *Journal of Male Feminism* 1 (1980): 8–11. Accessed July 25, 2020. https://www.digitaltransgenderarchive.net/files/5138jf05g.
Kessler, Suzanne J. and Wendy McKenna. *Gender: An Ethnomethodological Approach.* New York: John Wiley & Sons, 1978.
Kuhn, Thomas. *The Structure of Scientific Revolutions.* Chicago, IL: University of Chicago Press, 1968.
Laub, Donald R., and Norman Fisk. "A Rehabilitation Program for Gender Dysphoria Syndrome by Surgical Sex Change." *Plastic and Reconstructive Surgery* 53, no. 4 (1974): 388–403.
Levy-Lenz, Ludwig. Quoted on Rudolph R. Dorchen page of the Magnus-Hirschfeld-Gesellschaft website. Accessed July 23, 2021. https://www.hirschfeld.in-berlin.de/institut/en/personen/pers_34.html.

Lothstein, Leslie. *Female-to-Male Transsexualism: Historical, Clinical and Theoretical Issues.* Boston, MA: Routledge & Kegan Paul, 1983.

Mancini, Elena. *Magnus Hirschfeld and the Quest for Scientific Freedom.* New York: Palgrave Macmillan, 2010.

Mate-Kole, Charles. "Review of A. Bolin. In *Search of Eve: Transsexual Rites of Passage.*" *Archives of Sexual Behavior* 21, no. 2 (1992): 207–10.

McHugh, Paul R. "Psychiatric Misadventures." *American Scholar* 61, no. 4 (1992): 497–510.

———. "Surgical Sex: Why We Stopped Doing Sex Change Operations." First Things, 2004. Accessed July 24, 2020. https://www.firstthings.com/article/2004/11/surgical-sex.

Meerloo, Joost A. M. "Change of Sex and Collaboration with the Psychosis." *American Journal of Psychiatry* 124, no. 2 (1967): 263–64.

Meyer, Jon K., and Donna J. Reter. "Sex Reassignment: Follow-up." *Archives of General Psychiatry* 36, no. 9 (1979): 1010–15.

Meyerowitz, Joanne. *How Sex Changed: A History of Transsexuality in the United States.* Cambridge: Harvard University Press, 2002.

Milliken, A. Donald. "Homicidal Transsexuals: Three Cases." *Canadian Journal of Psychiatry* 27, no. 1 (1982): 43–6.

Money, John, and Clay Primrose. "Sexual Dimorphism and Dissociation in the Psychology of Male Transsexuals." *Journal of Nervous and Mental Disease* 147, no. 5 (1968): 472–86.

Money, John, and Florence Schwartz. "Public Opinion and Social Issues in Transsexualism: A Case Study in Medical Sexology." In *Transsexualism and Sex Reassignment*, edited by Richard Green and John Money, 253–69. Baltimore, MD: Johns Hopkins Press, 1969.

Ogas, Ogi. "Spare Parts: New Information Reignites a Controversy Surrounding the Hopkins Gender Identity Clinic." *City Paper* 18, no. 10 (March 9, 1994): 10, 12–15.

Oppenheim, Garrett. "The Holes in Meyer's Study." *Transition (Confide Counseling Services)* 11 (1979).

———. Meyer's Survey Draws Fire from Leading Authorities. *Transition (Confide Counseling Services)* 11 (1979).

Pauly, Ira B. "Female Transsexualism: Parts I & II." *Archives of Sexual Behavior* 3, no. 6 (1974): 487–07, 509–25.

———. "Female to Gay Male Transsexualism." Paper presented at the XI Harry Benjamin International Gender Dysphoria Association Symposium, Cleveland, OH, September 20–23, 1989.

———. "Gender Identity and Sexual Orientation." In *Current Concepts in Transgender Identity*, edited by Dallas Denny, 238–48. New York: Garland Publishing: 1998.

Person, Ethyl, and Lionel Ovesey. "The Transsexual Syndrome in Males: I. Primary Transsexualism." *American Journal of Psychotherapy* 28 (1974): 4–20.

———. "The Transsexual Syndrome in Males: II. Secondary Transsexualism." *American Journal of Psychotherapy* 28 (1974): 174–93.

Pierce, D., I. Pauly, and R. Matarrazzo. "The Psychosocial Characteristics of the Wives and Girlfriends of Female-to-Male Transsexuals." Proceedings of the 7th Harry Benjamin International Gender Dysphoria Conference, Lake Tahoe, NV, 1981, p. 73.

Raymond, Janice. *The Transsexual Empire: The Making of the SheMale.* Boston, MA: Beacon Press, 1979.

Roback, Howard B., and Leslie M. Lothstein. "The Female Mid-Life Sex Change Applicant: A Comparison with Younger Female Transsexuals and Older Male Sex Change Applicants." *Archives of Sexual Behavior* 15 (1986): 401–15.

Rohrer, Megan. "Lou Sullivan: Battling Gender Specialists." 1988 Accessed August 12, 20224. https://www.youtube.com/watch?v=SxgZNNX-v2g.

Rosenhan, David L. "On Being Sane in Insane Places." *Science* 179, no. 4070 (1973): 250–58. https//doi.org/10.1126/science.179.4070.250.

Rothblatt, Martine. *The Apartheid of Sex: A Manifesto on the Freedom of Gender.* New York: Crown Publishers, 1994.

Shuster, Stef M. *Trans Medicine: The Emergence and Practice of Treating Gender.* New York: New York University Press, 2021.

Siotos, Charlampos, Paula M. Neira, Brandyn D. Lau, et al. "Origins of Gender Affirmation Surgery: The History of the First Gender Identity Clinic in the United States at Johns Hopkins." *Annals of Plastic Surgery* 83, no. 2 (August 2019): 132–36.

Smith, Matthew Nitch. "The 24 Most Prestigious Universities in the World, According to *Times Higher Education*." Business Insider, May 10, 2016. Accessed July 8, 2020. https://www.businessinsider.com/the-24-best-universities-in-the-world-by-reputation.

Smith, Phoebe. *Phoebe.* Atlanta, GA: Self-published by the author, 1979. Reprinted as *From Sharecropper's Son to Who's Who in American Women: Phoebe Smith, Transsexual Pioneer*, 2014.

Steiner, Betty W. "Intake Assessment of Gender-Dysphoric Patients." In *Clinical Management of Gender Identity Disorder in Children and Adults,* edited by Ray Blanchard and Betty W. Steiner, 93–106. Washington, DC: American Psychiatric Press, 1990.

Stoller, Robert J. "Near Miss: 'Sex Change' Treatment and Its Evaluation." In *Eating, Sleeping, and Sexuality*, edited by M. R. Zales, 258–83. New York: Brunner/Mazel, 1982.

Stone, Allucquére Rosanne (as Sandy Stone). "The Empire Strikes Back: A Posttranssexual Manifesto." In *Body Guards: The Cultural Politics of Gender Ambiguity,* edited by Julia Epstein and Kristina Straub, 280–304. New York: Routledge, 1991. Accessed July 13, 2020. http://sites.middlebury.edu/soan191/files/2013/08/StoneEmpire1.pdf.

Stone, C. B. "Psychiatric Screening for Transsexual Surgery." *Psychosomatics* 18, no. 1 (1977): 25–27.

Times Higher Education. "World University Rankings 2020." Accessed July 8, 2020. https://www.timeshighereducation.com/world-university-rankings/2020/world-ranking#!/page/0/length/25/sort_by/rank/sort_order/asc/cols/stats.

Tornqvist, Ann. "Sweden's Shameful Transgender Sterilization Rule." *Salon*, November 2, 2011. Accessed July 25, 2020. https://www.salon.com/2011/11/02/sweden_transgender_sterilization/.

Walker, Paul A., Jack C. Berger, Richard Green, Donald R. Laub, Charles L. Reynolds Jr., and Leo Wollman. *Standards of Care: The Hormonal and Surgical Sex Reassignment of Gender Dysphoric Persons.* Baltimore: Harry Benjamin International Gender Dysphoria Association, 1979.

"What's Wrong with "Stanford?" *The Gateway* 3, no. 2 (August 1980): 3. Accessed July 25, 2020. https://www.digitaltransgenderarchive.net/files/0z708w53f.

Witkin, Rachel. "Hopkins Hospital: A History of Sex Reassignment." *Johns Hopkins Newsletter*, May 1, 2014. Accessed August 3, 2020. https://www.jhunewsletter.com/article/2014/05/hopkins-hospital-a-history-of-sex-reassignment-76004/.

12

TRANS RIGHTS AS CIVIL RIGHTS

Carolyn Wolf-Gould

During the civil rights era of the 1960s, groups of Americans suffering under systems of oppression rose in linked or disparate groups to fight for freedom and justice. While movements on racial equity, women's rights, and gay liberation feature prominently in the historical record, the fight for trans rights is rarely included. And yet, advances around civil and human rights for transgender and gender-diverse (TGD) citizens, including the right to inclusive healthcare, also emerged during this tumultuous period. While some TGD individuals and groups found support from adjacent liberation movements, others suffered rejection. The fight for the right to trans-inclusive and affirming healthcare remains rooted in the struggles of this time and subsequent decades—battles that continue to inflame and divide our country and healthcare system today. This chapter describes some of the events (and repercussions) that gave rise to trans rights, a liberation movement that compelled the development of inclusive healthcare practices.

McCARTHYISM AND THE LAVENDER SCARE

In the late 1950s, the government's fear of Communist infiltration engendered McCarthyism, a campaign that relentlessly attacked the character of governmental employees, largely based on unsubstantiated charges of communist collusion. These attacks also targeted those who deviated from heteronormative cultural values, triggering increased homosexual repression. In what has since been dubbed the Lavender Scare, the US Senate held hearings on homosexuals and "other sex perverts" who worked for the government, sparking the purge of thousands of government employees, an increase in police surveillance of LGBT+ communities, discharges from the military, and arrests for homosexual activities.[1] The lives and careers of scores of LGBT+ people were publicly destroyed, and many gay men focused on passing as heterosexual to ensure safety.

The homophile movement, the first gay civil rights movement in the United States, was formed in response to this repression; however, this first iteration tended to attract members from privileged white, upperclass, and educated backgrounds—particularly men who held traditional attitudes regarding masculinity. The homophiles and closeted homosexuals engaged in bitter debates about "swishes," gay men with feminine mannerisms that drew negative attention to their cause.[2] The American public watched, and although many were horrified by the purges, effeminate gay men absorbed the fact that swishing led to exposure, public shaming, and loss of employment, and they modified their behaviors accordingly. These assaults magnified suspicion, revulsion, and violence toward those assigned male at birth who not only demonstrated feminine expressions but also possessed feminine gender identities, pushing TGD women further into societal margins.

THE COMPTON'S CAFETERIA RIOTS AND THE STONEWALL UPRISING

While the Stonewall Uprising of 1969 galvanized the gay rights movement, the lesser-known San Francisco Compton's Cafeteria riots of 1966 marked the beginning of the transgender rights movement. Around this time, trans individuals and activists, emboldened by the Civil Rights Movement, began to speak out about their communities' specific, intersectional, social, and healthcare needs, drawing attention to disparities hitherto ignored or dismissed by society and healthcare systems. For the first time, transgender people who existed on the margins of society—street youth, sex workers—rose and organized to demand basic rights. When their individual efforts failed, they created their own organizations.

It started at Compton's.

In the 1960s, Compton's Cafeteria, a twenty-four-hour coffee shop in San Francisco's Tenderloin District, became the gathering place for the drag queens and transgender sex workers who earned their living hustling the nearby streets.[3] Rejected by their families and communities, these self-described "gutter girls"[4] were unable to find traditional employment. They gravitated to the Tenderloin because "we wanted to make a living and wanted to be loved."[5] The women met at Compton's to find comfort in community and escape harassment. Compton's staff periodically tipped off the police, who raided the cafeteria to arrest and imprison these women for the crime of female impersonation.

The Vietnam War and various civil rights movements had challenged traditional concepts regarding gender performance and roles. Men grew their hair long and wore love beads; women burned their bras and stepped out of the home for employment. The feminist movement empowered not only women but also lesbian and gay rights agendas. Gender roles shifted and expanded within a sociopolitical revolution that encouraged transgender people, including the women who gathered at Compton's, to embrace their identities. In 1964, in response to tumultuous social change, President Lyndon B. Johnson launched the Great Society with the intent to eliminate poverty and racial injustice. The War on Poverty included funding for community-based programs that provided education and job training for unemployed minorities, but these programs did not value or extend support to the Tenderloin women.

Civil rights activists demanded that discrimination against gender and sexual minorities be included in their agendas.[6] Responding to this call, San Francisco's Glide Memorial United Methodist Church developed a mission to support the disenfranchised of their community. Staff reached out to homophile groups and Tenderloin residents to encourage them to organize and advocate for their rights. LGBT+ youth formed Vanguard, an independent gay youth organization affiliated with Glide Church to educate themselves and the public that (1) being gay was natural and nothing to be ashamed of; (2) they were entitled to respect and equal rights and treatment; and (3) they could demonstrate for their right to equal treatment and to end discrimination.[7] Vanguard members picketed businesses that discriminated against LGBT+ patrons, including Compton's Cafeteria, where they faced discriminatory charges and time limits at tables.[8]

Historian Susan Stryker described the rebellion in the film *Screaming Queens: The Riot at Compton's Cafeteria*: "Management didn't like the uppity new political attitude some of its customers were starting to express. This friction lit the fuse that led directly to the Compton Riots."[9] During the next raid at Compton's, a cop grabbed a queen, who threw her coffee in his face, and pandemonium ensued.[10] The customers hurled saltshakers, cups, and plates, and shattered the restaurant's front windows. Patrons poured onto the street to fight the police. According to Stryker, "It was the first known incident of collective militant queer resistance to police harassment in US history."[11]

After the riot, the TGD people of the Tenderloin began work to change the rules that oppressed them. Lacking the white, heteronormative, economic, and class privilege of those like Christine Jorgensen, they found strength in community and agency through organization. They asserted their humanity, referring to themselves as healthy women in possession of diverse gender identities—not biologically muddled or mentally ill, as sex workers—not prostitutes. They worked with police officer Elliott Blackstone to change the laws that led to harassment, such as one that criminalized cross-dressing; they worked with physician Joel Fort, who founded the Center for Special Problems, and began issuing identification cards with an individual's identified gender and name, a process that enabled transsexuals to obtain training and jobs through government programs. The first gender clinic on the West Coast opened at Stanford in 1968, and although it was still difficult for the people in the Tenderloin to access this care, clinics like this one cemented the resolve of many to pursue medical transitions.[12] The general American public did not value or hear much about the TGD Tenderloin population; yet as these individuals acknowledged their self-worth and became activists, they planted seeds in the cultural soil, which eventually bloomed into current efforts to address diversity, equity, and inclusion in healthcare.

The more widely known Stonewall Uprising of 1969 moved the fight for LGBT+ rights into the national spotlight. In the 1960s, police systematically raided and harassed Greenwich Village gay bars known to be operating without New York State Liquor Authority licenses, which were typically withheld from gay bars.[13] The Stonewall Inn differed from other establishments in that it catered not only to the gay community but also to those LGBT+ people who were often rejected by this same community—the "drags, queens," and the young street youth.[14] On June 28, 1969, the police raided the Stonewall Inn, arrested the employees, and ordered its patrons to leave.[15] The customers filed outside to wait on the pavement, and when the cops emerged, threw pennies, beer cans, rocks, and even a parking meter at them, and then set the building on fire.[16] Skirmishes between hundreds of cops and thousands of LGBT+ protestors and bystanders lasted for six days, a wild confrontation that included the arrest of Mafia saloon owners, the use of fire hoses on crowds, a firebomb, loud songs warbled in high camp style, gay cheerleaders, kick-line dancing, and a drag queen bashing a cop on the head with her purse.[17] This spectacle lit the US news cycle with rainbow pyrotechnics, leading to a new sense of gay pride and an altered cultural consciousness.

The year 1969 marked a political awakening of the LGBT+ community in New York City, as well as intensive work to organize, advocate for human rights, and transform the politics of sexuality.[18] The Mattachine Society of New York, the Daughters of Bilitis, the East Coast Homophile Organization, the Gay Liberation Front, the Gay Activist Alliance, and other organizations (some of which had existed since the 1950s but had kept fairly low profiles) demanded gay civil rights, including the provision of legal and medical care.[19]

Yet transsexuals and transvestites even faced rejection in the context of LBGT+ activism. Cisnormative, classist, and racist cultural biases prevailed in homosexual spaces. At homophile events, lesbian, gay, and bisexual people complained that the transsexuals were too loud, badly dressed, the wrong color, low class, even prostitutes. This rejection inflicted deep wounds on TGD communities and fed national cultural anti-trans perceptions. Stung by this dismissal, TGD people began to carve out a separate liberation movement independent of LGBT+ rights. They established organizations that furthered their specific social and medical needs. In 1970, Sylvia Rivera and Marsha P. Johnson, disturbed by the health risks of young transvestites who supported themselves through sex work, organized Street Transvestite Action Revolutionaries, a collective to share support, food, and money; they also created a homeless shelter.[20] In 1969, Lee Brewster founded the Queens Liberation Front, a group that successfully fought anti-transvestism laws in New York. In 1964, Reed Erickson founded the Erickson Educational Foundation, the leading source of support for research, referrals, and public and professional education regarding gender dysphoria for the next twenty years.[21] This activism furthered the development of racially and economically diverse TGD communities and the realization that such communities could create powerful institutions and effect social change, including access to healthcare.

COMMUNITY ACTIVISM, THE AIDS EPIDEMIC, AND OVERLAPPING SYSTEMS OF OPPRESSION

The AIDS epidemic, which began in the 1980s, imposed a heavy burden on transgender women, especially Black women and/or those with low socioeconomic status, those whose rights had been previously championed by Johnson and Rivera.[22] To survive, members of this vulnerable population practiced high-risk behaviors, including sex work and substance use, putting them at risk for the virus.[23] Once diagnosed with HIV, they faced multiple barriers to care due to fear of rejection in medical facilities, lack of insurance, lack of money, lack of trans-competent clinicians, lack of programs designed for their needs, and persistent harassment in medical offices—creating a vicious circle of exposure, transmission, illness, and death. At the onset of the epidemic, clinicians and researchers conflated sexuality and gender identity, lumping transgender women into the same category as men who had sex with men; medical practitioners also excluded them from clinical trials. This process rendered their unique struggles and vulnerabilities invisible to public health efforts, and as a result, TGD women, unwilling or unable to seek care at HIV clinics that ignored their identities and specific health needs, continued to sicken and die.

As the HIV epidemic continued, clinicians and activist community members eventually recognized the need to respond to the unique needs of subsets of the TGD population. In 1989, Kimberlé Crenshaw, a pioneering scholar and writer on civil rights, Black feminist legal theory, race, racism, critical race theory, and the law, introduced her framework of intersectionality.[24] Under the rubric of Black, feminist theory, she argued that social identities (for instance, race, class, and gender) did not exist in separate compartments but rather in a fluid, intersecting manner.[25] For example, transgender women of color faced compounded oppression based on race, class, and gender, rendering them unseen to the medical or community assistance programs designed to serve those with less complex social identities. Crenshaw insisted that to address institutionalized discrimination, society must recognize an individual's multiple intersectional identities and consider how these identities together exacerbate oppression and limit access to care.

Healthcare professionals and the communities that they served also (slowly) began to study and discuss power relationships within medical institutions, especially gendered and racist policies that created additional barriers to care. In the following decades, medical and community groups began to challenge deficit models that suggested race and behavior led to educational and health are disparities,[26] instead identifying white supremacy culture as the leading cause of such disparities.

HIV programs began to focus on cultural assets that promoted community wellness. Public health organizations began to seek out the voices from subsets of the TGD community, those advocating for specific health needs. HIV clinics began offering hormone therapy to attract those requiring treatment or at risk for HIV. They provided mental health services, referrals for gender-affirming surgery, assistance with employment, and housing. They trained their clinicians in cultural competency and acknowledged the diversity within the trans community with targeted programs for specific groups. Medical and community programs also began to consider the importance of self-esteem and self-advocacy in the prevention of disease. Communities of color organized their own health interventions. For example, house and ballroom events not only offered a safe and celebratory venue for LGBT+ black and Latinx communities but also provided critical HIV education and programs to connect individuals with medical services.

WOMEN'S RIGHTS, TRANS RIGHTS, AND TRANS EXCLUSIVE RADICAL FEMINISTS

In the 1970s and 1980s, cisgender, female academics influenced by the women's rights and civil rights movements, began to contest the stereotypical and pathologizing expectations of the gender clinics and object to the research methods that defined transgender embodiment. White, cisgender men had published the early medical papers, and as feminist scholars increasingly entered academia, they employed radically different study techniques, including the sociocultural research tools of anthropologists and ethnomethodologists: participant observation, field immersion, and historical interviews. In contrast to those performing research in the gender clinics, the academics lacked the power to deny or further medical transition based on participant response. Not surprisingly, their studies yielded dramatically different results.

In 1976, sociologist Deborah Feinbloom published *Transvestites & Transsexuals*,[27] describing an astonishingly diverse community with a continuum of gender identities and expressions.[28] Her participants decried the cultural expectation that they conform to a gender binary with normative sexual orientations. Feinbloom detailed disparate family structures, some disorganized and dysfunctional, others loving and intact. She portrayed the experience of transgender men, who had been largely dismissed and ignored by the gender clinics. She defined a community with diverse educational experiences, professional talents, social and socioeconomic status, and an assortment of personalities. Some passed, and some did not; some found the concept of passing oppressive.[29] Some wished to present in normative feminine roles and attract men; others did not fuss with clothing or identified as feminist lesbians. Some successfully negotiated committed relationships and jobs; others suffered from family rejection and loss of employment. Many complained that the concept of sex reassignment did not consider the unique experience of women who grew up in male bodies. They explained that the reason for surgery was not, as assumed by the clinics, always about sex. Most desired surgery for the peace of having their gender identity align with their body. The only thing interviewees did have in common was the shared experience of transsexualism and the desire to learn about it, help themselves, and support one another. They had developed community.

In 1978, social psychologist Suzanne Kessler and sociologist Wendy McKenna published *Gender An Ethnomethodological Approach*,[30] positing that gender was not a biologic reality, but rather a social construction—the gender binary existed because of socially shared, taken-for-granted methods, which members used to construct reality, and varied across cultures.[31] They described the gender attribution process by which people classify someone as male or female based on learned rules for seeing two genders. In 1988, anthropologist Ann Bolin published *In Search of Eve*,[32] criticizing the assumption of transsexual homogeneity and the rigid eligibility criteria imposed by the gender clinics, arguing that it forced patients to lie to get treatment.[33] She debunked the idea that trans women universally experienced childhoods with dominant, overprotective mothers and absent fathers; effeminate childhoods; hated their penises; and were attracted only to men. She railed against literature that stigmatized transsexuality as a mental illness and was at first rejected for publication because the editors believed she must be a transsexual herself.[34] Transgender patients and activists, some influenced by their lived experiences and others by publications like these, resented the limited and pathologizing approach imposed by the medical community and began to demand systemic change. While most Americans did not read the texts or know about their ramifications, the culture's monolithic view of the transsexual experience slowly began to dissolve in some spaces, giving way to an emerging appreciation for the diversity of this human phenomenon.

In the 1970s, the lives of transgender women clashed with feminist philosophy and politics, a powerful and wrenching tension that escalated sociocultural transphobia but paradoxically led to the emergence of trans studies as a social and academic paradigm in the 1990s. In 1973, singer Beth Elliot, a transsexual woman, performed at the West Coast Lesbian Conference, inciting the anger of other participants, who felt "transsexual men" should not be allowed to infiltrate spaces intended for cisgender women.[35] The keynote speaker announced:

"I will not call a male 'she;' thirty-two years of suffering in the androcentric society, and of surviving, have earned me the title 'woman'; one walk down the street by a male transvestite, five minutes of his being hassled (which he may enjoy), and then he dares, he dares to think he understands our pain? No, in our mothers' names and in our own, we must not call him sister."[36] Conference participants brought the controversy home to their regional women's groups, where antipathy toward the transsexual community began to simmer and steam. Radical feminists and other women's groups argued for and against trans-inclusion in person, in print, and online, with one woman eventually coining the term trans exclusionary radical feminist (TERF) to describe those feminists who dismissed trans women as members of the sisterhood.[37]

In 1979, Janice Raymond brought the TERF's worldview to full boil with the publication of *The Transsexual Empire: The Making of the She-Male*,[38] a hostile polemic against transsexual women and the patriarchal medical empire that "constructed"[39] them. In her view, surgical transition, which she considered largely a male phenomenon, resulted only in the creation of artificial women due to the biologic imperative of the XY chromosomes and masculine cultural histories "unencumbered by the scars of patriarchy that are unique to a woman's personal and social history."[40] She maintained that transsexual surgeries, designed and performed by men for men, perpetuated centuries of sex-role oppression by molding women to meet men's rigid standards of femininity.[41] Raymond despised the transsexuals who conformed to masculine-defined feminine roles, but far worse in her mind was the transsexually constructed lesbian-feminist, who "attempts to possess women at a deeper level."[42] These individuals "insert themselves into the positions of importance and/or performance in the feminist community"[43] with obtrusively masculine behaviors that violate women and their spaces, an act she referred to as "rape."[44]

What is perhaps most remarkable about Raymond's diatribe is that it received admiring reviews from healthcare professionals. In the *New York Times*, psychiatrist Thomas Szasz called it, "flawless . . . an important achievement."[45] The National Center for Health Care Technology and Office of Health Technology commissioned Raymond to write a paper on the "social and ethical aspects of transsexual surgery" to inform their official reports, concluding that these procedures were controversial and expensive and considered experimental.[46] For decades, these documents influenced insurance companies, clinicians, hospital administrations, health policy analysts, and government administrators who banned coverage for transgender care. Christian conservatives later teamed up with TERFS, applying their vitriolic rhetoric to "protect women," positions that eventually led to the bathroom bans—laws that prohibited TGD people from using the restroom that aligned with their gender identity.[47] The American public listened, absorbed the anger, and added the term *she-male* to the cultural lexicon for disparaging trans women.

Feminist women's events, informed by ongoing complaints from the TERFs, responded to increasing organization and insistence on trans rights by developing trans exclusionary policies. The Michigan Womyn's Music Festival, Michfest, a feminist women's music festival held on private land annually from 1976 to 2015, hosted a "transformative . . . female utopia," a place where, for many, it was "the first or only time we've ever felt truly 100% safe from harassment, objectification, judgment, violence, rape."[48] In 1991, festival organizers asked Nancy Burkholder, a transgender woman,[49] to leave, maintaining that this event had been created by and for womyn-born womyn: ". . . [those] who were born as and have lived their entire life experience as womyn."[50] Trans activists protested the trans exclusionary practices and, the following year, established Camp Trans on a site across the road from the festival. They allied with festival subgroups, negotiated with Michfest organizers, and were eventually admitted.[51] Trans men, many of whom attended Michfest as dykes (and some of whom injected their first shots of testosterone at the festival), are largely ignored by historians of this event, as they often are to this day.[52]

In 2015, after artists and LGBT+ organizations boycotted the festival due to its continuing trans exclusionary policies, Michfest shut down, with its organizer announcing, "The Festival has been a crucible for nearly every critical cultural and political issue the lesbian feminist community has grappled with for four decades. Those struggles have been a beautiful part of our collective strength; they have never been a weakness."[53] American feminists reacted to news reports on the dispute and formed polarized opinions—ones that persist to this day—for or against the right for trans women to participate in women's spaces, use bathrooms that align with their gender, and on other trans-related issues such as the use of trans-inclusive medical language (that is, people with a cervix need PAP tests) and gender-affirming medical care for TGD youth.[54]

THE EMERGENCE OF TRANS STUDIES

In 1992, Sandy Stone published "*The Empire Strikes Back: A Posttranssexual Manifesto*,"[55] a response to Raymond's *The Transsexual Empire* and a work now regarded as the foundation of the academic field of trans studies. Raymond attacked Stone, a transgender woman, in *The Transsexual Empire* for presenting herself as female and working as a sound engineer in the Olivia Women's Music Collective. In *The Empire Strikes Back*, Stone explored the popular stories about transsexuals that replicated the stereotypical male view that in general, women wore dresses and makeup and fainted at the sight of blood—a position that bore a remarkable resemblance to the eligibility requirements of the gender clinics.[56] Stone astutely asserted: "The origin of the gender dysphoria clinics is a microcosmic look at the construction of criteria for gender. The foundational idea for the gender dysphoria clinics was first, to study an interesting and potentially fundable human aberration; second, to provide help, as they understood the term, for a 'correctable problem.'"[57] As an institution, gender clinics reinforced the idea that TGD people were not exactly people but rather a deviation, somehow not exactly human. Ultimately, the clinics were designed for research, largely performed by cisgender, white, male sexologists. In this medical model, clinicians defined *normal* with cisgender stereotypes, offering binary transitions to the lucky few who provided histories that conformed to the doctor's expected narratives. Researchers established these false narratives as truth in their literature, papers subsequently studied by TGD people who learned how they must present to receive care, perpetuating a cycle of deceit. Stone described the Stanford clinic "charm school," a grooming clinic that instructed trans women to behave according to the cultural expectations of male physicians.[58] She condemned the trope of transsexuals being "in the wrong body"[59] and argued that in the telling of these plausible histories, transsexuals became invisible, losing their voices and the ability to create or define their own narratives—ones that could fill the "intervening space in the continuum of sexuality."[60] She stated that the focus on passing led to a "denial of mixture"[61] and effacement of the previous gender, concluding: "So long as we, whether academics, clinicians, or transsexuals, ontologize both sexuality and transsexuality in this way, we have foreclosed the possibility of analyzing desire and motivational complexity in a manner which adequately describes the multiple contradictions of individual lived experience."[62]

Around the time of Stone's publication, increasing numbers of scholar-activists blasted the cultural status quo by exploring how investigators—who were often, but not exclusively, non-TGD—defined transgender embodiment through the lenses of colonization, language, race, and class. In 1991, Holly Boswell challenged a culture that polarized gender according to biology and defined transgenderism as a middle ground, an option beyond the existing, limited definitions for cross-dressers and transsexuals, one that instead offered a range of expressive choices for the nonbinary psyche—a concept now widely embraced.[63] Boswell entreated her community to be "more than our culture dictates . . . each of us, in our own small way, are makers of our culture. We can exercise that function by expressing our true selves—not by simply fulfilling our culture's expectations."[64] In 1992, Leslie Feinberg published *Transgender Liberation: A Movement Whose Time Has Come*,[65] a rallying cry to the trans community to reclaim its history, embrace its diversity, recognize the roots of oppression, and fight for a more just society. Feinberg argued that early communal societies often revered gender-diverse people but that the imposition of Christianity and patriarchal and capitalistic societies led to the oppression of women and those who lived outside gender norms. In 2006, Emi Koyama revisited the history of Michfest, this time with attention to an early proposal from Camp Trans protesters to allow only post-op transsexuals into the festival, a plan that discriminated against those who were unable to pay for surgical care, that is, the economically disadvantaged and transgender women of color.[66] She called out the white feminist and transgender activists who ranked oppression of women above all other forms by ignoring race, class, and ability. In 2010, American Indian scholar Deborah Miranda reclaimed the history of TGD Indigenous people by deconstructing the records of "gendercide" from early Spanish missionaries, describing how murder, renaming, regendering, and replacing the third gender *joyas* reimagined cultural beliefs and practices.[67] She entreated her community to reconstruct a "spiritual and community-oriented role for Two-Spirit people . . . as keepers of a dual or blended gender that holds male and female energy in various mixtures and keeps the world balanced."[68] In 2015, Monica Roberts asserted the contributions of early Black American transgender people, publishing previously untold stories to expand the range of cultural narratives.[69]

From these works and others, the field of transgender studies emerged. Stryker referred to the discipline as, "queer theory's evil twin," with "its own trajectory . . . and . . . the potential to address emerging problems in the critical study of gender and sexuality, identity, embodiment, and desire in ways that gay, lesbian, and queer studies have not always successfully managed."[70] British legal scholar and trans activist Stephen Whittle saluted this new discipline that "enabled trans men and trans women to reclaim the reality of their bodies, to create within them what they would, and to leave the linguistic determination of those bodies open to exploration and invention."[71] Most academics and Americans remained unaware of the birth of this new academic field and ignored the progressive voices of transgender scholars and activists; nonetheless, these revolutionary ideas percolated under the dominant cultural surface, creating space for the emergence of nonbinary/nontraditional gender identities and expressions and the development of medical care tailored to meet specific patient needs.

TRANS RIGHTS IN THE TWENTY-FIRST CENTURY

In the first two decades of the twenty-first century, the collective efforts of community members, community-based organizations, allies, lawyers, and scholars produced an explosion in TGD advocacy efforts, including access to healthcare. President Barack Obama passed the Affordable Care Act (with Article 1557, which prohibited discrimination on the basis of sexual orientation or gender identity in federally funded programs), the US Supreme Court ruled for same-sex marriage and against LGBT+–based discrimination in the workplace. In 2013, Patrisse Cullors, Alicia Garza, and Opal Tometi launched the Black Lives Matter movement, building power to intervene in violence inflicted on Black communities while simultaneously centering the leadership of Black women, queer, and trans people. These initiatives were met with a volatile, conservative backlash. American presidents sequentially flipflopped around pro- and anti-TGD legislation under presidents Barack Obama, Donald J. Trump, and Joe Biden. After Trump's presidential election in 2016, the American people faced rising authoritarianism, the packing of the courts with conservative judges, an increase in violent race-based and religion-based attacks by right-wing extremists, voter suppression, and the reversal of protections for LGBT+ citizens.

Despite, or perhaps because of the setbacks, increasing numbers of TGD people and their allies stepped into positions of power in academia, research, public health, mental health, and medicine. Healthcare medical education and delivery systems slowly, and with varying success, began to process new information about gender diversity, and more clinics and hospitals began to offer trans-affirming services, including new language and gender paradigms that enabled people with nonbinary gender identities to self-identify and advocate for appropriate medical treatment, including microdosing of hormones and nontraditional gender surgeries.

In 2007, Harvard physician Norman Spack began to prescribe GnRH analogs (pubertal blockers) and hormone therapy for TGD youth, using protocols developed in the Netherlands. His work triggered the admiration and dismay of subgroups within the medical community, the trans community, religious organizations, the government, and the American public. As research established the efficacy of TGD youth interventions, professional organizations endorsed these protocols, and clinics for youth opened across the United States.[72] Voices supporting and opposing the treatment of youth grew louder as the wider public response increasingly aligned with the divergent political views of the right and the left. Parents attested to the beneficial effect of the treatment for their youth; others fought to discredit the clinicians, families, schools, and organizations that sought to construct safe spaces for children. Critics proposed legislation to prohibit transgender children from using restrooms and locker rooms at school that correspond with their gender identity. Hate groups disguised themselves as professional associations, such as the American College of Pediatricians, to promote anti-LGBT+ junk science and conversion therapy.[73] In March 2021, the Arkansas Senate passed a bill banning access to pubertal blockers and hormones for TGD minors.[74] In 2022, dozens of states will consider anti-trans legislation including bills criminalizing medical care for TGD youth and restricting bathroom and locker room use and participation in sports.[75]

At the time of this writing (November 2022), a polarized American society remains divided on numerous social issues, including the necessity and right to trans-affirming healthcare and trans human rights. No other medical issue (except perhaps abortion) mobilizes such intense cultural involvement around medical decision making. Despite evidence-based data to support the efficacy of trans-affirming healthcare and the endorsement of important medical societies, sociocultural beliefs continue to influence and control decisions about healthcare and the healthcare rights of TGD people.

Yet in some states, for example New York, insurance coverage for trans-affirming healthcare is a basic right. In our hospital-owned clinic in rural upstate New York, where we fought long and hard to create a successful and affirming Gender Wellness Center within a family practice, there's a lift to the air, hints of spring. We have finally garnered institutional support for our program and insurance covers the costs of care for our patients.

In 2014, a photo of actress Laverne Cox graced the cover of *Time* magazine, next to the headline "The Transgender Tipping Point, America's Next Civil Rights Frontier."[76] In the article, Cox stated: "We are in a place now where more and more trans people want to come forward and say, 'This is who I am.' . . . More of us are living visibly, pursuing our dreams visibly, so people can say, 'Oh yeah, I know someone who is trans.' When people have points of reference that are humanizing, that demystifies difference."[77]

It is my hope that Cox's words also hold true for the provision of equitable medical care and that TGD people throughout the United States will someday say, "Oh yeah, I get excellent gender care in my primary care office, all covered by my insurance." Affirming medical offices serve as points of reference—they humanize, demystify difference. They signal to the American public the truth long fought for by activists: transgender people possess inherent humanity and dignity; they, too, have a right to gender-affirming healthcare, a privilege routinely offered to all cisgender people.

NOTES

1. Loftin, "Unacceptable Mannerisms."
2. Loftin, "Unacceptable Mannerisms."
3. Silverman and Stryker, *Screaming Queens.*
4. Silverman and Stryker, *Screaming Queens.*
5. Silverman and Stryker, *Screaming Queens.*
6. Silverman and Stryker, *Screaming Queens.*
7. Vanguard, "Vanguard History and Origins."
8. Vanguard, "Vanguard History and Origins."
9. Silverman and Stryker, *Screaming Queens.*
10. Silverman and Stryker, *Screaming Queens.*
11. Silverman and Stryker, *Screaming Queens.*
12. Silverman and Stryker, *Screaming Queens.* The clinic opened, but not because Stanford had any intention of providing gender care services. Stanford recruited Don Laub from Johns Hopkins, and he said was bringing his gender surgical practice with him. Stanford first rescinded this offer but reconsidered and allowed Laub to practice gender-affirming surgery until 1990, when they insisted that he no longer use any Stanford facilities to conduct this work. Personal communication with Jamison Green, June 22, 2021. Many transgender people were rejected by this clinic for not conforming to traditional narratives. See Sullivan, "Correspondence," and Levy, "Two Transsexuals Reflect."
13. Franke-Ruta, "An Amazing 1969 Account of the Stonewall Uprising."
14. Carter, *Stonewall*, 86.
15. Leitsch, "'Hairpin Drop Heard Around the World.'"
16. Leitsch, "'Hairpin Drop Heard Around the World.'"
17. Franke-Ruta, "An Amazing 1969 Account of the Stonewall Uprising."
18. Baumann, "Street Transvestite Action Revolutionaries."
19. Baumann, "Street Transvestite Action Revolutionaries."
20. Baumann, "Street Transvestite Action Revolutionaries"; Global Network of Sex Work Projects, "Street Transvestite Action Revolutionaries found STAR."

21. Devor, "Building a Better World for Transpeople."
22. Poteat, Reisner, and Radix, "HIV Epidemics." Although research during this time described HIV risks for sex workers and homosexual men, few studies looked at risks for transgender people or high-risk subsets of transgender people. The first systemic review and meta-analysis of HIV prevalence data for US transgender people was not published until 2008. Herbst et al., "Estimating HIV Prevalence." The authors identified only twenty-nine studies from 1990 to 2003 referencing data on HIV burden for transgender populations, and these papers only described disparities within Black transgender People Of Color communities. The early period of the HIV epidemic is defined by the *lack* of targeted research and healthcare for infected or at-risk trans populations.
23. Poteat, Reisner, and Radix, "HIV Epidemics," 2–3; Smart et al., "Transgender Women of Color," 164–65.
24. Crenshaw, "Demarginalizing the Intersection of Race and Sex"; Crenshaw, "Mapping the Margins."
25. Crenshaw, "Demarginalizing the Intersection of Race and Sex"; Crenshaw, "Mapping the Margins."
26. Malebranche and Nelson, *Interactions Between Culture*.
27. Feinbloom, *Transvestites & Transsexuals*.
28. Feinbloom, *Transvestites & Transsexuals*, 57–128, 146–244.
29. Feinbloom, *Transvestites & Transsexuals*, 223–44. Passing is when a transgender person is perceived as cisgender instead of their assigned sex at birth. Trans people who are not visibly transgender hold "passing privilege" and face less harassment and discrimination.
30. Kessler and McKenna, *Gender: An Ethnomethodological Approach*.
31. Kessler and McKenna, *Gender: An Ethnomethodological Approach*, vii–viii.
32. Bolin, *In Search of Eve*.
33. Bolin, *In Search of Eve*, 48–68.
34. Dallas Denny and Jamison Green, in communication with author, January 2021.
35. Goldberg, "What Is a Woman?"
36. Goldberg, "What Is a Woman?"
37. Smythe, "I'm Credited With Having Coined the word 'Terf.'"
38. Raymond, *The Transsexual Empire*.
39. Raymond, *The Transsexual Empire*, 99.
40. Raymond, *The Transsexual Empire*, 103, 114–16.
41. Raymond, *The Transsexual Empire*, 118–19.
42. Raymond, *The Transsexual Empire*, 99.
43. Raymond, *The Transsexual Empire*, 101.
44. Raymond, *The Transsexual Empire*, 103–4.
45. Szaz, "Male and Female Created He Them."

46. Williams, "Fact Checking Janice Raymond."
47. Michaelson, "Radical Feminists and Conservative Christians."
48. Anderson-Minshall, "Op-ed: Michfest's Founder Chose to Shut Down."
49. Burkholder had been attending Michfest annually for several years and was overheard telling someone she had transitioned many years prior; Jamison Green, in communication with author, September 2021.
50. Vogel, "Festival Reaffirms Commitment."
51. We've Been Around, "Camp Trans."
52. Green, personal communication with author, September 15, 2021. As our editorial group researched this book, we were continually struck by the relative historical erasure of transgender men in medical and general American cultural spheres. We have struggled, often unsuccessfully, to provide a balanced analysis, not only for transgender people of color but also for transgender men.
53. Ring, "This Year's Michigan Womyn's Music Festival Will Be the Last."
54. Souza, "Understanding TERFs."
55. Stone, "The 'Empire' Strikes Back."
56. Stone, "The 'Empire' Strikes Back," 9.
57. Stone, "The 'Empire' Strikes Back," 9.
58. Stone, "The 'Empire' Strikes Back," 10.
59. Stone, "The 'Empire' Strikes Back," 14–15.
60. Stone, "The 'Empire' Strikes Back," 9.
61. Stone, "The 'Empire' Strikes Back," 7.
62. Stone, "The 'Empire' Strikes Back," 15.
63. Boswell, "The Transgender Alternative," 29–31.
64. Boswell, "The Transgender Alternative," 30.
65. Feinberg, *Transgender Liberation.*
66. Koyama, "Whose Feminism Is It Anyway?"
67. Miranda, "Extermination of the Joyas."
68. See chapter 5 in this volume.
69. Roberts, "Black Trans History is Inspirational."
70. Stryker, "Transgender Studies," 212, 214.
71. Whittle, "Foreward," xii
72. See chapter 18 in this volume.
73. American College of Pediatricians, "Deconstructing Transgender Pediatrics"; Cretella, "Gender Dysphoria."
74. Yurcaba, "Arkansas Passes Bill."
75. Trans Legislation Tracker, "Tracking the Rise of Anti-Trans Bills in the U.S."
76. Steinmetz, "The Transgender Tipping Point."
77. Steinmetz, "The Transgender Tipping Point."

WORKS CITED

American College of Pediatrics. "Deconstructing Transgender Pediatrics." 2020. Accessed January 2020. https://acpeds.org/topics/sexuality-issues-of-youth/gender-confusion-and-transgender-identity/deconstructing-transgender-pediatrics.

Anderson-Minshall, Diane. "Op-ed: Michfest's Founder Chose to Shut Down Rather than Change with the Times." *Advocate*, April 24, 2015. Accessed January 2, 2021. https://www.advocate.com/commentary/2015/04/24/op-ed-michfests-founder-chose-shut-down-rather-change-times.

Baumann, Jason. "Street Transvestite Action Revolutionaries (STAR)." *1969: The Year of Gay Liberation*, New York Public Library's Online Exhibition Archive. Accessed January 2, 2021. http://web-static.nypl.org/exhibitions/1969/revolutionaries.html.

Bolin, Anne. *In Search of Eve*. Westport, CT: Bergin & Garvey, 1988.

Boswell, Holly. "The Transgender Alternative." *Chrysalis Quarterly* 1, no. 2 (1991): 29–31.

Carter, David. *Stonewall, The Riots that Sparked the Gay Revolution*. New York: St. Martin's Press, 2004.

Crenshaw, Kimberlé. "Demarginalizing the Intersection of Race and Sex: A Black Feminist Critique of Antidiscrimination Doctrine, Feminist Theory and Antiracist Politics." *University of Chicago Legal Forum* (1989): 139–67.

———. "Mapping the Margins: Intersectionality, Identity Politics, and Violence Against Women of Color." *Stanford Law Review* 43, no. 6 (1991): 1241–99.

Cretella, Michelle. "Gender Dypshoria in Children." American College of Pediatricians, January 2018. Accessed November 1, 2021. https://acpeds.org/position-statements/gender-dysphoria-in-children.

Devor, Aaron. "Building a Better World for Transpeople: Reed Erickson and the Erickson Educational Foundation." *International Journal of Transgenderism* 10, no. 1 (2007): 47–68.

Feinberg, Leslie. *Transgender Liberation: A Movement Whose Time Has Come*. New York: World View Forum, 1992.

Feinbloom, Deborah. *Transvestites & Transsexuals*. New York: Dell, 1976.

Franke-Ruta, Garance. "An Amazing 1969 Account of the Stonewall Uprising." *The Atlantic*, January 24, 2013. Accessed January 2, 2021. http://www.theatlantic.com/politics/archive/2013/01/an-amazing-1969-account-of-the-stonewall-uprising/272467/.

Global Network of Sex Work Projects. "Street Transvestite Action Revolutionaires found STAR House." History of of NSWP, 2014. Accessed January 2, 2021. https://www.nswp.org/timeline/1970/all.

Goldberg, Michelle. "What Is a Woman? The Dispute Between Radical Feminsim and Transgenderism." *The New* Yorker, July 28, 2014. Accessed January 2, 2021. https://www.newyorker.com/magazine/2014/08/04/woman-2.

Herbst, Jeffrrey, Elizabeth Jacobs, Theresa Finlayson, Vel McKleroy, Mary Neumann, and Nicole Crepaz. "Estimating HIV Prevalence and Risk Behaviors of Transgender Persons in the United States: A Systematic Review." *AIDS and Behavior* 12, no. 1 (2008): 1–17.

Kessler, Suzanne, and Wendy McKenna. *Gender: An Ethnomethodological Approach.* New York: John Wiley & Sons, 1978.

Koyama, Emi. "Whose Feminism Is It Anyway? The Unspoken Racism of the Trans Inclusion Depate." In *The Transgender Studies Reader*, edited by Susan Stryker and Steven Whittle, 698–705. New York: Routledge, 2006. Accessed January 1, 2021. http://eminism.org/readings/pdf-rdg/whose-feminism.pdf.

Leitsch, Dick. "'Hairpin Drop Heard Around the World.'" Stonewall: Riot, Rebellion, Activism and Identity, 1969. Accessed January 2, 2021. https://stonewallhistory.omeka.net/items/show/31.

Levy, Dawn. "Two Transsexuals Reflect on University's Pioneering Gender Dysphoria Program." *Stanford Report*, May 3, 2000. Accessed January 2, 2021. https://news.stanford.edu/news/2000/may3/sexchange-53.html.

Loftin, Craig. "Unacceptable Mannerisms: Gender Anxieties, Homosexual Activism, and Swish in the United States, 1945–1965." *Journal of Social History* 40, no. 3 (2007): 577–808.

Malebranche, D., and L. Nelson. *Interactions Between Culture, Race, and Sexuality in Health.* In *The GLMA Handbook on LGBT Health*, Vol. 1, edited by Vinvent Silenzio and Laura Erickson-Schroth, 39–59. Santa Barbara, CA: ABC-CLIO, 2019.

Michaelson, Jay. "Radical Feminists and Conservative Christians Team up against Transgender People." *Daily Beast*, September 4, 2016. Accessed May 11, 2021. https://www.thedailybeast.com/radical-feminists-and-conservative-christians-team-up-against-transgender-people.

Miranda, Deborah. "Extermination of the Joyas Gendercide in Spanish California." *GLQ: A Journal of Lesbian and Gay Studies* 16, no. 1–2 (2010): 253–84.

Poteat, Tonia, Sari Reisner, and Anita Radix. "HIV Epidemics among Transgender Women." *Current Opinion in HIV and AIDS* 9, no. 2 (2014): 168–73.

Raymond, Janice G. (1979) 1994. *The Transsexual Empire: The Making of the She-Male.* Boston, MA: Beacon Press.

Ring, Trudy. "This Year's Michigan Womyn's Music Festival Will Be the Last." *Advocate*, April 21, 2015. Accessed January 2, 2021. https://www.advocate.com/michfest/2015/04/21/years-michigan-womyns-music-festival-will-be-last.

Roberts, Monica. "Black Trans History is Inspirational." Transgender Law Center, February 25, 2015. Accessed January 2, 2021. https://transgenderlawcenter.org/archives/11401.

Silverman, Victor, and Susan Stryker. *Screaming Queens: The Riot at Compton's Cafeteria.* Directed by Victor Silverman and Susan Stryker and produced by Fameline, 2005. Performed by Ray Baxter, Elliot Blacksone, Aleshia Brevard, Felicia Elizondo, Ed Hansen, Lawrence Helman, Menzies, Molie, et al.

Smart, Benjamin, Lilli Mann-Jackson, Jorge Alonzo, et al. "Transgender Women of Color in the U.S. South: A Qualitative Study of Social Determinants of Health and Healthcare Perspectives." *International Journal of Transgender Health* 23, no. 1–2 (2022): 164–67.

Smythe, Viv. "I'm Credited With Having Coined the word 'Terf.' Here's How it Happened." *The Guardian*, November 28, 2018.

Souza, Luisa. "Understanding TERF's: Their History, Thought, and "Activism." Medium. October 30, 2019 Accessed August 12, 2024. https://luisa29.medium.com/understanding-terfs-their-history-thought-and-activism-896cbebc3e25.

Steinmetz, Katy. "The Transgender Tipping Point, America's Next Civil Rights Frontier." *Time*. June 9, 2014. Accessed August 12, 2024. https://time.com/135480/transgender-tipping-point/.

Stone, Sandy. "The 'Empire' Strikes Back: A Posttranssexual Manifesto." 1987. Accessed July 22, 2022. https://sandystone.com/empire-strikes-back.pdf.

Stryker, Susan. "Transgender Studies: Queer Theory's Evil Twin." *GLQ: A Journal of Lesbian and Gay Studies* 10, no. 2 (2004): 212–15.

Sullivan, Lou. "Correspondence from Lou Sullivan to Jude Patten." Digital Transgender Archives, June 26, 1985. Accessed January 1, 2021. https://www.digitaltransgenderarchive.net/files/0c483j46q.

Szaz, Thomas. "Male and Female Created He Them." *New York Times Archives*, June 10, 1979. Accessed August 12, 2024. https://www.nytimes.com/1979/06/10/archives/male-and-female-created-he-them-transexual.html.

Trans Legislation Tracker. "Tracking the Rise of Anti-Trans Bills in the U.S." n.d. Accessed August 12, 2024. https://translegislation.com/learn.

Vanguard. "Vanguard History & Origins." 1965. Accessed August 12, 2024. http://www.vanguard1965.com/.

Vogel, Lisa. "Festival Reaffirms Commitment to Womyn-Born Space." TransAdvocate. August 24, 1999. Accessed August 12, 2024. http://www.transadvocate.com/wp-content/uploads/2014/08/MichiganWomynsMusicFestival_FestivalReaffirmsCommitmentToWomyn-BornSpace_082499.pdf.

We've Been Around. "Camp Trans." YouTube, June 10, 2016. https://www.youtube.com/watch?v=Ca3erlRoGg8&t=19s.

Whittle, Stephen. "Foreword." In *The Transgender Studies Reader*, edited by Susan Stryker and Stephen Whittle, xi–xvi. New York: Routledge, 2006.

Williams, Cristan. "Fact Checking Janice Raymond: The NCHCT Report." The Trans Advocate. Accessed May 11, 2021. https://www.transadvocate.com/fact-checking-janice-raymond-the-nchct-report_n_14554.htm.

Yurcaba, Jo. "Arkansas Passes Bill to Ban Gender-Affirming Care for Trans Youth." *NBC News*, March 29, 2021. Accessed January 16, 2022. https://www.nbcnews.com/feature/nbc-out/arkansas-passes-bill-ban-gender-affirming-care-trans-youth-n1262412.

12.1. PROFILE: MARSHA P. JOHNSON (1945–1992)

Amanda Yijun Wang

"My life has been built around sex and gay liberation, being a drag queen, and sex work."

—Marsha P. Johnson, interviewed by Steve Watson

We remember Marsha P. Johnson, a self-identified transvestite, sex worker, and gay liberation/AIDS activist, as a pioneer in an era when sex workers and transgender women of color existed only on the margin of society. Born August 24, 1945, in Elizabeth, New Jersey, as Malcolm Michaels Jr., Johnson was the fifth of seven children to Malcolm Michaels Sr., a General Motors assembly line worker, and Alberta Claiborne, a housekeeper.[1] From a young age, Johnson enjoyed wearing girls' clothes but stopped after experiencing harassment by neighborhood boys and a sexual assault. Johnson's family did not accept her gender identity or sexuality.

After graduating high school in 1963, Johnson left for New York City with fifteen dollars in her pocket and a bag of clothes. After a brief stint waiting tables, she met street hustlers. With them, she dressed in feminine clothing and adopted the name Black Marsha and, later, Marsha P. Johnson. (Johnson from Howard Johnson's restaurant on 42nd St., and P for "Pay it no mind," her famously flippant answer to a judge who questioned her gender.)[2] Johnson worked the streets most of her life. She performed in drag with groups like the Hot Peaches and became a fixture on Christopher Street with her colorful dresses, heels, flamboyant jewelry, and the flower crowns she made after sleeping under tables in the Flower District.[3] In 1975, she served as the subject for two of Andy Warhol's paintings in his Ladies and Gentlemen collection.[4] She was quirky, charismatic, and generous, despite never having much of her own.[5] Raised as an Episcopalian, Johnson remained deeply religious throughout her life. Some considered her a saint.[6]

The Stonewall riots of June 28, 1969, marked the beginning of Johnson's activism. Accounts vary about exactly who did what and when during the Stonewall uprising, but popular mythology credits her as having thrown the first brick at police as they raided the bar.[7] Reports from the scene described Johnson amid a group of drag queens, ferociously fighting, screaming, swearing, and ultimately dropping a heavy bag from a lamppost to smash the window of a patrol car.[8] Johnson herself claimed, "After the Stonewall riot, that's when I started my little rioting."[9] She subsequently joined the Gay Liberation Front and the first Gay Pride March, taking to the streets annually thereafter. White gay men and lesbians, though, dominated the mainstream Gay Liberation Front, ostracizing transvestites like Johnson and Sylvia Rivera.[10] When the organizer of the Gay Pride March banned transvestites, Johnson and Rivera defiantly marched ahead of the parade with their peers.

In 1972, Johnson helped Rivera found the Street Transvestites Action Revolutionaries (STAR),[11] and they established STAR House, a safe home for transvestite street kids and sex workers.[12] She and Rivera hustled to provide food, shelter, and support for these youth, who were otherwise ignored, harassed, or arrested by men on the streets and police alike.[13] The original STAR house was in a run-down apartment building. It moved into a bus when money ran low and later disbanded due to lack of funds.

In 1980, after being homeless for most of her life, Johnson moved in with her friend and fellow LGBTQ activist, Randy Wicker, and nursed Wicker's partner Dave Combs as he died of AIDS. Johnson was also a member of Act Up, an AIDS activist organization, attending protests and gatherings. In a 1992 interview, she disclosed that she was HIV positive, suffered from mental illness, and had experienced numerous breakdowns.[14] During her mental health crises, she could be volatile and aggressive and was hospitalized at Bellevue Hospital multiple times.

Johnson died in 1992 at age forty-six under mysterious circumstances, her body found in the Hudson River. Though initially ruled a suicide, many suspected foul play due to frequent violence against sex workers and transgender women of color. A police investigation in 2002 reclassified her death as a drowning of unknown cause. In 2012, the Manhattan District Attorney reopened the case.[15]

In a 2012 documentary, Michael Lynch, a member of Hot Peaches, eulogized her thus: "She is one of the reasons that [kids today who are gay] are sitting in all their liberated glory. But Marsha paid the price for who she was."[16] Johnson faced harassment and violence on the streets. She claimed to have been arrested more than one hundred times and was even shot once in the late 1970s.[17] She once remarked that the police treated her like "the highest murderer in the world."[18] Despite her own struggles with medical and mental health problems, she repeatedly faced down this oppression. Johnson was one of the first to stand up for the safety and health of sex workers and trans women of color in New York City. Her boldness inspired others to live openly and demand respect, housing, and healthcare. Forgotten and mistreated in life, Johnson's now iconic story serves as a beacon in today's movement toward diversity, equity, and inclusion in healthcare.

NOTES

1. Chan, "Marsha P. Johnson."
2. Kasino, *Pay It No Mind.*
3. Gossett, *Happy Birthday Marsha.*
4. Zhang, "Artwork Spotlight."
5. Kasino, *Pay It No Mind.*
6. Jacobs, "DA Reopens Unsolved 1992 Case"
7. Carter, *Stonewall*, 298; O'Neill, "Who Threw the First Brick."
8. Carter, *Stonewall*, 188–89, 298.
9. Kasino, *Pay It No Mind.*
10. Johnson met Rivera in 1963, when she was seventeen and Rivera was twelve. In a 1995 interview, Rivera said Johnson was the first friend she made on 42nd Street; Kauffman, "ABOUT NEW YORK").
11. First called Street Transvestites Actual Revolutionaries.
12. Hunter and Robinson, "The Two Ms. Johnsons," 70.
13. Nothing, "Rapping with a Street Transvestite," 21–22, 26.
14. Calafell, "Narrative Authority," 27.
15. Jacobs, "DA Reopens Unsolved 1992 case."
16. Kasino, *Pay It No Mind.*
17. Chan, "Marsha P. Johnson."
18. Kasino, *Pay It No Mind.*

WORKS CITED

Calafell, Bernadette Marie. "Narrative Authority, Theory in the Flesh, and the Fight over the Death and Life of Marsha P. Johnson." *QED: A Journal in GLBTQ Worldmaking* 6, no. 2 (2019): 26–39.

Carter, David. *Stonewall: The Riots that Sparked the Gay Revolution.* New York: St. Martin's Press, 2004.

Chan, Sewell. "Marsha P. Johnson, a Transgender Pioneer and Activist." *New York Times*, March 8, 2018. Accessed August 20, 2024. https://www.nytimes.com/interactive/2018/obituaries/overlooked-marsha-p-johnson.html.

Gossett, Reina, dir. *Happy Birthday Marsha 'Pay It No Mind' Johnson.* Crunk Feminist Collective, 2013.

Hunter, Marcus Anthony, and Zandria F. Robinson. "The Two Ms. Johnsons." In *Chocolate Cities*, 67–76. Berkeley: University of California Press, 2018.

Jacobs, Shayna. "DA Reopens Unsolved 1992 Case Involving the 'Saint of Gay Life.'" *New York Daily News*, December 16, 2012. Accessed August 20, 2024. https://www.nydailynews.com/new-york/da-reopens-unsolved-1992-case-involving-saint-gay-life-article-1.1221742.

Kasino, Micahel, dir. *Pay It No Mind—The Life and Times of Marsha P. Johnson.* Redux Pictures, 2012. Accessed August 19, 2024. https://www.youtube.com/watch?v=rjN9W2KstqE&ab_channel=MichaelKasino.

Kaufman, Michael T. "ABOUT NEW YORK; Still Here: Sylvia, Who Survived Stonewall, Time and the River." *New York Times*, May 24, 1995. Accessed August 19, 2024. https://www.nytimes.com/1995/05/24/nyregion/about-new-york-still-here-sylvia-who-survived-stonewall-time-and-the-river.html?searchResultPosition=1.

Nothing, Ehn. "Rapping with a Street Transvestite Revolutionary: An Interview with Marsha P. Johnson." In *Street Transvestite Action Revolutionaries: Survival, Revolt, and Queer Antagonist Struggle*, 21–29. Untorelli Press, 2006. Accessed August 19, 2024. https://archive.org/details/untorelli_2013_transvestite/untorelli_2013_transvestite_print/mode/2up.

O'Neill, Shane. "Who Threw the First Brick at Stonewall? Let's Argue About it." *New York Times*, May 31, 2019. Accessed August 20, 2024. https://www.nytimes.com/2019/05/31/us/first-brick-at-stonewall-lgbtq.html.

Watson, Steve. "Pride Archives: Stonewall 1979: The Drag of Politics." *Village Voice*, June 15, 1979. Accessed August 20, 2024. https://www.villagevoice.com/2019/06/04/stonewall-1979-the-drag-of-politics/.

Zhang, Larry Luowei. "Artwork Spotlight: Andy Warhol's 'Ladies and Gentlemen.'" Grey Art Museum New York University. August 12, 2019. Accessed August 20, 2024. https://greyartgallery.nyu.edu/2019/08/artwork-spotlight-andy-warhols-ladies-and-gentlemen/.

12.2. PROFILE: SILVIA RIVERA (1951–2002): "THE ROSA PARKS OF THE MODERN TRANSGENDER MOVEMENT"

Teri Wilhelm and Carolyn Wolf-Gould

Sylvia Rivera, a now prominent transgender rights activist, was born to parents of Venezuelan and Puerto Rican descent in New York City on July 2, 1951, "in the morning in a taxi-cab in the old Lincoln Hospital parking lot."[1]

Shortly after her birth, her father abandoned her family. When Rivera was three, her mother committed suicide and attempted to kill Rivera at the same time.[2] Shunned and beaten by a grandmother who disapproved of her dark skin and feminine ways, Rivera ran away from home at age ten, joining New York City street life, where she panhandled, engaged in sex work, and found comfort in the drag community.[3]

In 1963, Rivera met Marsha P. Johnson at a Halloween party.[4] Rivera became dependent on Johnson, six years her senior, who served as her mentor. "Marsha taught Sylvia how to apply makeup, live on the street, and look out for trouble. She also encouraged Sylvia to love herself and her identity."[5]

In 1969, when Rivera was seventeen, she and Johnson participated in the Stonewall riots. While Rivera characterized the Stonewall Inn as a place that catered mostly to middle-class, white gay men, the marginalized street queens and street youth of color were at the bar and fought fiercely at the uprising. Although often credited with throwing the first Molotov cocktail by historians, Rivera denied this story, claiming, "I threw the second one. I did not throw the first one!"[6]

Rivera focused her attention on vulnerable trans street youth. She and Johnson housed them in their hotel rooms, once commenting that "you can sneak fifty people into two hotel rooms."[7] With money earned from hustling and sex work, Rivera and Johnson, who were in their late teens and early twenties, respectively, fed and clothed the more vulnerable youth. In 1970, Rivera approached Johnson with a vision of kinship and community, wanting to create a home to protect "her children." Together, they opened STAR House, the first shelter of its kind in the country.[8] Rivera cooked dinners for her kids and prayed to Saint Barbara, the patron saint of queer Latinos, before turning tricks in the streets to support them.[9] Rivera and Johnson didn't want the kids hustling and instead sent them out to perform "fingers for Jesus"—shoplifting—to keep food on the table.[10]

Although Stonewall motivated the gay community to pursue social justice and civil rights, most LGB people still disparaged the poor, transgender people of color, who Rivera identified as the most oppressed and most at risk. She and Johnson fought to end racial and gender-based violence against those like herself. Drawing on her experience as an activist in the civil rights movement, the women's movement, and protests against the Vietnam War, she engaged in political activism, railing against the oppression of gender normativity, police harassment, and class-based discrimination.[11] She had prior activist experience and high hopes for participation in the newly formed Gay Liberation Front and

Gay Activists Alliance, but she found herself shunned at meetings because of her race, gender expression, passionate speeches in broken English, and status as a street person.[12] Notably, Rivera worked on the campaign to pass the New York City Gay Rights Bill, only to discover later that politicians and gay activists removed gender protections from the bill to make it more likely to pass.

At the 1973 Gay Pride Rally in New York City, Rivera took the stage to the boos and jeers of the crowd and asked what this "white middle-class white club" was doing to ensure equal rights for all LGBT people, including those in jail.[13] She condemned the crowd: "I have been beaten. I have had my nose broken. I have been thrown in jail. I have lost my job. I have lost my apartment for gay liberation, and you all treat me this way? What the fuck's wrong with you all? Think about that!"[14] Later, at the podium, lesbian feminist Jean O'Leary denounced Rivera as a "man" who "caused a ruckus," stating that "men impersonating women insults women."[15] After this event, Rivera tried to commit suicide and left the movement.[16] Later that same year, STAR House closed due to waning community support, issues with legal occupancy, and nonpayment of rent.[17] Rivera moved upstate to Tarrytown, where she refrained from activism for two decades.

In 1992, Rivera returned to New York City, broken by years of homelessness and substance abuse, and squatted on the pier near where Johnson's body had been discovered. In 1997, she accepted an invitation to live at Transy House, a community home inspired by STAR House and founded in 1995 by Rusty Mae Moore and Chelsea Goodwin. Located in Park Slope, Brooklyn, Transy House became a "haven for all trans and gender-nonconforming people who had been kicked out of their homes, had dropped out of school, or were refused housing at men's and women's shelters."[18] With finding refuge, Rivera also returned to activism; she lived in Transy House until her death from liver cancer in 2002 at age fifty.[19]

Celebrating her life, a photograph of Rivera taken at the 2000 New York City Pride Parade hangs in the National Portrait Gallery in Washington, DC.[20] She smiles, head cocked to one side and hands linked with her partner, Julia Murray, on one side, and fellow activist Christina Hayworth, on the other. Oppressed and discounted during her lifetime, Sylvia lives posthumously as a civil rights icon who "changed queer and trans activism forever."[21] When contemporary organizations confront homelessness, racial discrimination, incarceration, addiction, sex work, the HIV epidemic, hunger, and healthcare for those TGD people most marginalized by society, they invoke Rivera's tireless advocacy and labor in her name. The Sylvia Rivera Law Project in

New York City "works to guarantee that all people are free to self-determine gender identity and expression, regardless of income or race, and without facing harassment, discrimination or violence."[22] A growing number of health departments and community-based organizations across the country now target those TGD communities most in need, offering services for health, housing, addiction, and legal assistance that didn't exist in Rivera's time.

And yet, it is still not enough. We must continue to harness Rivera's courage and vision, speak up, and ensure that all American citizens receive equitable treatment, including the right to inclusive healthcare.

NOTES

1. Marcus, "Sylvia Rivera—Part 1."
2. Gan, "'Still at the Back of the Bus.'"
3. Ellison, *Silvia Rivera and Marsha P. Johnson*.
4. Ellison, *Silvia Rivera and Marsha P. Johnson*.
5. New York Historical Society Museum & Library, "Life Story."
6. Goodman, "Sylvia Rivera Changed."
7. Feinberg, "Street Transvestite Action Revolutionaries."
8. New York Historical Society Museum & Library, "Life Story."
9. Brockell, "The Transgender Women at Sonewall."
10. Kuwabara, "At Star House"; Feinberg, "Street Transvestite Action Revolutionaries."
11. Gan, "'Still at the Back of the Bus.'"
12. Gan, "'Still at the Back of the Bus.'"
13. Love Tapes Collective, "L039A Jean O'Leary Speech"; Love Tapes Collective, "L020A Sylvia."
14. Love Tapes Collective, "L039A Jean O'Leary Speech"; Love Tapes Collective, "L020A Sylvia."
15. Love Tapes Collective, "L039A Jean O'Leary Speech"; Love Tapes Collective, "L020A Sylvia."
16. Gan, "'Still at the Back of the Bus.'"
17. Gan, "'Still at the Back of the Bus'"; Brockell, "The Transgender Women at Stonewall."
18. NYC LGBT Historic Sites, "Transy House."
19. Rothberg, "Sylvia Rivera (1951–2002)."
20. Perry, "Sylvia Rivera: Activist and Trailblazer."
21. Goodman, "Sylvia Rivera Changed."
22. Sylvia Rivera Law Project.

WORKS CITED

Brockell, Gillian. "The Transgender Women at Stonewall Were Pushed Out of the Gay Rights Movement. Now They are Getting a Statue in New York." *Washington Post*, June 12, 2019. Accessed September 19, 2021. https://www.washingtonpost.com/history/2019/06/12/transgender-women-heart-stonewall-riots-are-getting-statue-new-york/.

Ellison, Joy Michael. *Silvia Rivera and Marsha P. Johnson, Guiding Stars*. n.d. Accessed September 19, 2021. https://jmellison.net/if-we-knew-trans-history/sylvia-rivera-and-marsha-p-johnson-guiding-stars/.

Feinberg, Leslie. "Street Transvestite Action Revolutionaries: Lavender & Red, Part 73." *Workers World*, September 24, 2006. Accessed September 19, 2021. https://www.workers.org/2006/us/lavender-red-73/.

Gan, Jessi. "'Still at the Back of the Bus': Sylvia Rivera's Struggle." *Centro Journal* XIX, no. 1 (2007): 124–39. Accessed September 19, 2021. https://www.redalyc.org/pdf/377/37719107.pdf.

Goodman, Elyssa. "Sylvia Rivera Changed Queer and Trans Activism Forever." *them*, March 26, 2019. Accessed September 20, 2021. https://www.them.us/story/sylvia-rivera.

Kuwabara, Sessi. "At STAR House, Marsha P. Johnson and Sylvia Rivera Created a Home for Trans People." *VICE*, June 8, 2020. Accessed September 25, 2021. https://www.vice.com/en/article/z3enva/star-house-sylvia-rivera-marsha-p-johnson.

Love Tapes Collective. *L020A Sylvia, "Y'all Better Quiet Down" Original Authorized Video, 1973 Gay Pride Rally NYC*. 1973. Accessed September 26, 2021. https://www.youtube.com/watch?v=Jb-JIOWUw1o.

———. *L039A Jean O'Leary Speech at 1973 Gay Rally with Watermark*. 1973. Accessed September 25, 2021. https://www.youtube.com/watch?v=USWWUVEFLUU.

Marcus, Eric. "Sylvia Rivera—Part 1." Episode 1. *Making Gay History: The Podcast*. December 9, 1989. Accessed August 6, 2021. https://makinggayhistory.com/podcast/episode-1-1/.

New York Historical Society Museum & Library. "Life Story: Marsha P. Johnson (1945–1992)." n.d. Accessed September 20, 2021. https://wams.nyhistory.org/growth-and-turmoil/growing-tensions/marsha-p-johnson/.

NYC LGBT Historic Sites. "Transy House." 2016. Accessed September 6, 2021. https://www.nyclgbtsites.org/site/transy-house/.

Perry, Ana. "Sylvia Rivera: Activist and Trailblazer." Smithsonian, National Portrait Gallery. n.d. Accessed September 25, 2021. https://npg.si.edu/blog/welcome-collection-sylvia-rivera.

Rothberg, Emma. "Sylvia Rivera (1951–2002)." National Women's History Museum. March 2021. Accessed September 25, 2021. https://www.womenshistory.org/education-resources/biographies/sylvia-rivera.

Sylvia Rivera Law Project (website). Accessed September 28, 2021. htttps://srlp.org/.

Wilchins, Riki. "A Woman for Her Time." *The Village Voice*, February 26, 2002. Accessed August 28, 2021. https://www.villagevoice.com/2002/02/26/a-woman-for-her-time/.

12.3. PROFILE: DALLAS DENNY (1949–)

Kenneth Hubbell

Dallas Denny is an historian, scholar, community organizer, and activist for transgender healthcare and civil rights. In a career spanning four decades she has produced, curated, and disseminated scholarly research on transgender health and been a powerful voice advocating for the rights of trans patients to participate in the development of gender-affirming treatment models.

Denny was born August 18, 1949, in Asheville, North Carolina. In personal writings, she describes a youth spent fruitlessly seeking reliable information on transsexual issues, a body of knowledge to which she would ultimately become a major contributor.[1] In 1974, she completed her bachelor's in psychology and sociology at Middle Tennessee State University and went on to earn her master's in psychology from the University of Tennessee in 1979. During this period, she encountered for the first time the medical establishment's approach to trans patients: Vanderbilt University's transgender treatment program declined to treat her, as she was not sufficiently debilitated by her experience. She also began a decade-long career as a psychological examiner for the state of Tennessee.

Two transitions took place in Denny's life in the 1980s: She contacted the larger transgender community and took personal steps to affirm her gender. After an exchange of letters with Virginia Prince in 1980, she began researching the use of hormones through her access to academic libraries.[2] At age twenty-nine, when she was unable to find a provider, she began taking self-prescribed estrogens.[3] In 1987, she connected with the Society for the Second Self and the International Foundation for Gender Education. Through the International Foundation for Gender Education, she learned of the Montgomery Medical and Psychiatric Institute in Atlanta, Georgia, which offered a support group for transsexuals. In 1989, she relocated to Atlanta to participate in this group and began leading their sessions. This move also marked her transition to living as a woman; she changed her style of dress, underwent electrolysis, and found a provider to prescribe legal estrogens.

In 1990, her advocacy career blossomed. She founded the American Educational Gender Information Service, an organization dedicated to the curation and dissemination of educational materials for trans people. Denny launched *Chrysalis Quarterly*, a journal that published a wide range of articles on trans health topics. These articles provided information that was otherwise largely inaccessible to trans patients at the time, including overviews of medical and surgical options and their complications,[4] research on intersex conditions,[5] and descriptions of mental health concerns in the trans community.[6] She also wrote extensively on the gatekeeping model of gender-affirming care, critiquing the then prevalent view that trans patients must exhibit gross social and occupational dysfunction to qualify for care.[7]

In the 1990s, Denny emerged as a leading authority on transgender healthcare. In 1994, she published *Gender Dysphoria: A Guide to Research*,[8] the first book-length collection of research on transsexualism authored by a transgender person, and in 1998, she published *Current Concepts in Transgender Identity*[9]—an edited textbook detailing the surgeries, hormonal regimens, and counseling recommended for gender transitions. She also conducted surveys that defined the healthcare preferences and priorities of the transgender community and wrote critiques of the terminology employed by medical professionals in the treatment of patients.[10]

In the late 1990s, Denny called for American Educational Gender Information Service's transition to a digital platform and, by the early 2000s, was conducting much of her work virtually. Over the past twenty-plus years she has remained active in academic and political spheres, publishing more than twenty chapters in books on transgender topics and delivering dozens of keynote addresses for professional organizations.

Denny's leadership drove the development and distribution of detailed educational materials in an era when transgender individuals had little access to reliable information. As the academic field of transgender research matured, she worked to curate and advance the body of scholarly knowledge on transgender health and was a key advocate in ensuring that transgender voices, including the voices of transgender men, were respected in the development of treatment models.

NOTES

1. Denny, "NTL&A Dedication Ceremony Program Book 2004." *Transgender* has since largely replaced the word *transsexual*.
2. Denny and Prince, "First Contact."
3. Denny, "Beyond our Slave Names."

4. Denny, "The Care and Feeding of the Neovagina"; Green, "Getting Real about FTM Surgery"; Denny, "Sex Reassignment Surgery, Hormones, and Health."

5. Dreger, "Doctors Containing Hermaphrodites."

6. Tayleur, "Transsexuals and Addiction."

7. Denny, "The Politics of Diagnosis and a Diagnosis of Politics"; Denny, "No Regrets"; Denny, "How to Shop for Service Providers."

8. Denny, *Gender Dysphoria: A Guide to Research*.

9. Denny, *Current Concepts in Transgender Identity*.

10. Denny and Roberts, "Results of a Questionnaire on the Standards of Care"; Denny, "You Make Me Sick!"; Green, Denny, and Cromwell, "'What Do You Want Us to Call You?"

WORKS CITED

Denny, Dallas. *Current Concepts in Transgender Identity*. New York: Taylor & Francis, 1998.

———. "Dallas Denny: Beyond our Slave Names." Dallas Denny: Body of Work. October 2011. Accessed August 20, 2024. http://dallasdenny.com/Writing/2011/10/31/beyond-our-slave-names-1999/.

———. *Gender Dysphoria: A Guide to Research*. New York City: Garland, 1994.

———. "How to Shop for Service Providers." *Chrysalis Quarterly* 1, no. 2 (1991): 9–12. Accessed August 20, 2024. http://dallasdenny.com/Writing/wp-content/uploads/2013/12/Chrysalis-V.-1-No.-2-Summer-1991-aa10.pdf.

———. "No Regrets: The Standards of Care." *Chrysalis Quarterly* 1, no. 2 (1991): 13–16. Accessed August 20, 2024. http://dallasdenny.com/Writing/wp-content/uploads/2013/12/Chrysalis-V.-1-No.-2-Summer-1991-aa10.pdf.

———. "NTL&A Dedication Ceremony Program Book." March 25, 2004. Accessed August 20, 2024. http://dallasdenny.com/Writing/wp-content/uploads/2013/11/Dedication-of-the-National-Transgender-Library-Archivessmallpdf.com_.pdf.

———. "Sex Reassignment Surgery, Hormones, and Health." *Chrysalis Quarterly* 1, no. 1 (1991): 7–11. Accessed August 20, 2024. http://dallasdenny.com/Writing/wp-content/uploads/2013/12/Chrysalis-V.-1-No.-1-aa10.pdf.

———. "The Care and Feeding of the Neovagina." *Chrysalis Quarterly* 1, no. 4 (1992): 21–30. Accessed August 20, 2024. http://dallasdenny.com/Writing/wp-content/uploads/2014/01/Chrysalis-V.-1-No.-4-1992-Entiresmallpdf.com_.pdf.

———. "The Politics of Diagnosis and a Diagnosis of Politics: The University-Affiliated Gender Clinics, and How They Failed to Meet the Needs of Transsexual People." *Chrysalis Quarterly* 1, no. 3 (1992): 9–20. Accessed August 20, 2024. http://dallasdenny.com/Writing/wp-content/uploads/2013/12/Chrysalis-Quarterly-V.-1-No.-3-Winter-1992smallpdf.com_.pdf.

———. "You Make Me Sick! A Critique of the Psychological and Medical Literature of Transsexualism." Trans-Progressing Symposium, Fantasia Fair, Provincetown, MA, October 17–24, 2004. Accessed August 20, 2024. http://dallasdenny.com/Writing/2013/08/24/you-make-me-sick-2004/.

Denny, Dallas, and Jan Roberts. "Results of a Questionnaire on the Standards of Care of the Harry Benjamin International Gender Dysphoria Association." In *Gender Blending*, edited by Bonnie Bullough, Vern Bullough, and James Elias, 320–26. Amherst, NY: Prometheus Books, 1997. Accessed August 20, 2024. http://dallasdenny.com/Writing/2011/10/27/results-of-a-questionnaire-on-the-standards-of-care/.

Denny, Dallas, and Virginia Prince. "First Contact: My Letter to Virginia Prince and Reply." *Chrysalis Quarterly Online*. 1980. Accessed August 20, 2024. http://dallasdenny.com/Chrysalis/2013/08/21/first-contact/.

Dreger, Alice. "Doctors Containing Hermaphrodites: The Victorian Legacy." *Chrysalis Quarterly* 2, no. 5 (1997): 15–22. Accessed August 20, 2024. http://dallasdenny.com/Writing/wp-content/uploads/2013/12/Chrysalis-V.-2-No.-5-1997-1998-Intersex-Issuesmallpdf.com_.pdf.

Green, James. "Getting Real about FTM Surgery." *Chrysalis Quarterly* 2, no. 2 (1995): 27–32. Accessed August 20, 2024. http://dallasdenny.com/Writing/wp-content/uploads/2014/01/CQ-22-Entire-smallpdf.com_.pdf.

Green, Jamison, Dallas Denny, and Jason Cromwell. "'What Do You Want Us to Call You?': Respectful Language." *Transgender Studies Quarterly*, 5, no. 1 (2018): 100–10.

Tayleur, Christine. "Transsexuals and Addiction." *Chrysalis Quarterly* 1, no. 7 (1994): 11–14. Accessed August 20, 2024. http://dallasdenny.com/Writing/wp-content/uploads/2013/12/CQ-17-Spring-1994-Entiresmallpdf.com_.pdf.

12.4. PROFILE: JAMISON GREEN (1948–)

Teri Wilhelm

Jamison Green is an articulate and persuasive powerhouse in many communities. He is as comfortable in activist circles as he is in academic, legal, corporate, medical, and political circles. One of the transgender community's truest champions for healthcare advocacy, civil rights, and public policy reform, his voice is one of reason and thoughtfulness.

Born on November 8, 1948, in Oakland, California, Green was raised by adoptive parents who were supportive of his wide-ranging intellectual and athletic interests. He knew from an early age that he was different from the other boys and girls but had no language to articulate that difference. Despite his popularity among classmates and neighborhood children, he felt a tension between who he knew himself to be and his body all through elementary and secondary school. By the late 1960s, Green had come to think of himself as "cross-gendered."[1]

After receiving a Master of Fine Arts degree in 1972 for English/Creative Writing,[2] Green tested his physical strength by taking a job as a Bell Telephone Company cable splicer for three-and-one-half years. He was the first female-bodied person to succeed in that role. He then moved into technical writing, first in the legal and medical fields then documenting computer hardware and software. His natural leadership skills often led him to take on management roles then director and officer roles, where he set the vision for large teams. Throughout his career, however, the feeling of being cross-gendered continued to nag at Green and challenged his relationships where his female body seemed at odds with his masculine energy.

In 1987, while searching for advice about transitioning, Green, by fortunate accident, met Lou Sullivan, a trans man living in San Francisco. Sullivan had recently launched a support group and newsletter, both titled FTM, to help trans men find much-needed information and, perhaps, a community. Sullivan connected Green with Steve Dain, who at that time was the most publicly known trans man on the US west coast. Green pursued Dain as a mentor, although the two eventually became friends.

Green also continued to participate in Sullivan's group, FTM. Sullivan became ill from HIV-related causes and shortly before he died, Sullivan asked Green to continue his work. Sullivan died of complications of HIV/AIDS in March 1991.[3] Green supported and built on Sullivan's legacy, greatly expanding the readership of the organization's *FTM Newsletter*,[4] as well as the support group's membership.

Green made the conscious, brave decision (for the times) to live openly as a transgender man. He believed the burgeoning trans movement needed role models to share their stories and encourage others to do the same, asserting: "People need to know that we are here, that we exist, that it is okay to be us; because if they don't, then we'll always be strangers."[5] He spoke at every educational opportunity and testified at public, civil, and criminal proceedings on behalf of transgender people. He became the subject of numerous articles and documentaries, which leveraged his influence on public policy.

Green's efforts increasingly attracted attention in the United States and abroad.[6] During the 1990s, the FTM group incorporated. In 1994, as membership and need expanded, FTM evolved into FTM International (FTMI), a thriving nonprofit educational organization. Before the end of the decade, FTMI would be the largest transmasculine–focused organization in the world.[7]

In 1994, Green authored the nation's first citywide effort in San Francisco, California, to address discrimination and improve treatment of transgender people. Over a period of two years, he and fellow activists pressured the San Francisco Human Rights Commission to focus on the difficulties faced by transgender residents. The Commission eventually held a public hearing and appointed Green to write the report *Investigation into Discrimination Against Transgendered People*, which led to a nondiscrimination ordinance, police officer trainings, and ultimately (in 2001), removal of exclusions from one of the city's five employee health benefit plans.[8]

In 1995, after securing a five hundred dollar challenge[9] grant from Dallas Denny, FTMI created and held the first, large-scale conference for and about trans men in San Francisco. Under the guidance of then President Green,[10] nearly four hundred people attended from across the United States and from other continents, far more than the planning team originally expected.[11]

His desire to support the nascent transmasculine community led Green to learn about the Harry Benjamin International Gender Dysphoria Association (HBIGDA) and its standards of care for transgender people. At that time, he felt the organization's treatment objectives lacked focus and exhibited a bias toward practitioners' concerns over those of transgender patients.[12] Green has described his advocacy work as personal, explaining: "As a trans man dedicated to improving the quality of trans lives, I have a big stake in how trans people are represented, and misrepresented."[13] Inspired to make change, Green attended HBIGDA's 1997 conference; he and Denny submitted a paper they had coauthored, "Gender Identity and Bisexuality,"[14] and Green's presentation and his active engagement at the conference led to an invitation to join the organization as a supporting member. In 2002, the HBIGDA board decided to make Green a full member (eligible to vote and run for office), and in 2003, he was elected to serve a four-year term on the board of directors. That same year, he delivered the manuscript for *Becoming a Visible Man* to Vanderbilt University Press. The resulting book, published in 2004, earned the 2005 Sylvia Rivera Prize for Best Book in Transgender Studies. Over the next decade, Green became a well-regarded academic theorist in the field of medical policy.[15]

Relying on his deep knowledge of change management and trans activism, Green served for fifteen years on the HBIGDA/ World Professional Association for Transgender Health (WPATH)[16] Board of Directors, including two years and five months as president (February 2014–June 2016). He dedicated his time to writing internal and external policies to improve trans lives and to strengthen the organization, championing and initiating formal medical education led by experts, and working diligently to improve the standards of care.

While deeply engaged with WPATH, Green also served as member of the board of directors for the International Foundation for Gender Education,[17] the Transgender Law and Policy Institute,[18] and TransYouth Family Allies,[19] a parent-run educational group. He served on the Human Rights Campaign's Business Council from 2002 through 2007, eventually becoming a consultant to the organization's Workplace Equality Program.[20] Using his ability to heavily influence outcomes, Green became a vigorous advocate for the addition of criteria to measure trans-inclusive, employer-based health benefits in the Corporate Equality Index, the Human Rights Campaign's national benchmarking tool for encouraging LGBT workplace equality.[21] He also wrote a monthly column for PlanetOut.com from 2000 to 2005, and he appeared in numerous documentary films and in the initial episode of the sci-fi series *Sense8*.

From 2009 to 2013, Green worked as a policy analyst with JoAnne Keatley at the Center of Excellence for Transgender Health at the University of California San Francisco, where he spearheaded the effort to create the first University of California San Francisco Primary Care Protocol for Transgender Care, launched in 2011.[22] That same year, after seven years of study with British legal scholar Stephen Whittle, Green, at age sixty-two, earned a PhD in Law from Manchester Metropolitan University. He also became president-elect of WPATH, the first American trans person chosen to serve in that role in the organization's forty-plus year history.

In November 2018, Green transitioned out of his executive board role with WPATH, though he continues to serve as cochair of the ethics committee and on the faculty of WPATH's Global Education Institute. In 2020, Vanderbilt University Press released a second edition of *Becoming a Visible Man*. Green's efforts as an activist and scholar continue unabated. His commitment to advocating on behalf of the trans community shapes his vision for the future, one rooted in education:

> The trans movement is chaos now. I think social media has lifted up the individual at the cost of promoting understanding and connection to larger community and movement goals. We need to become part of the education system so we do not remain strangers to everybody. Medical schools need to be educated and to educate about LGBTQ+

people and about human sexuality much more than they do. Elementary schools need to acknowledge that people are different. It's not only boys and girls.[23]

NOTES

1. Green, *Becoming a Visible Man*, 18.
2. Academia, "Jamison Green."
3. Green, *Becoming a Visible Man*, 64–65.
4. University of Victoria FTM Newsletter Collection, collection details.
5. Doe, *Sexplanations*.
6. Funk, "Jamison Green."
7. Beemyn, "Transgender History in the United States."
8. Green and Brinkin, *Investigation into Discrimination*.
9. *FTM Newsletter*, Issue 32, 3.
10. Beemyn, "Transgender History in the United States," 28.
11. *FTM Newsletter*, Issue 32, 1.
12. Green, *Becoming a Visible Man*, 193.
13. McQuade, "Transgender Advocate Jamison Green."
14. Denny and Green, "Gender Identity and Bisexuality."
15. McQuade, "Transgender Advocate Jamison Green."
16. See chapter 14 in this volume for the history of the organization.
17. International Foundation for Gender Education, "International Foundation for Gender Education."
18. DBpedia. "About."
19. TransYouth Family Allies, "Who Are TransYouth Family Allies?"
20. Human Rights Campaign, "Workplace Equality Program."
21. Human Rights Campaign, *Corporate Equality Index*.
22. University of California San Francisco, "Center of Excellence for Transgender Health."
23. Green, interview with the author.

WORKS CITED

Academia. "Jamison Green." Accessed October 10, 2021. https://independent.academia.edu/GreenJamison.

Beemyn, Genny. "Transgender History in the United States." University of Massachusetts. n.d. Accessed October 17, 2021. https://www.umass.edu/stonewall/sites/

default/files/Infoforandabout/transpeople/genny_beemyn_transgender_history_in_the_united_states.pdf.

Bloom, Amy. "The Body Lies." *New Yorker*, July 18, 1994, 38.

DBpedia. "About: Transgender Law and Policy Institute." Accessed January 8, 2022. https://dbpedia.org/page/Transgender_Law_and_Policy_Institute.

Denny, Dallas, and Jamison Green. "Gender Identity and Bisexuality." In *Bisexuality: The Psychology and Politics of an Invisible Minority*, 84–102. Thousand Oaks, CA: SAGE, 1996.

Doe, Lindsay. *Sexplanations: An Interview with Jamison Green*. October 22, 2015. Accessed October 3, 2021. https://www.youtube.com/watch?v=m3Z7SlZqxpI.

FTM Newsletter, Issue 32 (October 1995). Accessed August 29, 2022. https://www.digitaltransgenderarchive.net/downloads/g445cd139.

Funk, Mason. "Jamison Green." Outwords, May 17, 2017. Accessed October 10, 2021. https://theoutwordsarchive.org/interview/green-jamison/.

GLSEN. "Unheard Voices: Stories of LBGT HIstory." June 2020. Accessed September 21, 2021. https://www.glsen.org/sites/default/files/2020-06/Jamison%20Green%20Backgrounder.pdf.

Green, Jamison. *Becoming a Visible Man.* Nashville, TN: Vanderbuilt University Press, 2020/2004.

Green, Jamison, and Larry Brinkin. *Investigation into Discrimination against Transgender People*. Human Rights Commission, City and County of San Francisco. September 1994. Accessed August 7, 2024. https://sf-hrc.org//sites/default/files/Documents/HRC_Publications/Articles/Investigation_into_Discrimination_Against_Transgendered_People.pdf.

Human Rights Campaign. *Corporate Equality Index*. Accessed November 5, 2021. https://www.hrc.org/resources/corporate-equality-index.

Human Rights Campaign. "Workplace Equality Program." Accessed November 5, 2021. https://www.thehrcfoundation.org/about/workplace-equality-program.

International Foundation for Gender Education. "International Foundation for Gender Education." Accessed January 8, 2022. http://ifge.org/index0.htm.

McQuade, Aaron. "Transgender Advocate Jamison Green Speaks about Policy Work and Education." Accessed August 7, 2024. https://web.archive.org/web/20111010050439/https://glaad.org/blog/transgender-advocate-jamison-green-speaks-about-policy-work-and-education.

Sosin, Kate. *Logo: NEWNOWNEXT.* October 29, 2018. Accessed August 10, 2024. https://web.archive.org/web/20200206133211/http://www.newnownext.com/jamison-green-trans-health-care-pioneer/10/2019/.

TransYouth Family Allies. "Who Are TransYouth Family Allies?" 2017. Accessed January 8, 2022. http://www.imatyfa.org/.

University of California San Francisco. "Center of Excellence for Transgender Health." Accessed January 8, 2022. https://prevention.ucsf.edu/transhealth.

University of Victoria, Transgender Archives, FTM Newsletter Collection. Accessed August 11, 2024. https://vault.library.uvic.ca/collections/d13ed5ae-6ea3-4cb8-b72a-4a5c794982b6.

Wright, Andy. "Open Up and Let Us In." *Medium*, September 22, 2015. Accessed October 10, 2021. https://medium.com/gender-2-0/open-up-and-let-us-in-4b2be99c1ebb.

13

THE EVOLUTION OF PROFESSIONAL ORGANIZATIONS AND STANDARDS OF CARE
An Inside-Outsider's Perspective

Jamison Green

In the 1960s, reports from the fields of psychology and sexology gripped the American psyche, partly because of the astounding revelations found in Alfred Kinsey's research roughly a decade previously[1] and partly because of the sexual revolution that, according to historian Maurice Isserman, arose from the conviction that erotic feelings should not be repressed but embraced as a normal part of life.[2] But in spite of the almost magical ability of modern science (a popular concept) to turn a man into a woman á la Christine Jorgensen, information about transgender and gender-diverse (TGD) people barely blipped on the cultural radar's big screen. Even in those days, it took a special kind of person to focus on the permutations of sex and gender.

In the 1950s, the prolific researcher and psychologist John Money emerged as that kind of special: intelligent, curious, determined, bold, and creative.

This is not to say he was admirable in every way; he was not. Not everyone who enters this field is destined for notoriety or greatness, but because of the contested nature of the topic, many manage to achieve their fifteen minutes of fame (which social media has now reduced to fifteen seconds every so often). But Money's character in those early days before his career imploded[3] exhibited a rare charismatic combination of qualities that drew people to him and opened minds to new ideas about human experience. Despite the later collapse of his reputation, Money's work and influence moved the field away from academic individualism on a rogue topic toward the development of academic collaboration and organization.

After Kinsey died in 1956, Money became the biggest name in the field of sexology. He mentored many up-and-coming young researchers, such as psychiatrist and (later) attorney Richard Green and psychologist Paul Walker, two of the future founders of the Harry Benjamin International Gender Dysphoria Association (HBIGDA; 1977–1979). Green (no relation to yours truly) went from Johns Hopkins to the University of California Los Angeles to work with psychiatrist Robert Stoller, and later, with Harry Benjamin in Benjamin's New York office, eventually settling in at Charing Cross Hospital in London. Walker also worked at the University of Texas, Medical Branch in Galveston, and later established a private practice in San Francisco, California.[4]

Green and Money possessed distinct personalities, but both were extremely intelligent. Not only did they know it, but they made sure everyone around them knew too. They could be insightful, inspiring, and in the next moment, condescending and insulting. I heard this from many who knew them, and personally experienced this behavior with Green. Still, the accomplishments of these cisgender men inspired deep admiration among their colleagues. Walker, also competent and accomplished, presented as a modest, personable man who encouraged queer and trans people like Lou Sullivan,[5] young clinicians like Lin Fraser, and future scholar and activists like Jude Patton and, by extension, me.

For both academic research and clinical career success, membership in professional societies serves many purposes. Such memberships bring together people who are interested in developing a field of study or practice. Professional societies foster research and education, and they can lobby for change in existing systems that need to adapt to new discoveries. Professional society membership has long been encouraged as a way of enhancing one's career prospects. Scholarly meetings provide opportunities to meet professional peers and mentors, rub elbows with leaders in the field, present one's research, and win awards, which lend prestige to one's curriculum vitae. Serving on a professional association's board of directors or committees allows individuals to develop working relationships with colleagues and directly influence the association, institution, or governmental policies. Such influence is difficult to achieve without the stamp of an academic or professional society, providing the clout individuals rarely achieve alone. In the burgeoning field of sexology, Money served in the World Association for Sexual Health and the Society for the Scientific Study of Sex. These organizations and their associated scholarly journals raised his own academic profile and the profiles of his graduate students, mentees, and other colleagues and slowly established the ground to support a new academic and clinical research society.

Building a professional society or association requires financial support. Some of the early trans-related research and publications of Benjamin, Money, Johns Hopkins surgeon Milton T. Edgerton, Green, Walker, physician Leo Wollman, psychiatrist Ira Pauly, and others received funding from the Erickson Educational Foundation (EEF), established by philanthropist and trans man Reed Erickson.[6] The EEF promoted the budding field of research on and treatment of transsexualism from 1964 to 1976. One of the Foundation's chief interests was "organizing, promoting, and funding symposia for the exchange of ideas and the cementing of research relationships."[7] EEF sponsored the first three international conferences concerned with trans people[8] and provided administrative support for the fourth such meeting in 1975, the first held in the United States.[9]

At the first convening in 1969, cosponsored by EEF and the Albany Trust of London, the symposium chairman, professor C. J. Dewhurst of Queen Charlotte's Hospital, London, posed a series of questions in his opening remarks—questions that remain vexing today for many trans people and the medical and mental health providers who work in this field:

> This Symposium is on Gender Identity, and all the problems which surround it. . . . Now, if we are going to discuss this . . . we are going to come across many, many questions that I hope will be answered during the course of this symposium. . . . What, for instance, do we know already of its origins? Under what circumstances does it arise? Are there certain consistent endocrine, or enzymatic, or chromosomal changes associated with it? What physical investigations are required in any patient who appears to be suffering from transsexualism or associated conditions? What investigations are likely to be helpful to allow us to learn more about the underlying sense of the condition?

How often, if ever, is there any physical ambiguity of sex to go with the confusion in the patient's mind? . . . And if we regard the condition as an abnormality, that would be cured by getting the patient to accept their true anatomical sex, can [we] say that this is ever possible? . . . Is a cure . . . ever possible? How should it be approached? At what age is it wise to take it very seriously? . . . It should be suggested [to pediatricians] that they must take the early manifestations of transsexualism very seriously indeed. If we do that, will we sometimes be taking it too seriously? Is there an age, after which we can say . . . cure is no longer possible, but we must do all we can to arrange for the patient to assimilate their desired sex as smoothly as possible? . . . If we are considering an individual for assimilation into a new sex, . . . what criteria are we to accept as to whether the patient should be accepted or rejected so far as surgery is concerned? Am I to be swayed when I see a patient, with whether I like them, whether they seem to fit well into a new sex, or are there other criteria . . . that will help me to decide the genuine from the spurious? What safeguards are required before we undertake surgery? What investigations should be employed? And what surgical complications exist, because undoubtedly there will be surgical complications. [And, to turn to the legal aspects:] What is the precise legal position of a patient before surgery is undertaken, if they dress, shall we say, as a woman and go out into the streets? After surgery has been undertaken what is the precise legal position? Is legal re-registration possible . . . is marriage legally possible? Is it successful? . . . Those were a number of questions and undoubtedly there will be more. . . . But I hope somehow, that most of them will be answered before the symposium is over.[10]

Fifty-six years later, these questions have yet to be fully answered, despite considerable effort by clinicians and community members and a significant body of research validating the *Standards of Care* (*SOC*).

Just prior to the planned 1977 convening held in Norfolk, Virginia, the EEF announced it would be closing its New York office and turning its attention to New Age spirituality.[11] The researchers were so alarmed by EEF's withdrawal of funding and administrative support that a core group organized an impromptu meeting to take place during the Norfolk symposium. By the end of that meeting, this group had chosen the members of the founding committee of the HBIGDA, "and Paul Walker was charged with drawing up articles of incorporation for the new organization."[12] Green wrote "Eight of us founded the . . . (HBIGDA) in 1978 [sic]. There was Harry, of course, and three surgeons, a psychologist, a general practitioner, and a sex-reassigned teacher."[13] Green's memory failed him: Patton was (as far as he could tell[14]) the only trans person present at that 1977 meeting and worked not as a teacher but as the co-director of Renaissance, a transsexual service organization. Although Benjamin may have indeed been present in Norfolk in 1977, he was never an officer or an active participant in HBIGDA activities or in the development of its *SOC*. However, two trans men, Erickson and Patton, contributed to the formation of the only professional medical and scientific organization to focus entirely on studying and assisting transgender people.

HBIGDA was officially incorporated and constituted in 1979. The members elected Patton to join the original founding committee of six doctors to "represent the consumers of scientific research and service on transsexualism."[15] As described in chapter 7, Patton's election generated controversy. Originally, the organization admitted only physicians, psychologists, and nurses, and Jude was not yet certified as either a marriage and family therapist or as a physician's assistant, though he would be so qualified in just a few years. The split vote to include him also exposed tensions within HBIGDA about the perceived inadvisability of including trans-identified people, who then were seen as only "consumers," as full members of a professional organization. By including "consumers of care," professional organizations risked being dismissed as unprofessional, as nothing more than consumer advocacy groups. The practice of sex reassignment in the late 1970s and into the 1980s was regarded as dubious and unsound by many physicians, and professionals outside of HBIGDA often shunned their colleagues who provided this care. Some professionals did not reveal the fact that they treated transgender people even to other physicians within their practices, and in some surgical journals, when surgeons published articles describing procedures performed on transgender patients, subsequent issues of the journals would contain complaints from other subscribers in the form of letters to the editor, asserting their displeasure that such content was given any editorial consideration at all. These fears lingered among some professionals through the first decade of the twenty-first century, even though qualified trans-identified physicians, psychologists, social workers, social scientists, and others in the health and legal fields related to transgender care were gradually becoming aware of the organization and seeking active membership. Notably, the membership application forms for

HBIGDA (now known as the World Professional Association for Transgender Health [WPATH]) have never asked an applicant to reveal their gender identity or medical history, only their professional qualifications. The early interest in selective trans inclusivity reflects awareness among the medical and mental health professionals who had sufficient experience with transgender patients/clients to know that transness in itself is not an impairment, and many accomplished trans people have the capacity to contribute to the professional knowledgebase and to the association's development. Prejudice against trans people simply because they have a transgender history does nothing to ensure scientific integrity in research or analysis; in fact, such prejudice inhibits both analysis and research and has effectively restrained advancement in the field.

HBIGDA changed its name to the WPATH in 2007. The spare organizational history presented on the wpath.org website[16] reflects the fact that overworked volunteers performed the work of managing and recording the organization's business, and the group received operational funding only through membership dues.[17] The roles of chairperson, president, and executive director evolved or sometimes fractured as new people took on these roles roughly every two years. Although the website once listed all presidents from 1979, board members receive no mention until 1993. At the time of this writing, the WPATH website lists only the current serving board of directors, officers, and staff, something this author hopes will be remedied before the end of the current decade.

Patton served on the original board of directors from 1979 through 1985 and again from 1997 through 2001, both times as a member of the Advocacy and Liaison Committee. He also served on the SOC Committee for versions 5 (1998) and 6 (2001) of that document. At this writing, he is chair of the Trans Aging & Older Adults Special Interest Group for the US Professional Association for Transgender Health (USPATH) regional organization, and he recently assisted the *SOC-8* Institutions Chapter committee. He also served on the Scientific Committee in planning WPATH's 2022 Scientific Symposium held in Montreal, Quebec, Canada, and the 2024 Symposium held in Lisbon, Portugal—the twenty-eighth convening since the first 1969 gathering in London. Patton received the WPATH Harry Benjamin Lifetime Distinguished Service Award at the 2022 event.

During Patton's last term on the HIBGDA board (1997–2001), gynecologist Sheila Kirk became the first trans-identified physician elected to serve as a director. Kirk also worked closely with the International Foundation for Gender Education, a transgender community service organization based in

Massachusetts, where she created health education materials for cross-dressers and transsexual people. In the 1990s, she opened the first transgender surgery clinic run by a trans-identified physician and surgeon. She also co-authored (with Martine Rothblatt) *Medical, Legal & Workplace Issues for the Transsexual* (1995) and (with Walter Bockting) *Transgender and HIV: Risks, Prevention, and Care* (2001). Kirk was elected HBIGDA's secretary-treasurer for the 2001–2003 term. Other trans women who have served on the HBIGDA/WPATH Board include Marsha Botzer (2009–2013), founder of the Ingersoll Gender Center in Seattle, Washington, and surgeon Marci Bowers, elected to the board in 2016. Bowers became the first trans woman-elected president of WPATH in 2020, occupying that office from 2022 to 2024. Three trans men have so far served as president: law professor Stephen Whittle, elected in 2005, serving 2007–2009; yours truly, elected in 2011, serving 2014–2016; and physician Asa Radix, elected in 2022, serving 2024–2026.

During the forty-five-plus years of the organization's existence, trans members have only recently held positions of authority or influence. As more trans people have earned degrees and joined professional ranks in associations and institutions of higher learning, we have made significant impacts in numerous fields. Historically, though, we trans people were often told, albeit indirectly, that we were not the experts in our own experience; we were just unfortunate people whose experience informed the research carried out by important, qualified, predominantly cisgender professionals. Not everyone within HBIGDA/WPATH felt that way; no association is a monolith, and many HBIGDA/WPATH members appreciated us as individuals and respected our knowledge and abilities. HBIGDA, from the start, established a committee charged with representing the consumer experience in raising issues for consideration in the *SOC* or to encourage research in areas the professionals hadn't previously considered. Still, TGD people, both close-up and far away from the professional circles, perceived the power dynamic and observed how some people leveraged organizational power more forcefully than others. Patton recalled feeling grateful to be invited to the 1975 meeting and unable to say a word to anyone else there (more from shyness than anything else), and he was completely surprised and honored to be named to the HBIGDA board in 1979.[18] Marsha Botzer, who attended her first HBIGDA meeting in 1985 in Minneapolis, Minnesota, remarked: "I remember what it felt like, sitting in the back of the room and listening to how they talked about us—the feeling of separation from the powers describing my identity. I was excited that these people were honestly trying to be helpful, but none of them actually lived our lives. The medicalized talk was so far from the realities I observed among the hundreds of trans people who were trying to get help."[19]

Clinicians who participated in HBIGDA meetings discovered opportunities for personal and professional growth. Fraser, a licensed psychotherapist since 1976, already had more than two hundred transgender clients in her San Francisco private practice when she attended the 1979 symposium—her first. "[Being there was] so exciting!" Fraser remembered. "And the *Standards of Care* were just what I needed; they were truly helpful and such an important guide. We were all trying to help people, at least I was, and I loved being able to meet other clinicians who were so creative, mavericks, pioneers, able to think out of the box, who wanted to help people and do something that matters!"[20] Fraser met Patton at that San Diego conference; she met Leah Schaeffer, who had worked in New York with Benjamin, and Shaefer's associate Christine Wheeler, both of whom would later serve as association officers; she met Virginia Prince and trans woman psychologist Ann Vitale; and of course, she met symposium hosts surgeon Donald Laub and psychiatrist Norman Fisk. Fraser was already well connected with the transgender population in San Francisco, having completed her internships at the public and community-based health centers Haight-Ashbury and Fort Help. Fascinated by the people she met, concerned about their well-being, and respectful of their self-awareness and lived experience, Fraser arrived at the conference anxious to make connections. HBIGDA provided networking opportunities not only with clinicians but also with trans people engaged in the work of improving their lives and the lives of others. Fraser later served as president of WPATH from 2011 to 2014, and she remains an active participant in the organization, with a particular interest in education and ethics.

In the 1990s, HBIGDA served as a magnet for individuals who wanted to usher in a new era of transgender community, civil rights, and affirming transgender care. Katherine (Kit) Rachlin was one of those who entered the organization determined to initiate change. In 1985, she had been working on a doctorate in applied research in organizational psychology when she met Johnny Science through friends in New York City. Science was just beginning to research the possibility of transition from female to male and shared with Rachlin the information he had accumulated from contact with Lou Sullivan, Rupert Raj, and in the 1990s, from me. Rachlin and Science together started the F2M Fraternity, a support group and information network "for FTM transsexuals, crossdressers, their partners, and interested helping professionals" at roughly the same time Sullivan launched his group, FTM in San Francisco.

The New York City F2M group ran from 1987 to 1995, ultimately supplanted by support groups at the Gender Identity Project of the LGBT Community Center of New York City, spearheaded by Barbara Warren. Rachlin facilitated the first groups for families and for partners of trans people in the Gender Identity Project.

The resources for transgender individuals in New York City and almost everywhere else in the early 1980s were oriented toward transfeminine individuals, and F2M was the first in New York to address the needs of transmasculine people. Hundreds of people came through the group over time, and Rachlin became aware of the disparity between how trans people—particularly transmasculine people—were discussed in the scientific literature and the real lives of the people she knew. After she completed her doctorate in applied research, she entered the postdoctoral respecialization program in clinical psychology at Teachers College, Columbia University, to obtain the equivalent of a doctorate in clinical psychology. Her goal was to impact the HBIGDA *SOC* by conducting research to document the experiences of transgender people in the community and to support improved access to healthcare for trans people. Unlike other psychologists of her generation who came to the field of transgender health because transgender patients entered their practice, Rachlin had already known a world of transgender people prior to becoming a psychotherapist and was already an advocate and trans-positive researcher. She may have been the first individual to become a clinical psychologist for the specific purpose of working with transgender people; she was definitely the first to declare that intention on admittance to the clinical psychology program at Teachers College in 1994.

Rachlin attended the HBIGDA conference in New York City in 1993 and became active in the organization, serving two terms on the board of directors of WPATH (2007–2011 and 2014–2018) during a period when the board was focused on the depathologization of transgender identity across the globe and increasing access to healthcare. She lobbied for input into *SOC-6* (2001), was a co-author of *SOC* versions 7 (2011) and 8 (2022), and founded the WPATH Graduate Student Initiative, which encourages young researchers and future clinicians.

Beginning in the 1990s, Rachlin published community-based research (many projects with TGD co-authors, including me) and was a frequent speaker at professional and community conferences, trying to build a bridge between the providers and consumers of transgender care.

Through working internationally within WPATH, Rachlin saw that the mission to serve people worldwide did not always meet the local needs of the communities in the United States. In particular, the United States had a strong tradition of consumer lobbies that many other nations did not. And the United States was developing a cohort of transgender professionals who were now ready to assume the reins of transgender medicine. They would need an organization that could elevate their voices while benefiting from the historical influence of WPATH. Rachlin purchased the URL, USPATH.org, in anticipation that the United States would need its own professional organization, one that reflected the transgender professionals who were ready to assume leadership of trans-affirming healthcare in the United States. Years later, under my presidency, WPATH established regional organizations, and Rachlin gave that URL to WPATH when USPATH was launched in 2017. Rachlin was also cochair of the committee to launch USPATH, serving in leadership until the US membership could elect its own board of directors. As I had designed the regional affiliate structure, the president of each regional affiliate organization automatically has a seat on the WPATH board.

Today there are many training programs and internships for social workers and psychologists who want to specialize in transgender health. Rachlin is distinguished as a cisgender advocate, practitioner–scholar who helped train generations of psychotherapists while bringing community voices into the scientific literature and supporting the advancement of transgender professionals. She has maintained a private psychotherapy practice in New York City since 1996 where she now focuses on helping gender-diverse people in mid and late life and their families and partners.

Every recognized medical specialty has its own standard of care. Without a standard of care and treatment criteria, professionals in any specialty would be reluctant to deliver care. The initial document was spare and to the point, assuming that persons who sought treatment for transsexualism (the diagnosis at that time) were seeking a direct and uncomplicated transition from one pole of the binary sex construct to its polar opposite. There were no references for clinicians to review for background, and there was no explanatory language. Many trans people found the treatment criteria recommended by the HBIGDA *SOC*[21] impossible, for example, the requirement of three or more months of expensive therapy with a psychiatrist or psychologist to be approved for hormone therapy (six months for surgery) and proof that the candidate had been preoccupied with the wish to be rid of one's genitals. Many were unable to find a knowledgeable and affordable psychiatrist willing to treat TGD people. The *SOC* required physical examinations, psychological examinations, in some cases IQ testing, and proof that individuals had been "successfully living in the genetically other sex role for at least one year." The *SOC* stated that "some experts on gender identity recommend that the time parameters listed . . . should be doubled, or tripled."[22] To trans people, this meant they could be held prisoner by their mental health provider, in a state of indefinite limbo.

Many TGD people felt that the worst requirement in the *SOC* was the Real Life Test. This appeared in Version 1 (1979) of *SOC*:

> **Principle 12.** The best indicator for hormonal and surgical sex-reassignment is how successfully the patient has been in living-out, full-time, vocationally and avocationally, in all social situations, the social role of the genetically other sex and how successful the patient has been in being accepted by others as a member of that genetically other sex. **Standard 4.** The initiation of hormonal sex-reassignment shall be preceded by a period of at least 3 months during which the patient lives full time in the social role of the genetically other sex. **Standard 5.** Non-genital sex-reassignment (facial, hip, limb, etc.) shall be preceded by a period of at least 6 months during which time the patient lives full time in the social role of the genetically other sex. **Standard 6.** Genital sex-reassignment shall be preceded by a period of at least 12 months during which time the patient lives full-time in the social role of the genetically other sex.[23]

The authors of the *SOC* removed the Real Life Test requirement in Version 2 (1980), recognizing the inherent impossibility of living in one's experienced gender without the necessary physical attributes (that is, it can be difficult—even dangerous—to try to live, for example, as a male if one has large breasts, or as a female if one has a large frame, a deep voice, and abundant facial and body hair). However, many TGD people and healthcare professionals believed then (and some may still believe) that trans people must run this gauntlet to prove they deserve access to transition-related care. In the 1970s, there were therapists and physicians who judged TGD applicants for treatment based on how feminine or masculine they appeared. The more convincingly they represented their "target gender," the more likely the clinicians anticipated a smooth ride for the person through transition. This archaic position represented a sexist, classist, and even racist bias toward conformity with stereotypical norms of gender-associated roles and physical characteristics. It was and remains patently unfair to transgender people. Clinicians within WPATH recognized these early oversights and evolved over the decades, recognizing the experience of trans people as valid, not as a mental illness or as a mystery. Reading the current highly interdisciplinary and thoughtful *SOC-8* (2022) is an educational experience. To address the need for clinicians trained in the flexible and affirming use of the *SOC*, WPATH established the Gender Education Initiative in 2013 so that healthcare professionals can become trained and certified in care informed by research and respect for TGD people.

Prior to 2012 and *SOC-7*, most physicians and therapists (few of whom encountered trans people—to their knowledge—in their practices) did not commonly read or abide by recommendations in the *SOC*. As insurance plans began to cover transition-related medical care (see Insurance Coverage section below), professionals received increasing requests for care and began to self-train. Through their research, they might discover the *SOC*. Even in the San Francisco Bay Area, where I transitioned (1988–1991), no one at the Sex Reassignment Program at Stanford University mentioned HBIGDA or the *SOC*—I think they felt these were an organization and a document for professionals, not patients. I was never required to undergo therapy or a Real Life Test; I just took the Minnesota Multiphasic Personality Inventory test and participated in three interviews: two with clinicians at Stanford and one with Walker in San Francisco. Over the next twenty years, I asked every medical provider who treated me for any condition if they had ever heard of HBIGDA or the *SOC* and they all said, "No." The *SOC* presented no obstacles to me, but I was glad it was there to provide guidance and legitimacy to my care.

Green attributed the Real Life Test to Money,[24] but other sources indicate that prior to the existence of the HBIGDA *SOC*, many clinicians believed that a trial period was the best way to determine if transition would be successful. Benjamin recommended a trial period in his 1966 book.[25] Erickson's educational foundation became one of the most effective purveyors of the Real Life Test concept among TGD people. One of EEF's publications, *Guidelines for Transsexuals*, a booklet widely circulated among trans people for years beyond the EEF's existence (and replicated by many other community-based organizations in their own informational campaigns), declared:

> Most gender identity clinics, and many physicians in private practice, require from six months to two years of cross-gender experience before recommending a patient for surgery. This may seem an excessively long period to you before you begin, but experience has shown that no other test is so effective in preventing the tragedy of a wrong

decision for surgery, the results of which are irreversible. On the other hand, there is no better means of laying the groundwork for every aspect of your new life, and strengthening your confidence for it, than this preparatory period.[26]

This statement, in conjunction with similar statements published in Green and Money's 1969 edited text, *Transsexualism and Sex Reassignment*, as well as journal articles that EEF reproduced and distributed to trans people, frequently emphasized Money's two-year Real Life Test or the concept of a trial period. Many trans people in the 1970s and 1980s, anxious for validation from the medical community, accepted this as a matter of course, while others, especially those who were unable to support themselves and pay for therapy to verify that they were meeting the trial period requirements, became frustrated and angry. Stories began to circulate through the trans community about mental health clinicians who abused these requirements to keep their own income stream flowing, though these characterizations are not necessarily accurate interpretations of a therapist's motivation for encouraging a client to continue treatment. Clients who enter treatment because they're told they must rather than because they want to learn something about themselves generally don't perceive the same value for the money they pay. And the mythology about the process of gender-related diagnosis, psychological care, and surgical procedures has persisted because people repeat stories they've heard as if they are uniform fact and generalizable to themselves and all similarly situated individuals. Certainly, throughout the US medical system, for many conditions and procedures, people have been asked to pay for services that they didn't think benefited them directly, whether they did benefit them or not. This doesn't mean that the practice is acceptable; it just means that sometimes medicine involves trial and error as much as it involves standardized processes. Open and clear communication and respect between clients/patients and healthcare professionals is almost always necessary to achieve the best possible results. And outside of a few major cities, therapists or physicians with experience in treating trans people were few and far between for most of the twentieth century, so tales of horror about trying to find someone to treat even the simplest of medical needs when applied to a transgender body (let alone trans-specific care) were ubiquitous and difficult to forget, keeping many people from seeking care before they were in extreme distress. Distress, regardless of its source, inevitably complicates the relationship between clinicians and patients/clients.

In the 1970s, 1980s, and into the 2000s, many legal entities in the United States often required proof of "bottom surgery" (genital reconstruction) or sterilization to change gender markers on identity documents. Insurance didn't pay for our treatment. Some therapists told us we had to lie about our past, our childhood, our relatives, everything, to receive treatment. Many of us gave up marriages, families, jobs, everything to be recognized as the man or woman we knew ourselves to be. These rules and expectations filtered into the mainstream culture and the consciousness of the average, isolated American trans person. But the homogenized story of who trans people were and how we transitioned or worked in concert with the medical community was not the real story of every individual trans person. Even as we wanted "the hormones" and/or "the surgery," even as we searched for clinicians who we felt comfortable with or whom we were willing to trust long enough to get the procedure we sought, some trans people have doubted much about what they were doing. Read the community-based newsletters or magazines from the 1980s or 1990s and see the complaints that endocrinologists didn't know anything about how hormones worked; some of us suspected that surgeons were experimenting on us, since we never completely understood how they modified our bodies, and often we were afraid to ask questions. Yet, we did what we felt we had to do to become ourselves. Some of us did trust the doctors, were grateful, and got along well with them; others were damaged in surgery, verbally abused in doctor's offices or therapeutic settings. There was no way to know what you were going to find in your relationship with a clinician or their front office staff. There was nowhere to go if something went wrong. We read the community newsletters, we traveled to other states, we looked for community among people we met on the street or in a bar or in an adult bookstore (where some transgender community publications were available in the mid-twentieth century). And the *SOC*, a document we could never see because it was not for us, hung over our heads, always somehow out of reach, telling us what we should do to deserve care.

LEGAL INTERSECTIONS

From the time of Magnus Hirschfeld, and Benjamin after him, the physicians who helped TGD people have recognized that legal issues are important for us. Not being treated as real human beings, not having photographic identification that matches our appearance, constantly being questioned about who or what we are is, frankly, one of the reasons many of us go to the trouble of a medical transition in the first place. Most wanted their identities confirmed, validated, and recognized, and their past forgotten. Both Hirschfeld and Benjamin, and many early gender programs in the 1970s and 1980s provided their clients with "passes" or "carry-letters" they could show to police or others who questioned them. The signature of a doctor and the assertion that we were under medical care didn't solve every problem, but in many cases, it did help keep folks out of trouble.

This medicalization of our existence serves as a double-edged sword. On one hand, it gives pause to people who think we are trying to deceive them, but on the other, it contributes to our being viewed as mentally ill. The problems stem from our society's stereotypes about the meaning and proper use of male and female bodies and the system of classification of all bodies according to sex. Misogyny plays a role, too, as male authorities who make the rules tend to classify female bodies as less valuable economically, yet more valuable reproductively and therefore more important to control. Male bodies that appear as or become women are particularly at risk for abuse or punishment for transgressing social norms.

Advancements around the intersection of law and medicine have helped many TGD people. Trans activists have used the law to secure legal recognition and to educate legislators, administrators, workplaces, medical personnel, law enforcement, school personnel, government agencies, prison administrators and staff, and students at every level. It would be ideal if people needed only education to make the world a better place for us. It would be ideal if human rights were more than a concept implying equity and equality, fairness, and freedom to be who we are—but in the United States, our laws don't recognize human rights concepts with the same weight as civil rights. Despite our Declaration of Independence, operationally our system of law is rooted in civil rights, rights granted by the state, parceled out to those who matter, those whose words are listened to, those who can buy influence.

Trans people have worked hard to make the legal system work for us because we believe we deserve equal rights, just as our foundational Declaration has promised us. Over the last fifty years, we have successfully fought our way into civil rights protections with name and sex designation changes on driver licenses or state IDs in nearly every state (many of which no longer require surgery or a doctor's certification),[27] passport application procedures that acknowledge lived gender even if the sex on the birth certificate doesn't match,[28] same-sex marriage[29] and Title VII workplace protections[30] that acknowledge gender identity and expression as a component of the category of sex. However, the recent Dobbs decision in the Supreme Court[31] has demonstrated that in our legal system precedent is no longer sacred.

Nevertheless, we work with what we've got and now find ourselves in the fortunate position of having many brilliant trans, queer, and cisgender attorneys and legislative advocates working to change the laws and policies that support our rights and identities. Although we've fought against required medical procedures and forced sterilization in exchange for legal recognition, we still need physicians and psychologists to help our attorneys educate legislators and judges about the challenges we face and our needs in a variety of settings. The WPATH and its *SOC* have proven to be powerful tools for obtaining and reinforcing our legal rights. WPATH members contribute to amicus briefs and serve as expert witnesses in scores of legal cases that bring medical care and transition-related care to state and federal prisoners, preserve parental rights of trans people, combat instances of workplace discrimination, thwart criminal prosecution for living while transgender, and support the medical necessity of transition-related care in states where trans people are being targeted by lawmakers who want to legislate us out of existence.

The law by itself cannot resolve all social problems, all inequities. Political will is necessary to change society. We must use all the tools available to drive evolution toward the realization of a diverse and thriving nation. From the first modern lawsuits that ruled against people like us in the 1960s and 1970s, we have persisted in the self-education and partnerships that enabled our community to come out of the shadows. Many of us now serve as leaders in the arts, sciences, medicine, education, and law. Our trans politicians are increasing in number. Many cis politicians now recognize our contributions to society and our rights to Life, Liberty, and the Pursuit of Happiness. We must nurture strong partnerships within our community to achieve the freedom, fairness, equality, equity, and safety we all deserve. As a community, we must speak out and educate to ensure that gender diversity is recognized as a common human experience, not an aberration. Every human being on this planet possesses a gender identity and should be free to express it. Our politicians, lawyers, physicians, and researchers must also speak out with appreciation of our challenges and our gifts to bridge the fear of difference that hinders our quest for our real equality and safety in the United States.

HBIGDA BECOMES WPATH

Back in the 1960s through the 1990s, some of us managed to find information in university and medical school libraries, assuming we could get inside and could locate the surgery journals or the *Archives of Sexual Behavior* in the stacks. A few psychiatry and sociology journals published articles about these rare people, mysterious people, transsexual people, in which the authors viewed us from a distance. The surgery journals published reports on genital reconstruction—most often vaginoplasty but occasionally something about phalloplasty or metoidioplasty. We read the Letters to the Editor in subsequent issues, noting the appalled reaction from other surgeons. They castigated the editors for publishing trash or disgusting material; they claimed the articles demeaned the journal by implying these procedures were reputable or desirable practices. They affirmed the widespread belief that treating transsexuals with respect and dignity constituted a waste of time and energy.

Rachlin joined HBIGDA in 1993, intending to improve the *SOC* so that the document better met the needs of transmasculine people, giving trans people greater agency, and by introducing into the medical literature the same language that trans people used to speak about themselves. She attended her first HBIGDA Scientific Symposium in New York in 1993. The *SOC-4* hadn't changed much since the original *SOC-1* text from 1979; other than removing the Real Life Test in 1980, the subsequent changes were mostly grammatical corrections and slight reorganizations of the text. Rachlin expressed surprise and delight when she found progressive cisgender clinicians and trans-identified people participating in the conference, speaking on panels, and presenting research. "Everyone was so welcoming and progressive, and they were very welcoming of health providers who were themselves transgender," Rachlin told me.[32] Attendees discussed affirming children's gender identity and expression, a topic most trans people avoided due to fear of persecution whether they supported or opposed the idea.

The 1995 HBIGDA meeting took place in Kloster Irsee, Germany. Neither Fraser nor Rachlin attended. Instead, they appeared at the more accessible 1997 meeting in Vancouver, British Columbia. This was also my first HBIGDA meeting. I had only recently discovered the organization, didn't know much about the *SOC*, or understood how this organization would be of help to me, an average trans person who was not a clinician or researcher.

Nonetheless, I arrived at the conference with an agenda. In 1994, I helped establish a nondiscrimination ordinance in the city and county of San

Francisco. I sought to convince the city government to remove exclusions for transsexual treatments from their employee health plans, since it appeared to me that all the treatments trans people needed were covered for people who were not trans (the term *cisgender* did not exist yet), and it was only when clinicians or the insurers discovered that a person was trans that they might deny access to care. This sounded like discrimination to me. I posited that it would not increase costs to remove these exclusions and provide medically necessary care to trans employees (we knew there were at least a dozen trans people then employed by the city and county). I knew my cause would benefit from physician allies, and what better place to find them than at the HBIGDA meeting? I contacted my colleague Dallas Denny to propose that I offer to present a paper she and I had co-authored (published in Beth Firesteins's book, *Bisexuality: The Psychology and Politics of an Invisible Minority*), and Dallas agreed. I wanted to attend the conference as a presenter, on equal footing with other participants. The HBIGDA scientific committee accepted my proposal, and I arranged to travel to Vancouver, staying with a local trans man activist to save money.

Like Rachlin, I found the HBIGDA meeting to be a welcoming place. I realized that I could listen and comment or question presenters respectfully, and even if I disagreed with them, they accepted me as a contributor to the conversation. At first, I felt intimidated by the famous people—like Richard Green from the University of California Los Angeles, Ira Pauly from the University of Nevada, and Kenneth Zucker from the Clarke Institute in Toronto—but I gradually recognized that I was responsible for my feelings of inferiority and could disavow them. I found that when I was calm, rational, and carried myself with confidence, participants respected me. Though sometimes they would misinterpret my intensity as either aggression or defensiveness, so I quickly learned to tone it down. In one session, I listened to an older cis male psychologist deliver a paper about how all the trans men he saw in his practice projected a brittle masculinity he associated with feminine attempts to pose as male. I raised my hand and calmly suggested that his interpretation might be a projection of his own beliefs about trans men combined with the reflection of his clients' unexpressed anger, concealed due to fear of his rejection. My statement was met with applause from other professionals. Later that day, I presented the paper that Denny and I had co-authored (with Denny in the audience), and afterward we both engaged in conversation with Pauly. This discussion led to our later research on how clinicians should respectfully refer to trans people.[33]

A dramatic interruption of the 1997 meeting staged by Transexual Menace and other trans-identified demonstrators complaining about the inaccessibility of the conference resulted in the protestors being "invited to stay and participate."[34] I discussed the aftermath of this event elsewhere;[35] suffice it to say, "[t]he basic ideological differences were demonstrated between those clinicians who seem[ed] to perceive [trans] people as damaged goods, versus those who see us has having agency in our own lives, and it seemed to me that most professionals were in the more supportive camp."[36] The chair of the Standards Committee invited me to provide recommendations to the committee concerning better attention to transmasculine needs and treatments, but my effort was ultimately ignored by the committee, though they did me the dubious honor of listing me (along with Denny) as a consultant to *SOC-5*, released in 1998.

At the 1999 HBIGDA meeting in London, Rachlin proposed that the board establish an ethics committee. President Richard Green approved the motion. Although the ethics committee was not particularly active for the first twenty years, an important shift happened with the *SOC* at that meeting. Trans clinicians Patton, Sheila Kirk, and Anne Lawrence, as well as sociologist Holly Devor (who was not yet out as trans but was certainly more than an ordinary ally), sat on the Standards of Care Committee. Patton and Devor requested a copy of the changes I had recommended for *SOC-5*, and the committee integrated nearly all of them into the *SOC-6*, released in 2001. This later version, however, still structurally aligned with *SOC-5*, which perpetuated the mental illness model predicated on the definition of *gender identity disorder* in the *Diagnostic and Statistical Manual* (*DSM*).

The 2001 HBIGDA conference in Galveston, Texas, occasioned a subtle but transformative change for the organization and for the trans community. At that meeting, the roughly 450 attendees listened to opening plenary presentations by three trans women, one cisgender man, and one trans man (me), all focused on "The Language of Gender Variance." Psychologist Walter Bockting, an up-and-coming leader in trans-focused psychology, HIV research, and a champion of trans voices in research and clinical professions moderated the session. Conference presenters included (1) Norwegian physician and sexologist Esben Esther Pirelli Benestad and her wife, psychologist and sexologist Elsa Almaas, speaking about "Transforming Concepts in Genderland"; 2) United Kingdom–based sociologist Richard Ekins discussing "Configurations of Ungendering: On the Emergence of Gender-Negating Identities"; (3) Rosalyne Blumenstein and Barbra Ann Perina, trans women from New York City, deliberating on "The Construction, De-construction and Re-construction of Gender Identity Mergers and the Power of Language"; and (4) me, on behalf of Denny, and anthropologist Jason Cromwell, speaking about "The Language of Gender Variance," research based on the questions Pauly had posed to Denny and me at the 1997 conference. In this ninety-minute session, each speaker offered perspectives about the harmful medicalization of trans terminology, the variety of identities in the trans community outside the medicalized gaze, and the anger we felt as a result of objectifying diagnoses and gatekeeping. We presented with customary conventions—not as a protest attack—to clearly and effectively communicate our positions. At first, we did not realize just how effective we'd been, but over the ensuing days of the conference, doctor after doctor showed overhead projector slides with the quotation marks around patients' names, pronouns, and body parts scribbled out and with pronouns changed to reflect their patient's experienced gender. Sometimes the doctors caught overlooked mistakes and stopped midsentence to apologize for using inaccurate or dehumanizing language. They were catching on.

Thus, in 2001, a sea change started within HBIGDA, a change that sprang from within the trans community, evidenced by the number of trans people who attended and presented, participating as clinicians, scholars, and other professional contributors to the fund of knowledge that would improve trans people's lives. Trans clinicians and scholars served on HBIGDA's Scientific Planning Committee, including cardiologist Rebecca Allison, law professor Stephen Whittle, gynecologist Sheila Kirk, and physician assistant Jude Patton, along with eight cisgender physicians, two psychologists, and one doctor of education. Trans individuals delivered thirty-three presentations on medical, mental health, legal, and social topics. These changes established an allyship between trans people and the growing number of researchers and clinicians who were interested in us as human beings, in our care, and in full equality for trans people.

Not everyone at HBIGDA felt positive about this evolution. Every year, some members chose not to renew their memberships because there were too many trans people involved. They feared the influence of patients and clients and worried that other professionals would judge the organization as unscientific, or just an advocacy group, easily dismissed in academic or professional circles. Several members of the board of directors objected to the proposal (which I was not aware of) that I be considered for full membership in HBIGDA, but they were overruled when it came to a vote. In 2002, much to my surprise, I received a letter informing me of my full membership. In

2003, after being elected to the board of directors, one of the prominent board members told me HBIGDA had lost members because of my election. I was as surprised by this remark as I had been when I received my notice of full membership, though this was not as happy a moment. I replied, "Gee, that's too bad; they're going to miss all the fun!"

In 2005, Whittle became the first trans person elected as president of HBIGDA. He would serve as president-elect for two years (beginning with the meeting held in 2005 in Bologna, Italy); be installed as president at the meeting in 2007 (held in Chicago); preside over the planning of the 2009 meeting in Oslo, Norway; pass the baton to the next president at the end of that meeting; and remain on the board, sharing his post-presidential wisdom for another two years. While he was still president-elect, the board realized that the world was changing, that trans people were becoming adept at securing their rights and asking for better services, more research, more autonomy. I believe the board realized this in part because of the success of the 2001 and 2003 (held in Ghent, Belgium) meetings, both of which involved more trans people and more discussion of legal and social topics than ever before, and because of the presence of Whittle and myself on the board. We were accomplished activists who had changed laws and policies at the local and national level in our respective countries. Whittle worked as a respected professor of law and an attorney; I lived as a lowly writer with an MFA in short fiction, supporting myself and my trans activism as a freelance corporate technical writer, department manager, and occasional voice actor. I was not the typical professional member of HBIGDA, but through running a support group for nearly a decade and doing global outreach and research, I knew the trans community, understood management and organizational development, and valued what I believed HBIGDA offered in terms of legitimizing trans-focused medical care, research, and support for legal rights. I knew the organization was not pulling its weight yet, but with proper encouragement, I believed it could. Whittle and I agreed there was no other organization in the United States or elsewhere with the longevity and potential for respect in the field of transgender health, and we needed the influence of those physicians, therapists, and researchers to change things for the better and to help increase the availability of trans-knowledgeable healthcare professionals globally.

In 2006, the board decided to hold a meeting in New York City because the business activity of the association had increased. An every-other-year business meeting (held in concert with the scientific symposia) was proving insufficient for managing the growing needs and interests of the members and the needs of TGD people. President Stan Monstrey, a surgeon from Belgium, engaged the services of past-president Professor Eli Coleman from the University of Minnesota to lead the board through a series of exercises designed to assess the strengths, weaknesses, opportunities, and threats faced by HBIGDA. We realized we needed to up our game; modernize our policies and objectives; increase our communications; and pay more attention to our influence in the legal arena, where, since 2001, we had been responding to legal cases through amicus briefs to educate the courts. Our senior members had been increasingly called to testify as experts on behalf of trans people in litigation. Psychiatrist George Brown and I developed mission and vision statements for the board to debate and accept, and Coleman took the bold step of proposing to change the organization's name. As I said at the time, "Our name needs to immediately communicate what we are focused on, and it's time to stop focusing on a diagnosis or a supposed disease condition and start focusing on the health and wellbeing of transgender people." Within an hour we collectively settled on the name World Professional Association for Transgender Health, WPATH, and someone in the room reserved the URL so we could one day build a website.

To officially change the name, we needed approval from a majority of the membership. This process took nearly a year, and some of the membership were offended, heartbroken, or furious that we would consider abandoning Benjamin and consigning his legacy to the dustbin of history. Richard Green threatened to sue the board members. "No!" I explained in materials prepared for the membership vote, "we will always honor Harry, we will always tell his story, we will always acknowledge his pioneering influence, but to communicate in today's marketplace, we must have a name that is more forward-thinking, that more clearly communicates our objective, our *raison d'etre*." The majority of the members agreed. The organization's ability to influence policy, impact litigation, and negotiate and collaborate with other national and global organizations such as the National Institutes of Health and the World Health Organization grew rapidly from that time forward.

In 2007, I was reelected to the WPATH board, and the same former leader told me we lost members because I was elected. I repeated my original retort with a smile. Rachlin also joined the board that year, and our leadership was collectively recognizing the need for a more proactive approach to transgender health. I proposed that WPATH publish a statement on medical necessity and insurance coverage in the United States. I developed a draft with the help of my associate, André Wilson, with whom I had been working since 2004 to remove exclusions for transition-specific treatments from insurance plans and to assist the Human Rights Campaign to raise the bar for trans inclusion in the *Corporate Equality Index*. The other board members debated the draft for six months, and in June 2008, WPATH published its first public policy statement.[37] This was followed by many statements on topics including identity recognition without surgery, the need to cease criminalization of cross-dressing, and other issues affecting the health of TGD people.

INSURANCE COVERAGE

Transgender people who seek medical support for their gender identity have struggled to pay for those treatments or procedures from the time that such interventions became available. Street hormones, back-alley surgeons, and silicone-pumping parties have been common since people discovered that these body modifications were possible in the mid-twentieth century. Before that time, people were able to transition only with the assistance of clothing and behavior modifications, which often made interaction with institutions and officials—including medical practitioners, even for ordinary health concerns—complicated, if not impossible. But by the mid-1970s when gender clinics were public knowledge, demand for full-service, legitimate medical care increased. Those who could afford to pay for medical services were often able to get what they wanted if they could find a physician or surgeon willing to help them. Those without economic means continued to suffer. Unfortunately, in the United States, most people obtain their health insurance through their employer, and with the discrimination trans people face, jobs are sometimes hard to find or to hold onto.

Health insurance in the United States is extremely complicated. Insurance companies are run by diverse human beings with diverse personalities, business goals, and beliefs about healthcare and how it should be administered. Each state in the United States has its own insurance commission (or similar body) with an elected or appointed insurance commissioner (depending on the state's constitution and self-imposed regulations). Even self-insured corporations that may self-determine what their plans will cover may have conflicts with the insurance company from which they procure their benefit plan and with which they contract to administer the plan and process every individual claim generated by the enrolled employees and their covered dependents.[38] It can be a nightmare to figure out what is covered, even when employers intend to be trans-competent and inclusive.[39]

Health insurance companies were not aware of transgender treatments being provided and billed in the 1950s through much of the 1970s, and some lucky people, with doctors who were willing to stand up for them if insurers pushed back, were able to get hormones and some surgeries paid for by their insurance carriers and, in some states, even Medicaid. But in 1980, Janice Raymond, the author of *The Transsexual Empire: The Making of the She-Male* produced a report[40] for the National Center of Health Care Technology, a division of the US Department of Health and Human Services (HHS), which led the entity now called Center for Medicare and Medicaid Services (CMS—then known as HCFA or Health Care Financing Administration) to issue a 1981 memorandum recommending "that transsexual surgery not be covered by Medicare at this time." HCFA published this National Coverage Determination language in the Federal Register on August 21, 1989, as part of its Coverage Issues Manual for Medicare contractors.[41] This was the nail in the coffin, leading to broad and often vaguely worded exclusions for transsexual surgery in virtually every public and private health benefits policy written by any insurer in the country. It also brought transsexualism to the attention of legislators who chose to reinforce this prohibition during debate on the American's with Disabilities Act, which was enacted in 1990, a great victory for disability communities and their advocates[42] but a resounding slap in the face of transgender people, as "the legislative history appears to confirm, that these exclusions [transvestism, transsexualism, gender identity disorders not resulting from physical impairments] were based on the moral opprobrium of two senior senators [Jesse Helms, R-NC and William L. Armstrong, R-CO], conveyed in the eleventh hour of a marathon day-long floor debate, who believed these conditions [and others then-associated with sexual perversion] to be undeserving of legal protection.[43]

Many contemporary articles dealing with insurance coverage for transgender health credit the Affordable Care Act (ACA), particularly Section 1557 of that Act, with the availability of insurance coverage for TGD people, but years of community-based activist work, beginning well before the Obama Administration, led to the inclusion of trans nondiscrimination and positive coverage for trans-related health matters in the ACA. At the third International Conference on Transgender Law and Employment Policy (1994),[44] workers' compensation insurance executive and trans woman Lisa Middleton presented a summary of health insurance issues and suggested strategies for alleviating them. She wrote: "To achieve reimbursement for medical procedures, including transgender procedures, a body of medical evidence must exist that defines accepted, standard and proven medical practice for a given condition. That is not an argument for any or all of the specific HBIGDA standards. It is an argument for <u>recognized standards</u> in the application of medical services to transgender people."[45] Middleton also noted that "a modern protocol includes the experiences of the patient."[46] I was present in the audience, and those words hit me hard. Not being an attorney, but having worked as a medical writer and having taught legal writing, I thought this problem was something I could try to take on. I wasn't sure how, but I thought HBIGDA would somehow be part of the process.

The next month in San Francisco, the city's Human Rights Commission formally accepted the report I had written[47] and asked me to help the city attorney draft protective legislation, which was the first to include Gender Identity and Expression. The law went into effect in January 1995, and I saw the opportunity to let the Human Rights Commission know that they were failing the city's transgender employees because they couldn't get appropriate medical care due to exclusions in the city's employee health benefits plans. This put them on alert. In 1996, two trans men complained during a public meeting about the lack of trans-competent health services and the lack of reimbursement through health insurance plans. My phone started ringing off the hook: the mayor's office was referring media calls to me to explain what the issues were. I was caught off guard, but opportunistically I jumped on the chance to push the city of San Francisco, as an employer, to do the right thing by its trans workers and remove the exclusions from their plans. It took four years of monthly meetings with city officials, putting up with their repeated attempts to defer our requests, silencing our attempts to offer evidence, and canceling the physicians and psychologists we brought in to testify about the need for exclusions to be excised. My contention was there would be no appreciable increase in costs if they covered trans-related care and also made it possible for trans people to get basic, routine, and emergency care without fear of being turned away by doctors and nurses who were afraid to treat them because they were afraid the services weren't covered (and they wouldn't be reimbursed for their services) or were afraid of touching a transgender body.

With the help of the majority of San Francisco's Board of Supervisors, in 2000 the city finally approved changing one of the five plans employees could select from, so there would be one plan that covered trans surgeries; this plan went into effect in 2001. It was another four years before we could get any actuarial information, usage data, or cost analysis. But what we finally got was very exciting. My theory was proven correct: the cost was not excessive; in fact, it was surprisingly low. The city had collected roughly five million dollars in premium payments but had spent roughly $156,000 in claims. They dropped the premium charge to $0.00. Other institutional plans followed, like the University of California, which offered trans-inclusive benefits for students, faculty, and staff at all ten campuses with no additional premium.

I took this information to the Human Rights Campaign Foundation in Washington, DC, the largest gay and lesbian advocacy group in the country. They launched the *Corporate Equality Index* in 2002 and were committed to keeping transgender issues vitally integrated into the requirements they placed on those companies that wanted to demonstrate their positive regard for LGBT workers. In 2004, I met André Wilson, a Graduate Student Union (GSU) organizer at the University of Michigan who was trying to make trans benefits part of the bargaining agreement that year. The GSU asked me to come to Ann Arbor and train the other GSU activists on trans issues so they could be comfortable convincing others to support the GSU platform. I brought Wilson into my work with the Human Rights Campaign Foundation Workplace Project. We went to every trans community–based conference and every LGBT medical conference we could talk our way into, presenting about the strategy of getting self-insured companies to demand their insurance carriers to remove exclusions and offer trans-positive benefits. And we trained managers, doctors, and administrators about the value and utility of the HBIGDA/WPATH *SOC*, which were getting better all the time, and which were starting to provide the evidence base for the effectiveness of trans-specific healthcare. Every year, more and more corporations were offering trans-inclusive care. We worked with researchers at the Williams Institute to document employers' satisfaction with the efforts they made on behalf of trans employees.[48] We presented to the California Department of Insurance and successfully motivated them to regulate plans sold in California to eliminate discrimination on the basis of trans status or gender identity.[49] We consulted with benefits managers at major companies, law firms, and universities and colleges across the country, all of whom were trying to do what was right by the growing number of transgender people they were seeing in their workforces, clientele, and student bodies. We encouraged the State Department to amend their passport requirements. We spoke with graduate students, lawyers, doctors, anyone who would listen as we told them how important it was that trans people have access to responsible, competent healthcare and transition-related care. We encouraged trans people everywhere to get involved in policy work, training, medicine, and law. We spoke with software engineers at Epic, a leading vendor of electronic medical records systems, warning them of the problems created by dividing decision trees and coding everything based on a designation of a patient's sex. We spoke with representatives of CMS. That private companies were successfully offering trans-inclusive coverage was a significant factor in encouraging CMS to evaluate their national coverage determination. Forensic psychologists and a variety of physicians who were WPATH members testified before departmental appeals board within HHS, and on May 30, 2014, the Medicare exclusion was lifted.[50] This opened the door to the researchers and policy folks within the Obama Administration, several of whom were trans themselves, to press for trans inclusion in the ACA.

We know these things take a long time. But when one is committed, one just keeps at it, a little bit at a time. And on August 16, 2022, judges for the Fourth Circuit Court of Appeals ruled transgender people are entitled to protections under the Americans with Disabilities Act,[51] based on the change in nomenclature from gender identity disorder to gender dysphoria, a better body of scientific knowledge about gender dysphoria and better *SOC*. One step at a time . . . we will prevail.

THE *SOC* EVOLVES

By 2007, Coleman had begun supervising work on what would become *SOC-7*. In 2009, the *International Journal of Transgenderism* published a critique of the nomenclature in the *SOC* by historian Nicholas Matte and sociologists Aaron Devor and Theresa Vladicka. The effort to redesign the *SOC* to be more educational and helpful to clinicians and trans people required five years to complete and included more than thirty contributors and nine primary authors, including myself and Botzer, who had been elected to the board in 2009. Several other trans professionals contributed to this version of the *SOC*, released in 2011 at the Scientific Symposium in Atlanta and widely hailed as a significant improvement. In the words of British trans activist Christine Burns, this version "stops telling trans people what they had to do to please the doctors, and now tells the doctors what they need to do to help trans people."[52] WPATH president Bockting helped set the stage for the association's efforts to deliver physician education to improve access to competent care, which some in leadership still believed could not be done. In 2011, Bockting passed the presidential gavel to Fraser, and I was installed as president-elect.

Also in 2011, the National Academies Press published the Institute of Medicine's first major report on the health of lesbian, gay, bisexual, and transgender people.[53] Bockting, Judith Bradford (Fenway Institute, Boston), and Robert Garofalo (Northwestern University, Feinberg School of Medicine) were among the members of the Committee on Lesbian, Gay, Bisexual, and Transgender Health Issues and Research Gaps and Opportunities who authored this seminal report that has since guided many research priorities that emphasize trans people's health. Bradford also mentored trans woman researcher Jessica Xavier, who went on to work inside the Health Resources and Services Administration (which runs the Ryan White HIV/AIDS Program), helping evaluate health research, building the relationships within influential institutions to help increase awareness of trans health issues. She also served on the HHS LGBT Coordinating Committee during the Obama administration, advocating for improved data collection methodology in federal health surveys to measure gender identity. Garofalo, in addition to his work as a Chicago pediatrician, is a co-author of WPATH *SOC* versions 7 and 8, and is also editor of the peer-reviewed journal *Transgender Health*.

WPATH members impacted the development of other organizations as well. Endocrinologists Walter Meyer, Vin Tangpricha, Louis Gooren, and Norman Spack, and professor of medical psychology Peggy Cohen-Kettenis helped endocrinologist Wylie Hembree develop the 2009 Endocrine Society Guidelines.[54] In 2017, the Endocrine Society published updated guidelines; eight of its ten authors were also members of WPATH. From 2009 until 2011, Allison served as the first trans woman president of GLMA: Health Professionals Advancing LGBTQ+ Equality. Cisgender psychiatrist and long-time trans champion Dan Karasic has been a constant advocate for diagnosis reform within the American Psychiatric Association (which controls the *DSM*), and other members of that organization also contributed to these efforts. In 2012, Karasic led a team of WPATH members (including myself, President Fraser, and immediate past president Bockting) in drafting WPATH's recommendation to remove the diagnosis of "gender identity disorder" from the *DSM* and replace it with "gender dysphoria," recognizing that trans people did not suffer from mental disorder because of their transness and that treatment could reduce distress (leaving their transness intact). *DSM-5*, released in 2014, took most of our recommendations into account. No longer did being transgender imply that one was mentally ill nor was a medicalized or "polar" transition the only treatment approach. The binary was no longer the only way, nor was surgery the only option.

Since its inception, the day-to-day work of the HBIGDA/WPATH organization was executed chiefly through the volunteer efforts of the officers and members of the board of directors. For nearly two decades, from 1997 to 2015, the administration and recordkeeping for the organization had been lovingly run with the institutional memory and tireless work of the board-appointed executive director, professor and psychologist Bean Robinson. From 2009, at the beginning of Bockting's term as president, Rachlin and I developed an internal policy and procedure manual to standardize administrative practices within the organization and prepare to move the organization toward expansion and more professional management. We continually maintained that document for about eight years.

The same period saw an increase in the number of amicus briefs we joined to protect the rights of trans people in prison, to allow trans people to use restrooms that matched their gender identity at work, and to claim expenses for gender-affirming surgery not covered by insurance as legitimate medical expenses for income tax reporting purposes.

In 2013, under President Fraser, WPATH worked with representatives of the World Health Organization to develop background for the forthcoming *International Classification of Diseases* revision 11 (adopted by the 72nd World Health Assembly and published in 2019; effective date January 1, 2022), which would remove "transsexualism" from the mental disorders chapter and place the diagnosis of "gender incongruence" in a planned new chapter on sexual health. The board also held a strategic planning session in which we declared education, research, and organizational development as priorities for the coming five years. We discussed the possibility of contracting with a professional association management firm to take the administrative burden away from underpaid staff and the volunteers who struggled to adapt to quickly increasing demands on the association and its growing membership. We completed preliminary work to identify potential firms, but few of them seemed interested in dealing with an association as small, underfunded, and controversial as ours. Still, we remained excited about the future. We pushed our meeting date to February 2014 to avoid the rainy season in Bangkok, the site of our first scientific symposium to be held in Asia, breaking the original model of alternating between Europe and the United States. We felt determined to reach out to the entire world, even if our reach remained tentative for lack of resources. Our membership continued to grow slowly, and we had little in the way of financial support or reserves to meet our expenses should conference attendance falter or membership renewals decline.

During Fraser's tenure as president, she supported Rachlin's proposal to establish the WPATH Graduate Student Initiative. The organization had previously made no accommodations for students in the field. In the 1990s and early 2000s, Rachlin saw the energy of young clinicians and researchers in the growing network of community conferences such as the FTM Conference of the Americas, True Spirit, Gender Odyssey, Southern Comfort, and the Philadelphia Trans Health Conference. She believed that WPATH would benefit from the influence of young professionals and researchers, many of whom were TGD. The young researchers would benefit as well from the affiliation and from having access to seasoned professionals and what was becoming a specialty within medicine and behavioral health. Within the board of WPATH this was not an easy sell, as some members of the board pushed back in the belief that the small professional organization striving for legitimacy should limit membership to those who had already achieved full professional status. Rachlin first co-chaired this effort with (then graduate student) Colt St. Amand and later with Luke Roy Allen. Through their determined work they produced an annual WPATH graduate student research symposium (held for many years in conjunction with the Philadelphia Trans Health Conference) and ushered in a new era of mentorship and young professional participation in WPATH, building talent for the future.

In 2014, a total of 525 people attended the WPATH Biennial Symposium in Bangkok—the largest meeting yet held. Fraser conducted an international, invitational working session to explore the idea of a global education initiative through which we assessed the prospects of delivering professional education using a human rights framework. A delegation of trans people from India attended, and many speakers gave voice to Asia's diverse range of trans communities. Fraser passed the gavel to me in Bangkok, and I asked Coleman to lead the effort to develop *SOC-8*. I also asked Fraser and Canadian psychiatrist and sexual health physician Gail Knudson to cochair the Global Education Initiative and begin to develop a volunteer faculty and a proposed curriculum to certify professionals in gender-affirming care through comprehension of the *SOC*.

We had been trying to change the name of WPATH's journal, the *International Journal of Transgenderism*, to the *International Journal of Transgender Health* since 2006, and the publisher Taylor & Francis required that we raise the impact factor and ensure a regular (rather than irregular) publication schedule before they would allow the change of title. Our lead journal editors, Walter Bockting (2005–2015) and Walter Bauman (2016–2022) worked hard to meet those requirements, and the publisher changed the journal's title in 2020, with issue one of volume twenty-one.

In 2015, the board agreed to engage Veritas Meeting Solutions as our medical association management service provider. Of all the firms we considered, Veritas was the only one willing to accommodate our meager budget and take on the significant challenges of supporting a controversial condition. During my presidency, we also developed the regional affiliate organizations to give different cultures and political systems an opportunity to address their own cultural issues and build their membership. We reduced membership dues, especially the dues for all student members and for professionals from economically disadvantaged countries. The Global Education Initiative began delivering training in November 2015. It's unlikely that we could have managed to develop the training program without the administrative expertise of the Veritas Meeting Solutions staff. This group has also grown, now managing more than twenty-five small medical associations. WPATH remains their most demanding client because of our rapid growth and the persistent controversies in the field.

Our 2016 meeting in Amsterdam drew more than one thousand participants. There, I passed the presidential gavel to Knudson. In 2018, Knudson convened our scientific symposium in Buenos Aires. During the COVID-19 pandemic, we met virtually in 2020 and expanded our training reach exponentially; the training initiative is now a Global Training Institute. WPATH's membership includes more than 3,600 individuals at this writing. In 2022, Bowers became our first trans woman president, and our symposium held in Montreal hosted 1,800 participants. Physician Asa Radix, one of the co-chairs to oversee the creation of *SOC-8*, was elected in 2022, and in October 2024, he will become the third trans man and first trans man medical doctor to lead WPATH.

The work never ceases. Even as we have made tremendous progress, the political right in the United States and around the world has used misinformation about transgender people to create moral panic, increasingly targeting transgender people and the professionals who serve them with discriminatory policies and criminalization. Leaders in the public square, legislative chambers, religious strongholds, and courtrooms across the world debate aspects of trans-related care, often refusing to hear testimony from trans people and their families or their physicians, demonstrating the serious need for ongoing support from professional organizations and robust standards of care.

I cannot express enough gratitude to those volunteer leaders and administrative personnel who worked ceaselessly to keep this association alive in the beginning and through the long development process, leading us to the more stable ground we stand on today. As a trans person who is not a clinician, I am grateful for the opportunity I had to serve and influence this development, and I'm proud to see the evolution of the *SOC*. *SOC-8*, released in September 2022, may still not be perfect, but the document, with more than one hundred contributors, substantial references, and truly evidence-based guidelines, moves the field another step forward. As noted in the abstract of *SOC-8*: "One of the main functions of WPATH is to promote the highest standards of health care for TGD people through the *Standards of Care (SOC)*. . . . The *SOC* is based on the best available science and expert professional consensus in transgender health."[55]

> The overall goal of the *SOC* is to provide clinical guidance for health professionals to assist transsexual, transgender, and gender nonconforming people with safe and effective pathways to achieving lasting personal comfort with their gendered selves, in order to maximize their overall health, psychological well-being, and self-fulfillment. This assistance may include primary care, gynecologic and urologic care, reproductive options, voice and communication therapy, mental health services (e.g., assessment, counseling, psychotherapy), and hormonal and surgical treatments. While this is primarily a document for health professionals, the *SOC* may also be used by individuals, their families, and social institutions to understand how they can assist with promoting optimal health for members of this diverse population."[56]

The group that started in 1979 as a handful of cis and trans clinicians and researchers has now become an institution where caring cisgender and trans healthcare professionals have a voice. It is where we have achieved the authority to uphold respect and integrity in our ongoing pursuit of health, human rights, and justice for TGD people. It's important to understand the history, and it's time to let go of the mythology and the rumors that swirled around the early versions of the *SOC*. It's time to reject the misinformation promulgated by politicians and fear mongers. Anyone who is truly interested in transgender health should spend some quality time digesting the wisdom in *SOC-8* getting to know the clinical experts and researchers and transgender people themselves. Evolution of knowledge is the process that science engages. It is always changing, never static, just like life, and the infinite diversity science works to understand.

NOTES

1. Pomeroy, *Dr. Kinsey and the Institute for Sex Research*, 3. Alfred Kinsey's two volumes *Sexual Behavior in the Human Male* (1948) and *Sexual Behavior in the Human Female* (1953) "brought sex out of the bedroom and into the world's parlor."
2. Isserman, *America Divided*; Pomeroy, *Dr. Kinsey and the Institute for Sex Research*, 138–40.
3. See chapter 11 in this volume.
4. Green, *Gay Rights and Trans Rights*, 147.
5. Sullivan, *We Both Laughed in Pleasure*, 250–55.
6. See chapter 10 in this volume.
7. See chapter 10 in this volume.
8. See chapter 10 in this volume.
9. See chapter 7 in this volume.
10. Dewhurst, "First International Symposia," 2–7.
11. See chapter 10 in this volume.
12. Devor, "International Symposia."
13. Green, *Gay Rights Trans Rights*, 147.
14. Patton, conversation with the author, August 28, 2022.
15. Walker, "Memorandum and Announcement."
16. See https://www.wpath.org/about/history.
17. Annual membership dues: $60 per year in 1979; $110 ($55 for students) per year in 2007; and $225 per year ($35 for students) and lower fees for residents of low- and middle-income countries and emeritus members in 2022 (since 2015). Membership had also grown from a few dozen in 1979–1980 to roughly five hundred in 2007.
18. See chapter 7 in this volume.
19. Botzer, conversation with the author, April 15, 2022.
20. Fraser, conversation with the author, August 15, 2022.
21. Copies of the first four versions of the HBIGDA *Standards of Care* are no longer easy to find. In preparing this chapter, I referred to copies in my possession. Readers interested in a more detailed point-by-point comparison and evolution of the *Standards of Care* from Version 1 to Version 8 are encouraged to read the analysis by Cross, "The WPATH Standards of Care."
22. This language appeared in the first, second, third, and fourth versions of the *SOC*. The fifth version specified the minimum criteria could be "raised" by individual

clinicians with respect to any client. The sixth version stated, "individual professionals and organized programs may modify them" and the seventh version stated, "individual health professionals and programs may modify them." Version 8 (2022) further evolved to state: "Individual health care professionals and programs may modify them in consultation with the TGD person. . . . The *SOC-8* are guidelines rooted in the fundamental rights of TGD people that apply to all settings in which health care is provided regardless of an individual's social or medical circumstances." *SOC-8*, pp. S6–S7. This linguistic evolution demonstrates the growing awareness of TGD autonomy and the justice TGD people deserve.

23. Harry Benjamin International Gender Dysphoria Association, *"Standards of Care, Version 1,"* 4.

24. Green, *Gay Rights Trans Rights*, 150.

25. Benjamin, *The Transsexual Phenomenon*, 137–38.

26. Erickson Educational Foundation, *Guidelines for Transexuals*, 3.

27. Movement Advancement Project, "Identity Document Laws and Policies."

28. US Department of State, "Gender Transition Applicants."

29. Obergefell v. Hodges.

30. Bostock v. Clayton County, Georgia.

31. Dobbs v. Jackson Women's Health Organization.

32. Rachlin, conversation with the author, August 14, 2022.

33. Green, Denny, and Cromwell, " 'What Do You Want Us to Call You?' " 100–10.

34. Green, "The Benjamin Conference,"14.

35. Green, "Unbending the Light," 509–18.

36. Green, "The Benjamin Conference," 14.

37. WPATH Clarification on Medical Necessity of Treatment, Sex Reassignment, and Insurance Coverage in the U.S.A., June 17, 2008, was replaced by an updated position statement issued December 21, 2016; additionally, a statement about medical necessity of electrolysis was issued July 15, 2016. Available at http://wpath.org/policies.

38. Smith, "The Complete History of Employer-Provided Health Insurance."

39. Kirkland, "Transition Coverage and Clarity," 208.

40. Raymond, "Paper Prepared for the National Center for Health Care Technology."

41. Williams, "Fact Checking Janice Raymond.

42. See White House, "Transcript of Statement by The President July 26, 1990."

43. See ADA Project, "Gender Dysphoria Discrimination," and Goren, "Understanding the ADA."

44. ICTLEP meetings were organized annually in Houston, Texas, from 1992 to 1997 by trans attorney Phyllis Frye. It was a training ground for a generation of trans activists and attorneys. For further information, see Long and Tuttle, *Phyllis Frye*.

45. Middleton, "Insurance and the Reimbursement," F-9.

46. Middleton, "Insurance and the Reimbursement," F-9.

47. Green, "Investigation into Discrimination."
48. Herman, "Costs and Benefits."
49. State of California Department of Insurance, "Economic Impact Statement," 4–6.
50. Green, "Transsexual Surgery May Be Covered by Medicare."
51. Migdon, "Americans with Disabilities Act Protects Transgender People."
52. Remarks by Christine Burns at the launch of *SOC-7* at the WPATH meeting held in Atlanta, Georgia, September 2011.
53. Institute of Medicine, *The Health of Lesbian.*
54. Hembree et al., "Endocrine Treatment of Transsexual Persons."
55. Coleman, et al., WPATH, *Standards of Care, 8th version*, S3.
56. Coleman, et al., WPATH, *Standards of Care, 8th version*, S5.

WORKS CITED

ADA Project. "Gender Dysphoria Discrimination." Accessed December 12, 2022. ada-lawproject.org/gender-dysphoria-discrimination.

Benjamin, Harry. *The Transsexual Phenomenon.* New York: Warner Books, 1966.

Blumenstein, Rosalyne. *Branded T.* Bloomington, IN: AuthorHouse, 2003.

Bostock v. Clayton County, Georgia, 590 U.S. No. 17-1618. 11th Circuit, 2020.

Campbell, Travis, and Yana van der Meulen Rodgers "Health Insurance Coverage and Health Outcomes among Transgender Adults in the United States." *Health Economics* 31, no. 6 (2022): 1–20. https://doi.org/10.1002/hec.4483. Accessed August 22, 2024.

Cannon, Loren. 2022. *The Politicization of Trans Identity: An Analysis of Backlash, Scapegoating, and Dog-Whistling from Obergefell to Bostock.* Lanham, MD: Lexington Books.

Coleman, Eli, Walter Bockting, Marsha Botzer, et al. "Standards of Care for the Health of Transsexual, Transgender, and Gender-Nonconforming People, Version 7." *International Journal of Transgenderism* 13, no. 4 (2012): 165–232. Accessed August 22, 2024. https://doi.org/10.1080/15532739.2011.700873.

Coleman, Eli, A. E. Radix, W. P. Bouman, et al. "Standards of Care for the Health of Transgender and Gender Diverse People, Version 8." *International Journal of Transgender Health* 23, no. S1 (2022): S1–259. Accessed August 22, 2024. https://doi.org/10.1080/26895269.2022.2100644.

Cross, Alexander. "The WPATH Standards of Care: Their History and Importance in Advocating for Transgender Health." Degree with honors (international affairs) thesis. University of Maine, 2023. Accessed October 29, 2023. https://digitalcommons.library.umaine.edu/cgi/viewcontent.cgi?article=1798&context=honors.

Currah, Paisley. *Sex Is as Sex Does: Governing Transgender Identity*. New York: New York University Press, 2022.

Currah, Paisley, Richard M. Juang, and Shannon Price Minter, eds. *Transgender Rights*. Minneapolis: University of Minnesota Press, 2006.

Denny, Dallas, and Jamison Green, "Gender Identity and Bisexuality." In *Bisexuality: The Psychology and Politics of an Invisible Minority*, edited by Beth A. Firestein, 804–102. Thousand Oaks, CA: Sage, 1996.

Devor, Aaron. "History of the Association." World Professional Association for Transgender Health, 2013. Accessed August 30, 2022. https://www.wpath.org/about/history.

———. "International Symposia." World Professional Association for Transgender Health, 2021. Accessed August 30, 2022. https://www.wpath.org/about/history/international-symposia.

Dewhurst, C. J. "First International Symposia, Opening Remarks." World Professional Association for Transgender Health, 1969. Accessed, August 30, 2022. https://www.wpath.org/media/cms/Documents/History/Symposium/1969/Prof%20Dewhurst%20Opening%20Remarks.pdf.

Dobbs v. Jackson Women's Health Organization 597 U.S. (2022). No 20.19-1392. 5th Circuit, 2022.

Erickson Educational Foundation. *Guidelines for Transexuals*. University of Victoria Transgender Archives Collection, Baton Rouge, LA, 1974. Accessed, October 9, 2022. http://archive.org/details/transgenderarchives/.

Goren, William. "Understanding the ADA." William D. Goren, J.D, LL.M. (blog), 2022. Accessed December 12, 2022. https://www.understandingtheada.com/?s=legislative+history+of+transsexualism+exclusion .

Green, James. "The Benjamin Conference: A Seedbed for Change." *FTM Newsletter*, Issue 39 (November 1997): 14.

———. "Investigation into Discrimination against Transgendered People." Archived with the San Francisco Human Rights Commission Documents, 1994. Accessed August 1, 2022. https://wayback.archive-it.org/org-571/20220601203622/https://sf-hrc.org/reports-research-investigations#LGBT%20and%20Intersex%20Communities.

———. "Transsexual Surgery May Be Covered by Medicare." *LGBT Health* 1, no. 4 (2014): 256–58.

Green, Jamison. "Unbending the Light: Changing Laws and Policies to Make Transgender Health Visible; Reflections of an Advocate." *Journal of Law, Medicine, and Ethics* 50, no. 3 (2022): 509–18.

Green, Jamison, Dallas Denny, and Jason Cromwell. "'What Do You Want Us to Call You?' Respectful Language." *Transgender Studies Quarterly* 5, no. 1 (2018): 100–10. Accessed August 22, 2024. https://doi.org/10.1215/23289252-4291812.

Green, Richard. *Gay Rights Trans Rights: A Psychiatrist/Lawyer's 50-Year Battle*. Agenda Book, 2018.

Green, Richard, and John Money, eds. *Transsexualism and Sex Reassignment*. Baltimore, MD: Johns Hopkins University Press, 1969.

Harry Benjamin International Gender Dysphoria Association. "*Standards of Care*: The Hormonal and Surgical Sex Reassignment of Gender Dysphoric Persons, version 1." 1979. Copy in author's possession.

———. "*Standards of Care*: The Hormonal and Surgical Sex Reassignment of Gender Dysphoric Persons, version 2." 1980. Copy in author's possession.

———. "*Standards of Care*: The Hormonal and Surgical Sex Reassignment of Gender Dysphoric Persons, version 3." 1981. Copy in author's possession.

———. "*Standards of Care*: The Hormonal and Surgical Sex Reassignment of Gender Dysphoric Persons, version 4." 1990. Copy in author's possession.

———. *The Standards of Care for Gender Identity Disorders: Fifth Version*. Dusseldorf: Symposium Publishing, 1998. Copy in author's possession.

———. *The Standards of Care for Gender Identity Disorders: Sixth Version*. Dusseldorf: Symposium Publishing, 2001. Copy in author's possession.

Hembree, Wylie C., Peggy Cohen-Kettenis, Henriette A. Delemarre-van de Waal, et al. "Endocrine Treatment of Transsexual Persons: An Endocrine Society Clinical Practice Guideline." *Journal of Clinical Endocrinology & Metabolism* 94, no. 9 (2009): 3132–54. Accessed August 22, 2024. https://doi.org/10.1210/jc.2009-0345.

Hembree, Wylie C., Peggy T. Cohen-Kettenis, Louis Gooren, et al. "Endocrine Treatment of Gender-Dysphoric/Gender-Incongruent Persons: An Endocrine Society Clinical Practice Guideline," *Journal of Clinical Endocrinology & Metabolism* 102, no. 11 (2017): 3869–903. Accessed August 22, 2024. https://doi.org/10.1210/jc.2017-01658.

Herman, Jody. 2013. "Costs and Benefits of Providing Transition-Related Health Care Coverage in Employee Health Benefits Plans." Los Angeles, CA: Williams Institute. Accessed December 13, 2022. https://williamsinstitute.law.ucla.edu/wp-content/uploads/Costs-Transition-Health-Plans-Sep-2013.pdf.

Institute of Medicine. *The Health of Lesbian, Gay, Bisexual, and Transgender People: Building a Foundation for Better Understanding*. Washington, DC: National Academies Press, 2011.

Isserman, Maurice. *America Divided*. New York: Oxford University Press, 2012.

Kirkland, Anna, Shauhin Talesh, and Angela K. Perone. "Transition Coverage and Clarity in Self-Insured Corporate Health Insurance Benefit Plans." *Transgender Health* 6, no. 4 (2020): 207–16. Accessed August 22, 2024. https://doi.org/10.1089/trgh.2020.0067.

Levasseur, Dru. 2015. "Gender Identity Defines Sex: Updating the Law to Reflect Modern Medical Science is the Key to Transgender Rights." *Vermont Law Review* 39 (2015): 943–1004.

Long, Michael G., and Shea Tuttle. *Phyllis Frye and the Fight for Transgender Rights*. College Station: Texas A&M University Press, 2022.

Matte, Nicholas, Aaron H. Devor, and Theresa Vladicka. "Nomenclature in the World Professional Association for Transgender Health's *Standards of Care*: Background and Recommendations." *International Journal of Transgenderism* 11, no. 1 (2009): 42–52.

Middleton, Lisa. "Insurance and the Reimbursement of Transgender Health Care." *Proceedings of the International Conference of Transgender Law and Employment Policy*, Appendix F. Houston, TX: ICTLEP, 1994, F-1–F-12. Accessed December 13, 2022. https://www.digitaltransgenderarchive.net/catalog?utf8=%E2%9C%93&f%5Bcollection_name_ssim%5D%5B%5D=International+Conference+on+Transgender+Law+and+Employment+Policy%3A+Annual+Proceedings+and+Newsletters&q=Third+Conference.

Migdon, Brooke. "Americans with Disabilities Act Protects Transgender People Judge Rules." Changing America, August 16, 2022. Accessed December 12, 2022. https://thehill.com/changing-america/respect/equality/3604307-americans-with-disabilities-act-protects-transgender-people-judge-rules/.

Movement Advancement Project, "Identity Document Laws and Policies." 2022. Accessed December 6, 2022. https://www.lgbtmap.org/equality-maps/identity_document_laws.

Obergefell v. Hodges, 576 U.S. (2015). No. 14-556. 6th Circuit, 2015.

Pomeroy, Wardell B. *Dr. Kinsey and the Institute for Sex Research*. New York: Harper & Row, 1972.

Raymond, Janice. "Paper Prepared for the National Center for Health Care Technology on the Social and Ethical Aspect of Transsexual Surgery." 1980. Obtained from http://www.gendercare.org/raymond.htm; no longer available. Copy in author's possession.

Raymond, Janice G. *The Transsexual Empire: The Making of the She-Male*. Boston, MA: Beacon Press, 1979.

Sharpe, Andrew. *Transgender Jurisprudence: Dysphoric Bodies of Law*. London: Cavendish, 2002.

Smith, Gabrielle. "The Complete History of Employer-Provided Health Insurance" PeopleKeep.com, 2021. Accessed December 11, 2022. https://www.peoplekeep.com/blog/the-complete-history-of-employer-provided-health-insurance#.

State of California, Department of Insurance. "Economic Impact Statement," 2012. Accessed December 11, 2022. http://transgenderlawcenter.org/wp-content/uploads/2013/04/Economic-Impact-Assessment-Gender-Nondiscrimination-In-Health-Insurance.pdf.

Sullivan, Lou. *We Both Laughed in Pleasure: The Selected Diaries of Lou Sullivan, 1961–1991*, edited by Ellis Martin and Zach Ozma. New York: Nightboat Books, 2019.

US Department of Health and Human Services. "About the Affordable Care Act." Accessed December 12, 2022. https://www.hhs.gov/healthcare/about-the-aca/index.html.

US Department of State—Bureau of Consular Affairs. "Gender Transition Applicants." Last updated April 19, 2024. Accessed December 6, 2022. https://travel.state.gov/content/passports/en/passports/information/gender.html.

Walker, Paul A. Memorandum and Announcement directed to "Persons interested in the Harry Benjamin International Gender Dysphoria Association." April 17, 1979. Accessed September 3, 2022. https://www.wpath.org/media/cms/Documents/History/Harry%20Benjamin/First%20HBIGDA%20Membership%20Request%20Letter%201979.pdf.

White House, Office of the Press Secretary. "Transcript of Statement By The President, July 26, 1990." Accessed August 22, 2024. https://www.archives.gov/research/americans-with-disabilities/transcriptions/naid-6037493-statement-by-the-president-americans-with-disabilities-act-of-1990.html.

Williams, Cristan. "Fact Checking Janice Raymond: The NCHCT Report." *The Trans Advocate*. Accessed December 11, 2022. https://www.transadvocate.com/fact-checking-janice-raymond-the-nchct-report_n_14554.htm.

World Health Organization. "*ICD-11*." 2019. Accessed August 22, 2024. https://icd.who.int/en/.

14

THE BIOLOGICAL UNDERPINNINGS OF GENDER IDENTITY

Carolyn Wolf-Gould and Joshua D. Safer

> The future may see more efforts to solve the riddle of the etiology of gender role disturbances. How much can be psychological? How much may be genetic, how much neuroendocrine? What would be the nature of a predisposition to transsexuality, and how much of a role does it play in the final clinical picture? Can the imprinting phenomenon, as observed in animals, find a parallel in humans? And to be personal once more, will I live long enough to see the answers to any of these questions?
>
> —Harry Benjamin, 1969

Sexologist Milton Diamond famously proclaimed, "Nature loves variety. Unfortunately, society hates it."[1] The animal kingdom exhibits abundant gender diversity—it's bursting with biological rainbows that challenge the evolutionary biologists who attempt to classify organisms into tidy, binary categories based on behaviors, methods of reproduction, and anatomical parts.[2] Members of some animal species change or crisscross between genders, possess intersex anatomies, express nontraditional (for humans) sex roles, exist in multiple gender families (that is, sunfish have three distinct male morphological categories and one female type[3]) and exhibit same-sex sexuality.[4] Stanford University biology professor Joan Roughgarden wrote, "Organisms flow across the bounds of any category we construct. In biology, nature abhors a category."[5] We humans listen, astonished, to descriptions of fish that change sex or stories about the male penguin pair who hatched an egg and raised their chick. We gaze at the gorgeous seahorse fathers gestating their young. These creatures encounter no stigma. In their world, diversity simply is what it is. Given the wondrous mix of the animal kingdom, is it any surprise that humans, too, express gender and sexual diversity?

Early medical research focused on describing and categorizing transgender and gender-diverse (TGD) people. Researchers asked: What is this phenomenon? What do we call it? In the early to mid-twentieth century, clinicians like Magnus Hirschfeld and Harry Benjamin labored to categorize those they encountered and then moved to a more practical problem: As medical providers, what is the appropriate response?

As exploratory technologies emerged, researchers asked increasingly nuanced questions about the etiology of gender and sexual diversity. The birth of the radioimmunoassay in the late 1950s[6] allowed scientists to measure circulating levels of hormones and ask: Are differences in gender identity and sexual orientation due to hormone levels? Microscopists developed increasingly powerful instruments and sophisticated tissue staining techniques to address another question: Are sexuality and gender diversity due to structural differences in the brain? In 1954, James Watson and Francis Crick modeled DNA's double helix, a discovery that led to sequencing techniques that unlocked genetic codes to reveal the action of proteins on human biology and behaviors. Is gender identity linked to a gene? Increasingly powerful twin studies defined inherited patterns of gender diversity. Is gender diversity inherited? In the 1960s, scientists began to explore the process of sex differentiation in utero, asking: Is gender identity established while still in the womb?[7] In 1977, magnetic resonance imaging (MRI) sliced the body like Wonder Bread to reveal detailed anatomical images, and in the 1990s, functional MRI enabled researchers to visualize blood flow to parts of the brain and examine our unspoken thoughts by asking: What connections are happening inside the brain?[8] An array of evolving techniques and technologies enabled scientists to test evolving hypotheses. Recently, the microscopic MRI extended the view of the functional MRI to the level of individual neurons and cell nuclei.[9] Scientists can now tag nuclei to explain the cellular origins of captured signals and map the lineage of cells. Soon, perhaps, they will identify additional pieces in gender diversity's etiological puzzle.

In the 1960s and 1970s, some psychoanalysts placed blame for transgressive gender expression (identified as a "disorder") on nurture—specifically, unhealthy parental practices (overbearing mother, absent father), psychic trauma, mental illness, and loss.[10] Early biomedical researchers did not directly reject psychological theories but emphasized possible biological predispositions.

In this chapter, we explore the history of efforts to understand the biological underpinnings of gender diversity. We describe some of the sentinel reports that have led to current understandings. We defer judgment on the strength and validity of the studies and focus instead on how the investigative questions evolved as emerging technology offered scientists new paths to explore. As you, the reader, wander these paths (some with dead ends), remember that these research efforts did not follow a logical, linear course but emerged instead from diverse hypotheses moving in scattered directions through a jungle of academic thought—a process profoundly shaped by the prevailing cultural winds of the time.

EPIDEMIOLOGIC RESEARCH

How many people are trans? Historical prevalence data chronicle the movement, primarily in Western countries, from viewing gender diversity as rare to recognizing that it's a relatively common phenomenon. The term *prevalence* refers to the proportion of a population who possesses a characteristic (or disease) within a specific time frame.[11]

In 1980, the *Diagnostic and Statistical Manual of Mental Disorders (DSM-III)* established diagnoses related to gender identity for the first time. These included "transsexualism and gender identity disorder of childhood" under the category of Psychosexual Disorders. The authors stated that the prevalence was "apparently rare."[12] Seven years later, the *DSM-III, Revised Edition*, stated that a "disturbance in gender identity is rare" and estimated the prevalence of transsexuality as "one in 30,000 for males and one in 100,000 for females."[13] At this time, few options existed for care, and nosology classified gender diversity as a mental illness. Only the desperate stood up to be counted.

Historically, prevalence data varied considerably depending on study methodology, diagnostic classification for gender diversity, and the year and country where the research took place.[14] Evolving nosology—for example, the evolving diagnoses of transsexualism, gender identity disorder, and gender dysphoria—muddied which individuals were included in a particular study.[15]

Data collected in cities and more trans-tolerant countries demonstrated higher prevalence rates than those documented in rural areas or intolerant countries. Older studies reported lower prevalence rates than newer studies, and comparisons of the two revealed changing sex ratios for those seeking care over time.

Apparently rare? Several quasi-epidemiological studies in the 1990s estimated prevalence by counting those who sought care at the few established gender clinics, which were primarily located in the Western world.[16] These papers described larger numbers of trans women requesting care compared to trans men, a ratio as high as 3:1. In 2015, Arcelus et al. performed a meta-analysis of twenty-one such epidemiologic studies, primarily from Europe, and found a prevalence rate of transsexualism of 4.6 per 100,000, or 1 in every 21,739 individuals, with a higher percentage of trans women (0.0068 percent) compared to that for trans men (0.0026 percent), and increasing prevalence rates in more recent studies.[17] The authors suggested their data be used only as a starting point, as their methodology failed to count those who did not seek care and relied on varied diagnostic criteria. Many TGD people, especially those further marginalized by fear of exposure, race, and socioeconomic status, did not attend the clinics.

Data from the United States include studies on information collected in electronic health records, again counting only those brave enough to self-identify as TGD in the health system. In 2015, the Centers for Medicare and Medicaid Services mandated that all electronic health record systems certified under the Meaningful Use Incentive Program demonstrate the capacity to collect data on sexual orientation and gender identity.[18] While health systems were not required to purchase or implement sexual orientation and gender identity data collection tools, some did, creating a new method for collecting statistics. These studies, conducted through the Veterans Administration Hospitals[19] and at Kaiser Permanente,[20] estimated prevalence in a range from 0.02 to 0.075 percent.

More recently, researchers surveyed representative samples of the US population, asking participants to self-identify according to their gender identity, a confidential process that also counted those not seeking care. A telephone survey in Massachusetts in 2007–2009 reported that 0.5 percent of adults identified as transgender.[21] A population-based study by the Williams Institute reported that 0.6 percent of US adults identified as transgender, with rates varying state by state and with increased prevalence in younger populations.[22] They established that 1.4 million US adults identified as trans, or roughly 1 in 200, which represents about the same number as those who identify as vegan.[23] Another population-based study in Flanders, Belgium, asked more nuanced questions designed to identify those with less binary or "gender ambivalent" identities through the use of scaled answers to statements like, "I feel like a man" or "I feel like a woman." They established a prevalence of 0.6–0.7 percent for gender incongruence and 1.9–2.2 percent for gender ambivalence.[24]

In the mid-2000s, epidemiologists began to report a significant change in the number of trans youth seeking care and a reversal of sex ratios. In 2016, surveillance data of high school students in Minnesota revealed the prevalence of a trans or gender-nonconforming identity at 2.7 percent.[25] In a Canadian pediatric gender clinic, the numbers of youth seeking care rose significantly and linearly between 1999 and 2013. From 1999 to 2005, the ratio of trans girls to trans boys seeking care was 2.11:1, and from 2006 to 2013, the ratio reversed to 1:1.76.[26] A 2017 survey of clinics in the United States, Europe, and South America reported that 63 percent of youth seeking care identified as transmasculine.[27]

The cumulative prevalence data, especially that collected recently, affirm that TGD people are neither rare nor uncommon and suggest that emerging cultural acceptance may further facilitate self-identification, thus increasing prevalence estimates. Also, being TGD does not equate with interest in treatment. The number of TGD people exceeds the number identified from those seeking care.

BIOMEDICAL RESEARCH: THE CONFLATION OF GENDER IDENTITY AND SEXUAL ORIENTATION

Early investigators often conflated gender identity with sexual orientation.[28] This research paradigm assumed that gender diversity was an expression of homosexuality rather than a separate phenomenon. As a legacy, much of the American population still fails to appreciate this distinction.

In the late nineteenth and early twentieth century, Eugen Steinach, an Austrian physiologist and colleague to Hirschfeld and Benjamin, identified hormonal substances that altered the development and behaviors of rodents. Although many of his theories were eventually dismissed, his research to identify hormonal substances and attempt to manipulate their effects on gender expression, gender-based behaviors, homosexuality, and aging provided a bedrock for later biomedical research.

Hirschfeld (1868–1935), the first to clearly define transsexualism as a distinct phenomenon, observed in his 1910 publication, *Die Transvestiten,* that his study group was not defined by same-sex attraction but instead by the drive to change gender.[29] He chose the term *transvestite*, from the Latin *trans* (across) and *vestis* (clothing), adding that he did not consider clothing "a dead thing," but rather "a form of expression of the inner personality as a valid symbol."[30] He stated, "If one wanted to stress the condition that it is not simply a matter of cross-dressing, but rather more of a sexual desire to change, then the word 'metamorphosis' would be better."[31] He did not believe the "transvestite drive [could] be made to disappear."[32]

With few biomedical technologies available apart from the existing observations on heritable conditions, Hirschfeld proposed a theory of intermediaries in which he separated the differences between the sexes into four groups, based on (1) sexual organs; (2) other physical characteristics; (3) sex drive; and (4) other emotional characteristics.[33] He asserted that all sexual characteristics existed in degrees on a spectrum and calculated the numbers of possible different combinations of all four groups. He proposed a total of 43,046,721 intermediary types, noting that this number represented roughly one-third of the world's population at that time.[34] Hirschfeld, ever prescient, wrote:

> Even if there is an internal or external influencing . . . sexual individuality as such with respect to body and mind is inborn, dependent upon the inherited mixture of manly and womanly substances, independent of externals; it is formed in advance by nature and is dormant in the individual long before it is awakened, forces its way into awareness, and develops. It is particularly subject to temporary, even periodic changes; develops consequently nevertheless, gradually increases; maintains itself at a certain level, then returns again, but maintains the same characteristic impressions in all essentials for the entire lifetime.[35]

In the period after Hirschfeld's death, researchers proposed psychological etiologies for homosexuality and gender diversity, but contemporary thinkers have returned to Hirschfeld's view of sexual and gender identities existing on a vast spectrum—now with specific biological theories to support this model.

Benjamin (1885–1986) also struggled to address the etiology of transsexualism, as evidenced in the chapter with this name in his 1966 book *The*

Transsexual Phenomenon.[36] Notably, Benjamin observed: "The possible origin of transsexualism is not discussed in the medical literature very often or in very much detail. Most frequently, there is a simple statement that the cause is unknown. Almost invariably, it is linked with that of transvestitism and sometimes with homosexuality, both giving rise to confusion." He described a field dominated by psychology and psychoanalysts, who "have little biological background and training. Some seem actually contemptuous of biological facts and persistently overstate psychological data, so much so that a distorted, one-sided picture of the problem under consideration results." Again, with limited biomedical technology, he could only speculate on possible biological causes. In his chapter, he considered the limited but emerging data in the fields of genetics and endocrinology. He discussed how psychological imprinting and childhood conditioning (forms of learning in early development) might contribute to transsexualism, particularly for those with an inherited predisposition for imprinting. With a nod to both nature and nurture, he concluded his chapter thus: "The chromosomal sex, supported and maintained by the endocrine, form the substance and the material that make up our sexuality. Psychoanalytical conditioning in early life would determine its final shape and individual function."

Late in the 1900s, scientists continued to conflate gender diversity and homosexuality. In 1990, American psychologist, Michael Gorman referred to "the ubiquitously held conviction that homosexuality represents 'femininity' in men, and 'masculinity' in women."[37] Researchers continued to seek evidence of female brain differentiation in gay men and male brain differentiation in lesbians, and most investigators failed to report on gender identity outside the context of sexual orientation. By the turn of century, in the late 1990s and early 2000s, numerous authors published small and sometimes contradictory studies claiming an association of gender identity and sexual orientation with birth order, finger length ratios, and handedness.[38]

NATURE VERSUS NURTURE

The realization that gender identity may be determined as early as in the womb occurred only recently.[39] From the 1970s to the 1990s, John Money (1921–2006), a New Zealand-born American psychologist and sexologist, championed the theory that gender identity was learned, not inherent. He believed infants were born tabula rasa, that environmental forces molded gender identity—how one was raised—and that one's psychosexual development occurred in response to the appearance of one's genitals.[40] At Johns Hopkins, he consulted on intersex cases for years, observing that those surgically altered did well in their assigned gender.[41] In 1966, he set out to prove his theory with an irresistible opportunity—a surgical mishap involving David Reimer (1965–2004, named Bruce at birth[42]), an identical twin. Ironically, Money's notorious study on nature versus nurture—research that profoundly changed existing treatment paradigms for intersex babies and TGD people—did not involve intersex or transgender people.

In 1966, during a routine circumcision for phimosis at eight months of age, the surgeon accidentally ablated Bruce's penis, rendering it flush with the abdominal wall.[43] In light of this tragedy, the parents canceled Brian's (1965–2002, Bruce's identical twin) planned circumcision for the same problem; ultimately, Brian's phimosis resolved spontaneously as he grew. In 1967, Bruce's parents, frantic with worry, traveled from Winnipeg, Canada, for consultation with Money to ask how best to help their child find health, happiness, and a place in the world. Money advised the parents to surgically castrate Bruce and raise him as a girl. Over the next two decades, as Money periodically reported on the success of this twin study (and other research), he became one of the most prominent sexologists in the world.

With the Reimer family, Money insisted on a strict program of feminine acculturation for Bruce, which included complete secrecy about his recorded gender at birth and rigid attention to gender roles. The parents renamed the infant Brenda, referred to him exclusively with feminine pronouns, and dressed him as a girl. At twenty-two months, Brenda underwent bilateral orchiectomy with surgical construction of a rudimentary vulva, and in adolescence, his physicians prescribed estrogen therapy to induce feminine puberty.[44]

Money described Brenda's healthy engagement with her assigned gender. He asserted that "she" conformed to stereotypical feminine gender roles. She helped in the kitchen, urinated sitting down, and asked for Christmas dolls. He quoted Brenda's mother, who did her best to construct a reality in which Brenda's behavior and identity was not a mistake: "One thing that really amazes me is that she is so feminine. I've never seen a little girl so neat and tidy. . . . She is very proud of herself, when she puts on a new dress, or I set her hair . . . she just loves to have her hair set . . . could sit under the drier all day long to have her hair set. She just loves it."[45] But Brenda was, in fact, not a model of femininity. Brenda's mother also noted Brenda's tomboyish behavior, stating, "I teach her . . . to be polite and quiet."[46] Money described the twin experiment in the medical literature as a success[47] until the point that the Reimer twins were lost to follow-up.

Inside and outside Johns Hopkins's ivory tower, Money's fame grew from this work. Feminists latched onto his theory to reverse the practice of attributing societal sex roles to sex-based brain differences. *Time* reported, "This dramatic case . . . provides strong support . . . that conventional patterns of masculine and feminine behavior can be altered. It also casts doubt on the theory that major sex differences, psychological as well as anatomical, are immutably set by the genes at conception."[48] The apparent malleability of gender identity encouraged surgeons and parents to continue with early surgical interventions for intersex babies, who were often assigned female genitalia because it was simpler to construct a vagina than a penis. Parents then raised these children in their surgically assigned gender roles. For transgender people, Money's work implied that their gender identity could be manipulated by conversion therapies, parenting techniques, or societal pressure.

But all was not well with Brenda Reimer, who became increasingly dysfunctional. Unbeknown to the public and the academic community, Brenda's experience differed from that portrayed by Money in the literature. As a girl child, Brenda's classmates relentlessly teased her for her boyish ways. Brenda dropped out of school in her early teens, refused to visit Johns Hopkins to see Money, and experienced recurrent suicidal thoughts and depression. At age fourteen, after Reimer voiced to his psychiatrist that he did not feel like a girl, his father confessed the truth to the boy and told him his story. Reimer socially transitioned to male and renamed himself David, which gave him some comfort, although he continued to struggle with dark moods and explosive anger.

Diamond (1934–2024), a professor of anatomy and reproductive biology at the University of Hawaii at Mānoa, held opposing views to Money. Diamond believed gender identity was inborn rather than learned.[49] From 1994 to 1995, Diamond and Keith Sigmundson (a psychiatrist and member of David's clinical team in Winnipeg) repeatedly interviewed David, his wife, and his mother, and in 1997, published, with David's blessing, a truthful account of David's experience.[50] Nine months later, *Rolling Stone* published journalist John Colapinto's account of the case.[51] Colapinto's book *As Nature Made Him* followed in 2000.[52] Although Diamond and Sigmundson's account had appeared in a medical journal with limited circulation, it reached millions when it was reported in newspapers and as a *New York Times* bestseller. Colapinto revealed allegations by the Reimer family of bizarre and unethical sexual behavior required by Money when the twins made visits, so Money could monitor young Brenda's adaptation to the feminine role. Money, his story exposed, faced a flurry of attacks on his integrity, honesty, and ethics—he had covered up and misrepresented information about David—accusations that permanently damaged his reputation and place in history.[53]

David continued to battle with depression, anger, and in 2002, the death of his brother by suicide. At age thirty-eight, on May 4, 2004, David drove to a grocery store parking lot in his hometown and with a sawed-off shotgun took his own life.[54] After David's death, Diamond and his colleague, University of Hawaii legal scholar Hazel Glenn Beh, challenged the authority of the doctors and parents who sought to normalize the ambiguous genitalia of intersex infants, claiming that shame, anxiety, repugnance, or parental guilt foreclosed the right of the infant to live according to their gender identity.[55] Cheryl Chase (also known as Bo Laurent) began to speak out on intersex rights in the mid-1990s, having founded the Intersex Society of North America in 1993, an advocacy organization that also argued against early genital surgery.[56] Treatment paradigms for intersex babies began to change at this time.[57]

While the Reimer case involved two cisgender youth, David's social story paralleled many of the experiences of TGD men.[58] He did not behave like other girls and was teased when his masculine gender signals were at odds with his feminine dress. He felt out of synch with his body, was unable to be who others wished him to be, and was unable to please them. With his testes and phallus removed as a child, he required exogenous testosterone to masculinize his body and would require extensive surgery. Reimer's tale is now told to demonstrate the immutability of gender identity and frequently trotted out in discussions on etiology.

Other studies followed that also documented the inability to modify gender identity through medical interventions. For example, in 2004, the *New England Journal of Medicine* published a paper from Johns Hopkins describing the surgical treatment of infants with cloacal exstrophy (that is, a portion of the large intestine lies outside the body at birth, with two halves of the bladder connected to it; in boys, the penis is short and flat with an exposed urethra and sometimes split into two halves) by creating female genitalia (the more straightforward surgery) on individuals with XY chromosomes.[59] To the surprise of the study's authors and despite an aggressive program with both surgery and rearing consistent with a medically assigned feminine gender identity, a majority of the treated XY individuals ultimately identified as male.

Most early researchers also believed sex-typical behavior, childhood play, and toy choices were learned socially and involved a process of cognitive development leading to sex-related behavior. In 2009, Gerianne Alexander et al. reported that at six to eight months of age, girls preferred to look at dolls and boys were fixated on trucks.[60] In 2010, Melissa Hines reported that at birth, female infants preferred to look at human faces, while boy infants preferred to watch mechanical mobiles.[61] These studies suggested that not only gender identity but also gender-based behavior, develop in utero.

HORMONAL INFLUENCES ON GENDER IDENTITY

The production of sex steroids in the 1930s and the development of the radioimmunoassay in the 1950s allowed researchers to manipulate and measure circulating levels of sex hormones in the body and explore the process of sexual differentiation in utero. In 1959, C. H. Phoenix et al. published the first of these studies, reporting that after administering exogenous testosterone to pregnant guinea pigs, the offspring demonstrated masculine anatomical and behavioral changes.[62] Subsequent research established that in humans, sexual differentiation begin at six to twelve weeks gestational age when the production of testosterone (determined by the Y chromosome) and its conversion to dihydrotestosterone lead to the formation of the penis and scrotum.[63] The absence of androgens (masculinizing hormones) or the lack of androgen receptors determines the formation of the vagina, even in an individual with a Y chromosome. Sexual organization of the brain happens in the second half of pregnancy when the presence or absence of testosterone affects changes in the developing brain. The sex-linked genes controlling this process induce variable expression of proteins, leading to fluctuations in hormone levels—a phenomenon that confers sexually dimorphic features as continuous variables on the masculine-feminine spectrum.[64] In the three months after birth, individuals with a Y chromosome sustain another testosterone surge, and the presence or absence of (or the inability of the body to process) this hormonal peak induces further differentiation of the developing brain. At puberty, the hormonally organized, dimorphic brain structures established in utero become activated by circulating sex hormones generated by the gonads. The differentiation of the body and the brain at separate points in time suggests a mechanism for gender identity variability with the vast spectrum of possibilities first noted by Hirschfeld.[65]

Studies involving people with intersex conditions or *differences of sexual development*[66] contributed to our understanding of how the hormonal milieu and functional differences in hormone receptors direct the development of gender identity. For example, research on individuals with complete androgen insensitivity syndrome revealed that gender identity and sexual orientation can be influenced by the direct effect of testosterone on the developing brain.[67] In complete androgen insensitivity syndrome, mutations in the androgen receptor gene render cells insensitive to circulating testosterone, and fetuses with XY chromosomes develop feminine genitalia and are usually (not always) heterosexual with a feminine gender identity.

A genetically XY fetus with 5-alpha-reductase deficiency, a condition in which XY individuals have testes but do not produce sufficient dihydrotestosterone, develops feminine external genitalia with a large clitoris and undescended testes. These individuals possess functioning androgen receptors but little to no dihydrotestosterone. Parents may raise these infants as girls, but when puberty hits, an endogenous testosterone surge from the testes compensates for the lack of dihydrotestosterone to induce masculinization of the body, significant growth of the clitoris, and testicular descent. The youth may then choose to live as men.[68]

Congenital adrenal hyperplasia (CAH) refers to a group of genetic conditions affecting the adrenal glands, leading to the overproduction of androgens.[69] Individual signs and symptoms depend on the age of diagnosis, the variant of CAH, and the chromosomal genotype. Female infants with a virilizing form of congenital adrenal hyperplasia that results in exposure to high levels of prenatal androgens showed increases in male-typical behavior (for instance, physical aggression) and a reduction in what is labeled female-typical behaviors (for instance, empathy).[70] A meta-analysis of 250 patients with CAH revealed that 5.2 percent of those raised female suffered from severe problems with gender identity and had a higher percentage of transsexualism than the general population of chromosomal females.[71] Psychologist Pasterski et al. measured gender identity and gender roles in chromosomal girls with high prenatal exposure to androgens due to classic CAH and found that 12.8 percent of those surveyed exhibited cross-gender identification compared to 0 percent in unaffected controls.[72] A third study examined moderate to severe types of CAH (salt wasting, non-classic variant, and simple virilizing CAH) and concluded that the three types demonstrated mild, moderate, and severe behavioral masculinization.[73] Combined, these three studies suggest that prenatal exposure to high levels of androgens may influence gender identity.

Other scientists investigated how early hormonal influence played a role in the emergence of psychiatric disorders, which differ in frequency between sexes.

Examples include autism spectrum disorder, obsessive-compulsive disorder, and Tourette syndrome, which are more commonly diagnosed in boys. In 2016, psychiatrist Aron Janssen explored the link between autism spectrum disorder and being transgender and reported that youth with a diagnosis of autism spectrum disorder were 7.76 times more likely to state they wished to be the opposite sex than the comparison group.[74] Such models have contributed to the idea that different levels of and/or sensitivity to prenatal hormones might affect the development of sex-related variation and human behavior, hinting at a possible mechanism for the association of being transgender and autism.

GENETIC INFLUENCES ON GENDER IDENTITY

In 1953, American biologist James Watson and English physicist Francis Crick modeled the three-dimensional structure of DNA, a landmark event that led to our understanding of DNA replication and the encoding of specific proteins by the nucleic acids that dictate gene expression.[75] In the subsequent decades, researchers developed techniques for the gene sequencing of DNA and RNA molecules, starting with short oligonucleotides and eventually mapping the entire human genome.[76] The order of nucleic acids in polynucleotide chains not only determines the biochemical and hereditary properties of all organisms (their expression and behaviors) but also allows scientists to reconstruct their evolutionary history and identify inherited traits. With these tools, researchers began to investigate whether gender identity was encoded within the genome. Genes not only control hormone production and the responsiveness of hormone receptors but also exert a direct effect on behavioral and brain sex differences.

TWIN AND FAMILY STUDIES

In 1875, Victorian scientist Francis Galton[77] first recognized that the study of twins served as a powerful method for estimating genetic and environmental effects.[78] Statisticians later latched onto twin studies to investigate how genetic factors contribute to the development of gender identity and/or gender incongruence, analyzing data from monozygotic (identical) twins, who share identical additive and nonadditive (that is, interactions between alleles within and across genes) genetic effects, and dizygotic (fraternal) twins, who share approximately fifty percent of additive and twenty-five percent nonadditive genetic effects.[79] They employed statistical methods to separate genetic and environmental effects. Family studies similarly contributed information about genetic traits, with varying degrees of shared genetic material.

In the 1970s, sexologists began to report cases of twins and families with discordance or co-occurrence of transsexualism and speculate on the role of heredity in gender identity.[80] In 1971, sexologist/psychiatrists Richard Green and Robert Stoller described two pairs of monozygotic twins with discordant gender identities.[81] Psychiatrists C. Hyde and J. C. Kenna reported a monozygotic twin pair who were concordant for transsexualism and explosive personality disorder but discordant for schizophrenia.[82] Psychiatrist B.D. Hore and colleagues described two Chinese siblings assigned male at birth who expressed feminine gender identities early in life.[83]

As increasing numbers of case reports filled the literature, researchers began to conduct large-scale studies of twins and families, searching for patterns of heritability—defined as the "proportion of phenotypic variation that arises from genetic influences."[84] The studies attempted to separate genetic influence from environmental influences, both shared and unshared, within their cohorts. In 2002, psychologist Frederick Coolidge and colleagues published one of the first studies to estimate the heritability of gender identity disorder in ninety-six monozygotic and sixty-one dizygotic same-sex child and adolescent twins. Data obtained through parental questionnaires revealed that 2.3 percent of the sample demonstrated what the investigators called "gender identity disorder symptoms," with a high estimated heritability of 0.62.[85] In 2011, sexologist Gunter Heylens and colleagues conducted a literature review of the concordance of gender identity disorder in twins and found a thirty nine percent concordance in monozygotic twins.[86] Both same-sex dizygotic twins and opposite-sex twins in this study were discordant for gender identity disorder. Similarly, family studies also demonstrate increased heritability rates in family members with shared genes. A Spanish family study found the probability that a sibling of a transsexual was also a transsexual was higher than the expected range, based on prevalence data on transsexualism in Spain.[87]

More recently, researchers conducted meta-analyses of existing twin studies for greater statistical power. A meta-analysis is a systematic method for combining pertinent qualitative and quantitative data from multiple studies to find common results and identify trends. In 2018, geneticist Tinca Polderman and colleagues published a meta-analysis of eleven large twin studies that reported heritability estimates for gender diversity.[88] They concluded that family and twin studies offered significant and consistent evidence for the role of innate genetic factors in the development of gender identity, "a negligible role for shared environmental factors" (that is, environmental influences shared by individuals in a population) and a small potential role for unique environmental factors" (that is, environmental influences experienced uniquely by each individual). They reported heritable estimates for gender identity in the range of thirty to sixty percent, similar to that of behavioral and personality traits.

GENETIC POLYMORPHISMS AND THE POLYGENIC THRESHOLD MODEL

A candidate gene is a gene associated with a particular disease or phenotype.[89] Because of the association, researchers may suspect it is the cause of the disease or phenotype. Family studies found increased rates of homosexuality among siblings and the maternal uncles of gay men, and for decades, geneticists have searched unsuccessfully for a "gay gene," a collection of nucleotides that encoded sexual orientation to explain this phenomenon.[90] Similarly, no one has identified a single candidate gene responsible for gender identity. But after the development of gene sequencing tools, researchers began to search for polymorphisms (small or large differences in the DNA sequences among individuals or groups who are more prevalent in a certain phenotype) in transgender people compared to cisgender controls.

Scientist Richard Dawkins offered this metaphor to demonstrate the complex nature of genetic determinism and counsel against the simplistic notion of a candidate gene:

> I like to use the analogy of a big sheet hanging from the ceiling by a thousand rubber bands. The shape of the sheet symbolizes the developing body. The rubber bands don't just hang vertically—they crisscross in a great tangle. Now imagine that the tensions in the rubber bands symbolize the genes, so you can represent a mutation by cutting one band. If you do cut a rubber band, the balance of tensions will shift, and this change will affect the shape of the whole sheet. The message is that genes don't have effects in isolation.... [G]enes do not have a one-to-one correspondence with effects.[91]

Dutch geneticist Tinca Polderman and colleagues endorsed the polygenic threshold model, which asserts that many genes contribute to, but do not determine, complex traits.[92] Hundreds or thousands of genetic variants (not a single gene) contribute to the development and expression of specific traits, each with a small but additive effect that may also be influenced by nongenetic factors, such as the environment. They maintained that this framework changed the conceptualization of autism spectrum disorders by recognizing that some people who carry many associated genetic variants demonstrate many autistic traits, while others carry few associated genetic variants and display few autistic traits. They hypothesized that gender identity also fit this model, believing everyone naturally lands on some point(s) of the spectrum, corresponding to their genetic load.

Spanish psychologist Rosa Fernández and colleagues discovered no difference in the karyotype of transgender people but found polymorphisms in the gene for the beta estrogen receptor and ESR1 gene in transgender men.[93] Australian researcher Madeleine Foreman and colleagues extracted genomic DNA from blood and saliva to investigate the possible link of sex hormone signaling genes to gender dysphoria.[94] They genotyped DNA to identify polymorphisms in twelve sex-signaling genes and found a significant association between specific alleles (that is, one of two or more versions of a gene) and gender dysphoria. Transgender women were more likely to have allele combinations that affected the androgen receptor. The authors proposed that these alleles and genotypes demasculinized or feminized their transfeminine subjects. Swedish physiologist and pharmacologist Susanne Henningsson and colleagues published a small study demonstrating differences in a CA repeat polymorphism in intron 5 of the estrogen receptor beta gene, a CAG repeat sequence in the first axon of the androgen receptor gene, and a tetranucleotide repeat polymorphism in intron 4 of the aromatase gene between trans women and cisgender male controls.[95] Chinese geneticist Fu Yang and colleagues reported rare mutations in the RYR3 gene in transgender women compared to cisgender men.[96]

In 2011, American neurobiologist Tuck Ngun and colleagues maintained that sexual differentiation was not just hormonally mediated but that direct genetic effects arising from the expression of the X and Y genes in nongonadal cells also resulted in sex differences.[97] In mice, the absence or presence of the SRY region of the Y chromosome had a direct genetic effect on the development of gonadal tissue and sexual differentiation in nongonadal tissue.

KARYOTYPES

Before 2010, some treatment centers subjected transgender patients to a variety of baseline biomedical and psychological tests.[98] In such centers, this included a karyotype (determination of an individual's collection of chromosomes) to exclude chromosomal abnormalities as a basis for being transgender.[99] In 2011,

Dutch endocrinologist Inoubli and colleagues described the karyotypes of 368 transsexual individuals and found no karyotype linked to transsexualism.[100] They recommended dispensing with costly karyotype testing unless an individual exhibited signs or symptoms that suggested a disorder of sexual development.

EPIGENETICS

Genetic research led to the field of epigenetics, the study of how behaviors and the environment change the way genes function.[101] Epigenetic influences do not change the DNA sequence but may alter how genes are expressed. These influences turn genes "on" or "off" by determining which proteins are produced. For example, diet, exercise, and smoking cause epigenetic changes that affect genetic expression and make us variably susceptible to infections or cancer. Epigenetic changes determine which of our cells (which contain the same DNA) differentiate into cells for the heart, the skin, or the brain and determine how we age. Some epigenetic changes are permanent, and some change in response to our behaviors and environment. While the complex mechanisms for epigenetic change are beyond the scope of this chapter, the changes involve the addition of a chemical group to the DNA (DNA methylation), the wrapping of DNA around proteins called histones (histone modification), and the attachment of noncoding RNA to control gene expression. Researchers have described epigenetic modifications associated with homosexuality and suggest that these mechanisms account for discordance in sexual orientation in monozygotic twins.[102] Numerous publications demonstrate that epigenetic mechanisms affect the development of sex differences and behaviors in rodents.[103] Could epigenetic modifications, with their variability of expression, explain the wide spectrum of gender identities in humans as well?[104] These studies are limited by lack of access to the brain during research and difficulty in deriving causality due to genetic and environmental heterogeneity.[105] These and similar studies present small but additive advances to our understanding of the genetic influences on gender diversity.

NEUROANATOMICAL INFLUENCES ON GENDER IDENTITY

Several postmortem studies of human brains used evolving microscopy techniques to identify dimorphic structural sex differences in the hypothalamus related to gender identity. In 1995, Dutch neurobiologist Jiang-Ning Zhou and colleagues demonstrated striking anatomical differences in the size and neuron number in the central nucleus of the bed nucleus of the stria terminalis (BSTc, sometimes referred to as the extended amygdala, is linked to sexual behavior) between cisgender men and women.[106] The cisgender men possessed a larger volume BSTc than cisgender women and, interestingly, trans women matched the volume of cisgender women.[107] A second study examined neuronal differences in the BSTc and found cisgender men had almost twice as many somatostatin neurons as cisgender women.[108] Transgender women possessed similar numbers of neurons as cisgender women, and the single transgender man examined had numbers similar to cisgender men.

In 2008, a third study demonstrated similar findings on the same research material regarding the interstitial nucleus of the anterior hypothalamus 3 (INAH3).[109] Researchers found similar volume and number of neurons in the INAH3 for transgender and cisgender women along with dissimilarity compared to cisgender men. The above reported a single transmasculine subject had INAH3 volume similar to cisgender men. The neuronal growth in these studies seemed to have arisen during development and was not the result of circulating hormones. These studies suggested gender identity might result from the differentiation of sexually dimorphic brains.

CONCLUSION

Despite significant scientific advancements that enhance our biological understanding of this (now understood to be) relatively common human experience, many of the same theories purporting a psychological cause for gender diversity that Hirschfeld and Benjamin encountered in the last century (that is, parenting, socialization, grooming) still drive decisions that negatively impact TGD people and the clinicians who serve them today. Yet, as evidence about a biological etiology unfolds, the ethical mission of TGD healthcare remains straightforward and unchanged.

As clinicians, we vow to provide customized, patient-centered, evidence-based, and comprehensive care to meet individual needs. We take steps to create office space that is inclusive to diverse people with intersectional identities. We work to repair the medical systems that create barriers to affirming care. We train ourselves to alleviate human suffering with proven medical interventions that offer relief. As clinicians for TGD people, we must exemplify the attitudes that drive societal change. In doing so, we bow to the variability and mystery of the human experience and celebrate the diversity of life on this wondrous planet.

NOTES

1. This quote, widely attributed to Milton Diamond, appears on his website at the Pacific Center for Sex and Society, within the University of Hawai'i, Manoa.
2. Roughgarden, *Evolution's Rainbow*, 13–14.
3. Roughgarden, *Evolution's Rainbow*, 78–81.
4. Roughgarden, *Evolution's Rainbow*, Chapters 2–9, 22–158.
5. Roughgarden, *Evolution's Rainbow*, 14.
6. Goldsmith, "Radioimmunoassay."
7. Phoenix et al., "Organizational Action"; Swaab and Garcia-Falgueras, "Sexual Differentiation of the Human Brain."
8. Glover, "Overview of Functional Magnetic Resonance Imaging"; Somers, "Head Space."
9. Lee et al., "Magnetic Resonance Microscopy."
10. Coates, Friedman, and Wolfe, "The Etiology of Boyhood Gender Identity Disorder"; Herman, "Gender Identity Disorder in a Five-Year-Old Boy."
11. Phelan, Cruz-Rojas, and Reiff, "Genes and Stigma." Historically, researchers and clinicians have pathologized transgender people with medical language. The term *prevalence* is more often used to describe rates of disease rather than human characteristics; it's use in the medical literature implies not only that gender diversity is an illness but also that gender identity is identifiable, fixed, and simple to quantify—none of which are true. As historians, we chose to use the word *prevalence* in this volume (as well as other outdated terms, such as *transsexual, transgenderism*, and *gender identity disorders*) to reflect the language researchers employed to report their work at different points in time. We invite you to consider how the use of this term and others used in the scientific reports described in this chapter impacted medical and cultural beliefs about gender diversity.
12. American Psychiatric Association, *Diagnostic and Statistical Manual of Mental Disorders*, 3rd ed., 263.
13. Zucker, "Epidemiology of Gender Dysphoria"; American Psychiatric Association, *Diagnostic and Statistical Manual of Mental Disorders*, 3rd ed., revised, 1.
14. Arcelus et al., "Systemic Review and Meta-Analysis."
15. Arcelus et al., "Systemic Review and Meta-Analysis."
16. Bakker et al., "The Prevalence of Transsexualism in the Netherlands"; Wilson, Sharp, and Carr, "The Prevalence of Transsexualism in Scotland"; Van Kesteren, Gooren, and Megens, "An Epidemiological and Demographic Study."

17. Arcelus et al., "Systemic Review and Meta-Analysis."
18. National LGBT Health Education Center, "Collecting Sexual Orientation and Gender Identity Data."
19. Blosnich et al., "Prevalence of Gender Identity Disorder"; Kauth et al., "Health Differences."
20. Quinn et al., "Cohort Profile."
21. Conron et al., "Transgender Health in Massachusetts."
22. Flores et al., "How Many Adults Identify as Transgender."
23. Zucker, "Epidemiology of Gender Dysphoria."
24. Van Caenegem et al., "Prevalence of Gender Nonconformity in Flanders, Belgium."
25. Eisenberg et al., "Emotional Distress."
26. Aitken et al., "Evidence for an Altered Sex Ratio."
27. Steensma, Cohen-Kettenis, and Zucker, "Evidence for a Change in the Sex Ratio"; de Graaf et al., "Data from the Gender Identity Development Service in London"; Skordis et al., "ESPE and PES International Survey."
28. Gooren, "The Biology of Human Psychosexual Differentiation."
29. Hirschfeld, *Die Transvestiten* and *Transvestites*.
30. Hirschfeld, *Transvestites*, 124.
31. Hirschfeld, *Transvestites*, 234.
32. Hirschfeld, *Transvestites*, 234.
33. Hirschfeld, *Transvestites*, 215–236.
34. Hirschfeld, *Transvestites*, 227.
35. Hirschfeld, *Transvestites*, 233.
36. Benjamin, *The Transsexual Phenomenon*, 43.
37. Gorman, "Male Homosexual Desire," 61.
38. Green and Young, "Hand Preference, Sexual Preference"; Watson and Coren, "Left-Handedness in Male-to-Female Transsexuals"; Kraemer et al., "Finger Length Ratio (2D:4D)" and "Finger Length Ratio (2D:4D) in Adults"; Wallien et al., "2D:4D Finger-Length Ratios"; Blanchard and Sheridan, "Sibship Size"; Blanchard et al., "Birth Order and Sibling Sex Ratio"; Schagen et al., "Sibling Sex Ratio."
39. Swaab, Wolff, and Bao, "Sexual Differentiation of the Human Hypothalamus."
40. Diamond and Sigmundson, "Sex Reassignment at Birth."
41. Green, *Becoming a Visible Man*, 200.
42. To underscore David's confusing experience, we chose to use the name and pronouns assigned to or by David Reimer at various points in this history. We use David's chosen name and pronouns after the age in which he stated his preference.
43. Money and Ehrhardt, *Man and Woman*, 118; Diamond and Sigmundson, "Management of Intersexuality."
44. Diamond and Sigmundson, "Sex Reassignment at Birth."
45. Money and Ehrhardt, *Man and Woman*, 119–20.
46. Money and Ehrhardt, *Man and Woman*, 122.

47. Money and Ehrhardt, *Man and Woman*, 118–23.
48. *Time*, "The Sexes: Biological Imperatives."
49. Diamond, "A Critical Evaluation."
50. Diamond and Sigmudson, "Sex Reassignment at Birth."
51. Colapinto, "The True Story of John/Joan."
52. Colapinto, *As Nature Made Him*.
53. Dallas Denny and Jamison Green, personal communication with the authors, provided assistance for this section.
54. Diamond and Sigmundson, "Sex Reassignment at Birth."
55. Beh and Diamond, "David Reimer's Legacy."
56. Intersex Society of North America, "Cheryl Chase (Bo Laurent)."
57. Diamond and Sigmundson, "Management of Intersexuality."
58. Green, *Becoming A Visible Man*, 2nd ed., 201–03.
59. Reiner and Gearhart, "Discordant Sexual Identity."
60. Alexander, Wilcox, and Woods, "Sex Differences in Infants."
61. Swaab and Garcia-Falgueras, "Sexual Differentiation of the Human Brain"; Phoenix et al., "Organizational Action."
62. Phoenix et al., "Organizational Action."
63. Swaab and Garcia-Falgueras, "Sexual Differentiation of the Human Brain"; Swaab, Wolff, and Bao, "Sexual Differentiation of the Human Hypothalamus."
64. O'Hanlan, Gordon, and Sullivan, "Biological Origins of Sexual Orientation and Gender Identity."
65. Swaab and Garcia-Falgueras, "Sexual Differentiation of the Human Brain."
66. Historically, medical terminology has also pathologized intersex individuals who, until recently, were diagnosed with *disorders of sexual development*. Although not universally accepted in the field, many now employ the less pathologizing term *differences of sexual development*.
67. Mazur, "Gender Dysphoria and Gender Change"; Wisniewski et al., "Complete Androgen Insensitivity Syndrome."
68. Imperato-McGinley et al., "Androgens and the Evolution of Male-Gender Identity"; Swaab, Wolff, and Bao, "Sexual Differentiation of the Human Hypothalamus."
69. National Institutes of Health, "Congenital Adrenal Hyperplasia."
70. Hines, "Sex-Related Variation."
71. Dessens, Slijper, and Drop, "Gender Dysphoria and Gender Change."
72. Pasterski et al., "Increased Cross-Gender Indetification."
73. Meyer-Bahlburg et al., "Gender Development in Women."
74. Janssen, Huang, and Duncan, "Gender Variance among Youth."
75. Watson and Crick, "Molecular Structure of Nucleic Acids."
76. Heather and Chain, "The Sequence of Sequencers."

77. Gillham, "Sir Francis Galton and the Birth of Eugenics." Galton, the half-cousin to Charles Darwin, later initiated the eugenics movement.

78. Gillham, "Commentary: Francis Galton."

79. Polderman et al., "The Ideological Contributions to Gender Identity and Gender Diversity."

80. Stoller and Baker, "Two Male Transsexuals in One Family"; Sabalis et al, "The Three Sisters"; McKee, Roback, and Hollender, "Transsexualism in Two Male Triplets"; Hyde and Kenner, "A Male MZ Twin Pair"; Hore et al., "Male Transsexualism"; Green and Stoller, "Two Monozygotic (Identical) Twin Pairs."

81. Green and Stoller, "Two Monozygotic (Identical) Twin Pairs."

82. Hyde and Kenner, "A Male MZ Twin Pair."

83. Hore et al., "Male Transsexualism."

84. Polderman et al., "The Biological Contributions to Gender Identity and Gender Diversity," 98.

85. Coolidge, Thede, and Young, "The Heritability of Gender Identity Disorder."

86. Heylens et al., "Gender Identity Disorder in Twins."

87. Gómez-Gil et al., "Familiarity of Gender Identity Disorder."

88. Polderman et al., "The Biological Contributions to Gender Identity and Gender Diversity."

89. National Institutes of Health, "Candidate Gene."

90. Bailey and Pillard, "Genetics of Human Sexual Orientation."

91. Coutu, "What Is Science Good For?"

92. Visscher et al., "10 Years of GWAS Discovery"; Polderman et al., "The Biological Contributions to Gender Identity and Gender Diversity," 97–8.

93. Fernández et al., "Analysis of Four Polymorphisms" and "The Genetics of Transsexualism."

94. Foreman et al., "Genetic Link between Gender Dysphoria and Sex Hormone Signaling."

95. Henningsson et al., "Sex Steroid-Related Genes."

96. Yang et al., "Genomic Characteristics of Gender Dysphoria Patients."

97. Ngun et al., "The Genetics of Sex Differences in Brain and Behavior."

98. Weyers et al., "Long-Term Assessment of the Physical, Mental, Sexual Health among Transsexual Women."

99. Inoubli et al., "Karyotyping."

100. Inoubli et al., "Karyotyping."

101. McCarthy et al., "The Epigenetics of Sex Differences in the Brain"; Khoury, "Epigenetics and Public Health."

102. O'Hanlan, Gordon, and Sullivan, "Biological Origins of Sexual Orientation and Gender Identity"; Ngun and Vilain, "The Biological Basis of Sexual Orientation";

Rice, Friberg and Gavrilets, "Homosexuality as a Consequence" and "Homosexuality via Canalized Sexual Development."

103. Szyf, "The Epigenetics of Perinatal Stress"; McCarthy and Nugent, "At the Frontier of Epigenetics"; McCarthy and Nugent, "Epigenetic Contributions to Hormonally-Mediated Sexual Differentiation of the Brain"; McCarthy et al., "The Epigenetics of Sex Differences in the Brain"; Forger, "Epigenetic Mechanisms in Sexual Differentiation."

104. O'Hanlan, Gordon, and Sullivan, "Biological Origins of Sexual Orientation and Gender Identity."

105. Szyf, "The Epigenetics of Perinatal Stress."

106. Zhou et al., "A Sex Difference in the Human Brain"; Kruijver et al., "Male-to-Female Transsexuals Have Female Neuron Numbers."

107. Zhou et al., "A Sex Difference in the Human Brain."

108. Kruijver et al., "Male-to-Female Transsexuals Have Female Neuron Numbers."

109. Garcia-Falgueras and Swaab, "A Sex Difference in the Hypothalamic Uncinate Nucleus."

WORKS CITED

Aitken, Madison, Thomas D. Steensma, Ray Blanchard, et al. "Evidence for an Altered Sex Ratio in Clinic-Referred Adolescents with Gender Dysphoria." *Journal of Sexual Medicine* 12, no. 3 (2015): 756–63.

Alexander, Gerianne M., Teresa Wilcox, and Rebecca Woods. "Sex Differences in Infants' Visual Interest in Toys." *Archives of Sexual Behavior* 38, no. 3 (2009): 427–33.

American Psychiatric Association. *Diagnostic and Statistical Manual of Mental Disorders*. 3rd ed. Washington, DC: American Psychiatric Association, 1980.

American Psychiatric Association. *Diagnostic and Statistical Manual of Mental Disorders*. 3rd ed., revised. Washington, DC: American Psychiatric Association, 1987.

Arcelus, Jon, Walter Pierre Bouman, Wim Van Den Noortgate, et al. "Systematic Review and Meta-Analysis of Prevalence Studies in Transsexualism." *European Psychiatry* 30, no. 6 (2015): 807–15.

Bailey, J., and Richard Pillard. "Genetics of Human Sexual Orientation." *Annual Review of Sex Research* 6 (January 1995): 126–50.

Bakker, Abraham, Paul J. M. van Kesteren, Louis J. G. Gooren, and Pieter D. Bezemer. "The Prevalence of Transsexualism in the Netherlands." *Acta Psychiatrica Scandinavica* 87, no. 4 (1993): 237–38.

Beh, Hazel Glenn, and Milton Diamond. "David Reimer's Legacy Limiting Parental Discretion." *Cardozo JL & Gender* 12 (2005): 5. Accessed August 14, 2024. http://heinonline.org/hol-cgi-bin/get_pdf.cgi?handle=hein.journals/cardw12&section=8.

Benjamin, Harry. "Introduction." In *Transsexualism and Sex Reassignment*, edited by Richard Green and John Money, 1–10. Baltimore, MD: Johns Hopkins Press, 1969.

———. *The Transsexual Phenomenon*. New York: Julian Press, 1966.
Blanchard, Ray, and Peter M. Sheridan. "Sibship Size, Sibling Sex Ratio, Birth Order, and Parental Age in Homosexual and Nonhomosexual Gender Dysphorics:" *Journal of Nervous and Mental Disease* 180, no. 1 (1992): 40–47. https://doi.org/10.1097/00005053-199201000-00009.
Blanchard, Ray, Kenneth J. Zucker, Petty T. Cohen-Kettenis, Louis J. G. Gooren, and J. Michael Bailey. "Birth Order and Sibling Sex Ratio in Two Samples of Dutch Gender-Dysphoric Homosexual Males." *Archives of Sexual Behavior* 25, no. 5 (1996): 495–514.
Blosnich, John R., George R. Brown, Jillian C. Shipherd, Michael Kauth, Rebecca I. Piegari, and Robert M. Bossarte. "Prevalence of Gender Identity Disorder and Suicide Risk among Transgender Veterans Utilizing Veterans Health Administration Care." *American Journal of Public Health* 103, no. 10 (2013): e27–32.
Coates, Susan, Richard C. Friedman, and Sabrina Wolfe. "The Etiology of Boyhood Gender Identity Disorder: A Model for Integrating Temperament, Development, and Psychodynamics." *Psychoanalytic Dialogues* 1, no. 4 (1991): 481–523.
Colapinto, John. *As Nature Made Him*. New York: HarperCollins, 2000.
———. "The True Story of John/Joan." *Rolling Stone*, December 11, 1998.
———. "Gender Gap." *Slate*, June 3, 2004. Accessed August 14, 2024. https://slate.com/technology/2004/06/why-did-david-reimer-commit-suicide.html.
Connellan, Jennifer, Simon Baron-Cohen, Sally Wheelwright, Anna Batki, and Jag Ahluwalia. "Sex Differences in Human Neonatal Social Perception." *Infant Behavior and Development* 23, no. 1 (2000): 113–18.
Conron, K. J., G. Scott, G. S. Stowell, and S. J. Landers. "Transgender Health in Massachusetts: Results from a Household Probability Sample of Adults." *American Journal of Public Health* 102, no. 1 (2012): 118–22. https://doi.org10.2105/AJPH.2011.300315.
Coolidge, Frederick L., Linda L. Thede, and Susan E. Young. "The Heritability of Gender Identity Disorder in a Child and Adolescent Twin Sample." *Behavior Genetics* 32, no. 4 (2002): 251–57.
Coutu, Diane. "What Is Science Good For? A Conversation with Richard Dawkins." *Harvard Business Review*, January 1, 2001. https://hbr.org/2001/01/what-is-science-good-for-a-conversation-with-richard-dawkins.
Dessens, Arianne B., Froukje M. E. Slijper, and Stenvert L. S. Drop. "Gender Dysphoria and Gender Change in Chromosomal Females with Congenital Adrenal Hyperplasia." *Archives of Sexual Behavior* 34, no. 4 (2005): 389–97.
Diamond, Milton. "A Critical Evaluation of the Ontogeny of Human Sexual Behavior." *Quarterly Review of Biology* 40, no. 2 (1965): 147–75. https://doi.org/10.1086/404539.
———. "Pacific Center for Sex and Society." University of Hawaii, 2020. September 23, 2020. http://www.hawaii.edu/PCSS/.

Diamond, Milton, and H. Keith Sigmundson. "Management of Intersexuality: Guidelines for Dealing with Persons with Ambiguous Genitalia." *Archives of Pediatrics & Adolescent Medicine* 151, no. 10 (1997a): 1046–50.

———. "Sex Reassignment at Birth: Long-Term Review and Clinical Implications." *Archives of Pediatrics & Adolescent Medicine* 151, no. 3 (1997): 298–304.

Eisenberg, Marla E., Amy L. Gower, Barbara J. McMorris, G. Nicole Rider, and Eli Coleman. "Emotional Distress, Bullying Victimization, and Protective Factors among Transgender and Gender Diverse Adolescents in City, Suburban, Town, and Rural Locations." *Journal of Rural Health* 35, no. 2 (2019): 270–81.

Feder, Ellen K. "Disciplining the Family: The Case of Gender Identity Disorder." *Philosophical Studies: An International Journal for Philosophy in the Analytic Tradition* 85, no. 2–3 (1997): 195–211.

Fernández, Rosa, Enrique Delgado-Zayas, Karla Ramírez, et al. "Analysis of Four Polymorphisms Located at the Promoter of the Estrogen Receptor Alpha ESR1 Gene in a Population with Gender Incongruence." *Sexual Medicine* 8, no. 3 (2020): 490–500.

Fernández, Rosa, Isabel Esteva, Esther Gómez-Gil, et al. "The Genetics of Transsexualism." In *Gender Identity: Disorders, Developmental Perspectives and Social Implications*, 117–22. Hauppauge: Nova Science, 2014.

Flores, Andrew R., Jody L. Herman, Gary J. Gates, and Taylor N. T. Brown. "How Many Adults Identify as Transgender in the United States?" Williams Institute, 2016. http://williamsinstitute.law.ucla.edu/wp-content/uploads/How-Many-Adults-Identify-as-Transgender-in-the-United-States.pdf.

Foreman, Madeleine, Lauren Hare, Kate York, et al. "Genetic Link between Gender Dysphoria and Sex Hormone Signaling." *Journal of Clinical Endocrinology & Metabolism* 104, no. 2 (2019): 390–96.

Forger, Nancy G. "Epigenetic Mechanisms in Sexual Differentiation of the Brain and Behaviour." *Philosophical Transactions of the Royal Society B: Biological Sciences* 371, no. 1688 (2016): 20150114.

Garcia-Falgueras, A., and D. F. Swaab. "A Sex Difference in the Hypothalamic Uncinate Nucleus: Relationship to Gender Identity." *Brain* 131, no. 12 (2008): 3132–46.

Gillham, Nicholas W. "Commentary: Francis Galton, Twins and Intelligence." *International Journal of Epidemiology* 41, no. 4 (2012): 920–22. doi:10.1093/ije/dys098.

———. "Sir Francis Galton and the Birth of Eugenics." *Annual Review of Genetics* 35, no. 1 (2001): 83–101.

Glover, Gary H. "Overview of Functional Magnetic Resonance Imaging." *Neurosurgery Clinics of North America* 22, no. 2 (2011): 133–39. 10.1016/j.nec.2010.11.001

Goldsmith, S. J. "Radioimmunoassay: Review of Basic Principles." *Seminars in Nuclear Medicine* 5, no. 2 (1975): 125–52. https://doi.org/10.1016/s0001-2998(75)80028-6.

Gómez-Gil, Esther, Isabel Esteva, M. Cruz Almaraz, Eduardo Pasaro, Santiago Segovia, and Antonio Guillamon. "Familiality of Gender Identity Disorder in Non-Twin Siblings." *Archives of Sexual Behavior* 39, no. 2 (2010): 546–52.

Gooren, Louis. "The Biology of Human Psychosexual Differentiation." *Hormones and Behavior*, 50, no. 4 (2006): 589–601. https://doi.org/10.1016/j.yhbeh.2006.06.011.

Gorman, Michael R. "Male Homosexual Desire: Neurological Investigations and Scientific Bias." *Perspectives in Biology and Medicine* 38, no. 1 (1994): 61–81.

Graaf, Nastasja M. de, Polly Carmichael, Thomas D. Steensma, and Kenneth J. Zucker. "Evidence for a Change in the Sex Ratio of Children Referred for Gender Dysphoria: Data from the Gender Identity Development Service in London (2000–2017)." *Journal of Sexual Medicine* 15, no. 10 (2018): 1381–83.

Green, Jamison. *Becoming a Visible Man*. Nashville, TN: Vanderbilt University Press, 2004.

———. *Becoming a Visible Man*. 2nd ed. Nashville, TN: Vanderbilt University Press, 2020.

Green, Richard, and Robert J. Stoller. "Two Monozygotic (Identical) Twin Pairs Discordant for Gender Identity." *Archives of Sexual Behavior* 1, no. 4 (1971): 321–27.

Green, Richard, and Robert Young. "Hand Preference, Sexual Preference, and Transsexualism." *Archives of Sexual Behavior* 30, no. 6 (2001): 565–74.

Heather, James M., and Benjamin Chain. "The Sequence of Sequencers: The History of Sequencing DNA." *Genomics* 107, no. 1 (2016): 1–8. https://doi.org/10.1016/j.ygeno.2015.11.003.

Henningsson, Susanne, Lars Westberg, Staffan Nilsson, et al. "Sex Steroid-Related Genes and Male-to-Female Transsexualism." *Psychoneuroendocrinology* 30, no. 7 (2005): 657–64.

Herman, Stephen P. "Gender Identity Disorder in a Five-Year-Old Boy." *Yale Journal of Biology and Medicine* 56, no. 1 (1983): 15.

Heylens, Gunter, Griet De Cuypere, Kenneth J. Zucker, et al. "Gender Identity Disorder in Twins: A Review of the Case Report Literature." *Journal of Sexual Medicine* 9, no. 3 (2012): 751–57.

Hines, Melissa. "Sex-Related Variation in Human Behavior and the Brain." *Trends in Cognitive Sciences* 14, no. 10 (2010): 448–56.

Hirschfeld, Magnus. *Die Transvestiten*. Berlin: Alfred Pulvermacherm, 1910. Accessed August 14, 2024. https://www.digitaltransgenderarchive.net/files/6395w7174.

———. *Transvestites: The Erotic Drive to Cross Dress*. Translated by Michael Lombardi-Nash. New York: Prometheus Books, 1991.

Hore, B. D., M. Phil, F. V. Nicolle, B. Chir, and J. S. Calnan. "Male Transsexualism: Two Cases in a Single Family." *Archives of Sexual Behavior* 2, no. 4 (1973): 317–21.

Hyde, C., and J. C. Kenna. "A Male MZ Twin Pair, Concordant for Transsexualism, Discordant for Schizophrenia." *Acta Psychiatrica Scandinavica* 56, no. 4 (1977): 265–73.

Imperato-McGinley, Julianne, Ralph E. Peterson, Teofilo Gautier, and Erasmo Sturla. "Androgens and the Evolution of Male-Gender Identity among Male Pseudohermaphrodites with 5α-Reductase Deficiency." *New England Journal of Medicine* 300, no. 22 (1979): 1233–37.

Inoubli, Adrien, Griet De Cuypere, Robert Rubens, et al. "Karyotyping, Is It Worthwhile in Transsexualism?" *Journal of Sexual Medicine* 8, no. 2 (2011): 475–78.

Intersex Society of North America. "Cheryl Chase (Bo Laurent)." Accessed August 14, 2024. https://isna.org/about/chase/.

Janssen, Aron, Howard Huang, and Christina Duncan. "Gender Variance among Youth with Autism Spectrum Disorders: A Retrospective Chart Review." *Transgender Health* 1, no. 1 (2016): 63–68.

Kauth, Michael R., Terri L. Barrera, F. Nicholas Denton, and David M. Latini. "Health Differences among Lesbian, Gay, and Transgender Veterans by Rural/Small Town and Suburban/Urban Setting." *LGBT Health* 4, no. 3 (2017): 194–201.

Khoury, Mulin J. "Epigenetics and Public Health: Why We Should Pay Attention." Genomics & Precision Health Blog Archive, Center for Disease Control. October 9, 2014. Accessed August 14, 2024. https://blogs.cdc.gov/genomics/2014/10/09/epigenetics/.

Kraemer, Bernd, Thomas Noll, Aba Delsignore, Gabriella Milos, Ulrich Schnyder, and Urs Hepp. "Finger Length Ratio (2D: 4D) and Dimensions of Sexual Orientation." *Neuropsychobiology* 53, no. 4 (2006): 210–14.

———. "Finger Length Ratio (2D: 4D) in Adults with Gender Identity Disorder." *Archives of Sexual Behavior* 38, no. 3 (2009): 359–63.

Kruijver, Frank P. M., Jiang-Ning Zhou, Chris W. Pool, Michel A. Hofman, Louis J. G. Gooren, and Dick F. Swaab. "Male-to-Female Transsexuals Have Female Neuron Numbers in a Limbic Nucleus." *Journal of Clinical Endocrinology & Metabolism* 85, no. 5 (2000): 2034–41.

Lee, Choong H., Niclas Bengtsson, Stephen M. Chrzanowski, Jeremy J. Flint, Glenn A. Walter, and Stephen J. Blackband. "Magnetic Resonance Microscopy (MRM) of Single Mammalian Myofibers and Myonuclei." *Scientific Reports* 7, no. 1 (2017): 1–9.

Mazur, Tom. "Gender Dysphoria and Gender Change in Androgen Insensitivity or Micropenis." *Archives of Sexual Behavior* 34, no. 4 (2005): 411–21.

McCarthy, Margaret M. and Bridget M. Nugent. "At the Frontier of Epigenetics of Brain Sex Differences." *Frontiers in Behavioral Neuroscience* 9 (2015): 221.

———. "Epigenetic Contributions to Hormonally-Mediated Sexual Differentiation of the Brain." *Journal of Neuroendocrinology* 25, no. 11 (2013): 1133–40.

McCarthy, Margaret M., Anthony P. Auger, et al. "The Epigenetics of Sex Differences in the Brain." *Journal of Neuroscience* 29, no. 41 (2009): 12815–23.

McKee, Embry A., Howard B. Roback, and Marc H. Hollender. "Transsexualism in Two Male Triplets." *American Journal of Psychiatry* 133 (1976): 334–37.

Meyer-Bahlburg, Heino F. L., Curtis Dolezal, Susan W. Baker, Anke A. Ehrhardt, and Maria I. New. "Gender Development in Women with Congenital Adrenal Hyperplasia as a Function of Disorder Severity." *Archives of Sexual Behavior* 35, no. 6 (2006): 667–84.

Money, John, and Anke A. Ehrhardt. *Man and Woman, Boy and Girl: Differentiation and Dimorphism of Gender Identity from Conception to Maturity*. Oxford: Johns Hopkins University Press, 1972.

National Institutes of Health. "Candidate Gene." National Human Genome Research Institute, updated July 21, 2022. Accessed November 24, 2021. https://www.genome.gov/genetics-glossary/Candidate-Gene.

National Institutes of Health. "Congenital Adrenal Hyperplasia." Genetic and Rare Diseases Information Center (GARD), updated November 8, 2021. Accessed November 21, 2021. https://rarediseases.info.nih.gov/diseases/1467/congenital-adrenal-hyperplasia.

National LGBT Health Education Center. "Collecting Sexual Orientation and Gender Identity Data in Electronic Health Records: Workshop Summary." 2013. https://doi.org/10.17226/18260.

Ngun, Tuck C. and Eric Vilain. "The Biological Basis of Human Sexual Orientation: Is There a Role for Epigenetics?" *Advances in Genetics* 86 (2014): 167–84.

Ngun, Tuck C., Negar Ghahramani, Francisco J. Sánchez, Sven Bocklandt, and Eric Vilain. "The Genetics of Sex Differences in Brain and Behavior." *Frontiers in Neuroendocrinology* 32, no. 2 (2011): 227–46.

O'Hanlan, Katherine A., Jennifer C. Gordon, and Mackenzie W. Sullivan. "Biological Origins of Sexual Orientation and Gender Identity: Impact on Health." *Gynecologic Oncology* 149, no. 1 (2018): 33–42.

Pasterski, Vickie, Kenneth J. Zucker, Peter C. Hindmarsh, et al. "Increased Cross-Gender Identification Independent of Gender Role Behavior in Girls with Congenital Adrenal Hyperplasia: Results from a Standardized Assessment of 4- to 11-Year-Old Children." *Archives of Sexual Behavior* 44, no. 5 (2015): 1363–75. https://doi.org/10.1007/s10508-014-0385-0.

Phelan, Jo C., Rosangely Cruz-Rojas, and Marian Reiff. "Genes and Stigma: The Connection between Perceived Genetic Etiology and Attitudes and Beliefs about Mental Illness." *Psychiatric Rehabilitation Skills* 6, no. 2 (2002): 159–85.

Phoenix, C. H., R. W. Gay, A. A. Gerall, and W. C. Young. "Organizational Action of Prenatally Administered Testosterone Propionate on the Tissues Mediating Mating Behavior in the Female Guinea Pig." *Endocrinology* 65 (1959): 369–82.

Polderman, Tinca J. C., Baudewijntje P. C. Kreukels, et al. "The Biological Contributions to Gender Identity and Gender Diversity: Bringing Data to the Table." *Behavior Genetics* 48, no. 2 (2018): 95–108.

Quinn, Virginia P., Rebecca Nash, Enid Hunkeler, et al. "Cohort Profile: Study of Transition, Outcomes and Gender (STRONG) to Assess Health Status of Transgender People." *BMJ Open* 7, no. 12 (2017): e018121.

Reiner, William G., and John P. Gearhart. "Discordant Sexual Identity in Some Genetic Males with Cloacal Exstrophy Assigned to Female Sex at Birth." *New England Journal of Medicine* 350, no. 4 (2004): 333–41.

Rice, William R., Urban Friberg, and Sergey Gavrilets. "Homosexuality as a Consequence of Epigenetically Canalized Sexual Development." *Quarterly Review of Biology* 87, no. 4 (2012): 343–68.

———. "Homosexuality via Canalized Sexual Development: A Testing Protocol for a New Epigenetic Model." *Bioessays* 35, no. 9 (2013): 764–70.

Roughgarden, Joan. *Evolution's Rainbow: Diversity, Gender, and Sexuality in Nature and People.* Berkley: University of California Press, 2013.

Sabalis, Robert F., Allen Frances, Susan N. Appenzeller, and Willie B. Moseley. "The Three Sisters: Transsexual Male Siblings." *American Journal of Psychiatry* 131, no. 8 (1974): 907–09.

Schagen, Sebastian E. E., Henriette A. Delemarre-van de Waal, Ray Blanchard, and Peggy T. Cohen-Kettenis. "Sibling Sex Ratio and Birth Order in Early-Onset Gender Dysphoric Adolescents." *Archives of Sexual Behavior* 41, no. 3 (2012): 541–49.

Skordis, Nicos, Gary Butler, Martine C. de Vries, Katharina Main, and Sabine E. Hannema. "ESPE and PES International Survey of Centers and Clinicians Delivering Specialist Care for Children and Adolescents with Gender Dysphoria." *Hormone Research in Paediatrics* 90, no. 5 (2018): 326–31. https://doi.org/10.1159/000496115.

Somers, James. "Head Space." *The New Yorker*, December 6, 2021. Accessed August 14, 2024. https://www.newyorker.com/magazine/2021/12/06/the-science-of-mind-reading.

Steensma, Thomas D., Peggy T. Cohen-Kettenis, and Kenneth J. Zucker. "Evidence for a Change in the Sex Ratio of Children Referred for Gender Dysphoria: Data from the Center of Expertise on Gender Dysphoria in Amsterdam (1988–2016)." *Journal of Sex & Marital Therapy* 44, no. 7 (2018): 713–15.

Stoller, Robert J. and Howard J. Baker. "Two Male Transsexuals in One Family." *Archives of Sexual Behavior* 2, no. 4 (1973): 323–28.

Swaab, Dick F., and Alicia Garcia-Falgueras. "Sexual Differentiation of the Human Brain in Relation to Gender Identity and Sexual Orientation." *Functional Neurology* 24, no. 1 (2009): 17–28.

Swaab, Dick F., Samantha E. C. Wolff, and Ai-Min Bao. "Sexual Differentiation of the Human Hypothalamus: Relationship to Gender Identity and Sexual Orientation." *Handbook of Clinical Neurology* 181 (2021): 427–43.

Szyf, Moshe. "The Epigenetics of Perinatal Stress." *Dialogues in Clinical Neuroscience* 21, no. 4 (2019): 369.

Time. "The Sexes: Biological Imperatives." January 8, 1973. Accessed August 14, 2024. https://time.com/archive/6844366/the-sexes-biological-imperatives/.

Van Caenegem, Eva, Katrien Wierckx, Els Elaut, et al. "Prevalence of Gender Nonconformity in Flanders, Belgium." *Archives of Sexual Behavior* 44, no. 5 (2015): 1281–87.

Van Kesteren, Paul J., Louis J. Gooren, and Jos A. Megens. "An Epidemiological and Demographic Study of Transsexuals in the Netherlands." *Archives of Sexual Behavior* 25, no. 6 (1996): 589–600.

Visscher, Peter M., Naomi R. Wray, Qian Zhang, et al. "10 Years of GWAS Discovery: Biology, Function, and Translation." *American Journal of Human Genetics* 101, no. 1 (2017): 5–22. https://doi.org/10.1016/j.ajhg.2017.06.005.

University of Hawai'i, Manoa. Pacific Center for Sex and Society. Updated March 22, 2024. Accessed August 15, 2024. http://www.hawaii.edu/PCSS/.

Wallien, Madeleine S. C., Kenneth J. Zucker, Thomas D. Steensma, and Peggy T. Cohen-Kettenis. "2D: 4D Finger-Length Ratios in Children and Adults with Gender Identity Disorder." *Hormones and Behavior* 54, no. 3 (2008): 450–54.

Watson, Diane B., and Stanley Coren. "Left-Handedness in Male-to-Female Transsexuals." *JAMA* 267, no. 10 (1992): 1342–42.

Watson, J. D., and F. H. C. Crick. "Molecular Structure of Nucleic Acids." *Landmarks in Medical Genetics: Classic Papers with Commentaries* 171, no. 51 (2004): 216.

Weyers, Steven, Els Elaut, Petra De Sutter, et al. "Long-Term Assessment of the Physical, Mental, and Sexual Health among Transsexual Women." *Journal of Sexual Medicine* 6, no. 3 (2009): 752–60.

Wilson, Philip, Clare Sharp, and Susan Carr. "The Prevalence of Gender Dysphoria in Scotland: A Primary Care Study." *British Journal of General Practice* 49, no. 449 (1999): 991–92.

Wisniewski, Amy B., Claude J. Migeon, Heino F. L. Meyer-Bahlburg, et al. "Complete Androgen Insensitivity Syndrome: Long-Term Medical, Surgical, and Psychosexual Outcome1." *Journal of Clinical Endocrinology & Metabolism* 85, no. 8 (2000): 2664–69. https://doi.org/10.1210/jcem.85.8.6742.

Yang, Fu, Xiao-hai Zhu, Qing Zhang, et al. "Genomic Characteristics of Gender Dysphoria Patients and Identification of Rare Mutations in RYR3 Gene." *Scientific Reports* 7, no. 1 (2017): 8339. https://doi.org/10.1038/s41598-017-08655-x.

Zhou, Jiang-Ning, Michel A. Hofman, Louis J. G. Gooren, and Dick F. Swaab. "A Sex Difference in the Human Brain and Its Relation to Transsexuality." *Nature* 378, no. 6552 (1995): 68–70.

Zucker, Kenneth J. "Epidemiology of Gender Dysphoria and Transgender Identity." *Sexual Health* 14, no. 5 (2017): 404–11.

14.1. PROFILE: EUGEN STEINACH (1861–1944) AND HIS CLINICAL TRIALS

Carolyn Wolf-Gould

Eugen Steinach (1861–1944) performed the first sex reassignment surgeries in Vienna on infant rats and guinea pigs. In 1894 and 1910, he published reports on his castration of rodents and the grafting of ovaries into the males and testes into the females.[1] He observed that not only did the male rodents with ovarian grafts develop the physical characteristics of females, including smaller size and lactating mammary tissue, but they also behaved like females, displaying feminine mating behaviors and suckling young. Similarly, the female rodents with testicular grafts exhibited masculine mating behaviors and grew to the size of typical males, with glossy masculine fur and build, as well as "indifferent" mammary tissue. Those grafted with both ovarian and testicular grafts grew large, masculine bodies with developed mammary tissue and sexual behavior that alternated between masculine and feminine.

This study presented an astonishing finding: sexual characteristics and behaviors could be altered by surgical procedures. Steinach concluded that although sex was determined by genetic factors, sexual development and dimorphism were controlled by secretions from the sex glands.[2] Yes, ludicrous today, but the scientists who extrapolated from this data at that time assumed that homosexuality was due to the lack of proper sexual differentiation of the sex glands and that homosexual behaviors could be cured by glandular manipulation. Steinach encouraged urologist Robert Lichtentstern to treat three homosexual men by removing one native testicle and implanting a properly functioning one from a heterosexual donor.[3]

The Steinach procedure didn't work; the men remained gay. Steinach confronted a rock in his research road, a dead end. But no matter. With a mind lit by possibility, he pursued the work that was nearer and dearer to his own biologic concerns: the emerging field of rejuvenation—and the quest for a fountain of youth. The desire for rejuvenation is a powerful force; most seniors yearn for their young, vigorous bodies, bodies that better align with their personal identities. Most elders (including Steinach) don't feel old in the soul and are irked by the aging process.

Steinach believed the hormonal state of senility was similar to that of a prepubertal castrate. Both possessed ineffectual glandular tissue.[4] In elders, the physiologic manifestations of sex regressed as they aged: their bodies got shorter, they became less muscular, their gonads withered, and they lost the desire to have sex. Often it was hard to tell an old man from an old woman. He wondered, as with castrates, could he reverse the aging process through glandular manipulation?

Once again, he started with rodents and the hypothesis that by ligating the vas deferens (that is, performing a vasectomy), the testes would produce fewer Leydig cells, those related to spermatogenesis, and induce hypertrophy in the hormone-producing interstitial cells. It worked! Three weeks after his aging and lethargic rats underwent a vasectomy, they were transformed into vigorous rats with prodigious sexual energy.

Steinach convinced Lichtentstern to secretly vasectomize three human subjects during urologic surgery for unrelated conditions.[5] One was a forty-four-year-old man with premature senility and the physical signs and symptoms of aging: fatigue, dull skin, muscle weakness, and weight loss. Six months after the procedure, the subject began to gain weight and appear more vigorous,

Figure 14.1.1. Seventy-year-old man (a) before and (b) two months after the Steinach Operation. *Source*: Courtesy of the Wellcome Library, London. Public domain.

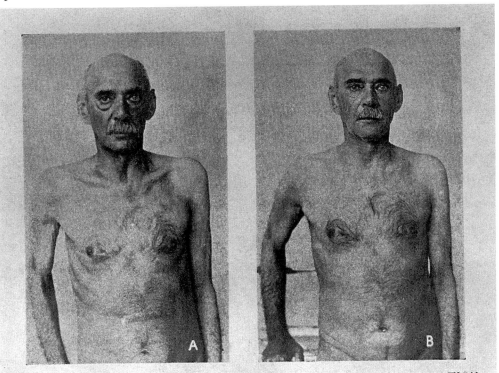

(a) SEVENTY YEAR OLD PATIENT BEFORE THE STEINACH OPERATION
(b) TWO MONTHS AFTER THE STEINACH OPERATION
(Ufa Steinach-Film)

and by eighteen months he looked like a youthful man at the peak of virility.[6] Photographs reveal a doddering elder transformed into a strongman.

Harry Benjamin, an enthusiastic supporter, performed more than four hundred Steinach operations in his practice in the United States and collaborated with Steinach to develop diathermy, a procedure to "Steinach" women using X-rays to destroy the germinal ovarian cells.[7] Soon, aging men and women lined up to be Steinached for rejuvenation. Stories regarding the success of the Steinach operation spread among doctors and patients throughout the Western world. The newspapers filled with gossipy stories of stodgy millionaires running amorously amok after being Steinached and Russian princesses selling their jewels to fund the procedure.[8] Famous people were Steinached. Sigmund Freud went under the knife, hoping the procedure would delay the recurrence of his oral cancer.[9] The American novelist Gerthrud Atherton announced she felt thirty years younger.[10] After his surgery, the poet William Butler Yeats went through what he referred to as his second puberty, a wildly prolific period of publication and oodles of affairs with younger women.[11] In tribute to Steinach, the Dublin newspapers nicknamed Yeats "The Gland Old Man."[12]

Ultimately, it became clear that the Steinach operation had at best only a sensationalized placebo effect. Although individuals sang its praise, as a rule, it did not reverse aging or improve sexual vigor. The procedure was relegated to the realm of quackery, along with organotherapy, "monkey ball" grafts, and other discredited rejuvenation procedures.[13] As the operation fell out of favor, Steinach faced mockery.

Judged through the lens of the twenty-first century, Steinach's research violated ethical principles and promoted bizarre and stigmatizing theories, but his work to identify the sex glands and their hormonal secretions advanced the field of endocrinology and ultimately led to the first human sex reassignment surgeries. Although he never received the Nobel Prize in Physiology, he was nominated six times between 1921 and 1938.[14] And while he also never found the fountain of youth, subsequent work based on his research enabled researchers to identify and produce the sex hormones testosterone and estradiol. Hormonal therapy is now the standard of care for gender dysphoria.

With hormone therapy, transitioning people also describe second puberties, ones that realign and, yes, *rejuvenate* the mind, body, and spirit. Perhaps Steinach discovered rejuvenation after all—even a fountain of hope—just not the sort he sought. While modern protocols for ethical research are meant to ensure that people no longer serve as guinea pigs, with the ongoing development of new technologies, such as puberty blockers and surgical techniques, it's important to note that many transgender and gender-diverse people still feel they are treated as experimental subjects.

NOTES

1. Sengoopta, "'Dr Steinach Coming to Make Old Young!'"
2. Sengoopta, "'Dr Steinach Coming to Make Old Young!'"
3. Meyerowitz, *How Sex Changed*, 17.
4. Sengoopta, "Rejuvenation" and "'Dr Steinach Coming to Make Old Young!'"
5. Sengoopta, "Rejuvenation," "The Modern Ovary," and "'Dr Steinach Coming to Make Old Young!'"
6. Steinach, *Sex and Life*.
7. Sengoopta, "The Modern Ovary."
8. Sengoopta, "The Modern Ovary"; Stipp, *The Youth Pill*, 6–8.
9. Sengoopta, "'Dr Steinach Coming to Make Old Young!'"
10. Sengoopta, "'Dr Steinach Coming to Make Old Young!'"
11. Stipp, *The Youth Pill*, 6–8; Lock, "'O That I Were Young Again.'"
12. Stipp, *The Youth Pill*, 6–8; Lock, "'O That I Were Young Again.'"
13. Sengoopta, "'Dr Steinach Coming to Make Old Young!'"
14. Sengoopta, "'Dr Steinach Coming to Make Old Young!'"

WORKS CITED

Lock, Stephen. "'O That I Were Young Again': Yeats and the Steinach Operation." *British Medical Journal (Clinical Research Ed.)* 287, no. 6409 (1983): 1964.

Meyerowitz, Joan. *How Sex Changed*. Cambridge: Harvard University Press, 2009.

Sengoopta, Chandak. "'Dr Steinach Coming to Make Old Young!': Sex Glands, Vasectomy and the Quest for Rejuvenation in the Roaring Twenties." *Endeavour* 27, no. 3 (2003): 122–26.

———. "The Modern Ovary: Constructions, Meanings, Uses." *History of Science* 38, no. 4 (2000): 425–88.

———. "Rejuvenation and the Prolongation of Life: Science or Quackery?" *Perspectives in Biology and Medicine* 37, no. 1 (1993): 55–66.

Steinach, Eugen. *Sex and Life. Forty Years of Biological and Medical Experiments*, edited by J. Loebel. London: Viking Press, 1940.

Stipp, David. *The Youth Pill: Scientists at the Brink of an Anti-Aging Revolution*. New York: Penguin, 2010.

14.2. "BORN THIS WAY" DATA: BIOLOGICAL VALIDATION OR CULTURAL OPPRESSION?

Carolyn Wolf-Gould

While diversity is a biological norm, stigma is purely a social phenomenon, and it is stigma, not gender diversity, that creates barriers to healthcare for transgender and gender-diverse (TGD) people—barriers that in turn lead to poor outcomes. The fear and revulsion heaped on TGD individuals throughout history induced in them shame, guilt, and self-loathing. This minority stress, coupled with lack of access to care and institutionalized discrimination, created a circular, self-perpetuating discriminatory storm that continues to traumatize the entire community. Over time, TGD people have wondered, "Why am I like this?" Many still question their sanity; others search for ways to understand, explain, and justify their experience. Some believe identifying a clear, biological etiology would validate their existence.

The fundamental question percolating beneath all historical exploration on gender diversity has been, "What is the cause?" Subsequent investigations launched epic disputes about the roles of nature versus nurture. These arguments drove behavioral and biomedical research, the development of healthcare protocols, the reinforcement of cultural perceptions, and legislative actions that perpetuated perceived norms.

In the 1960s and 1970s, psychoanalysts placed blame for this "disorder" on nurture—specifically, unhealthy parental practices (overbearing mother, absent father), psychic trauma, mental illness, and loss.[1] Early biomedical researchers did not directly reject psychological theories but emphasized possible biological predispositions. Even now, papers describing the biological underpinnings of gender identity eventually smack into unanswered questions and circle back to the inarguable thesis that (1) the etiology of gender identity is complex and (2) it rests in the interstices between biology, psychology, and the social environment.

Many TGD people and clinicians, despite incomplete evidence, assert their belief in a biological etiology due to commonalities in the trans experience and its persistence through time and place. In 1994, while challenging biological theories on sexual orientation, psychiatrist and scientist William Byne wrote, "The salient question about biology and sexual orientation is not whether biology is involved, but how it is involved. All psychological phenomena are ultimately biological."[2] Others, like neurobiologists Dick Swaab, Samantha

Wolff, and Ai-Min Bao, promote certainty of a biological origin, claiming in 2021: "All the genetic, postmortem, and in vivo scanning observations support the neurobiological theory about the origin of gender dysphoria. . . . There is no evidence that one's postnatal social environment plays a crucial role in the development of gender identity or sexual orientation."[3]

As the theories on the etiology of gender diversity emerged so too did the societal acceptance or rejection of TGD people and their access to healthcare. Pediatric endocrinologist Stephen Rosenthal stated: "[T]he goal of reviewing such studies is not to develop a 'litmus test' to confirm a person's gender identity, nor to uncover a mechanism that can be 'fixed' to prevent gender diversity. Rather, by shedding light on the role of biology in gender identity development, it is hoped that such knowledge can lead to de-stigmatization, greater acceptance, and improved quality of life for individuals with diverse gender identities."[4]

At this moment in history, a divisive political climate has once again called into question basic human rights for TGD people, including the right to healthcare. While numerous professional bodies, informed by evidence-based data, attest to the medical necessity of social, hormonal, and surgical transition, decisions about the right to this care are politicized, adjudicated in courtrooms, and debated by legislative bodies. Once again, many TGD people ask, "Would biological validation for our existence reduce stigma and ensure better care?" Increasingly, evidence points toward a biological etiology, but the volume and disparate nature of the data resist our attempt to pack it neatly into a box, tie it up with a bow, and present it as simple fait accompli. The body of work attesting to a biological cause crosses research disciplines and is usually published in academic journals in a language inaccessible to most of the public—including those who design healthcare systems or address social issues.

CONSEQUENCES OF IDENTIFYING A BIOLOGICAL ETIOLOGY FOR GENDER IDENTITY

Attribution theory predicts that forces seen as beyond a person's control (that is, biology) will be viewed in a more positive light than behaviors judged to be within a person's control.[5] Society places no blame on people with Alzheimer disease or breast cancer but stigmatizes those with conditions having a perceived social component, such as obesity, HIV, mental illness, and sexual and gender diversity. Evidence shows that education on research demonstrating biological etiologies may reduce stigma and negative stereotypes by reducing blame ascribed to the affected individuals.[6] American researchers Benjamin Goldstein and Francine Roselli proved that endorsement of a biological model for depression was associated with increased empowerment, a preference for psychotherapy, and decreased stigma.[7] Education of clinicians and the general public about the biological consequences of opioid addiction reduces the tendency to view opioid use disorders as a moral weakness and encourages engagement with medication-assisted treatment programs and lifesaving buprenorphine therapy.[8] And likewise, tests showed lesbians who believed sexual orientation was inborn rated lower scores for internalized stigma.[9]

However, other studies demonstrate that biological essentialism is a double-edged sword. Educational efforts may fail to improve attitudes, perpetuate existing stigma, or raise new specters that cause unintentional harm.[10] Psychologists Guy Boysen and David Vogel found that educational efforts to reduce negative attitudes about homosexuality were profoundly affected by preexisting attitudes.[11] Education on biological causes led only to changes in intensity of the original attitude; those with a positive attitude showed increased acceptance, and those with preexisting negative attitudes developed decreased acceptance and further polarization. Messaging on obesity as a disease rather than as a condition based on unhealthy behaviors decreased blame and anti-fat prejudice but also strengthened the belief in the unchangeable nature of weight, thus increasing anti-fat prejudice. Research scientist Jo Phelan and colleagues found that individuals who believed schizophrenia was caused by genetic factors were less likely to blame the individual but were also less likely to think the person could improve with appropriate help.[12] Biological explanations for human conditions create an "us vs. them" attitude that defines affected individuals through a deficit model, emphasizing distortions from established norms.[13] The identification of biological etiologies for unwelcome behaviors implies that affected individuals are unpredictable, dangerous, and best to avoid. Many view biological conditions as less responsive to treatment, more persistent, more serious, and less likely to resolve over time.

While clear biological evidence for the etiology of gender identity might in some ways validate the trans experience, some trans advocates argue against using the born-this-way argument to ensure the human rights of transgender people. For decades, LGBT activists have employed this slogan as a rallying cry in the case for legal equality, political change, and cultural acceptance.[14] In 2011, Lady Gaga released her defiant queer anthem, "Born This Way," and co-founded the Born This Way Foundation, inspiring a new set of Starbucks drinks and a line of beauty products.[15] But others argue the truth is more complicated.[16] Bioethicist Tia Powell and colleagues maintain that in the current political climate—in which biological evidence is often dismissed—the idea that gender identity is innate, immutable, or unassociated with choice relies on imperfect logic and the limitations of scientific inquiry and fails to provide a strong base for transgender rights.[17] The claim that gender identity is innate conflicts with evidence that gender identity is complex, develops and may change over time, and incorporates an array of behaviors, thoughts, feelings, and personal experiences. The complexity of the biological evidence renders it vulnerable to political attack. There are limits to what science can explain in a world also shaped by religious doctrine, political agendas, and cultural forces.

The implication that gender identity is immutable negates the fact that even factors under genetic control (such as hair color or patterns of baldness) change over time and may be influenced by the environment. Individual gender identities evolve in a myriad of ways over a lifetime. We now recognize that all aspects of gender exist on a spectrum and that gender identity and expression may be mutable. Many interpret born-this-way to indicate a lack of choice, a concept that fails to acknowledge the choices TGD people do make about expression and identity. University of Utah professor Lilly Martinez maintained that sexual orientation is sometimes a choice, citing evidence that an individual's experience with same-sex attraction may be fluid and change over time;[18] however, words like *choice* have been and continue to be used to oppress sexual minorities.[19] Yet the implication that one has no choice can promote a sense of helplessness or lack of agency rather than recognizing and celebrating gender diversity. Why should the dignity and rights of transgender people rest on a simplistic trope rooted in such unstable ground?

ETHICAL FRAMEWORKS FOR RESEARCH AND CLINICAL PRACTICE

Given the impulse to validate trans identity through biological research, we run the risk of overestimating the role of science in effecting social change.[20] Research efforts must acknowledge that biological essentialism does not ensure acceptance or equity. A study of heterosexual beliefs about sexual orientation demonstrated that acceptance of the born-this-way theory for sexual orientation did not predict tolerance.[21] Presuming that a simple biological cause could be found—a gene for gender identity, for example, or a specific anatomical landmark in the brain—would that gene or landmark confirm the existing pathological perspective, that gender diversity is a problem requiring medical treatment? Would surgeons develop procedures to remove the causal part of the brain? Would expectant parents screen for and eliminate fetuses with a transgender genetic trait? Would biological evidence lead to arbitrary standards and further gatekeeping about who would be considered trans enough to merit medical interventions? Just like psychological theories, biological theories have been and will continue to be weaponized by those with religious or political agendas. Trans activist Dana Beyer maintained, "When you know something to be true about yourself, you expect others to take your word for it, respect your dignity, and not subject you to an MRI."[22] In his article on the biological evidence for sexual orientation, Byne Mused: "Perhaps more importantly, we should also be asking ourselves why we as a society are so emotionally invested in this research. Will it—or should it—make any difference in the way we perceive ourselves and others or how we live our lives and allow others to live theirs? Perhaps the answers to the most salient questions in this debate lie not within the biology of human brains but rather in the culture those brains have created."[23]

Given the complex cultural response to arguments on biological essentialism, Dutch researcher Polderman and colleagues stressed the importance of centering research on the etiology of gender identity within a community-engaged research framework.[24] This framework values community participation from those most likely to be impacted by the research and is more likely to reflect the values, priorities, and experiences of the community.[25] The model exists on a continuum with increasing levels of influence and responsibility, from community-informed research on one end (community members advise on study design, reporting, and dissemination), to community-involved research in the middle (community members collaborate on project efforts), to community-directed research on the far end (where community members drive all aspects of investigating and disseminating research questions.) While in previous decades, researchers prohibited the involvement of TGD people in research, fearing they would bias investigations,[26] research organizations now prioritize and reward studies that engage the participation of community stakeholders.[27] The history of transgender medical practices attests to the irreparable bias created by the exclusion of TGD voices from research processes. The community-engaged framework ensures that those with lived experience—in this case, those who have experienced the validation or oppression caused by born-this-way arguments—contribute to the process of asking the questions and interpreting biological data that directly contributes to societal change.

CONCLUSION

As humans, we are curious about the world around us, about where we came from, about why we behave the way we do. It's clear that our individual experiences and cultures also drive the depth and breadth of our curiosity and the goals and outcomes of our efforts to learn. In the United States, the debates between nature (what is "real" or "natural," or for some, "ordained by God") and nurture (what is contrived or controlled by individuals, either the self or parents or other influential figures in an individual's life) have raged continuously, long before the Scopes Monkey Trial[28] in 1925 challenged Tennessee law that prohibited the study of Darwin's theory of evolution in public schools because it contradicted the Bible. Similar debates continue today in the form of anti-LGBT and anti-transgender legislative attempts to control what teachers can say in the classroom, who participates in athletics, what healthcare providers can do, and how individuals may express themselves. Despite significant scientific advancements, we still swim in a river driven by powerful historical currents beset with societal oxbows, resistant to change. Even cold empirical data eventually settle into the interstices of biology, psychology, and the social environment, where it lies vulnerable to disparate interpretation. The discovery of a biological cause for gender diversity will only offer validation to TGD people when their human experiences are culturally acknowledged, not disparaged.

NOTES

1. Coates, Friedman, and Wolfe, "The Etiology of Boyhood Gender Identity Disorder"; Feder, "Disciplining the Family"; Herman, "Gender Identity Disorder in a Five-Year-Old Boy."
2. Byne, "The Biological Evidence Challenged," 50.
3. Swaab, Wolff, and Bao, "Sexual Differentiation of the Human Hypothalamus," 427.
4. Rosenthal, "Challenges in the Care of Transgender and Gender-Diverse Youth," 3.
5. Boysen and Vogel, "Biased Assimilation and Attitude Polarization."
6. Polderman et al., "The Biological Contributions."

7. Goldstein and Rosselli, "Etiological Paradigms of Depression."
8. Olsen and Sharfstein, "Confronting the Stigma of Opioid Use Disorder."
9. Morandini et al., "Born This Way."
10. Canadian Health Services Research Foundation, "Myth: Reframing Mental Illness."
11. Boysen and Boysen and Vogel, "Biased Assimilation and Attitude Polarization."
12. Phelan, Cruz-Rojas, and Reiff, "Genes and Stigma."
13. Canadian Health Services Research Foundation, "Myth: Reframing Mental Illness."
14. Dastagir, "Born This Way'?"
15. Dastagir, "Born This Way'?"; Lady Gaga, "Born This Way"; Martinez, "Professor Strikes down 'Born This Way' Argument"; US Trans Survey, "2022 U.S. Trans Survey."
16. Martinez, "Professor Strikes down 'Born This Way' Argument"; Dastagir, "Born This Way'?"; Powell, Shapiro, and Stein, "Transgender Rights as Human Rights."
17. Powell, Shapiro, and Stein, "Transgender Rights as Human Rights."
18. Martinez, "Professor Strikes down 'Born This Way' Argument."
19. Dastagir, "Born This Way'?"
20. Barasch, "Biology Is Not Destiny."
21. Grzanka, Zeiders, and Miles, "Beyond 'Born This Way?'"
22. Beyer, "Professor Mickey Diamond."
23. Byne, "The Biological Evidence Challenged," 55.
24. Polderman et al., "The Biological Contributions."
25. Ferris, "Involving Community Members in Evaluation" and "Using a Framework for Community-Engaged Research."
26. Denny, "You Make Me Sick!" and "Writing Ourselves (1995)."
27. Wilkins et al., "Community Representatives' Involvement"; Patient-Centered Outcomes Research Institute, "About PCORI."
28. Linder, "State v. John Scopes."

WORKS CITED

Barasch, Alex. "Biology Is Not Destiny, Seeking a Scientific Explanation for Trans Identity Could Do More Harm than Good." *Washington Post*, June 27, 2018. Accessed August 14, 2024. https://www.washingtonpost.com/news/posteverything/wp/2018/06/27/feature/seeking-a-scientific-explanation-for-trans-identity-could-do-more-harm-than-good/.

Beyer, Dana. "Professor Mickey Diamond: 'Nature Loves Variety; Unfortunately, Society Hates It.'" *HuffPost Contributor Platform*, September 2, 2017. Accessed August 14, 2024. https://www.huffpost.com/entry/professor-mickey-diamond_b_11820398.

Boysen, Guy A., and David L. Vogel. "Biased Assimilation and Attitude Polarization in Response to Learning about Biological Explanations of Homosexuality." *Sex Roles* 57, no. 9 (2007): 755–62.

Byne, William. "The Biological Evidence Challenged." *Scientific American* 270, no. 5 (1994): 50–55.

Canadian Health Services Research Foundation. "Myth: Reframing Mental Illness as a 'Brain Disease' Reduces Stigma." *Journal of Health Services Research & Policy* 18, no. 3 (2013): 190–92.

Coates, Susan, Richard C. Friedman, and Sabrina Wolfe. "The Etiology of Boyhood Gender Identity Disorder: A Model for Integrating Temperament, Development, and Psychodynamics." *Psychoanalytic Dialogues* 1, no. 4 (1991): 481–523.

Dastagir, Alice. "Born This Way'? For Many in LGBT Community, It's Way More Complex." *USA Today*, June 15, 2017. Accessed August 14, 2024. https://www.usatoday.com/story/news/2017/06/16/born-way-many-lgbt-community-its-way-more-complex/395035001/.

Denny, Dallas. "Writing Ourselves (1995)." *TransSisters: Journal of Transsexual Feminism* 8 (October 2011): 38–39. Accessed August 14, 2024. http://dallasdenny.com/Writing/2011/10/05/writing-ourselves/.

———. "You Make Me Sick!" Presented at the Trans-Progressing Symposium, Provincetown, MA, 2004. Accessed August 14, 2024. http://dallasdenny.com/Writing/2013/08/24/you-make-me-sick-2004/.

Feder, Ellen K. "Disciplining the Family: The Case of Gender Identity Disorder." *Philosophical Studies: An International Journal for Philosophy in the Analytic Tradition* 85, no. 2–3 (1997): 195–211.

Ferris, Melanie. "Involving Community Members in Evaluation." Wilder Research, 2018. Accessed August 14, 2024. https://www.wilder.org/sites/default/files/Community-InvolvedResearchHandout_12-18.pdf.

Ferris, Melanie. "Using a Framework for Community-Engaged Research." Wilder Foundation, December 14, 2018. Accessed August 14, 2024. https://www.wilder.org/articles/using-framework-community-engaged-research.

Goldstein, Benjamin, and Francine Rosselli. "Etiological Paradigms of Depression: The Relationship between Perceived Causes, Empowerment, Treatment Preferences, and Stigma." *Journal of Mental Health* 12, no. 6 (2003): 551–63.

Grzanka, Patrick R., Katharine H. Zeiders, and Joseph R. Miles. "Beyond 'Born This Way?' Reconsidering Sexual Orientation Beliefs and Attitudes." *Journal of Counseling Psychology* 63, no. 1 (2016): 67.

Herman, Stephen P. "Gender Identity Disorder in a Five-Year-Old Boy." *Yale Journal of Biology and Medicine* 56, no. 1 (1983): 15.

Lady Gaga. *Lady Gaga—Born This Way* (official music video). YouTube, 2011. Accessed August 14, 2024. https://www.youtube.com/watch?v=wV1FrqwZyKw.

Linder, Douglas O. "State v. John Scopes ("The Monkey Trial")." n.d. University of Missouri Kansas City. Accessed August 14, 2024. http://law2.umkc.edu/faculty/projects/ftrials/scopes/evolut.htm.

Martinez, Lilly. "Professor Strikes down 'Born This Way' Argument for Homosexuality." *The Badger Herald* (blog), February 10, 2017. Accessed August 14, 2024. https://badgerherald.com/news/2017/02/10/professor-strikes-down-born-this-way-argument-for-homosexuality/.

Morandini, James S., Alexander Blaszczynski, Daniel S. J. Costa, Alexandra Godwin, and Ilan Dar-Nimrod. "Born This Way: Sexual Orientation Beliefs and Their Correlates in Lesbian and Bisexual Women." *Journal of Counseling Psychology* 64, no. 5 (2017): 560.

Olsen, Yngvild, and Joshua M. Sharfstein. "Confronting the Stigma of Opioid Use Disorder—and Its Treatment." *JAMA* 311, no. 14 (2014): 1393–94.

Patient-Centered Outcomes Research Institute. "About PCORI." Accessed October 28, 2021. https://www.pcori.org/about/about-pcori.

Phelan, Jo C., Rosangely Cruz-Rojas, and Marian Reiff. "Genes and Stigma: The Connection between Perceived Genetic Etiology and Attitudes and Beliefs about Mental Illness." *Psychiatric Rehabilitation Skills* 6, no. 2 (2002): 159–85.

Polderman, Tinca J. C., Baudewijntje P. C. Kreukels, Michael S. Irwig, et al. "The Biological Contributions to Gender Identity and Gender Diversity: Bringing Data to the Table." *Behavior Genetics* 48, no. 2 (2018): 95–108.

Powell, Tia, Sophia Shapiro, and Ed Stein. "Transgender Rights as Human Rights." *AMA Journal of Ethics* 18, no. 11 (2016): 1126–31.

Rosenthal, Stephen M. "Challenges in the Care of Transgender and Gender-Diverse Youth: An Endocrinologist's View." *Nature Reviews Endocrinology* 17 (2021): 581–91.

Swaab, Dick F., Samantha E. C. Wolff, and Ai-Min Bao. "Sexual Differentiation of the Human Hypothalamus: Relationship to Gender Identity and Sexual Orientation." *Handbook of Clinical Neurology* 181 (2021): 427–43.

US Trans Survey. "2022 U.S. Trans Survey." Accessed March 2, 2017. http://www.ustranssurvey.org/.

Wilkins, Consuelo H., Mark Spofford, Neely Williams, et al. "Community Representatives' Involvement in Clinical and Translational Science Awardee Activities." *Clinical and Translational Science* 6, no. 4 (2013): 292–96. https://doi.org/10.1111/cts.12072.

15

DEVELOPING MEANINGFUL TRANSGENDER HEALTH RESEARCH
A Journey toward Social Justice

George R. Brown and Carolyn Wolf-Gould

The history of transgender medical research is rife with accounts of desperate people requesting experimental care and clinician-researchers trialing protocols and procedures without adequate concern for participant well-being, consent, or safety. In the late nineteenth and early to mid-twentieth centuries, this activity led to a body of literature that systematically denigrated, pathologized, and derided gender-diverse people.[1] Contemporary research has moved toward honoring the lived experience of transgender and gender-diverse (TGD) individuals and establishing a health-based understanding of gender diversity as a normal human experience. Before it was fashionable for young clinicians to engage in any type of work with gender nonconforming people, I (the first author of this chapter) conducted boots-on-the-ground clinical research to improve transgender healthcare in the late twentieth and the early twenty-first centuries. In this chapter, I describe my professional experience and contributions: first by researching on the margins of clinical care and later as the first clinician-researcher to analyze big data with a comparison group for a population of people otherwise invisible to healthcare systems and their databases. Notably, much of my work focuses on clinical care and research with transgender veterans and transgender people who are incarcerated. I will illustrate the principles of translational research and, drawing on my advocacy work, explain why clinician-researchers must often take the additional step of translating research through the US court system to effect systemic change.

MY CLINICAL GENEALOGY: BUILDING ON HARRY BENJAMIN'S LEGACY

From our twenty-first century perch, it is easy to pass judgment on our predecessors for their flawed ethical principles and behaviors. These researchers worked with minimal knowledge of the subject matter, operated under nascent rules for scientific engagement, and lived within a society defined by inequity and prejudice toward gender, sexual, and racial minorities. Their work advanced the field but tainted our culture, specifically reinforcing formidable barriers to healthcare, including minority stress, stigma, institutionalized discrimination, and lack of access to medical care for TGD people.

Harry Benjamin himself recognized the pitfalls and travails of conducting research in this field, citing these difficulties in his seminal work from 1966, *The Transsexual Phenomenon*: "There is a challenge as well as a handicap in writing a book on a subject that is not yet covered in the medical literature. Transsexualism is such a subject. . . . The challenge lies in the novelty of these observations and in the attempt to describe clinical pictures and events without preconceived notions, with no axes to grind, and with no favorites to play."[2] The relevance of Benjamin's statement today is uncanny. Despite advances in healthcare and research, sociocultural ignorance of the TGD community persists, exacerbated by continued social stigma and overt social inequities. In some ways, today's world is strikingly similar to that of the early champions for trans-specific care. Clinician-researchers like me—and those within the TGD community—must continue to explain transgender identity and related subjects, translating these topics for clinical, sociocultural, political, and legal audiences. Recently, as part of a litigation process to advocate for equal rights for transgender people in the United States (for instance, access to transgender healthcare and appropriate bathroom facilities), I was asked to write expert opinions on the meaning of the words *sex* and *gender identity*. Here we are, more than fifty-five years after Benjamin's publication of *The Transsexual Phenomenon*,[3] and we are *still* trying to define both sex and gender in our culture, healthcare institutions, and highest courts.

In 2018, at the World Professional Association for Transgender Health's Biannual Symposium in Buenos Aires, Argentina, we celebrated the fiftieth anniversary of Benjamin's groundbreaking book. Every researcher, teacher, advocate, scholar, and clinician involved in advancing this field owes a debt of gratitude to Benjamin, on whose shoulders we stand. He already had a long, distinguished medical career in Europe and the United States before he decided to take on the taboo of changing sex in our binary Western culture. He was in what he called "the evening of his life," and he cared little about the criticism of colleagues, the press, and society. His work as the most prolific clinician-researcher for transgender people led to the establishment of the field of transgender healthcare in the United States. Benjamin popularized the terms *transsexualist* and *transsexual*, regretting the former and embracing the latter. After his death, Richard Green heralded him as the father of transsexualism.[4] I obtained my copy of *The Transsexual Phenomenon* in 1988. It was out of print and hard to come by even then.

Benjamin not only cared for the transsexual people who requested treatment in his office but also studied their lives, recorded their stories, and sought to understand the etiology of transsexualism. His views were out of step for his time. He recommended kind and compassionate medical care, including the provision of hormone therapy and surgical procedures to address the suffering of transgender people. Benjamin believed in a constitutional or biological etiology for gender diversity, rejecting the prevalent mental illness–based theories that blamed family dynamics or disease as the cause. Research on the etiology of gender diversity remains controversial; many view research findings as politically dangerous or fear they will be weaponized against TGD people.

In 1966, Benjamin described the politics within this emerging field and how divergent political positions were offered or received among his colleagues and within segments of American culture. Politics have played and continue to play a large role in the planning and delivery of research and healthcare for TGD people. Many clinicians and patients find the field as stifling now as it was in 1966. The absence of data to support transgender health services has contributed in important ways to the current shortages in delivery and funding. Payors have labeled gender-affirming procedures elective or cosmetic due to the scarcity of high-quality research that demonstrates they are effective treatments for gender dysphoria. What has passed as research has often been nothing more than a pronouncement of expert opinions, a retrospective or cross-sectional study limited to a small clinical setting, an anecdotal observation, or a case report.[5] Anecdotes will never be data, and yet much clinical work in this field has been informed only by anecdotal reports and case series with no control or comparison groups.

Censorship of transgender research has been rampant in medical and psychiatric journals despite the quality of work submitted. The American Psychiatric Association and its publication, the *American Journal of Psychiatry*, repeatedly ignored my manuscripts throughout the 1990s, often without the courtesy of a review: "We have chosen not to review your manuscript because the topic is not of general interest to our readership." I have witnessed, both then and now, the repression and censorship of open discussion in academic settings for various reasons, including rejection of the topic as unpleasant, uncommon, or unimportant; this repression has weakened the field. Conversely, I have done the hard, tedious work of reviewing research by those who challenge me and, at times, shock me by what they may say. Yet I do not suggest we silence these voices, as the field can lose critical thinking and innovation. Diversity of opinion is critical to moving a field forward, particularly in the absence of evidence-based data to resolve important research questions.

Although Benjamin was shunned for his work and often faced hostile medical audiences, he chose to welcome such disagreement in the service of moving the field forward. Benjamin was no stranger to duress or repression, particularly in the 1960s, but he still found his calling. The New York State County Medical Society's Division of Professional Misconduct sanctioned him for providing carry letters to patients; these were documents that offered a modicum of safety to citizens whose gender expression did not match their legal sex.[6] New York officials threatened to prosecute and forced Benjamin to stop providing these letters. As a younger man, Benjamin displayed professional courage by working to understand and assist commercial sex workers, another source of professional scorn.[7]

By 1964, Benjamin had amassed a considerable amount of research on thirty-one transsexual patients who had undergone some form of gender-affirming surgery, often in overseas locations due to the stigma of such work in the United States.[8] By the time of his death in 1986 at the age of 101, and despite the derision he received for his work, Benjamin had evaluated 1,560 transgender patients, meticulously collecting their data.[9] Imagine what

Benjamin could have done with access to computers, software, and electronic medical records.

I am one of the physician-scholars who followed in Benjamin's footsteps. I, too, have devoted my career to the understanding and care of TGD people. I have also faced attacks and hostile audiences and have tried to muster similar courage to move forward. Today, some professionals in the field still confront persecution, including the ridicule and personal attacks that bedeviled Benjamin's career. TGD people are regularly dismissed as disordered or irrelevant by those in the medical field, and this derision may also extend to the clinicians who serve them. These attacks have lowered the level of academic inquiry by silencing politically unpopular ideas, but they have also stimulated civil, scientific discourse on the competing theories that have evolved.

This chapter recounts my life's work to empathically understand those with trans identities, turn observations into practical research, and develop large databases with the potential to translate this research into tangible improvements in the lives of TGD persons and their families. I dedicate this account to the thousands of TGD people and their significant others, those who trained *me* with their stories and tears and spent their valuable time participating as research volunteers over three decades of work. I also dedicate this chapter to my mentors, those who served as academic and military supervisors during my medical and psychiatric training. Not one of them supported my interest in transgender health. Instead, they uniformly advised, "If you follow this path, it will dead-end your career. Why waste your promising career on this little niche that will never amount to anything?" I ignored their advice and followed my passions, a path that opened me to a world of meaningful work and powerful, personal connections.

MY CAREER: CONVERTING RESEARCH INTO TANGIBLE GAINS

I am often asked why I chose to focus on clinical care and research in the field of transgender health. While in medical school in 1979, I interviewed my first patient, who happened to be a transgender woman. She was an army veteran who transitioned in the 1970s. I listened and was deeply moved by her stories of discrimination, abuse, rejection, homelessness, and inability to find knowledgeable healthcare providers. As I searched for clinical information to help me care for this woman, I discovered the paucity of data available to inform clinical care. I collected all the English language publications on gender dysphoria, filling two slim manila folders in my file cabinet. This anthology of the available research was accessible only to those with academic libraries and a pocketful of nickels to feed the Xerox machines for copies—assuming the machines were functioning.

In the late twentieth century, transgender people sought care from clinicians who might (or might not) have had access to this paltry stack of articles—and those lucky enough to access healthcare had to pay cash, as private and public payers denied gender-affirming care, deeming it cosmetic or experimental. Transgender people had no legal protections around housing, education, or employment. Incarcerated transgender people had no access to care. After the publication of the Harry Benjamin International Gender Dysphoria Association's *Standards of Care, Version 1*, in 1979, the time was ripe for clinics to begin prospective, collaborative studies on treatments and outcomes—but such research did not truly begin until decades later.

In 1983, I was accepted for a psychiatry residency at the University of California at San Francisco and at Stanford University, places that interested me due to the presence of a few faculty members active in the emerging field of transgender healthcare. But the fine print in my military scholarship contract required me to train in the US Air Force, so I set off to begin my psychiatry residency as an Air Force officer in Dayton, Ohio. Once on base, I suddenly and unexpectedly found myself caring for TGD, active-duty troops and veterans in various stages of transition, with no mentors or experienced clinicians to advise me. These individuals were desperate for care but feared their military doctors would turn them in to the authorities, which would result in immediate discharge and loss of earned benefits.[10] I was required by military regulations to report these patients, but instead, I chose to serve as a psychiatrist, not a policeman. I worked quietly with these individuals, assuring them I would not turn them in. I arranged gender-affirming hormone therapy for some. I provided support to their spouses when asked. I listened to their stories, and I diligently wrote them down, following the model of Benjamin so many years before.

In 1980, the American Psychiatric Association published the *Diagnostic and Statistical Manual of Mental Disorders, Third Edition* (*DSM-III*), which for the first time included the diagnosis of transsexualism.[11] Despite concerns regarding how this document pathologized the community, the *DSM-III* provided a legitimate path for some of us to develop early research questions and collaborate.

Mental health clinicians and researchers now possessed a common language, despite its flaws. In 1988, I published my first paper from my collected military data.[12] I told the stories of transgender women in uniform, many of whom reported that they joined the hostile environment of the armed services "to become a real man" or die trying.[13] I described how gender-questioning young adults assigned male at birth struggled to cope with the unbearable stress of gender dysphoria with this "flight into hypermasculinity."[14] This observation was just a hypothesis, but one we later confirmed with a much larger report on the experiences of numerous active-duty transgender women and veterans.[15]

In the mid-1980s, I attempted another study, this one questioning how my fellow military officers serving as psychiatrists, psychologists, and social workers handled the complex issues inherent in working with sexual and gender minorities in the stifling environment of military medicine. Although this anonymous study would be the first of its kind, my Air Force superiors blocked my efforts and discouraged me from pursuing any further research in this highly stigmatized area. Prevented from doing this work aboveboard, I instead dove underground for data. I met with transgender people attending support groups that met in the basements of Ohio and on the rural ranches of Texas. I attended social networking and support conventions around the country, sponsored by and for transgender citizens, and sometimes their partners or spouses. I worked with trans-identified people and their spouses outside of the clinical settings where most of the existing research had been performed. I helped organize some of the largest social and educational events for trans-identified people and their significant others, including, for example, the Texas T Parties of the late 1980s and early 1990s—highly successful events with hundreds of people attending from around the country. I provided free workshops and asked for research volunteers at these and many other community events (such as the annual Be All weekends in the Midwest and Crossport events in southern Ohio), all in an era before we had access to the internet—a critical tool that now greatly simplifies research methods.

Over several years, I interviewed each of the 188 individuals who participated in one of my early studies to destigmatize transgender identity. This type of hands-on approach is largely a technique of the past in the medical field, with one-on-one interviews replaced by online survey instruments, which unfortunately enable researchers to conduct research without ever having to get to know their anonymous subjects; researchers also assume those who participate online are truly from the population of interest. Despite my unconventional research methods, a lack of funding, and the absence of modern-day internet survey methods, in 1966, I published the first large paper depathologizing trans-identified people and challenging the assumption they were all highly disturbed with personality disorders.[16] My findings surprised other clinicians. Even Paul Walker, a founder of the Harry Benjamin International Gender Dysphoria Association, believed most people with gender dysphoria suffered from one or more personality disorders. My work, done in nonclinical settings, found otherwise. Like cisgender people, transgender people do not all possess personality disorders.

In 1991, after the first Gulf War, I left the Air Force and sought employment at a rural, academically affiliated veterans' hospital in Appalachia. In my interviews for the position, I proposed to establish the first public Veteran's Health Administration (VHA) clinic for transgender veterans. I planned to begin by offering endocrine, psychiatric, and housing support for transgender veterans. To my surprise, the VHA hired me and supported my plan. I hoped this clinic would not only provide much needed care but also serve as a base for my research. We opened our doors in 1994, and shortly thereafter established the first unisex bathroom in Eastern Tennessee, an enormous achievement for this conservative region. Veterans flocked to my clinic from across the United States. One flew from California to Tennessee to obtain gender-affirming hormonal therapy from me, as she could not find anyone in California who would take on her case. Some retired veterans even moved from Europe to Tennessee to live near our services. We also developed a study on voice therapy for trans women, the first of its kind in any military or VHA setting. I offered care, gained experience, and began to consider research questions.

However, support for research in this field correlates with the contemporary political climate, and in 1995, the Tennessee winds were not in our favor. Conservative US Senator Fred Thompson[17] forced us to close when he learned about our clinic and research. He declared it illegal to prescribe hormones to veterans and ordered an investigation of me and my clinic. He told my boss he didn't want "those faggots being treated in my VHA hospital."[18] Despite both VHA and East Tennessee State University Institutional Review Board approval for this study, my superiors forced us to abandon the research. I was nearly fired due to this investigation, and the VHA prohibited me from offering medical care to veterans to change gender, according to existing directives. Never mind that I could do nothing to change anyone's gender—the nuances of sex and gender were beyond the ken of the investigators. I was reluctantly exonerated by the investigators, and a report was filed to that effect. The investigators failed to find evidence that I was prescribing gender-affirming hormones, apparently because they were inept at searching the nascent computerized records system that existed at that time.

In 2011, under the Obama administration, the VHA reversed its longstanding ban on the provision of most interventions for gender dysphoria. This policy change not only allowed for transgender healthcare in each of the VHA's 450-plus facilities but also mandated that transgender veterans receive at least a partial package of benefits in all major VHA facilities.[19] Suddenly, transgender veterans who had been legally denied access to transgender healthcare at any Veteran Affairs (VA) hospital were entitled (at least in theory) to receive gender-affirming hormones, voice therapy, formal psychiatric evaluations, presurgical evaluations and referral letters, and postoperative surgical care in all VA facilities. Given the dearth of knowledge and talent concerning transgender health within VHA at that time, I was one of the first people called to develop national policies and the national formulary for transgender veteran healthcare—quite a turnaround from my censure of the 1990s.

My professional and institutional role positioned me to transform the VHA transgender healthcare system from the inside. Whereas the inspector general's office had previously suspended my research protocol, I was now actively encouraged to conduct large-scale studies of healthcare disparities among transgender veterans. As one of a few clinician-researchers with experience in the field, I was also promoted to a leadership role in the VHA Central Office at the new Office of Health Equity in Washington, DC, and was granted access to the Veterans Health Database, dating back to 1996. The sudden change in the political climate enabled me to perform big data research by accessing twenty years of electronic health records for millions of veterans, including medical, mental health, and pharmacy data. The VHA had been on the leading edge in the development of computerized health records, and I was now able to reap those benefits on behalf of transgender veterans.

Electronic health records now offer the promise of rapid access to large volumes of medical information, a research trove about which Benjamin could only have dreamt. In the mid-1970s, the US VHA was one of the first large healthcare systems to develop a national electronic medical record, but it was not until the mid-1990s that the system was sophisticated enough to ask meaningful clinical research questions to inform clinical practice. In 2015, several researchers gathered in Washington, DC, to perform an environmental scan of the field and develop a State of the Science paper, which was published in *Current Opinion in Endocrinology, Diabetes, and Obesity* in February 2016.[20] In this paper, we concluded that there was insufficient large-scale research conducted with transgender people; serious gaps existed in important areas, including the sources of major health disparities, optimal hormonal treatment regimens, and systematic long-term studies to provide evidence-based guidance for treatments (including follow-up care).

THE BODY OF MY WORK AND ITS PRACTICAL SIGNIFICANCE FOR TGD PERSONS

Well after founding the Mountain Home VHA Gender Clinic in Tennessee in 1994, I established the Mountain Home Transgender Veteran Research Protocol in 2012 as the principal investigator, assisted by a single data analyst. This time lag was largely due to lack of VHA support for the provision of care for trans veterans and research on sexual or gender minorities. I quietly continued my work during this era but had no access to datasets any larger than 120 individuals. With the radical federal government change in approach to sexual and gender minorities effected under the Obama administration, which included my promotion to a research leadership position in the newly formed VHA Office of Health Equity, I was able to develop a research protocol that involved access to a nationwide VA database of all veterans who had ever been seen for clinical care at any of the more than 420 facilities since 1996. Due to its sensitive content, it took nearly a year to obtain what amounted to a top-secret security clearance before I could access this dataset. Under this protocol, I gathered results from a series of investigations conducted with 5,135 veterans with a diagnosis of *gender dysphoria* or the antiquated term *gender identity disorder*. Our work departed from prior studies due to the size of the cohort, the use of clinical data, and our ability to access national electronic health records to design studies with large numbers of matched cisgender control subjects. We conducted a series of studies based on this cohort—the first large, controlled studies of transgender people and their health in the United States. We focused on suicidal behavior, completed suicides, all-cause mortality, health and mental health disparities, breast cancer, racial disparities, incarceration issues, and changes in system-wide pharmacy use. I will briefly describe a few of these studies and offer additional highlights from this body of work.

Our first study looked specifically at suicidal behaviors.[21] We expected the rate to be higher in transgender veterans but did not anticipate the extent of this finding. We documented evidence of suicidal behaviors in trans veterans that were up to twenty times higher than that of the general population of American veterans. Because this study did not include directly asking veterans about their experiences (this would not have been possible) but did include information from actual medical records, our findings likely underreported the true extent of suicidal behaviors.

In the next study, we looked at hard endpoints: documented death from any causes, with completed suicides as a component.[22] We documented each death in our population in a nationally recorded cause of death database. We considered the likelihood that suicide might be underreported in our data, as suicide is often not recorded as such by coroners and medical examiners. Our results were notable for higher numbers of trans veterans with death due to accidents/suicides, as well as for infectious diseases (the latter representing the significant overrepresentation of HIV/AIDS in this population). We examined the data on suicide separately and confirmed that nearly five percent of the transgender group died from suicide by the ten-year follow-up point, for a crude rate of 82 per 100,000. Of note was the significantly younger age of suicide for the transgender veterans compared to the general veteran control group. A follow-up study of suicide data we published in 2021 confirmed this finding, with completed suicide rates twice as high in the transgender veteran group compared to cisgender veterans aged eighteen to thirty-nine.[23]

In a third study, we used our database to examine the risk of breast cancer for transgender patients, particularly those assigned male at birth who transitioned later in life, with or without the use of feminizing hormone therapy.[24] Trans women may take estrogens for decades, and clinicians and patients are understandably concerned about cancer risk over time. Researchers Louis Gooren, Henk Asscheman, Paul Van Kesteren, and their colleagues conducted the pioneering work of collecting the long-term hormone-related mortality and morbidity data in the Netherlands in studies that began over twenty years ago.[25] Our study was not as long in duration as their work, but our cohort included a larger group of at-risk patients. Within our group of 5,135 transgender veterans, we confirmed ten cases of breast cancer—seven in transgender men, two in transgender women, and one in an individual assigned male at birth with a diagnosis of transvestic fetishism.[26] Just over half of the sample group had received hormone therapy from within the VHA system and an unknown percentage from other sources. It is not possible in any study to reliably know the doses of hormones that individuals have taken given that many patients obtain hormones from street sources before, during, or after they have been prescribed gender-affirming hormones by a clinician if they are fortunate enough to have this access to healthcare. Our statistics showed no increased risk of breast cancer in trans women or trans men. This study confirmed data from the Netherlands research, which showed that breast cancer was not common and evidenced rates similar to the cisgender controls in our cohort. We still need studies with longer duration and larger cohorts to better clarify this risk, but these two large data studies are reassuring to trans women who take estrogens as part of their transition.

Our fourth study examined mental health and medical outcome disparities in our transgender cohort.[27] We used the VHA's large electronic health record database and all the coded diagnoses for more than 5,100 transgender veterans comparing them with more than 15,000 cisgender veteran controls matched for age, race, and other characteristics (a one-to-three matched cohort study). The largest disparity between trans veterans and controls was the incidence of HIV/AIDS, which was five times more likely in the trans veterans—a staggering increase. Other notable findings included a seventy percent increased chance of cardiac arrest and at least a fifty percent higher risk of hypertension, ischemic heart disease, obesity, and tobacco use for transgender veterans. We documented disparities for traumatic brain injuries, possibly due to the higher propensity of transgender veterans who served in active combat roles, often as volunteers. (Many volunteered for more dangerous duties than were assigned, making it more likely that they would sustain head trauma.) We showed substantially higher rates of diabetes, cerebral vascular disease, heart attacks, and congestive heart failure in trans veterans compared to cisgender controls. Only two conditions did not differ significantly between transgender veterans and controls: end-stage renal disease and cirrhosis.

We also found an increase in most of the psychiatric conditions that we studied. Transgender veterans were almost five times more likely to suffer from depression. Alcohol abuse—even when compared to the general veteran population with a substantial burden of addictions—was seventy percent more likely among transgender veterans.

The fifth study we conducted was the first large-scale, controlled study of racial health disparities in transgender persons.[28] In our cohort of 5,135 trans veterans, 387 were non-Hispanic Black and 4,120 were non-Hispanic White. While it had been reported that trans people of color were particularly disadvantaged and were likely to possess a greater burden of disease, no controlled study existed. We compared the two groups to look for significant medical and/or mental health disparities. We found striking differences in the prevalence of medical and mental health conditions, with Black trans veterans suffering a substantially increased burden of disease than their White veteran comrades, despite ostensibly similar access to healthcare. Black trans veterans were almost twice as likely to be diagnosed with alcohol abuse, nearly seven times more likely to be living with HIV/AIDS, and over three times as likely to have end-stage renal disease. Clinically and statistically significant increases in disease burden were also noted for benign prostatic hyperplasia, congestive heart failure, hypertension, serious mental illness, and tobacco use. Black trans veterans were nearly twice as likely to have a history of incarceration and to have experienced homelessness. Compared to Black trans veterans, White trans veterans were somewhat more likely to have depression, hypercholesterolemia, and obesity.

Lastly, I will touch on some unpublished but important work from this big data study. The delivery of transgender healthcare often occurs in systems, and in the VHA, our system was not prepared for the 2011 mandate to provide trans-specific healthcare for veterans. The new edict could not quickly eliminate the long-standing barriers that prevented transgender people from accessing care within a broken system. Examples of barriers to care included long wait times for appointments, long driving distances, and a nationwide lack of clinician expertise. A system reflects the policies and incentives in place, and before 2011, the VHA discouraged clinicians from learning about or providing transgender healthcare.

As part of our research, we used our database to determine whether veterans were able to access the newly mandated health benefits. First, we described a steep rise in the number of transgender patients diagnosed in the VHA.[29] This rise had begun some years prior but developed a steep upward slope after the VHA changed its policies regarding transgender healthcare in 2011. Our data reflected the unmet health needs of transgender veterans, proving that if you build a system that includes trans-specific support and care, they will come. The trend shown below has continued well past 2013, and it is now likely that the VA is the largest provider of transgender healthcare of any integrated healthcare system in the United States.

To investigate whether this increased rate of diagnoses translated into transgender veterans gaining access to trans-specific healthcare, we looked at the numbers of prescriptions for estrogen, testosterone, and spironolactone written in the VHA over the past fifteen-plus years. We found a striking increase for all three medications after the mandate. We also found higher increases for hormone use than for the acquisition of new gender dysphoria diagnoses, suggesting that existing patients were now accessing the VHA system for hormone therapy.

Table 15.1. Prevalence and Incidence of Transgender-Related Diagnoses in the Veterans Health Administration: United States, Fiscal Years 2006–2013

Fiscal Year	New Transgender Diagnoses	Deaths	Total Transgender Diagnoses	VHA Population	Incidence* (95% CI)	Prevalence* (95% CI)
2006	226	3	226	6,438,734	3.5 (0.0, 7.2)	3.5 (0.0, 7.2)
2007	223	4	446	6,574,157	3.4 (0.0, 7.0)	6.8 (1.7, 11.9)
2008	231	9	673	6,846,503	3.4 (0.0, 7.0)	9.8 (3.7, 16.0)
2009	272	10	936	7,147,546	3.8 (0.0, 7.6)	13.1 (6.0, 20.2)
2010	341	15	1267	7,381,314	4.6 (0.4, 8.8)	17.2 (9.0, 25.3)
2011	384	26	1636	7,552,783	5.1 (0.7, 9.5)	21.7 (12.5, 30.8)
2012	463	28	2073	7,666,940	6.0 (1.2, 10.9)	27.0 (16.8, 37.2)
2013	522	16	2567	7,809,269	6.7 (1.6, 11.8)	32.9 (21.6, 44.1)

Note: From Kauth, Michael, Jillian Shipherd, Jan Lindsay, John Blosnich, George Brown, and Kenneth Jones. "Access to Care for Transgender Veterans in the Veterans Administration Hospital." *Research and Practice* 104, S4 (2014): S25–54. CI = confidence interval; VHA = Veterans Health Administration.

Source: Kauth et al., "Access to Care for Transgender Veterans."

*Per 100,000 patients.

We further hypothesized that if gender-dysphoric people were able to access appropriate hormone treatment in systems that previously denied them care (that is, VHA patients before 2011), the need for medications for anxiety and depression would decrease. Doctors often treated the symptoms of gender dysphoria—anxiety, depression, and sleep disturbances—rather than the gender dysphoria itself (an ill-advised and usually ineffective approach). Our data on VHA patients before 2011 demonstrated that after gender-dysphoric patients gained access to gender-affirming hormone therapies, they had substantial reductions in the use of the antidepressants and notable reductions in the use of prescription sleeping pills.[30] The graphs below show the rapid

Figure 15.1 Changes in prescriptions before and after change in VHA Transgender Health Benefits. *Source*: Created by the author.

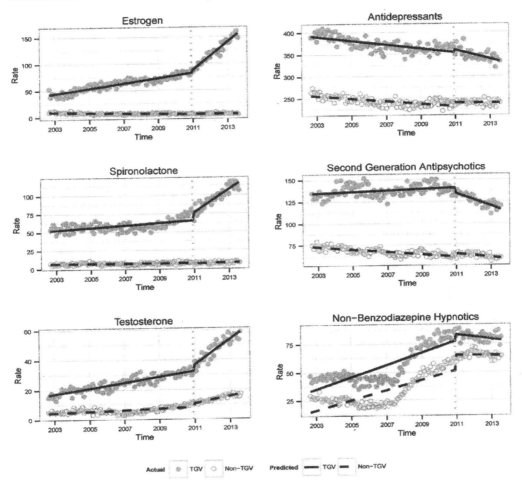

increases in prescriptions for transgender veterans for estrogen, spironolactone, and testosterone after the VHA directive of 2011, with an associated reduction across the same population in the use of antidepressants, antidepressant adjuncts (second-generation antipsychotics are used for this purpose), and nonbenzodiazepine hypnotics, like zolpidem.

Other highlights from the Mountain Home Transgender Project demonstrated that data obtained with our large cohort of transgender veterans supported uncontrolled survey data reports in the field, including for example, the higher suicidality and depression reported by respondents to national surveys like those conducted by the National Center for Transgender Equality.[31] Our big data studies in the VA confirmed the existence of widespread medical and mental health disparities for transgender individuals when compared to cisgender controls.[32] Our results established that transgender patients were three times more likely to be diagnosed with a mood disorder compared to cisgender controls, possibly due to untreated gender dysphoria. Transgender status for veterans also conferred higher rates of homelessness, incarceration, and military sexual trauma history, as well as financial instability and substantial racial health disparities.[33] Another large database study conducted after our studies reported similar results with a predominantly nonveteran American population.[34] The evolution of transgender research toward larger datasets and larger questions means that such work can then, in theory, serve as a needs assessment to spur policy changes in healthcare systems toward large-scale provisions for care.

OUT OF THE CLINIC AND INTO THE COURTROOM: TRANSLATIONAL RESEARCH AND THE RESEARCHER-ADVOCATE

Recently, the National Institutes of Health has promoted a new priority: translational research. The purpose of such research is to translate basic research findings into interventions with a rapid clinical utility to create better methods for the diagnosis, treatment, and prevention of disease. The goal is to bridge the gap—from the lab to the patient's bedside—by quickly transforming research findings into practical applications. Although a Medline search indicates that the term *translational research* appeared as early as 1993, there were only a few references to this concept in the medical literature during the 1990s, mostly regarding cancer research. The National Center for Advancing

Translational Sciences was established within National Institutes of Health in December 2011, the same year that the VA changed its policies in favor of providing transgender healthcare to veterans. For years, this new center focused its translational research on drugs, tests, and tissue chips; there were no initiatives related to the provision of transgender healthcare. Furthermore, while clinical research has the potential for rapid utility in clinical settings, translation cannot occur effectively if the individuals requiring medical attention cannot access treatment. The best research on gender-affirming hormone therapy—the aforementioned studies included—is useless to trans veterans or incarcerated transgender people if they face insurmountable barriers to care.

In the field of transgender health, the gap between research and care requires more than new clinical treatment protocols; institutional, structural, and legal barriers dictate the distance between the lab and the patient's bedside. We must affect institutional and structural change to accelerate access to care. Thus, translational research in this field (which I believe started well before the National Institutes of Health prioritized this concept) cannot be effective without concurrent policy and legal change—a process that not only obtains but also sustains civil rights for transgender people. To better capture the realities, I have redefined the term *translational research* to include bridging the gap from research to health *care*, *access*, and *rights*.

Given that the provision of transgender healthcare is intimately associated with healthcare access and rights, many clinicians, myself included, find that providing care in this field necessitates fighting for the rights of our patients in court. In 1988, while serving as a captain in the Air Force, I was called to testify as an expert witness in the first of more than seventy court cases involving discrimination and barriers to care for transgender people. In this case, I spoke on behalf of an active-duty officer with seventeen years of exemplary military service who had been outed by a neighbor. A neighbor took a picture of this off-duty officer dressed as a woman going to church on Sunday and then turned over the grainy print to the military police. I testified against the base commander, a brigadier general, who stated his intent to throw this officer out of "his" Air Force.

At that time, I had inadequate courtroom experience and no big data studies to support my arguments; I failed to pierce the ignorance and bias in that military courtroom. In military tribunals, the commanding officer not only can serve as the judge but he can also personally select the jury from a group of senior officers under his direct supervision. The general employed this process to remove my patient from active duty and strip her of all military benefits. As I grieved the outcome, I recognized the biggest barrier trans people face: the institutional and structural discrimination that prevents their access to care and basic rights. I decided that I must use my research not only to inform medical practice but also to change the laws and practices that denied equitable access to care.

As I continued my clinical and research work with transgender veterans, I also became involved in the plight of incarcerated transgender people who were denied access to safe living quarters and stripped of, or denied access to, transition-related healthcare. Although it is difficult to conduct research in prisons, over a twenty-five-year period, I interviewed a considerable number of incarcerated transgender women, including three on death row and several others who were serving life in prison without the possibility of parole. In a separate approach to this issue, by combining access to the VHA database with my interest in assisting imprisoned transgender people, I conducted the largest study of health disparities in the justice system involving people with gender dysphoria that included a prospective look at the effects of incarceration on health.[35] This, too, was a study with matched cisgender controls who had not been jailed or imprisoned and also included a control group of transgender veterans who had not been justice-involved. Trans veterans were more likely to be justice-involved than their cisgender controls (2.88% vs 1.38 %; $p <$ .0001). Compared to justice-involved cisgender veterans, the justice-involved transgender veterans were more likely to have a history of homelessness (67% vs 80%; $p < .05$) and to have reported sexual trauma while serving in the military (12% vs 23%; $p < .01$). Significant health disparities were also noted for the trans veterans compared to the controls for depression, hypertension, obesity, posttraumatic stress disorder, serious mental illness, and suicidal ideation/attempts. Transgender veterans were more likely to have brushes with the law, including incarceration, than their matched cisgender control veterans, and they also displayed ongoing health disparities after release from prison. Being in jail is generally a toxic experience for anyone, but transgender inmates suffer more from trauma than cisgender inmates, with higher rates of medical as well as mental illness.

I completed another study with transgender inmates from thirty-five states by correspondence analysis and revealed that of all the indignities and trauma faced by inmates in prisons, the lack of access to transgender healthcare was, by far, their number one concern, even higher than distress about prison rape.[36] Without access to gender-affirming care and with no hope of release, some inmates resorted to autocastration to eliminate their source of testosterone.[37]

Autocastration carries a significant risk for death by exsanguination and is rarely seen outside of the prison context.

Based on these experiences, my research, and the developing literature from other prison settings, I included recommendations in fifth, sixth, and seventh versions of the *World Professional Association for Transgender Health's Standards of Care*. The fifth version, published in 1998, was the first to include a section on the provision of transgender health care for incarcerated persons.[38]

Historically, grant organizations have ignored research questions in this field, creating additional barriers to evidence- and population-based care by withholding essential funding. Of note, other than partial salary support for two years of my thirty-five years of research, I completed my work and publications without research grants or monetary support. We need more high-quality research and more researchers to perform the heavy lifting this research requires. The common refrain of "no funding" should not be a barrier. Sometimes the resources must come from within.

We must mind these gaps, both the distance between research and provided care and the absence or neglect of research about marginalized populations like the TGD community. A gulf exists, too, between existing research (sometimes of doubtful quality or statistical power) and pointed, quality research that can drive systemic change to ensure basic rights to healthcare, equal access to employment, housing, and the right to serve one's country in uniform. The lack of high-quality evidence in support of gender-affirming care does not mean that those treatments are poor options; in many cases, the available gender-affirming treatment protocols offer the best available care, regardless of the accompanying research.

THE WEAPONIZATION OF RESEARCH

Individuals, religious organizations, insurance companies, state and federal law, and institutional policies routinely weaponize[39] existing research gaps to deny transgender people access to or the right to healthcare. In the United States, third-party payers employ capitation[40] to provide less care in medical systems by disallowing care that is not supported by rigorous research. The prison system provides another example: inmate medical care providers—state-owned and contracted—have denied access to gender-affirming hormonal therapy for incarcerated people, citing the lack of data regarding long-term safety of these off-label medications. Such prevarication is an excuse, as these treatments have been used successfully for more than sixty years, and the same arguments are not used for other treatments, for instance, vaccinations for SARS-Cov-2 or for any medication that has been marketed for less than fifty years.

A lack of data is not the same as having negative data. True, few researchers in trans health have rigorously documented the long-term effects and side effects of the commonly used treatments[41] thereby providing those with the intent to deny care an opportunity; those who seek to deny healthcare access have weaponized this gap. Their reward? Payers deliver less care and pocket the savings generated by care denials. It is a vicious circle established over decades of time: denial of care based on scant research data, as well as insufficient funding and institutional support for large studies on trans health, result in continued inertia, inadequate data, and ongoing denials of care.

The exploitation of research gaps for economic principle and profit represents one strategy of weaponization; the second willfully misinterprets and misapplies existing research, regardless of its caliber. One of the most weaponized papers in transgender health—and a highly respected one—is a 2011 Swedish study, "Long-Term Follow-up of Transsexual Persons Undergoing Sex Reassignment Surgery."[42] The authors found that after sex reassignment, transsexuals had higher risks of mortality, suicidal behavior, and psychiatric problems than the general population, thus concluding that although sex reassignment alleviated gender dysphoria, it did not necessarily suffice as the best treatment to address long-term psychiatric problems. The authors recommended improved psychiatric and medical care for this patient group.

Those seeking to deny access to care misinterpreted this Swedish report by claiming that the provision of treatment for gender dysphoria damages transgender people, and therefore it should not be provided. While the authors of the Swedish studies (my colleagues) vigorously object to this interpretation, I see this paper routinely touted by the opposing counsel and experts in court to justify denial of care to transgender people. Experts in trans healthcare are currently, as I write this today, testifying in US courts to this effect, seeking to withhold lifesaving and life-affirming treatments from trans adolescents and adults alike. Rather than condemn gender-affirming surgery, though, the Swedish paper legitimately asserts that mental health issues are common in those who seek such surgery and that surgery is not—and does not claim to be—a panacea for all mental and medical health disparities experienced by people who have endured a lifetime of gender dysphoria and its societal and familial implications. As the paper suggests, some patients who undergo gender-affirming surgeries may still benefit from postoperative mental healthcare delivered by a knowledgeable, supportive clinician.

I, too, can weaponize my research and the extant literature to attack the bogus argument that "do no harm" means "do nothing at all." Such misguided logic results from the faulty translation of clinical research—or of nonexistent studies. Advocates must employ responsible, accurate translation of research and call out those who misinterpret existing studies to deny medically necessary care for transgender people. For example, I fought in court for the rights of transgender inmates to access transition-related care,[43] citing my paper that documented how inmates attempted autocastration after prolonged treatment denials, as well as my big data paper that demonstrated the devastating effect of treatment denials on incarcerated transgender people.[44] This strategy was an effective use of research in multiple cases on behalf of inmates: laws changed and transgender inmates accessed care. We must continue to ethically weaponize research results to reverse the laws and institutional policies that block access to healthcare, employment, and societal benefits for transgender people.

Calculated misuse of research to perpetuate harm against transgender people continues today, with clinicians and politicians alike working to deny TGD people access to healthcare and other basic rights. The plight of trans athletes is one of the more recent attacks,[45] along with Texas' attempts to criminalize transgender care for trans teens as child abuse.[46] In such a hostile environment, it is not surprising that some transgender persons are hesitant to participate in research on trans phenomena, particularly studies on the etiology of gender diversity. However, in my experience over three decades, I have been impressed by the willingness of trans people to selflessly volunteer their time and talents in the interests of moving this field forward. Notably, I am grateful for their voluntary efforts to help me teach others, including large audiences of lay and medical people, in ways that I could never effectively do alone.

CONCLUSION

Benjamin established the field of transgender health by caring for people, amassing a collection of clinical observations, and writing them up as research. He had no mainstream or academic institutional grant support, computers, or electronic health records, and he faced significant resistance from the medical and nonmedical communities of the day. I have also lacked grant support and have faced the derision of colleagues, supervisors, and employers, but ultimately, I have been fortunate in my ability to add to the clinical research that informs medical care and to successfully challenge institutionalized barriers to care.

At this time, priorities for transgender outcomes research must include the determination of healthcare disparities and comorbid health conditions over the lifespan, along with the effects of mental health, medical, and surgical interventions on morbidity and mortality.[47] We must pursue rigorous, ethical research with the intent to broaden healthcare access and rights for all transgender people, be they veterans or people who are incarcerated, or any other group of TGD people. Benjamin himself recognized the sociocultural challenges inherent in his life's work but remained bolstered by the promise of clinical research: "Breaking a tabu always stirs quick emotions. . . . The forces of nature, however, know nothing of this tabu, and facts remain facts. . . . There is hardly a word in the English language comparable to the word 'sex' in its vagueness and in its emotional content."[48] Armed with these facts, we can create a national system for the provision of affirming and competent care for transgender Americans. And we can continue to honor Benjamin's work, as well as other affirming voices in the field—including TGD people themselves.

NOTES

1. Feldman et al., "Priorities for Transgender Medical and Health Care Research."
2. Benjamin, *The Transsexual Phenomenon*, 4.
3. Benjamin, *The Transsexual Phenomenon*; Tebbe and Budge, "Research with Trans Communities."
4. Green, "The Three Kings."
5. Feldman et al., "Priorities for Transgender Medical and Health Care Research."
6. Personal communication with psychiatrist and transactivist Leah Shaffer.
7. Benjamin and Masters, *Prostitution and Morality*.
8. Benjamin, "Nature and Management of Transsexualism."
9. Wheeler and Shaefer, "Historical Overview of Harry Benjamin's First 1500 Cases."
10. It is not well known by the public or by military service members that, unlike in civilian practice, there is no confidentiality for military patients seen by mental health care practitioners on military bases. Active-duty psychiatrists take an oath as officers as well as the Hippocratic Oath, which are in direct conflict with respect to protecting sensitive information that patients may share during therapy sessions. Transgender

identity and behavior, including any form of cross-dressing in off-duty time, were grounds for administrative separation (not medical separation) as unfit for duty, with forfeiture of any accrued benefits they would have received, such as a pension if they had served twenty years or more.

11. *Diagnostic and Statistical Manual of Mental Disorders, Third Edition.*
12. Brown, "Transsexuals in the Military."
13. Brown, "Transsexuals in the Military," 529.
14. Brown, "Transsexuals in the Military," 531.
15. McDuffie and Brown, "Seventy Veterans with Gender Identity Disturbances."
16. Brown et al., "Personality Characteristics."
17. In addition to being a politician, attorney, lobbyist, insurance salesman, and columnist, Thompson was an actor and radio personality. His television and cinema work includes roles in, among others, *The Hunt for Red October*, *Die Hard 2*, *Flight of the Intruder*, *Law & Order*, and *The Good Wife*.
18. Personal communication, as told to me, first author, by my Medical Center Director Carl Gerber, MD, PhD, 1995.
19. Kauth et al., "Access to Care for Transgender Veterans"; Department of Veterans Affairs, *Veterans Health Administration Directive 2011-024*; Department of Veterans Affairs, *Veterans Health Administration Directive 2013-003*.
20. Feldman et al., "Priorities for Transgender and Medical and Health Care Research."
21. Blosnich et al., "Prevalence of Gender Identity Disorder."
22. Blosnich et al., "Mortality Among Veterans."
23. Boyer et al., "Suicide, Homicide."
24. Brown and Jones, "Incidence of Breast Cancer."
25. Gooren, "A Ten-Year Safety Study"; Gooren, Giltay, and Bunck, "Long-Term Treatment of Transsexuals"; Gooren et al., "Breast Cancer Development"; Asscheman, Gooren, and Ecklund, "Mortality and Morbidity in Transsexual Patients"; Asscheman et al., "A Long Term Follow-up Study of Mortality"; Van Kesteren et al., Mortality and Morbidity in Transsexual Subjects."
26. Given the lack of experience and diagnostic acumen of most clinicians in this field, we found it to be the case that many of those diagnosed with transvestic fetishism were individuals with gender dysphoria, as confirmed by a thorough review of their records.
27. Brown and Jones, "Mental Health and Medical Health Disparities"; Brown and Jones, "Racial Health Disparities"; Blosnich et al., "Mental Health of Transgender Veterans"; Elders et al., "Medical Aspects of Transgender Military Service"; Blosnich et al., "Impact of Social Determinants"; Bukowski et al., "Exploring Rural Disparities"; Brown and McDuffie, "Health Care Policies"; Kauth et al., "Access to Care for Transgender Veterans."

28. Brown and Jones, "Racial Health Disparities."
29. Kauth et al., "Access to Care for Transgender Veterans."
30. Brown and Jones, unpublished data 2015.
31. James et al., *The Report of the 2015 U.S. Transgender Survey.*
32. Brown and Jones, "Mental Health and Medical Health Disparities."
33. Brown and Jones, "Incidence of Breast Cancer"; Brown and Jones, "Mental Health and Medical Health Disparities"; Brown and Jones, "Racial Health Disparities."
34. Quinn et al., "Cohort Profile."
35. Brown and Jones, "Health Correlates of Criminal Justice Involvement."
36. Brown, "Qualitative Analysis of Transgender Inmates."
37. Brown, "Autocastration and Autopenectomy."
38. Brown, "Qualitative Analysis of Transgender Innmates"; Brown and Jones, "Health Correlates of Criminal Justice Involvement"; Brown, "Recommended Revisions."
39. According to Oxford University Press, the verb *weaponize* means "adapt for use as a weapon."
40. Regardless of how much medical care someone needs, *capitation* refers to a fixed, annual price per patient, that is, payment covered by the third-party payer on behalf of the insured.
41. Bear in mind, as I have previously identified in this paper, that such research has also been discouraged and underfunded for decades.
42. Dhejne et al., "Long-Term Follow-Up of Transsexual Persons"; Kosilek v. Maloney, 221 F. Supp. 2d 156 (D. Mass. 2002).
43. Kosilek v. Maloney, 221 F. Supp. 2d 156 (D. Mass. 2002); Keohane v. Jones, 4:16-cv-511 (D. Fla. 2016); De'Lonta v. Angelone, 330 F.3d 630 (4th Cir. 2003); Gammett v. Idaho State Board of Corrections, No. CV05-257, 2007 U.S. Dist. 66456 (D. Idaho).
44. Brown and McDuffie, "Health Care Policies"; Brown, "Qualitative Analysis of Transgender Inmates"; Brown, "Autocastration and Autopenectomy."
45. Newberry, "Trans Athletes Are a Non-Issue"; Newberry, "Column: FINA ban Casts Storm Clouds on Transgender Athletes."
46. Abbott, Letter to the Honorable Jaime Masters.
47. Feldman et al., "Priorities for Transgender Medical and Health Care Research."
48. Benjamin, *The Transsexual Phenomenon*, 5–6.

WORKS CITED

Abbott, Greg. Letter to the Honorable Jaime Masters, Commissioner, Texas Department of Family and Protective Services. February 22, 2022. Accessed April 23, 2022. https://gov.texas.gov/uploads/files/press/O-MastersJaime202202221358.pdf.

Asscheman, Henk, Erik J. Giltay, Jos A. J. Megens, Michael A. A. van Trotsenburg, and Louis J. Gooren. "A Long Term Follow-up Study of Mortality in Transsexuals Receiving Treatment with Cross-Sex Hormones." *European Journal of Endocrinology* 164, no. 4 (2011): 635–42.

Asscheman, Henk, Louis J. Gooren, and P. L. Ecklund. "Mortality and Morbidity in Transsexual Patients with Cross-Gender Hormone Treatment." *Metabolism* 38, no. 9 (1989): 869–73.

Benjamin, Harry. "Nature and Management of Transsexualism, with a Report on 31 Operated Cases." *Western Journal of Surgery, Obstetrics and Gynecology* 72 (1964): 105–11.

———. *The Transsexual Phenomenon.* New York: Julian Press, 1966.

Benjamin, Harry, and Robert E. L. Masters. *Prostitution and Morality: A Definitive Report on the Prostitute in Contemporary Society and an Analysis on the Causes and Effects of the Suppression of Prostitution.* New York: Julian Press, 1964.

Blosnich, John, George Brown, Jillian Shipherd, Michael Kauth, Rebecca I. Piegaro, and Robert M. Bossart. "Prevalence of Gender Identity Disorder and Suicide Risk among Transgender Veterans Utilizing Veterans Health Administration Care." *American Journal of Public Health* 103, no. 10 (2013): e27–32.

Blosnich, John, George Brown, Sybil Wojcio, Kenneth Jones, and Robert M. Bosarte. "Mortality among Veterans with Transgender-Related Diagnoses in the Veterans Health Administration, FY 2000–2009." *LGBT Health* 1, no. 4 (2014): 269–76.

Blosnich, John, Mary Marsiglio, Melissa Dichter, et al. "Impact of Social Determinants of Health on Medical Conditions Among Transgender Veterans." *American Journal of Preventive Medicine* 52, no. 4 (2017): 491–98. Accessed 12 12, 2020. https://www.researchgate.net/profile/George_Brown10/publication/313269590_Impact_of_Social_Determinants_of_Health_on_Medical_Conditions_Among_Transgender_Veterans/links/5ce3eaa7299bf14d95abf55e/Impact-of-Social-Determinants-of-Health-on-Medical-Conditions.

Blosnich, John, Mary Marsiglio, Sasha Gao, et al. "Mental Health of Transgender Veterans in US States with and without Discrimination and Hate Crime Legislation." *American Journal of Public Health* 106, no. 3 (2016): 354–540.

Boyer, Taylor, Ada Youk, Ann Haas, et al. "Suicide, Homicide, and All-Cause Mortality among Transgender and Cisgender Patients in the Veteran's Health Administtration." *LGBT Health* 8, no. 3 (2021): 173–80.

Brown, George. "Qualitative Analysis of Transgender Inmates' Correspondence: Implications for Departments of Correction." *Journal of Correctional Health Care* 20, no. 4 (2014): 334–42.

———. "Recommended Revisions to the World Professional Association for Transgender Health's *Standards of Care* Section on Medical Care for Incarerateed Persons with Gender Identity Disorder." *International Journal of Transgenderism* 11, no. 2 (2009): 133–39.

———. "Transsexuals in the Military: Flight into Hypermasculinity." *Archives of Sexual Behavior* 17, no. 6 (1988): 527–37.

———. "Autocastration and Autopenectomy as Surgical Self-Treatment in Incarcerated Persons with Gender Identity Disorder." *International Journal of Transgenderism* 12, no. 1 (2010): 31–39.

Brown, George, and Kenneth Jones. "Health Correlates of Criminal Justice Involvement in 4,793 Transgender Veterans." *LGBT Health* 2, no. 4 (2015): 297–305.

———. "Incidence of Breast Cancer in a Cohort of 5,135 Transgender Veterans." *Breast Cancer Research and Treatment* 149, no. 1 (2015): 191–98.

———. "Mental Health and Medical Health Disparities in 5135 Transgender Veterans Receiving Healthcare in the Veterans Health Administration: A Case-Control Study." *LGBT Health* 3, no. 2 (2016): 122–31.

———. "Racial Health Disparities in a Cohort of 5,135 Transgender Veterans." *Journal of Racial and Ethnic Health Disparities* 1 (2014): 257–66.

Brown, George, and Everett McDuffie. "Health Care Policies Addressing Transgender Inmates in Prison Systems in the United States." *Journal of Correctional Healthcare* 15, no. 4 (2009): 280–91. Accessed December 12, 2020. https://www.researchgate.net/profile/George_Brown10/publication/26698949_Health_Care_Policies_Addressing_Transgender_Inmates_in_Prison_Systems_in_the_United_States/links/53e90a360cf28f342f3e60b4.pdf.

Brown, George, Thomas Wise, Paul Costa, Jeffrey Herbst, Peter Fagan, and Chester Schmidt. "Personality Characteristics and Sexual Functioning of 188 Cross-dressing Men." *Journal of Nervous and Mental Disease* 184, no. 5 (1996): 265–73.

Bukowski, Leigh, John Blosnich, Jillian Shipherd, Michael Kauth, George Brown, and Adam Gordon. "Exploring Rural Disparitites in Medical Diagnosis among Veterans with Transgender-Related Diagnoses Utilizing Veterans Health Administration Care." *Medical Care* 55, no. 9 (2017): 97–103.

Department of Veterans Affairs. *Veterans Health Administration Directive 2011-024: Providing Health Care for Transgender and Intersex Veterans.* June 9, 2011. Accessed August 7, 2022. VA National Policy on Trans Care 2011.pdf.

Department of Veterans Affairs. *Veterans Health Administration Directive 2013-003: Providing Health Care for Transgender and Intersex Veterans.* February 8, 2013. Accessed August 7, 2022. VA National Policy on Trans Care 2013.pdf.

Dhejne, Cecilia, Paul Lichtenstein, Marcus Boman, Anna L. V. Johansson, Niklas Långström, and Mikael Landén. "Long-Term Follow-Up of Transsexual Persons Undergoing Sex Reassignment Surgery." *PLoS One* 6, no. 2 (2011): 1–8.

Diagnostic and Statistical Manual of Mental Disorders, Third Edition. Washington, DC: American Psychiatric Association, 1980.

Elders, M. Joycelyn, George Brown, Eli Coleman, Thomas Kolditz, and Alan Steinman. "Medical Aspects of Transgender Military Service." *Armed Forces and Society* 41, no. 2 (2014): 1–22. Accessed December 11, 2020. https://www.researchgate.net/profile/

George_Brown10/publication/266423271_Medical_Aspects_of_Transgender_Military_Service/links/54328ee70cf22395f29c2794/Medical-Aspects-of-Transgender-Military-Service.pdf.

Feldman, Jamie, George Brown, Madeline B. Deutsch, et al. "Priorities for Transgender Medical and Health Research." *Current Opinion in Endocrinology, Diabetes, and Obesity* 23, no. 2 (2016): 180–87.

Gooren, Louis J. "A Ten-Year Safety Study of the Oral Androgen Testosterone Undecanoate." *Adrology* 15, no. 3 (1994): 212–15.

Gooren, Louis J., Erik J. Giltay, and Mathijs C. Bunck. "Long-Term Treatment of Transsexuals with Cross-Sex Hormones: Extensive Personal Experience." *Journal of Clinical Endocrinology and Metabolism* 93, no. 1 (2008): 19–25.

Gooren, Louis J., Michael A. A. van Trotsenburg, Erik J. Giltay, and Paul J. van Diest. "Breast Cancer Development in Transsexual Subjects Receiving Cross-Sex Hormone Treatment." *Journal of Sexual Medicine* 10, no. 12 (2013): 3129–34.

Green, Richard. "The Three Kings: Harry Benjamin, John Money, Robert Stoller." *Archives of Sexual Behavior* 38, no. 4 (2009): 610–13.

Ihlenfeld, Charles. "A Memorial for Harry Benjamin." *Archives of Sexual Behavior* 17, no. 1 (1988): 1–33.

James, Sandy E., Jody L. Herman, Susan Rankin, Mara Kiesling, Lisa Mottett, and Ma'ayan Anafi. *The Report of the 2015 U.S. Transgender Survey.* Washington, DC: National Center for Transgender Equality, 2016.

Kauth, M. R., and J. C. Shipherd. "Transforming a System: Improving Patient-Centered Care for Sexual and Gender Minority Veterans." *LGBT Health* 3, no. 3 (2016): 177–79. https://doi.org/10.1089/lgbt.2016.0047.

Kauth, Michael, Jillian Shipherd, Jan Lindsay, John Blosnich, George Brown, and Kenneth Jones. "Access to Care for Transgender Veterans in the Veterans Administration Hospital." *Research and Practice* 104, S4 (2014): S253–54.

Kruijver, Frank P. M., Jiang-Ning Zhou, Chris W. Pool, Michel A. Hofman, Louis J. Gooren, and Dick F. Swaab. "Male-to-Female Transsexuals Have Female Neuron Numbers in a Limbic Nucleus." *Journal of Clinical Endocrinology & Metabolism* 85, no. 5 (2000): 2034–41.

McDuffie, Everett, and George Brown. "Seventy Veterans with Gender Identiy Disturbances: A Descriptive Study." *International Journal of Transgenderism* 12, no. 1 (2010): 21–30.

Meyer, Jon, and Donna Reter. "Sex Rassignment: Follow-up." *Archives of General Psychiatry* 36, no. 9 (1979): 1010–15. https://www.adirondackdailyenterprise.com/opinion/columns/2021/03/trans-athletes-are-a-non-issue-but-discrimination-is-real/.

Newberry, Paul. "Column: FINA Ban Casts Storm Clouds on Transgender Athletes." AP News, June 20, 2022. Accessed August 3, 2022. https://apnews.com/article/winter-olympics-sports-discrimination-swimming-mens-868eec56e9799ba3e70431d65c6b6dd1.

———. "Trans Athletes Are a Non-Issue, But Discrimination Is Real." *Adirondack Daily Enterprise*, March 27, 2021. Accessed August 3, 2022.

Oxford University Press. *Oxford Languages.* Accessed March 5, 2021. https://languages.oup.com/google-dictionary-en/.

Quinn, Virginia P., Rebecca Nash, Enid Hunkeler, et al. "Cohort Profile: Study of Transition, Outcomes and Gender (STRONG) to Assess Health Status of Transgender People." *BMJ Open* 7, no. 12 (2017): e01812. https://doi.org/10.1136/bmjopen-2017-018121.

Tebbe, Elliot A., and Stephanie L. Budge. "Research with Trans Communities: Applying a Process-Oriented Approach to Methodological Considerations and Research Recommendations." *Counseling Psychologist* 44, no. 7 (2016): 996–1024. https://doi.org/10.1177/0011000015609045.

Van Kesteren, Paul J., Henk Asscheman, Jos A. Megens, and Louis J. Gooren. "Mortality and Morbidity in Transsexual Subjects Treated with Cross-Sex Hormones." *Clinical Endocrinology* 47, no. 3 (1997): 337–42.

Wheeler, Connie C., and Leah Shaefer. "Historical Overview of Harry Benjamin's First 1500 Cases." Presented at the Proceedings of the Harry Benjamin International Gender Dysphoria Association, Tenth International Symposium on Gender Dysphoria. Amsterdam, Netherlands, 1987.

15.1. BY US AND FOR US: BRINGING ETHICS INTO TRANSGENDER HEALTH RESEARCH

Noah Adams, Ruth Pearce, Jaimie F. Veale, Asa Radix, Amrita Sarkar, and Dani Castro

In 2017, we published "Guidance and Ethical Considerations for Undertaking Transgender Health Research and Institutional Review Boards Adjudicating this Research." We did so to address ethical lapses that we observed in the field of transgender health.[1] Subsequently, research teams around the world began to cite and adhere to our suggested guidelines for ethical research practices.

When we first identified the need for this publication, no similar English-language ethical guidelines existed for transgender health research, and as a result, researchers often engaged in unscrupulous practices—for example, the requirement that transgender people participate in research to receive healthcare was, and unfortunately still is, far too common. Such unethical practices include instances where the only option for transitional healthcare is at clinics where clients feel unable to decline to participate in studies conducted as part of the program's research mandate.[2] Another core concern was the existence of clinical research that obtained ethical approval despite being entirely disconnected from transgender people's interests and needs. Recently, researchers suspended a study that sought to intentionally "trigger 'gender dysphoria' by taking photographs of [transgender] participants in . . . unitards."[3] This study had received institutional review board approval but was halted only after community members voiced significant public concern.

Our project to establish ethical research guidelines began in the wake of several incidents that took place at the World Professional Association for Transgender Health's Biennial Symposium in 2016. Several institutional review board–approved research presentations demonstrated unethical practices. In one case, an academic poster included pictures of transgender individuals without their permission.[4] Another poster displayed scientifically questionable information about surgery on intersex infants; gratuitous pictures of these infants accompanied the text, with no regard to the potential future effect of these photos on the child's well-being.

Noah Adams led the effort to prepare and circulate an early draft of our ethical transgender research guidelines for comment. Our authors solicited and processed professional and community input to create recommendations that break down professional/community boundaries—both within and beyond transgender communities. We formalized our guidelines through international collaboration between members of the newly formed Transgender Professional Association for Transgender Health.[5] We are particularly grateful to coauthors Dani Castro and Amrita Sarkar for their guidance in using cultural humility to work across differences. This process, while difficult, was key to the creation of our guidelines.

Our guidelines sought to provide clear tools and advice for clinical researchers and their institutional review boards and ethics committees and to encourage research teams to think critically about research design and trans-specific ethical issues. Ultimately, we proposed the following guidelines for conducting ethical transgender research.

1. Whenever possible, research should be grounded, from inception to dissemination, in a meaningful collaboration with community stakeholders.

2. Language and framing of transgender health research should be nonstigmatizing.

3. Research findings should be disseminated within the trans community.
4. The diversity of the transgender and gender-diverse community should be accurately and sensitively reflected.
5. Informed consent must be meaningful, without coercion or undue influence.
6. The protection of participant confidentiality should be paramount.
7. Alternate consent procedures should be considered for transgender and gender-diverse minors.
8. Research should align with current professional standards that refute conversion, reorientation, or reparative therapy.
9. Institutional review boards should guard against temptation to avoid, limit, or delay research on this subject.

Our guidelines also offer an opportunity to challenge institutional review boards,[6] which tend to suggest that transgender-identified researchers are unable to conduct transgender health research objectively.[7] Transgender academics have often been marginalized within or entirely excluded from this field and viewed as a dependent group in need of protection and firm guidance.[8] In fact, while developing these guidelines, we observed that transgender health research has historically been "captured" by a particular segment of cisgender, gay, white, and/or male academic researchers.[9] Much transgender health research follows from these long-standing precepts. In response, our recommendations clarify that transgender-identified researchers can conduct ethical, objective studies and may even bring a particular expertise to the process.[10]

In addition to establishing trans perspectives in the foreground of transgender research, our guidelines have become a touchstone for those who wish to ensure such research is conducted ethically. After our 2017 publication, others issued additional recommendations, including Ben Vincent's "Studying Trans: Recommendations for Ethical Recruitment and Collaboration with Transgender Participants in Academic Research";[11] *The Canadian Professional Association for Transgender Health's Ethical Guidelines* (under development concurrently with ours);[12] and *The European Professional Association for Transgender Health's Research Policy*.[13] Bioethicist Florence Paré has also written extensively on multiple aspects of ethics in transgender healthcare,[14] and in 2018, a member of our team, Ruth Pearce, delivered a podcast on the subject.[15]

Our work has advanced discussions on transgender research, helping move transgender healthcare from the margins toward the mainstream by focusing on how research ethics impact transgender health research and researchers. In a time when transgender health research is increasing in both quantity and the degree to which it is mainstream, these guidelines address concerns that transgender people are now becoming over-researched, often unethically. In fact, our guidelines attest to the fact that transgender health research has reached a critical mass. Special attention to the historical and current ethics of this profession is increasingly important, given that we have moved so quickly from an under-researched to an over-researched population. Perhaps now, more than ever, it is important to maintain an awareness of ethical lapses in transgender health research.

NOTES

1. Adams et al., "Guidance and Ethical Considerations."
2. Denny, "The Politics of Diagnosis."
3. Stempniak, "UCLA."
4. The first author viewed these poster presentations in question at the 2016 World Professional Association for Transgender Health in Amsterdam, Netherlands.
5. Adams et al., "Guidance and Ethical Considerations." The Transgender Professional Association for Transgender Health is an international organization for transgender-identified and/or intersex individuals engaged or working in transgender healthcare, whether in a paid or voluntary capacity.
6. Also known as research ethics boards or ethical review boards, these groups are tasked with reviewing and approving institutional research to ensure that it is ethical.
7. United Nations Development Programme, *Implementing Comprehensive HIV and STI Programmes*. The TRANSIT Tool on *Implementing Comprehensive HIV and STI Programmes with Transgender People: Practical Guidance for Collaborative Interventions* is another example of an international guideline created primarily by transgender people. For further discussion on this topic, see Reicherzer, Shavel, and Patton, "Examining Research"; Pearce, "(Im)possible Patients."
8. Jamison Green spoke movingly about the moment in which transgender people gained access to a 1997 World Professional Association for Transgender Health Conference in a recent *Wired* article, Stahl, "Prisoners, Doctors, and the Battle Over Trans Medical Care." By doing so, they changed the course of the organization and transgender healthcare.
9. See Ansara and Hegarty, "Cisgenderism in Psychology," for a discussion of the impact of "networks or 'invisible colleges'" that create an outsized impact in their field through in-group promotion and citation in transgender health.

10. Adams et al., "Guidance and Ethical Considerations," 167–68.
11. Vincent, "Studying Trans."
12. Canadian Professional Association for Transgender Health, *CPATH Ethical Guidelines*.
13. European Professional Association for Transgender Health, *Research Policy*.
14. Ashley, *Florence Ashley*.
15. Pearce, "Clinical Research."

WORKS CITED

Adams, Noah, Ruth Pearce, Jaimie Veale, et al. "Guidance and Ethical Considerations for Undertaking Transgender Health Research and Institutional Review Boards Adjudicating this Research." *Transgender Health*, 2, no. 1 (2017): 165–75. https://doi.org/10.1089/trgh.2017.0012.

Ansara, Y. Gavriel, and Peter Hegarty. "Cisgenderism in Psychology: Pathologizing and Misgendering Children from 1999 to 2008." *Psychology & Sexuality* 3, no. 3 (2012): 137–60. https://doi.org/10.1080/19419899.2011.576696.

Ashley, Florence. *Florence Ashley*. 2021. Accessed April 12, 2021. https://www.florenceashley.com/.

Canadian Professional Association for Transgender Health. *CPATH Ethical Guidelines for Research Involving Transgender People & Communities*. 2019. Accessed July 9, 2021. https://cpath.ca/wp-content/uploads/2019/08/CPATH-Ethical-Guidelines-EN.pdf.

Denny, Dallas. "The Politics of Diagnosis and a Diagnosis of Politics." *Transgender Tapestry* 98 (2002): 17–27. Accessed July 9, 2021. http://dallasdenny.com/Writing/2013/10/05/the-politics-of-diagnosis-and-a-diagnosis-of-politics-1991/.

European Professional Association for Transgender Health. *European Professional Association for Transgender Health Research Policy*. 2020. Accessed July 9, 2021. http://epath.eu/wp-content/uploads/2020/02/EPATH-Research-Policy.pdf.

Pearce, Ruth. "Clinical Research with Trans Patients: A Critique." *Dr Ruth Pearce* (blog), December 18, 2018. Accessed July 9, 2021. https://ruthpearce.net/2018/12/18/clinical-research-with-trans-patients-a-critique/.

Pearce, Ruth. "(Im)possible Patients? Negotiating Discourses of Trans Health in the UK." PhD diss., University of Warwick, 2016. University of Warwick Publications Service & WRAP. Accessed March 6, 2021. http://wrap.warwick.ac.uk/88285/.

Reicherzer, Stacee, Sherece Shavel, and Jason Patton. "Examining Research Issues of Power and Privilege Within a Gender-Marginalized Community." *Journal of Social, Behavioral, and Health Sciences* 7, no. 1 (2013): 79–97.

Stahl, Aviva. "Prisoners, Doctors, and the Battle over Trans Medical Care." *Wired*, 2021. Accessed July 9, 2021. https://www.wired.com/story/inmates-doctors-battle-over-transgender-medical-care/.

Stempniak, Marty. "UCLA Suspends Brain Imaging Study Amid 'Grave Concerns' from LGBTQ Advocates." Radiology Business, 2021. Accessed July 9, 2021. https://www.radiologybusiness.com/topics/leadership-workforce/ucla-suspends-brain-imaging-study-lgbtq-advocates.

United Nations Development Programme, IRGT: A Global Network of Transgender Women and HIV, United Nations Population Fund, UCSF Center of Excellence for Transgender Health, Johns Hopkins Bloomberg School of Public Health, World Health Organization, Joint United Nations Programme on HIV/AIDS, United States Agency for International Development. *Implementing Comprehensive HIV and STI Programmes with Transgender People: Practical Guidance for Collaborative Interventions*. New York: United Nations Development Programme, 2016. Accessed August 14, 2024. https://www.unfpa.org/sites/default/files/pub-pdf/TRANSIT_report_UNFPA.pdf.

Vincent, Benjamin W. "Studying Trans: Recommendations for Ethical Recruitment and Collaboration with Transgender Participants in Academic Research." *Psychology & Sexuality* 9, no. 2 (2018): 102–16.

15.2. TRANSGENDER VETERANS AND THE VETERANS HEALTH ADMINISTRATION

Jillian Shipherd

Despite a series of Department of Defense (DOD) regulations prohibiting open service, transgender and gender-diverse (TGD) people have always served in the US military. Even before prohibitions were lifted, an estimated 150,000 transgender military veterans lived in the United States.[1] Between June 2016 and April 2019, a policy change under the Obama administration allowed transgender military personnel to openly serve and receive transition-related care,[2] but on July 26, 2017, then-President Donald Trump canceled this policy via tweet: "After consultation with my Generals and military experts, please be advised that the United States Government will not accept or allow transgender individuals to serve in any capacity in the US Military. Our military must be focused on decisive and overwhelming victory and cannot be burdened with the tremendous medical costs and disruption that transgender in the military would entail."[3] After enacting this military ban, enlistees could only serve in the military in the sex assigned at their birth. In early 2021, the Biden administration reversed the ban, once again allowing TGD people to openly join the military.[4] Currently, TGD individuals may enlist and serve in their experienced gender as long as they have undergone at least eighteen months of hormone therapy.[5]

The Veterans Health Administration (VHA) is a federal agency separate from the DOD and has its own policies. Given that VHA patients and many of the staff have served in the military, it is no surprise that the DOD culture regarding the exclusion of TGD people has influenced the VHA. While TGD veterans have always received general medical care through the VHA, it took institutional leaders and physicians like George Brown to establish the right to access trans-specific services at VHA facilities.

Good policy serves as the foundation for cultural change. In 2011, the VHA issued Directive 1341(2), which guaranteed access to healthcare based on one's self-identified gender identity, including inpatient room assignments, access to restrooms, and the use of preferred pronouns and name during medical visits and in medical records.[6] Directive 1341(2) established the expectation that VHA facilities and staff will create inclusive environments for TGD patients. TGD veterans may receive general healthcare, transition-related hormone therapy and counseling, prosthetics to support transition goals, vocal coaching, and fertility counseling.

The VHA also provides presurgical evaluations and postoperative care following gender-affirming surgery, including revisions for surgical complications but, at present, does not offer these initial surgical procedures. In June 2021, the Secretary of Veterans Affairs announced the start of a rule change process to remove these gender-affirming surgical exclusions from the VHA medical benefits package. This process, which includes a period for public commentary, will take time, but if it is successful, TGD veterans may soon be able to access comprehensive transition-related healthcare.

Changing the culture of healthcare at the VHA requires education and advocacy in addition to policy mandates. To address systemic discrimination, the VHA now provides LGBTQ+ Veteran Care Coordinators on-site in their hospitals to educate staff and address any issues TGD veterans may encounter. The VHA offered a live virtual course in transgender healthcare that almost nine hundred VHA clinicians attended.[7] VHA promotes online educational programs on culturally competent care, including twelve brief trainings about topics relevant to TGD care (now publicly available).[8] Clinicians also have the ability to consult (with patient consent) with an expert interdisciplinary team through the electronic medical record on questions regarding a TGD veteran's treatment plan.[9] In 2020, the VHA launched a telehealth program to improve access to speech and language pathologists with specialized training in vocal coaching for transition purposes. All of these strategies for care were built on a foundation of improving access to clinicians trained in LGBTQ+ health, such as those trained through the LGBTQ+ Health Fellowships. These fellowships are now available at ten VHA hospitals and are training a new generation of mental health providers.[10]

Since an Obama-era mandate in 2011, when the VHA reversed long-standing policy on banning most interventions for gender dysphoria, the VHA has evolved to better serve the unique healthcare needs of TGD veterans—and the agency continues to be leader in TGD healthcare. Notably, in the last decade, VHA has become one of the largest providers of clinical care to TGD patients in the United States.

NOTES

1. Gates and Herman, "Transgender Military Service," 1.
2. Department of Defense, *Transgender Service in the U.S. Military*.
3. Trump (@realDonaldTrump), "After consultation."
4. Department of Defense, "DOD Announces Policy Updates."
5. Department of Defense, "Medical Standards."
6. Department of Veteran Affairs, *Providing Health Care*.
7. Shipherd et al., "Interdisciplinary Transgender Veteran Care," 54–62.
8. Department of Veteran Affairs, "VHA Train."
9. Shipherd, Kauth, and Matza, "Nationwide Interdisciplinary E-Consultation," 1008–12; Kauth et al., "Teleconsultation," 1012–18.
10. Department of Veteran Affairs, "LGBTQ+ Veteran Training."

WORKS CITED

Department of Defense. "DOD Announces Policy Updates for Transgender Military Service." March 31, 2021. https://www.defense.gov/Newsroom/Releases/Release/Article/2557220/dod-announces-policy-updates-for-transgender-military-service/. Accessed August 20, 2024.

Department of Defense. "Medical Standards for Military Service: Appointment, Enlistment, or Induction." April 30, 2021. Accessed August 20, 2024. https://commons.wikimedia.org/wiki/File:DoD_Instruction_6130.03,_Volume_1_-_Medical_Standards_for_Military_Service_(April_2021).pdf.

Department of Defense. *Transgender Service in the U.S. Military*. September 30, 2016. Accessed August 20, 2024. https://dod.defense.gov/Portals/1/features/2016/0616_policy/DoDTGHandbook_093016.pdf.

Department of Veterans Affairs. "LGBTQ+ Veteran Training." Patient Care Services. Accessed September 24, 2021. Accessed August 20, 2024. https://www.patientcare.va.gov/LGBT/LGBT_Veteran_Training.asp.

———. *Providing Health Care for Transgender and Intersex Veterans*. VHA Directive 1341(2). June 26, 2020. Accessed August 20, 2024. https://www.va.gov/vha-publications/ViewPublication.asp?pub_ID=6431.

———. "Welcome to VHA Train." VHA Train. Accessed September 24, 2021. Accessed August 20, 2024. https://www.train.org/vha/welcome.

Gates, Gary J., and Jody L. Herman. "Transgender Military Service in the United States." Accessed August 20, 2024. https://williamsinstitute.law.ucla.edu/wp-content/uploads/Trans-Military-Service-US-May-2014.pdf.

Kauth, Michael R., Jillian C. Shipherd, Jan A. Lindsay, Susan Kirsh, Knapp Herschel, and Lexi Matza. "Teleconsultation and Training of VHA Providers on Transgender Care: Implementation of a Multisite Hub System." *Telemedicine and e-Health* 21, no. 12 (2015): 1012–18.

Shipherd, Jillian C., Michael R. Kauth, Anthony F. Firek, et al. "Interdisciplinary Transgender Veteran Care: Development of a Core Curriculum for VHA Providers." *Transgender Health* 1, no. 1 (2016): 54–62.

Shipherd, Jillian C., Michael R. Kauth, and Alexis Matza. "Nationwide Interdisciplinary E-Consultation on Transgender Care in the Veterans Health Administration." *Telemedicine and e-Health* 22, no. 12 (2016): 1008–12.

Trump, Donald (@realDonaldTrump). "After consultation with my generals and military experts." Twitter, July 26, 2017.

Section IV

ESTABLISHING THE INTERDISCIPLINARY FIELD OF TRANSGENDER HEALTH WITHIN THE MEDICAL MAINSTREAM

Over the last forty years, transgender healthcare evolved into an established, if not always respected, interdisciplinary field within the mainstream medical field. In chapter 16, clinicians Asa Radix, Zil Goldstein, and Alexander Harris chronicle the evolution of hormonal care in the United States.

In chapter 17, Carolyn Wolf-Gould details the development of the surgical procedures that change the body to match the mind. This chapter opens with a short piece by Jamison Green, who asks, "So, why change your body?" Following this chapter, physician Amy Block profiles the story of Elmer Belt, an early US surgeon who quietly performed some of the earliest recorded gender-affirming surgeries in the United States.

In chapter 8, Dallas Denny, Jamison Green, and Hansel Arroyo trace the history of developments in psychiatric and psychological theory that eventually led to affirmative mental healthcare models. In chapter 18, psychologist Diane Ehrensaft examines the development of the gender-affirmative model for TGD youth from its inception in the Netherlands to current day practices across the United States. In two commentaries following this chapter, clinicians David Diamond, Tresne Hernandez, and Blumoff Greenberg describe the development of their clinics, which specialize in medical care for transgender and gender-diverse (TGD) youth.

In chapter 19, speech and language pathologists Jack Pickering and Terren Lansdaal discuss the development of voice modification services for TGD people, and in chapter 20, Denny and electrologist Yuki Arai reveal historical practices for hair removal and replacement.

Section IV profiles several TGD people who helped advance medical, surgical, and community-based care. Jeanne Hoff, who took over Harry Benjamin's New York practice on his retirement in 1979, served as the first known transgender person to run a trans-centric medical practice in the English-speaking world. In California, JoAnne Keatley found her way, after years of street life, to assisting in the development of organizations that addressed substance use, HIV prevention, human rights, and primary care for TGD people. In 2021, physician Rachel Levine, the first openly transgender person to hold an office that requires confirmation by the US Senate, became the seventeenth Assistant Secretary for Health, inspiring many health professionals and policy makers to improve healthcare access for TGD people. Alan Hart's profile describes the first transgender person in the United States to receive supportive care from a physician who eventually provided the first gender-affirming hysterectomy. Pioneering surgeons Christine McGinn and Marci Bowers are also described within section IV, as is trans speech and language pathologist Terren Lansdaal who muses on his conflicted feelings on his work around voice modification therapy.

16

THE EVOLUTION OF HORMONAL CARE IN THE UNITED STATES

Asa Radix, Zil Goldstein, and Alexander B. Harris

More than 1.3 million transgender and gender-diverse (TGD) adults live in the United States today.[1] During the last few decades, transgender populations have become increasingly visible within US culture, and researchers have drawn attention to the numerous healthcare disparities TGD people face, including barriers to gender-affirming medical services. In 2015, a large cross-sectional survey in the United States demonstrated that although approximately fifty percent of the TGD people queried used gender-affirming hormone therapy, others were unable to access treatment due to financial or insurance barriers, lack of access to knowledgeable medical providers, or discrimination in healthcare settings.[2] This chapter reviews the history of the provision of hormonal care for TGD individuals in the United States from the 1950s to the present, with a focus on the evolution of standards of care (SOC), which resulted in improved access to this critical medical intervention.

Before the availability of commercially produced estrogens and testosterone in the 1930s,[3] transgender individuals who wanted to change their appearance had few opportunities. Laws in more than thirty states outlawed cross-dressing; some jurisdictions enforced these regulations as late as the 1970s.[4] Gender-affirming surgeries were not commonly performed in the United States until the 1960s, when Johns Hopkins University opened the first gender clinic to offer a range of surgical services.[5] The provision of hormone therapy radically transformed transgender healthcare by providing a path for individuals to change important physical characteristics: the development of breasts and hips with estrogen and growth of facial hair, muscularity, and the deepening of the voice with testosterone.

In the 1930s, after the development and marketing of sex hormones, transgender individuals began to use testosterone and estrogen for gender transition. Michael Dillon, a British transgender man and physician, medically transitioned with testosterone in 1938.[6] In 1952, American Christine Jorgensen underwent hormonal transition and gender-affirming surgery in Denmark.[7] The media stir surrounding her experiences led to greater awareness of transgender issues and an increase in the number of transgender people seeking information and care.[8] In 1962, the University of California Los Angeles Medical Center opened the Gender Identity Research Clinic under the leadership of psychiatrist Robert Stoller, who advocated for assessment and delivery of hormones to adolescents and adults.[9] Shortly after, in 1966, Johns Hopkins University established its gender identity clinic that offered gender-affirming surgery,[10] although the first "complete sex reassignment procedure" was performed there in 1965.[11] Dozens of other clinics soon arose throughout the country.[12]

Despite the proliferation of gender clinics, providers across the United States prescribed hormones without standardization or guidelines. In 1966, Harry Benjamin, a sexologist, endocrinologist, and pioneer in the provision of hormonal care for transgender people, published *The Transsexual Phenomenon* in which he described his experiences working with transgender individuals, including 141 on estrogen and 16 on androgen therapy.[13] Available hormone preparations at the time included oral testosterone propionate and methyltestosterone (androgens), as well as several estrogen preparations, including estradiol undecylate, estradiol valerate, diethylstilbestrol, conjugated estrogens (Premarin), the oral contraceptives ethinylestradiol (Estinyl), and mestranol/norethynodrel (Enovid).[14] Benjamin noted, "As to the particular estrogenic preparations and dosages to be employed . . . there are so far very few leads in the medical literature."[15]

CLINICAL PRACTICE GUIDELINES IN TRANSGENDER HEALTH

In 1979, a group of psychologists, psychiatrists, and surgeons, chaired by psychologist Paul Walker, formed the Harry Benjamin International Gender Dysphoria Association (HBIGDA). That same year, this organization issued the first version of the *Standards of Care: The Hormonal and Surgical Sex Reassignment of Gender Dysphoric Persons* (*SOC*).[16] This document provided clinicians with a standardized approach to the assessment of and treatment for individuals who requested hormonal therapy and gender-affirming surgery. To date, there have been eight versions of the *SOC*. In 2007, HBIGDA renamed itself the World Professional Association of Transgender Health (WPATH), four years before the release of the *SOC-7* in 2011. Version 8 was released in 2022.

In the absence of clinical trials and high-quality studies, earlier HBIGDA/WPATH SOCs were based predominately on expert opinion and clinical consensus.[17] Despite the lack of clear evidence-based data, the SOCs provided best practice recommendations to assist clinicians in delivering safe and consistent care. The gradual acceptance of the WPATH *SOC* by insurance companies, academic centers, clinicians, and health systems (a multiyear effort that began roughly in 2001 after *SOC-6* was published) improved access to gender-affirming hormones and surgeries.[18] Medical societies, professional organizations, health centers, and national organizations have also developed their own guidelines for the provision of hormone therapy. In the United States, these include the Endocrine Society's clinical practice guidelines[19] and the University of San Francisco's primary care protocols.[20] Other professional guidelines closely align with the WPATH *SOC*.[21]

KEY TENETS OF GENDER-AFFIRMING HORMONE THERAPY

Contemporary clinical practice guidelines for gender-affirming hormone therapy focus on patient-centered affirming care, with the objective of establishing a hormonal environment consistent with an individual's embodiment goals and gender identity. For people assigned male at birth, options for feminizing therapy include estrogens and, for those with testes, androgen blockers to inhibit testosterone production. In the past, clinicians prescribed ethinyl estradiol and conjugated estrogens, but these preparations were associated with high rates of venous thromboembolism and are no longer recommended.[22] Considerable variability exists in hormone regimens, due to hormone availability in different countries, treatment costs, and insurance coverage. Today, most regimens employ estradiol, available in oral, intramuscular, transdermal, and subcutaneous forms.[23] Available androgen blockers include spironolactone, finasteride, dutasteride, bicalutamide, gonadotropin-releasing hormone analogs, and cyproterone acetate (the latter only available outside the United States).[24] Clinicians choose androgen blockers by taking into account age, cost, concurrent medication use, and medical conditions. Those assigned female at birth may choose between intramuscular, subcutaneous, transdermal, intranasal, and oral testosterone preparations; most elect either transdermal or parenteral routes.[25] Guidelines recommend starting hormones at a low dose and titrating up until hormone levels are in the usual physiologic range or otherwise consistent with the individual's embodiment goals.

Recently, as increasing numbers of individuals with nonbinary gender identities seek care, clinicians have begun to assess individual treatment goals and prescribe with these goals in mind—a new area in transgender health not yet addressed in clinical guidelines.[26] For example, to reduce the symptoms of gender dysphoria without a noticeable (or minimal) change to appearance, some people prefer low doses of hormones or microdosing. Nonbinary individuals are more likely to request regimens that result in an androgenous appearance or have specific requests, such as feminization without breast development or partial masculinization (that is, stopping treatment once their voice is the desired pitch without developing a full beard).

PROVISION OF HORMONAL CARE IN GENDER CLINICS AND BEYOND

GENDER CLINICS: CARE ON THE BASIS OF MENTAL HEALTH

Over time, different kinds of medical providers began to initiate and monitor hormonal care in different subspecialty settings. In the 1960s, only a few physicians willingly prescribed hormone therapy for patients. The development and expansion of gender clinics a decade later in the United States and Europe (foremost, the Vrije Universiteit in Amsterdam) allowed hormonal care to reach thousands of individuals; however, in these institutions, the provision of hormone care was almost exclusively overseen by endocrinologists.[27]

The early WPATH SOCs reflected the specialization of transgender medicine; the majority of the authors were psychiatrists, psychologists, endocrinologists, and surgeons. Prior to the publication of the seventh version, the WPATH *SOC* recommended that before starting hormonal interventions, individuals undergo a period of real-life experience of at least three months and an evaluation with a psychotherapist for at least three months, including the procurement of letter of recommendation from said provider. This model of care worked well in academic centers where there was no shortage of specialty care, as well as in gender clinics that were predominately established within or alongside departments of psychiatry; however, this model did not work well in settings with fewer resources, such as community health centers.

COMMUNITY HEALTH CENTERS: FROM SPECIALTY TO PRIMARY CARE

The shift from a specialty and mental health–driven model to one in which hormone care became an accepted part of primary care began in the 1990s. Community health centers and other clinics with a mission to care for underserved populations spearheaded this primary care model for hormone treatment. For example, the Tom Waddell Health Center opened a clinic ("Transgender Tuesdays"[28]) in 1993 in San Francisco, California, to respond to the AIDS epidemic and recognized the need to address HIV prevention and treatment for transgender people. The center partnered with local transgender activists and organizations such as the Tenderloin AIDS Resource Center, Brothers' Network, Asian AIDS Project (now API Wellness Center), Proyecto Contra-Sida Por Vida, and FTM International to increase accessibility to hormonal care for the transgender community members (predominately transgender women) who regularly obtained illicit hormones without medical monitoring.[29] By 2001, the Tom Waddell Health Center transgender team was providing their treatment protocols to other interested parties, including clinicians, policy makers, and community activists, and were actively seeking feedback to increase their knowledge base.[30]

Throughout the late 1990s and early 2000s, US-based community health centers dedicated to serving LGBTQ communities and people living with HIV/AIDS began to follow the Tom Waddell Health Center's model, integrating gender-affirming hormonal care and HIV care into primary care practices.

Examples of LGBTQ-focused community health centers include Callen-Lorde in New York; the Mazzoni Center in Philadelphia; Whitman-Walker in Washington, DC; and Fenway Health Services in Boston. Unlike academic centers, these health centers often lacked access to psychotherapists, endocrinologists, and other subspecialists. In response, they created hormone protocols that allowed more flexible approaches to hormone initiation and eliminated the requirement of mental health evaluations and real-life experience. The clinicians based this integrated, gender-affirming and HIV primary care response (dubbed the "informed consent model") on harm reduction and a patient-centered approach.[31] The WPATH *SOC-6*[32] first mentioned this alternative approach as optional in 2001, and by 2011, WPATH had fully endorsed the informed consent model in the *SOC-7*.[33] This pivotal change, one that happened only in the last decade, moved trans health from an exclusive focus on care based on mental health and psychotherapy toward less pathologizing diagnostic and treatment models.

Callen-Lorde Community Health Center began providing hormone therapy to TGD clients in the 1990s and published its first hormone protocol in 2001, with a revision in 2014. The Center currently offers a primary care-based, integrated approach to hormonal care. The primary care clinician may clear an individual for hormone therapy during the initial medical visit, after appropriate assessment and laboratory testing.[34] During the initiation of hormone therapy, the clinician offers patients connections to behavioral health services, case management, health insurance enrollment, gender-affirming surgery navigation, legal assistance, and external referrals as needed.

The Mazzoni Center originated from Philadelphia Community Health Alternatives, an advocacy-driven organization formed in response to the AIDS epidemic. In 2003, the Mazzoni Center opened a transgender-inclusive primary care practice, incorporating trans-specific care into the primary care setting. The Mazzoni Center served as one of the first community health centers in the United States to offer an informed consent model without psychotherapy as a prerequisite to hormone initiation.

Whitman-Walker in Washington, DC, began offering clinical services to transgender patients in 2005 and authored their own internal informed consent hormone protocols in 2010, also offering an integrated approach to hormone treatment within a primary care setting.

Fenway Health initiated their Transgender Task Force in 1997 and formalized their standalone Transgender Health Program in 2004, initially offering mental health counseling, a hormone readiness assessment, and hormone therapy initiation and maintenance.[35] Clinicians at Fenway Health shifted to an informed consent model of care in 2007, modeling their program after the Mazzoni Center, which, despite being smaller than Fenway Health, maintained a patient base nearly four times larger than Fenway's Transgender Health Program. Current Fenway Health protocols require completion of biopsychosocial history completed by a medical provider, complete with screening lab tests before initiating hormone therapy and possible (not required) referral to a mental health provider. This process is expected to require anywhere from two to four visits to the clinic.[36] Many clinicians now perform these steps with one office appointment. All of the above approaches to clinical assessment fall within *SOC* guidelines.

EVOLUTION OF HORMONE CARE AT PLANNED PARENTHOOD

At the turn of the century, the Planned Parenthood Federation of America (PPFA) stepped up to become another organization that expanded access to hormone therapy. Planned Parenthood's decentralized structure allowed local affiliates to decide independently whether to offer transgender health services, in addition to their core, mission-driven reproductive health services.

Delivery of transgender healthcare at a Planned Parenthood clinic started in 1998 in Iowa. Joseph Freund, a family medicine physician, saw the first trans patient and identified the need to provide care to this underserved community.[37] At that time, PPFA recognized and supported this practice but had not yet developed tools to support affiliates working in transgender health.

In the early 2000s, Jen Hastings, another family medicine physician, joined forces with the local diversity center and a community advisory board and began offering hormone therapy at the Westside Planned Parenthood Clinic in Santa Cruz, California (part of Planned Parenthood Mar Monte). In 2007, the inaugural *Medical Standards and Guidelines* group collaborated with the PPFA and Planned Parenthood affiliate staff, including Hastings and Deborah Smith, to publish the first PPFA Medical Standards and Guidelines, which included the provision of transgender healthcare. This document continues to guide practices at Planned Parenthood affiliates. At present, the *PPFA Medical Standards and Guidelines* recommend integrating transgender health throughout all areas of practice and include a chapter outlining hormone care and pubertal suppression.

In the early 2000s, many Planned Parenthood affiliates began working with local transgender communities to champion training for new affiliates in transgender health. Training included not only guidance for medical providers but also the recommendation to collaborate with the trans community and human resources personnel to ensure Planned Parenthood affiliate policies protected transgender people at work. Planned Parenthood affiliates that engaged in this work in the early 2000s offered robust policy and educational resources, positioning Planned Parenthood to meet the explosion of demand for trans-specific care throughout the 2010s. The *PPFA Medical Standards and Guidelines*, in conjunction with PPFA training opportunities and needs assessments, allowed for the expansion of transgender health services at Planned Parenthood affiliates.[38] According to Maureen Kelly, the current manager for Affiliate Training and Learning Design at PPFA, 67 Planned Parenthood–affiliated health centers offered hormone therapy in 2016; 328 Planned Parenthood–affiliated health centers offered this care in 2020.

NEW HORMONE CARE DELIVERY MODELS

In 2010, the federal Affordable Care Act prohibited discrimination based on gender identity, subsequently requiring health providers and payors to include access to transgender health services and necessary insurance.[39] Despite improved reimbursement and the scaling up of gender-affirming care delivered through community health centers, hospital-based clinics, and entities such as Planned Parenthood, many transgender people still find it difficult (and sometimes impossible) to find knowledgeable providers who are sensitive to the psychosocial and medical needs of transgender people.[40] As a result, one in ten transgender individuals has self-treated with hormones without medical oversight or a prescription.[41]

Today, health educators, concerned with the knowledge deficit, advocate for the inclusion of transgender medicine in medical and nursing curricula.[42] Advocates and activists also call for increased access to primary care and research on best practices to connect transgender people with these primary care services.[43] Although evidence demonstrates that transgender people increasingly access care through mainstream settings (e.g., more than six thousand transgender patients currently receive care through Kaiser Permanente across Georgia, Northern California, and Southern California),[44] many transgender people still face insurmountable barriers to hormone therapy in medical settings.

Telehealth has helped close some care gaps for TGD individuals. In the mid-2010s, clinicians began to offer telehealth services to promote transgender health access, particularly in rural settings, eliminating the need for long patient commutes. Recently, several additional for-profit companies began to deliver telehealth, including Folx Health, Queer Med, and Plume.[45] These companies are trans led or employ trans clinicians, increasing the likelihood of welcoming and affirming services. With the onset of the COVID-19 pandemic in 2020, community-based and hospital-based health centers also started providing telehealth services.[46] Patients express satisfaction with gender-related telehealth,[47] although challenges exist, such as liability associated with the delivery of care over state lines, the inability to conduct physical examinations, the lack of internet access for many patients, and financial barriers to the telehealth companies that require monthly payment plans, which may not be reimbursed by insurance plans.

CONCLUSION

The delivery of hormone therapy evolved with improvements in evidence-based research, the development of clinical practice guidelines, and improved clinician education about trans-specific care and the unique needs of transgender people. Telehealth services, in addition to the existing traditional brick-and-mortar health services increase access to gender-affirming care, particularly in areas of the United States that lack trans-competent clinicians. Changes in legislation, including the Affordable Care Act,[48] have improved coverage for transgender healthcare. Together, these factors have increased access to gender-affirming health services and started the process of bringing trans-specific healthcare from the margins to mainstream medical practice.

NOTES

1. Herman, Flores, and O'Neill, "How Many Adults and Youth Identify as Transgender in the United States?" 1.

2. James et al., *The Report of the 2015 U.S. Transgender Survey*, 92–130; Safer et al., "Barriers to Healthcare for Transgender Individuals."

3. Kohn et al., "The History of Estrogen Therapy," 3; Nieschlag and Nieschlag, "Endocrine History," 5.

4. Redburn, "Before Equal Protection."

5. Meyerowitz, *How Sex Changed*, 218–19.

6. Kennedy, "20th Century Boy."
7. Jorgensen, *Christine Jorgensen*.
8. Reicherzer, "Evolving Language."
9. Money, "The Concept of Gender Identity Disorder"; Reicherzer, "Evolving Language"; Stoller, "A Biased View."
10. Meyerowitz, *How Sex Changed*, 219.
11. Money and Schwartz, "Public Opinion and Social Issues," 255.
12. Hastings and Blum, "A Transsexual Research Project." See also chapter 11 in this volume.
13. Benjamin, *The Transsexual Phenomenon*.
14. Benjamin, *The Transsexual Phenomenon*.
15. Benjamin, *The Transsexual Phenomenon*, 121.
16. Each edition of the *SOC* is denoted by its corresponding numeral, that is, *SOC-1*, *SOC-2*, and so on. Walker et al., "Standards of Care."
17. Deutsch et al., "What's in a Guideline?"
18. Deutsch et al., "What's in a Guideline?"; Goldenberg et al., "State-Level Transgender-Specific Policies." See also chapter 13 in this volume. This was a multi-year effort that began roughly in 2001, after *SOC-6* was published. These efforts are described in chapter 13.
19. Hembree et al., "Endocrine Treatment of Gender-Dysphoric."
20. Deutsch, *Guidelines for the Primary and Gender-Affirming Care*.
21. See also chapter 14 in this volume.
22. Kotamarti et al., "Risk for Venous Thromboembolism."
23. Tangpricha and den Heijer, "Oestrogen and Anti-Androgen Therapy."
24. Hembree et al., "Endocrine Treatment of Gender-Dysphoric"; Tangpricha and den Heijer, "Oestrogen and Anti-Androgen Therapy."
25. Deutsch, *Guidelines for the Primary and Gender-Affirming Care*; Hembree et al., "Endocrine Treatment of Gender-Dysphoric."
26. Cocchetti et al., "Hormonal Treatment Strategies."
27. Money, "The Concept of Gender Identity Disorder"; Reicherzer, "Evolving Language"; Wiepjes et al., "The Amsterdam Cohort."
28. Sheets, "Transgender Tuesdays"; Freeman, "Transgender Tuesdays: A Clinic in Tenderloin"; San Francisco Department of Public Health, "Our Services."
29. Tom Waddell Health Center, *Protocols for Hormonal Reassignment*; Erickson-Schroth, "Trans Bodies, Trans Selves;" Sheets, "Transgender Tuesdays"; Stryker, *Transgender History*.
30. Tom Waddell Health Center Transgender Team, "Memorandum," 1.
31. Deutsch, "Use of the Informed Consent Model."
32. Harry Benjamin International Gender Dysphoria Association, *Standards of Care*.
33. World Professional Association for Transgender Health, *Standards of Care*; Coleman, et al., "Standards of Care for the Health of Transsexual."

34. Callen-Lorde Community Health Center, *Protocols for the Provision of Hormone Therapy*; Reisner et al., "Integrated and Gender-Affirming."

35. Martorelli, *History of the Fenway Transgender Health Program*.

36. Reisner et al., "Integrated and Gender-Affirming"; Thompson et al., *Medical Care of Trans and Gender Diverse Adults*. See also, https://fenwayhealth.org/wp-content/uploads/TH-39-Gender-Affirming-Hormone-Therapy-for-Adults-Brochure-Final-Web.pdf.

37. Freund, "Moments in Transgender Healthcare."

38. Porsch et al., "An Exploratory Study."

39. Baker, "The Future of Transgender Coverage."

40. Radix et al., "Satisfaction and Healthcare Utilization"; Safer et al., "Barriers to Healthcare."

41. Stroumsa et al., "Insurance Coverage and Use of Hormones," 3.

42. Korpaisarn and Safer, "Gaps in Transgender Medical Education."

43. Bruessow and Poteat, "Primary Care Providers' Role"; Clark et al., "Primary Care Access and Forgone Care"; Edmiston et al., "Opportunities and Gaps in Primary Care"; Ziegler et al., "'Primary Care Is Primary Care.'"

44. Getahun et al., "Cross-Sex Hormones and Acute Cardiovascular Events," 208.

45. Asaad et al., "Telemedicine in Transgender Care"; FOLX; Hamanvik et al., "Telemedicine and Inequities in Health Care Access"; Plume, "Gender-Affirming Hormone Therapy from Anywhere"; Queer Med, "Gender-Affirming Care for Transgender and Nonbinary Individuals."

46. Grasso et al., "Gender-Affirming Care without Walls."

47. Apple et al., "Acceptability of Telehealth"; Sequeira et al., "Transgender Youths' Perspectives," 1208.

48. It must be noted, though, that the power of the Affordable Care Act (ACA) to preserve access to care for TGD people through the Act's nondiscrimination section 1557 remains hotly contested. The US Department of Health and Human Services (HHS) issued the following statement in 2021: "Consistent with the Supreme Court's decision in Bostock and Title IX, beginning May 10, 2021, OCR will interpret and enforce Section 1557's prohibition on discrimination on the basis of sex to include: (1) discrimination on the basis of sexual orientation; and (2) discrimination on the basis of gender identity. This interpretation will guide OCR in processing complaints and conducting investigations but does not itself determine the outcome in any particular case or set of facts." However, a more recent update noted: "On May 16, 2022, the court in Christian Employers Alliance v. EEOC [US Equal Opportunity Commission], No. 1:21-cv-00195 (D.N.D.), issued a preliminary injunction against HHS [US Department of Health and Human Services] and EEOC. The preliminary injunction prohibits HHS from interpreting or enforcing Section 1557 of the ACA and any regulations against the plaintiffs' present or future members in a manner that would require them to provide, offer, perform, facilitate, or refer for gender transition services or in a manner

that restricts or compels their speech on gender identity issues." At the time of this writing, this case has not been fully adjudicated.

WORKS CITED

Apple, Danielle E., Elle Lett, Sarah Wood, et al. (2021). "Acceptability of Telehealth for Gender-Affirming Care in Transgender and Gender Diverse Youth and Their Caregivers." *Transgender Health* 7, no. 2 (2022): 159–64.

Asaad, Malke, Aashish Rajesh, Krishna Vyas, and Shane D. Morrison. "Telemedicine in Transgender Care: A Twenty-First–Century Beckoning." *Plastic and Reconstructive Surgery* 146, no. 1 (2020): 108e–9e. https://journals.lww.com/plasreconsurg/Fulltext/2020/07000/Telemedicine_in_Transgender_Care__A.56.aspx.

Baker, Kellan E. "The Future of Transgender Coverage." *New England Journal of Medicine* 376, no. 19 (2017): 1801–04. https://doi.org/10.1056/NEJMp1702427.

Baumgardner, Mika, and Arlene Reynolds, comp. "University of California Los Angeles LGBTQ History Timeline." Accessed October 25, 2021. https://lgbtq.ucla.edu/file/ac66fa0b-b106-46d8-97ff-6a2b0b33fa4e.

Benjamin, Harry. *The Transsexual Phenomenon*. New York: Julian Press, 1966.

Bruessow, Diane, and Tonia Poteat. (2018). "Primary Care Providers' Role in Transgender Healthcare." *Journal of the American Academy of PAs* 31, no. 2 (2018): 8–11.

Callen-Lorde Community Health Center. *Protocols for the Provision of Hormone Therapy*. 2014. Accessed September 13, 2024. https://callen-lorde.org/graphics/2018/04/Callen-Lorde-TGNC-Hormone-Therapy-Protocols.pdf.

Christian Employers Alliance v. EEOC, No. 1:21-cv-195 (D.N.D., May 16, 2022).

Clark, Beth A., Jaimie F. Veale, Devon Greyson, and Elizabeth Saewyc. "Primary Care Access and Foregone Care: A Survey of Transgender Adolescents and Young Adults." *Family Practice* 35, no. 3 (2018): 302–06.

Cocchetti, Carlotta, Jiska Ristori, Alessia Romani, Mario Maggi, and Alessandra Daphne Fisher. "Hormonal Treatment Strategies Tailored to Non-Binary Transgender Individuals." *J Clin Med* 9, no. 6 (2020). https://doi.org/10.3390/jcm9061609.

Coleman, Eli, Walter Bockting, Marsha Botzer, et al. "Standards of Care for the Health of Transsexual, Transgender, and Gender-Nonconforming People, Version 7." *International Journal of Transgenderism* 13, no. 4 (2012): 165–232.

Deutsch, Madeline, ed. *Guidelines for the Primary and Gender-Affirming Care of Transgender and Gender Nonbinary People*. 2nd ed. UCSF Gender Affirming Health Program, Department of Family and Community Medicine. San Francisco: University of California San Francisco, 2016. Accessed September 13, 2024. https://transcare.ucsf.edu/guidelines.

Deutsch, Madeline B. "Use of the Informed Consent Model in the Provision of Cross-Sex Hormone Therapy: A Survey of the Practices of Selected Clinics." *International

Journal of Transgenderism 13, no. 3 (2012): 140–46. https://doi.org/10.1080/15532739.2011.675233.

Deutsch, Maddie B., Asa Radix, and Sari Reisner. "What's in a Guideline? Developing Collaborative and Sound Research Designs that Substantiate Best Practice Recommendations for Transgender Health Care." *AMA Journal of Ethics* 18, no. 11 (2016): 1098.

Edmiston, E. Kale, Cameron A. Donald, Alice Rose Sattler, J. Klint Peebles, Jesse M. Ehrenfeld, and Kristen Laurel Eckstrand. "Opportunities and Gaps in Primary Care Preventative Health Services for Transgender Patients: A Systemic Review." *Transgender Health* 1, no. 1 (2016): 216–30. https://doi.org/10.1089/trgh.2016.0019.

Erickson-Schroth, Laura. *Trans Bodies, Trans Selves: A Resource for the Transgender Community*. Oxford University Press, 2014.

FOLX [website]. Accessed October 4, 2021. https://www.folxhealth.com/.

Freeman, Mark. *Transgender Tuesdays: A Clinic in the Tenderloin*. 2012. YouTube (documentary). Accessed September 13, 2024. https://www.youtube.com/watch?v=g_-2qLW2O7Y.

Freund, Joe. "Moments in Transgender Healthcare 2004–2018: One Family Doctor's Perspective." *Journal of Critical Thought and Praxis* 7, no. 2 (2018).

Getahun, Darios, Rebecca Nash, W. Dana Flanders, et al. "Cross-sex Hormones and Acute Cardiovascular Events in Transgender Persons: A Cohort Study." *Annals of Internal Medicine* 169, no. 4 (2018): 205–13. https://doi.org/10.7326/m17-2785.

Goldenberg, Tamar, Sari L. Reisner, Gary W. Harper, Kristie E. Gamarel, and Rob Stephenson. "State-Level Transgender-Specific Policies, Race/Ethnicity, and Use of Medical Gender Affirmation Services among Transgender and Other Gender-Diverse People in the United States." *Milbank Quarterly* 98, no. 3 (2020): 802–46. https://doi.org/10.1111/1468-0009.12467.

Grasso, Chris, Juwan Campbell, Emily Yunkun, et al. "Gender-Affirming Care Without Walls: Utilization of Telehealth Services by Transgender and Gender Diverse People at a Federally Qualified Health Center." *Transgender Health* 7, no. 2 (2022): 135–43.

Hamanvik, Ole-Petter R., Shailesh Agarwal, Christopher G. Ahnallen, Anna L. Goldman, and Sari L. Reisner. "Telemedicine and Inequities in Health Care Access: The Example of Transgender Health." *Transgender Health* 7, no. 2 (2022): 113–16.

Harry Benjamin International Gender Dysphoria Association. *Standards of Care for Gender Identity Disorders*. 6th Version. 2001.

Hastings, Donald W., and J. A. Blum. "A Transsexual Research Project at the University of Minnesota Medical School." *Lancet* 87, no. 7 (1967): 262–64.

Health and Human Services, Office for Civil Rights (OCR). "Section 1557 of the Patient Protection and Affordable Care Act." July 22, 2010. Accessed August 7, 2022. https://www.hhs.gov/civil-rights/for-individuals/section-1557/index.html.

Hembree, Wylie C., Peggy T. Cohen-Kettenis, Louis Gooren, et al. "Endocrine Treatment of Gender-Dysphoric/Gender-Incongruent Persons: An Endocrine Society* Clinical Practice Guideline." *Journal of Clinical Endocrinology & Metabolism* 102, no. 11 (2017): 3869–903. https://doi.org/10.1210/jc.2017-01658.

Herman, Jody L., Andrew R. Flores, and Kathryn K. O'Neill. "How Many Adults and Youth Identify as Transgender in the United States?" Williams Institute, UCLA School of Law. 2022. Accessed September 13, 2024. https://escholarship.org/content/qt4xs990ws/qt4xs990ws.pdf.

James, Sandy E., Jody L. Herman, Susan Rankin, Mara Keisling, Lisa Mottet, and Ma'ayan Anafi. *The Report of the 2015 U.S. Transgender Survey*. Washington, DC: National Center for Transgender Equality, 2016.

Jorgensen, Christine. *Christine Jorgensen: Personal Autobiography*. New York: P. S. Eriksson, 1967.

Kennedy, Pagan. "20th Century Boy, In the 1930s, the Word 'Transsexual' Didn't Exist in the English Language. So Laura Dillon Had to Label Herself." *Bitch Media*, November 20, 2018. Accessed September 13, 2024. https://www.bitchmedia.org/article/laura-dillon-transgender-man.

Kohn, Grace E., Katherine M. Rodriguez, James Hotaling, and Alexander W. Pastuszak. "The History of Estrogen Therapy." *Sexual Medicine Review* 7, no. 3 (2019): 416–21. https://doi.org/10.1016/j.sxmr.2019.03.006.

Korpaisarn, S., and J. D. Safer. "Gaps in Transgender Medical Education Among Healthcare Providers: A Major Barrier to Care for Transgender Persons." *Reviews in Endocrine and Metabolic Disorders* 19 (2018): 271–75. https://doi.org/10.1007/s11154-018-9452-5.

Kotamarti, Vasanth S., Nicolas Greige, Adee J. Heiman, Ashit Patel, and Joseph A. Ricci. "Risk for Venous Thromboembolism in Transgender Patients Undergoing Cross-Sex Hormone Treatment: A Systematic Review." *Journal of Sexual Medicine* 18, no. 7 (2021): 1280–91. https://doi.org/https://doi.org/10.1016/j.jsxm.2021.04.006.

Martorelli, Thomas, ed. *History of the Fenway Transgender Health Program*. Boston, MA: Fenway Health, 2015. Accessed September 20, 2021. https://fenwayhealth.org/wp-content/uploads/COM-2159-transgender-history_booklet-1.pdf.

Meerwijk, Esther L., and Jae M. Sevelius. "Transgender Population Size in the United States: A Meta-Regression of Population-Based Probability Samples." *American Journal of Public Health* 107, no. 2 (2017): 216. https://doi.org/10.2105/AJPH.2016.303578a.

Meyerowitz, Joanne. *How Sex Changed: A History of Transsexuality in the United States*. Cambridge: Harvard University Press, 2002.

Money, John. "The Concept of Gender Identity Disorder in Childhood and Adolescence After 39 Years." *Journal of Sex & Marital Therapy* 20, no. 3 (1994): 163–77.

Money, John, and F. Schwartz. "Public Opinion and Social Issues in Transsexualism: A Case Study in Medical Sociology." In *Transsexualism and Sex Reassignment*, edited by Richard Green and John Money, 253–69. Baltimore, MD: Johns Hopkins University Press, 1969.

Nieschlag, Eberhard, and Susan Nieschlag. "ENDOCRINE HISTORY: The History of Discovery, Synthesis and Development of Testosterone for Clinical Use." *European Journal of Endocrinology* 180, no. 6 (2019): R201–12. https://doi.org/10.1530/eje-19-0071.

Plume. "Gender-Affirming Hormone Therapy from Anywhere." Accessed October 4, 2021. https://getplume.co/.

Porsch, Lauren M., Ila Dayananda, and Gillian Dean. "An Exploratory Study of Transgender New Yorkers' Use of Sexual Health Services and Interest in Receiving Services at Planned Parenthood of New York City." *Transgender Health* 1, no. 1 (2016): 231–37.

Queer Med. "Gender-Affirming Care for Transgender and Nonbinary Individuals." Accessed October 4, 2021. https://queermed.com/.

Radix, Anita E., Corina Lelutiu-Weinberger, and Kristi E. Gamarel. "Satisfaction and Healthcare Utilization of Transgender and Gender Non-Conforming Individuals in NYC: A Community-Based Participatory Study." *LGBT Health* 1, no. 4 (2014): 302–08. https://doi.org/10.1089/lgbt.2013.0042.

Redburn, Kate. "Before Equal Protection: The Fall of Anti-Crossdressing Laws and the Origins of the Transgender Legal Movement 1964–1980." April 30, 2018. Accessed September 13, 2024. https://ssrn.com/abstract=3199904.

Reicherzer, Stacee. "Evolving Language and Understanding in the Historical Development of the Gender Identity Disorder Diagnosis." *Journal of LGBT Issues in Counseling* 2, no. 4 (2008): 326–47.

Reisner, Sari L., A. Radix, A., and Mattie B. Deutsch. "Integrated and Gender-Affirming Transgender Clinical Care and Research." *Journal of Acquired Immune Deficiency Syndrome* 72 (2016): S235–42. https://doi.org/10.1097/qai.0000000000001088.

Safer, Joshua D., Eli Coleman, Jamie Feldman, et al. "Barriers to Healthcare for Transgender Individuals." *Current Opinion in Endocrinology, Diabetes, and Obesity* 23, no. 2 (2016): 168–71. https://doi.org/10.1097/med.0000000000000227.

San Francisco Department of Public Health. "Our Services: Information About the Transgender Clinic." Accessed August 7, 2022. https://www.sfdph.org/dph/comupg/oservices/medSvs/hlthCtrs/TransgenderHlthCtrInfo.asp

Sequeira, Gina M., Kacie M. Kidd, Robert W. S. Coulter, et al. "Transgender Youths' Perspectives on Telehealth for Delivery of Gender-Affirming Care." *Journal of Adolescent Health* 68, no. 6 (2021): 1207–10. https://doi.org/https://doi.org/10.1016/j.jadohealth.2020.08.028.

Sheets, Debra. "Transgender Tuesdays: A Clinic in the Tenderloin, by Mark Freeman." *Journal of Gerontological Social Work* 57, no. 2–4 (2014): 413–15. https://doi.org/10.1080/01634372.2013.837308.

Stoller, Robert J. "A Biased View of 'Sex Transformation' Operations." *Journal of Nervous and Mental Disease* 149, no. 4 (1969): 312–17.

Stroumsa, Daphna, Halley P. Crissman, Vanessa K. Dalton, Giselle Kolenic, and Caroline R. Richardson. "Insurance Coverage and Use of Hormones Among Transgender Respondents to a National Survey." *Annals of Family Medicine* 18, no. 6 (2020): 528–34. https://doi.org/10.1370/afm.2586.

Stryker, S. *Transgender History: The Roots of Today's Revolution*. 2nd ed. New York: Seal Press, 2017.

Tangpricha, V., and Martin den Heijer. "Oestrogen and Anti-Androgen Therapy for Transgender Women." *Lancet: Diabetes and Endocrinology* 5, no. 4 (2017): 291–300. https://doi.org/10.1016/s2213-8587(16)30319-9.

Thompson, J., R. Hopwood, S. deNormand, and T. Cavanaugh, T. *Medical Care of Trans and Gender Diverse Adults*. Boston, MA: Fenway Health, 2021.

Tom Waddell Health Center. *Tom Waddell Health Center Protocols for Hormonal Reassignment of Gender*. Revised May 7. 2013. Accessed August 7, 2022. https://www.sfdph.org/dph/comupg/oservices/medsvs/hlthctrs/transgendprotocols122006.pdf.

Tom Waddell Health Center Transgender Team. "Memorandum." *Protocols for Hormonal Reassignment of Gender*, 1–14. August 14, 2001. Accessed August 7, 2022. http://www.spectrumwny.org/info/sf_protocols.pdf.

Walker, Paul A., Jack C. Berger, Richard Green, Donald Laub, Charles L. Reynolds, and Leo Wollman. "Standards of Care: The Hormonal and Surgical Sex Reassignment of Gender Dysphoric Persons." *Annals of Plastic Surgery* 13, no. 6 (1984): 476–81.

Wiepjes, Chantal M., Nienke M. Nota, Christel J. M. de Blok, et al. "The Amsterdam Cohort of Gender Dysphoria Study (1972–2015): Trends in Prevalence, Treatment, and Regrets." *Journal of Sexual Medicine* 15, no. 4 (2018): 582–90. https://doi.org/https://doi.org/10.1016/j.jsxm.2018.01.016.

Witkin, Rachel. "Hopkins Hospital: A History of Sex Reassignment." *Johns Hopkins Newsletter*, May 1, 2014. Accessed October 25, 2021. https://www.jhunewsletter.com/article/2014/05/hopkins-hospital-a-history-of-sex-reassignment-76004.

World Professional Association for Transgender Health. *Standards of Care for the Health of Transsexual, Transgender, and Gender Nonconforming People*. 7th Version. 2012. Accessed September 13, 2024. https://www.wpath.org/publications/soc.

Ziegler, Erin, Ruta Valaitis, Jennifer Yost, Nancy Carter, and Cathy Risdon. "'Primary Care Is Primary Care': Use of Normalization Process Theory to Explore the Implementation of Primary Care Services for Transgender Individuals in Ontario." *PLOS One* 14, no. 4 (2019): e0215873.

Zurada, Aanna, Sonja Salandy, Wallisa Roberts, Jerzy Gielecki, Justine Schober, and Marios Loukas. "The Evolution of Transgender Surgery." *Clinical Anatomy* 31, no. 6 (2018): 878–86. https://doi.org/10.1002/ca.23206.

16.1. PROFILE: JEANNE HOFF (1938–2023)

Noah Adams

Jeanne Hoff was notable for being the first known transgender person to run a trans-centric medical practice in the English-speaking world. Born in 1938, Hoff received a Master of Science from Yale in 1961, a medical degree from Columbia in 1963, and a PhD in solid-state chemistry from the University College of London in 1971.[1] While still a medical student, she also copublished a paper on kidney disease.[2] Hoff subsequently trained in psychiatry at the Washington University School of Medicine.[3] Prior to her gender transition, she worked as a pathologist in New York City at the Harry Benjamin Foundation while simultaneously completing her residency in psychiatry. Her work with the foundation was presented in a television program that aired in 1976.[4] In 1978, Hoff returned for a second interview to describe her transition. This program, a frank and largely respectful discussion of her experience, took place on the eve of her vaginoplasty and included video footage from this surgery.[5] The production won an Ohio State Broadcasting award and its producer Madeline Argot received an Emmy nomination.[6]

Hoff took over Harry Benjamin's New York City practice in 1979, after Benjamin's chosen successor, Charles Ihlenfeld, resigned to pursue a psychiatric residency.[7] She immediately reviewed Benjamin's case files and followed up with all his patients. Hoff is remembered for her passion and care for her patients' well-being, work with transgender children, and advocacy around the case of an African American transgender woman who had been psychiatrically imprisoned since the age of fifteen due to her gender identity.[8] She also inspired at least one former trans patient to become a doctor himself.[9] Punk icon Jayne County remembers Hoff for her role in helping her understand her wish to transition.[10] Hoff also publicly confronted psychiatrist Charles Socarides about his pathologizing views regarding homosexuality at his presentations in New York City[11] and later opined that he was a "captive of the psychoanalytic school . . . and tried to use elements of that theory . . . [to] cause a great deal of suffering to parents and gays alike. . . . He never seems to have made the adjustment to data, objective study, or the demise of his psychoanalytic faith-based system."[12]

Hoff ultimately left her New York City practice in the 1980s and moved to California, where she worked through the latter half of the 1990s as a

Figure 16.1.1. Jeanne Hoff. *Source*: From the Collections of the Kinsey Institute, Indiana University. All rights reserved.

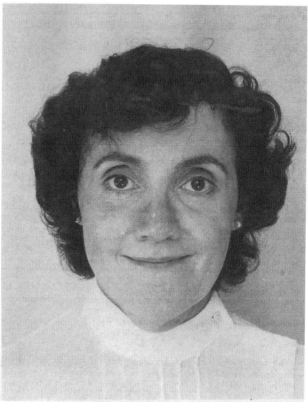

psychiatrist in the San Quentin prison system.[13] She spent the ensuing years contributing to the betterment of transgender and nontransgender mental healthcare in private practice and ultimately retired in the early to mid-2000s. In 2013 Hoff gifted her archives to the Kinsey Institute for Research in Sex, Gender, and Reproduction at Indiana University.[14]

From her beginnings in and eventual assumption of Benjamin's New York practice to her ground-breaking media work in which she first explained her work and later her own transition, Hoff was consistently at the forefront of transgender healthcare, perhaps especially when it meant calling out those in positions of power. She died of Parkinson disease at her home in San Francisco on October 26, 2023, at the age of 85.[15] She was a pioneer in the truest sense.

NOTES

1. *Washington University School of Medicine Bulletin*, 81; Cowan, "Jeanne Hoff (1938–)."
2. Kissane and Hoff, "Quantitative Histochemistry."
3. Brawley, "St. Louis LGBT."
4. Hoff, Bergen, and Fields, "Not for Women Only."
5. Hoff, Redgrave, and Fields, "Becoming Jeanne."
6. Kinsey Institute for Sex, Gender, and Reproduction, "Jeanne Hoff Archive."
7. Gill-Peterson, *Histories of the Transgender Child*, 171; Cowan, "Jeanne Hoff (1938–)."
8. Gill-Peterson, *Histories of the Transgender Child*, 160.
9. Gill-Peterson, *Histories of the Transgender Child*, 193.
10. County and Smith, *Man Enough to be a Woman*, 119–20.
11. Humm, "Socarides."
12. Humm, "Socarides."
13. Cowan, "Jeanne Hoff (1938-)"; Casey, "Gay Catholics"; Transparent California, "Jeanne Hoff."
14. Cowan, "Jeanne Hoff (1938-)."
15. Green, "Jeanne Hoff."

WORKS CITED

Brawley, Steven Lewis. "St. Louis LGBT History Project Timeline 1900–1960s." St. Louis LGBT History Project. Accessed May 5, 2021. http://www.stlouislgbthistory.com/timeline/1900-1960s.html.

Casey, Kathleen. "Gay Catholics Hear Transsexual's Story." *Asbury Park Press*, 11:B4 (October 1978). Accessed May 8, 2021. https://www.newspapers.com/clip/7291402/jeanne-hoff-md-wu/.

County, Jayne, and Rupert Smith. *Man Enough to Be a Woman*. London: Serpent's Tail, 1995.

Cowan, Zagria. "Jeanne Hoff (1938-) Psychiatrist." A Gender Variance Who's Who, September 20, 2013. Accessed May 5, 2021. https://zagria.blogspot.com/2013/09/jeanne-hoff-1938-psychiatrist.html#.XhbhsKHLc7Q.

Gill-Peterson, Julian. *Histories of the Transgender Child*. London: University of Minnesota Press, 2018.

Green, Penelope. "Jeanne Hoff, Pioneering Transgender Psychiatrist, Dies at 85." *New York Times*, December 18, 2023. Accessed August 20, 2024. https://www.nytimes.com/2023/12/18/us/jeanne-hoff-dead.html.

Hoff, Jeanne, Polly Bergen, and Frank Fields. "Not For Women Only." Aired 1976 on NBC. Produced by Madeline Amgott. Accessed May 8, 2021. https://web.archive.org/web/20140709111520/www.kinseyinstitute.org/library/jeannehoff.html.

Hoff, Jeanne, Lynn Redgrave, and Frank Fields. "Becoming Jeanne . . . A Search for Sexual Identity." Aired June 30, 1978 on NBC. Produced by Madeline Amgott. Accessed May 8, 2021. Accessed August 20, 2024. https://web.archive.org/web/20140709111520/www.kinseyinstitute.org/library/jeannehoff.html.

Humm, Andy. "Socarides, Leading Anti-Gay Shrink, Dies." *Gay City News*, January 4, 2005. Accessed May 5, 2021. https://www.gaycitynews.com/news-briefs-41/.

Kinsey Institute for Research in Sex, Gender and Reproduction. "Jeanne Hoff Archive." Accessed May 5, 2021. https://web.archive.org/web/20140709111520/www.kinseyinstitute.org/library/jeannehoff.html.

Kissane, John M., and Eugene Hoff. "Quantitative Histochemistry of the Kidney. 11. Enzymatic Activities in Glemeruli and Proximal Tubules in Aminonucleoside Nephrosis in Rats." *Journal of Histochemistry & Cytochemistry* 10, no. 3 (1962). Accessed April 5, 2022. https://doi.org/10.1177/10.3.259.

Transparent California. "Jeanne Hoff." 2017. Accessed May 8, 2021. https://transparentcalifornia.com/pensions/2015/calpers/jeanne-hoff/.

Washington University. *Washington University School of Medicine Bulletin: 1971-1972*. 1971. Accessed May 8, 2021. https://core.ac.uk/download/pdf/70377986.pdf.

16.2. PROFILE: JOANNE KEATLEY (1951-)

Teri Wilhelm

While searching for words to describe the life and motivations of activist JoAnne Keatley, I return repeatedly to the aphorism, "A rising tide lifts all boats."[1] Keatley worked tirelessly at first to raise her own boat and then selflessly returned to her beginnings as a professional to elevate the lives of transgender people—especially women of color—in the United States and throughout the world. Her life experiences and academic achievements enabled her to live in two worlds: that of a streetwise, homeless, immigrant child and that of a strategist, policy maker, and researcher focused on furthering the field of transgender healthcare.

Keatley possesses an American story that began in Mexico City in 1951. She was born into extreme poverty and identified as male then later immigrated to America at age seven. More than a year prior to her own crossing the border, Keatley's mother left the young family of five to seek a new life in America. After a lengthy absence and with little contact, her mother unexpectedly returned with a male companion and a plan to bring her children to the United States. "I came as an undocumented person," Keatley said. "Mom came back to Mexico with her American boyfriend to gather her little chicks. [She] put us in the back of a car and drove up north. We crossed the border in Corpus Christi, Texas, and didn't have documents for a couple of years."[2] In 1961, her mother accumulated enough resources to allow her return to Mexico once again and reenter the United States legally, thereby obtaining the necessary documents for her family to live, attend school, and work in the United States.

Social factors that lead many immigrant families toward more traditional views also influenced Keatley's family. They sharply scorned her feminine behavior, driving her out of the family home. She lived on the streets of San Francisco and, at age fourteen, without much understanding of the process and with poor English language skills, began to openly express the desire for gender transition. Over the next decade, Keatley embraced street life, drug abuse, and sex work to stay alive and to support her little-understood dreams of a gender transition.

In her late twenties, after receiving a benefactor's support for a medical transition, Keatley left the streets, stopped using drugs, and began to consider her education and life goals. She admitted that language was an enormous barrier: "I had the drive, street smarts, and natural intelligence, but couldn't understand grammar."[3] She began remedial learning, tested out of some requirements, then applied to City College in Los Angeles. After struggling through several difficult semesters as a first-generation student, she enrolled at San Jose State College, where she later became a presidential scholar. Shortly thereafter, Keatley attended the University of California Berkeley to study social work with a focus on families, communities, and groups, earning her master's degree in 1999.

As a University of California Berkeley, graduate student, Keatley engaged in research projects concerned with the health of transgender women, particularly HIV care, focusing on how transphobia and stigma led to disproportionate healthcare disparities. The project garnered the notice of a professor from the University of California San Francisco Tooru Nemoto, who led the first federally funded project on substance abuse and HIV prevention for transgender women of color. Inspired by the National Institute on Drug Abuse program, Keatley joined Nemoto's team and assisted in the development of federally subsidized, direct intervention programs for the San Francisco transgender community. She and the team designed drop-in centers and partnered with substance abuse and criminal justice professionals to encourage transgender people involved in drug use or sex work to engage with HIV prevention services, mental health services, and substance abuse treatment programs.[4]

In the late 1990s, Keatley would help open the Transgender Resource and Neighborhood Space, America's first drop-in space specifically created for transgender people. The program continues today with the name Trans Thrive,[5] and it serves as a nationally recognized model for safe drop-in centers that offer community support and connection to services.

Growing less enthusiastic for macrolevel social work and more enticed by a direct services approach, in 2007 she contributed to the launch of the Center of Excellence for Transgender Health at the University of California San Francisco,[6] a renowned interdisciplinary center for direct service, training, research, and advocacy. She organized a team of clinicians who developed evidence-based guidelines for transgender care, emphasizing primary care as a focus. Recognizing her work as substantive and impactful, staff at the Centers for Disease Control and Prevention, the National Institutes of Health, and the White House began to regularly call on Keatley to offer advice and insight regarding the provision of services for the transgender community.

At present, Keatley serves as the Chair of Governance for the Innovative Response Globally for Transgender Women and HIV, a global network working to build international organizational capacity to promote the human rights of transgender women around HIV/AIDS and to improve public health outcomes by working with nongovernmental organizations.[7] She also continues to work and be influential for the nongovernment organization Trans Education and Action Capacity for Health and expects to extend this organization's work to Peru and Nepal. She hopes that the transgender community will "respond to our own needs, in our own way, with our own people, with interventions designed in such a way to uniquely meet the needs of transgender people."[8]

Since 2016, Keatley continues to work beyond her retirement on special projects for the University of California San Francisco. Nowadays, she is inspired by transgender youth: "Their awareness and resilience are much greater than mine as a child. They want to educate themselves, study gender, and make space for their dreams and aspirations."[9] Keatley is proud to have opened doors and created opportunities for other trans health professionals. This particularly extends to her work in creating youth-focused training curricula for the Substance Abuse and Mental Health Services Administration and the Center for Substance Abuse Treatment. Keatley acknowledges that transgender healthcare has moved forward during her career, but when she listens to harsh politicians and their anti-trans rhetoric, she notes, "It is quite disheartening. There is still much to be done."[10]

NOTES

1. Kennedy, "Remarks in Heber Springs."
2. Keatley, Interview.
3. Keatley, Interview.
4. Keatley, Interview.
5. San Francisco Community Health Center, "Trans: Thrive."
6. University of California San Francisco, "Center of Excellence."
7. IRGT, "IRGT: Governance."
8. Keatley, Interview.
9. Keatley, Interview.
10. Keatley, Interview.

WORKS CITED

IRGT. "IRGT: A Global Network of Trans Women and HIV." Accessed August 6, 2024. https://irgt.org/. [No longer available.]

IRGT. "IRGT Governance: Joanne Keatley Chair." Accessed August 6, 2024. https://irgt.org/irgt-governance/.

Keatley, Joanne. Interview by Teri Wilhelm, March 1, 2021.

Kennedy, J. F. "Remarks in Heber Springs, Arkansas, at the Dedication of Greers Ferry Dam." The American Presidency Project, October 3, 1963. Accessed November 1, 2021. https://www.presidency.ucsb.edu/node/236260.

San Fransisco Community Health Center. "Trans: Thrive." Accessed October 22, 2021. https://sfcommunityhealth.org/program/trans-thrive/.

University of California San Francisco. "Center of Excellence for Transgender Health." Accessed October 22, 2021. https://prevention.ucsf.edu/transhealth.

Vidinsky, Kate. "Joanne Keatley: Championing Equity in Care for Transgender Community." *Campus News: University of California San Francisco*, June 21, 2016. Accessed August 30, 2021. https://www.ucsf.edu/news/2016/06/403316/joanne-keatley-championing-equity-care-transgender-community.

16.3. PROFILE: ADMIRAL RACHEL LELAND LEVINE (1957–)

Dallas Denny

On February 13, 2021, US President Joe Biden nominated Rachel Levine for the federal position Assistant Secretary for Health in the US Department of Health and Human Services.[1] On March 17, the US Senate Committee on Health,

Education, Labor, and Pensions voted thirteen to nine to send her nomination to the US Senate for a vote. On March 24, the Senate voted fifty-two to forty-eight to confirm her nomination. All Senate Republicans voted to reject the nomination except for Lisa Murkowski of Alaska and Susan Collins of Maine.[2] Levine has served since March 26, 2021, as the seventeenth Assistant Secretary for Health. She is the first openly transgender person to hold an office that requires confirmation by the US Senate.[3] She also serves as head of the US Public Health Service Commissioned Corps.[4]

Levine would soon create history again. On October 19, 2021, when she was promoted to the rank of four-star admiral in the US Navy, she became the first openly transgender officer to serve at that high rank in the US uniformed services.[5]

Levine was born in Wakefield, Massachusetts. Both of her parents were lawyers. She attended Hebrew School and graduated from the Belmont, Massachusetts Hill Boy's School. She subsequently earned degrees from Harvard College and Tulane University School of Medicine and completed her residency in pediatrics and a fellowship in adolescent medicine at New York City's Mt. Sinai Medical Center.[6] In 1993, Levine began working as faculty at the Penn State College of Medicine, where she served as the director of Pediatrics and Adolescent Medicine at the Poly-Clinic Medical Center.[7] From 1996 to 2015, she directed Pediatric Ambulatory Services and Adolescent Medicine at the Penn State Hershey Medical Center, where she oversaw development of the adolescent and young adult eating disorder program. She also worked as the faculty adviser for the university's LGBT student group and as the LGBT affairs liaison at Penn State Hershey's Office of Diversity.[8]

She served as physician general for the Commonwealth of Pennsylvania from 2015, and Pennsylvania Secretary of Health from March 2018, until her nomination for Assistant Secretary at Health and Human Services.[9] In her position as Pennsylvania Secretary of Health, Levine led the commonwealth's response to the COVID-19 crisis from its outbreak until January 2021. She drew both praise and criticism related to her handling of the COVID-19 crisis in Pennsylvania.[10] She has published widely in the medical literature on topics including gender dysphoria, genetics, and strategies for medical training about eating disorders and opioids.[11]

Levine publicly transitioned in 2008–2011: "Around 2008, she started to grow out her hair and in 2010 she came out as transgender. Her transition was slow and deliberate, as well as full of research. She slowly came out to her close family, and lastly to her elderly mother, who was nothing but accepting and full of love for her daughter."[12]

During her tenure in Pennsylvania, Levine was ridiculed because of her transgender status. On July 22, 2020, Governor Tom Wolf released a statement in response to an incident at Bloomsburg Fair in which he said:

> Dr. Levine is a distinguished and accomplished public servant. She is committed to keeping Pennsylvanians safe and healthy, even those who direct hate-fueled attacks at her. I'm proud of the work she has done in her five years serving Pennsylvanians, and her success at leading our commonwealth during the COVID-19 crisis is a testament to her intelligence and work ethic.
>
> Hate has no place in Pennsylvania, even in the smallest transphobic joke, action, or social media post. I'm calling upon all Pennsylvanians to speak out against hateful comments and acts, including the transphobia directed at Dr. Levine and all Transgender people in our great commonwealth.[13]

Levine's high position in the administration of President Joe Biden subjected her to further harassment. During her confirmation hearings, Senator Rand Paul (Republican from Kentucky) characterized gender-affirming surgery as genital mutilation and accused her of supporting "surgical destruction of a minor's genitalia."[14] Representative Jim Banks (Republican from Indiana) tweeted, regarding Levine's promotion, "The title of first female four-star officer gets taken by a man."[15] His Twitter account was subsequently suspended.[16] Levine continues to experience transphobic attacks. For example, on March 17, 2022, Twitter flagged a post by Texas Attorney General Ken Paxton for violating its rules about hateful conduct when Paxton referred to Levine as a man.[17]

Levine, an extraordinarily accomplished woman who chose to live authentically, inspires us to improve access to inclusive healthcare for all US citizens.

NOTES

1. Diamond and Schmidt, "Rachel Levine, Historic Transgender Nominee, confirmed as Assistant Health Secretary."
2. US Senate, "Question," 2021.

3. Srikanth, "Rachel Levine Could Be the First Transgender Official."
4. Casey, "Dr. Rachel Levine Is Now First Trans 4-Star Admiral in U.S. History."
5. Casey, "Dr. Rachel Levine Is Now First Trans 4-Star Admiral in U.S. History."
6. Brandman, "Rachel Levine."
7. Brandman, "Rachel Levine."
8. Equality Forum, "LGBT History Month."
9. Wolf, "Gov. Wolf Issues Statement on Hate"; Brandman, "Rachel Levine"; Equality Forum, "LGBT History Month."
10. Rubinkam, "Biden Picks Rachel Levine."
11. PennState, "Penn State Research Team Advances Health Equity in Pennsylvania." Accessed August 6, 2024. https://www.psu.edu/news/academics/story/penn-state-research-team-advances-health-equity-pennsylvania/.
12. Zezima, "Meet Rachel Levine."
13. Wolf, "Gov. Wolf Issues Statement on Hate."
14. Avery and Yurcaba, "Rand Paul Criticized."
15. Lange, "Rep. Jim Banks Faces Criticism." Banks's tweet was not accurate. The first female four-star officer was Ann Elizabeth Dunwoody, who, on November 14, 2008, earned a promotion to four-star general in the US Army. See also, Tyson, "Army Promotes Its First Female Four-Star General."
16. Kesslin, "Rep. Jim Banks Suspended."
17. Huber, "Twitter flags AG Paxton's Tweet."

WORKS CITED

Avery, Dan, and Jo Yurcaba. "Rand Paul Criticized for Trans "Gender Mutilation" Remarks in Rachel Levine hearing. *NBC News*, February 26, 2021. Accessed May 31, 2022. https://www.nbcnews.com/feature/nbc-out/rand-paul-criticized-trans-gender-mutilation-remarks-rachel-levine-hearing-n1259004.

Brandman, Mariana. "Rachel Levine." n.d. National Women's History Museum. Accessed October 11, 2022. https://www.womenshistory.org/education-resources/biographies/rachel-levine.

Casey, John. "Dr. Rachel Levine is Now First Trans 4-Star Admiral in U.S. History." *Advocate*, October 19, 2021. Accessed May 28, 2022. https://www.advocate.com/news/2021/10/19/dr-rachel-levine-now-first-trans-4-star-admiral-us-history.

Diamond, Dan, and Samantha Schmidt. "Rachel Levine, Historic Transgender Nominee, Confirmed as Assistant Health Secretary." *Washington Post*, March 24, 2021. Accessed October 11, 2022. https://www.washingtonpost.com/health/2021/03/24/rachel-levine-confirmed/.

Department of Health and Human Services. "Admiral Rachel L. Levine, Assistant Secretary for Health (ASH)." March 8, 2022. Accessed October 11, 2022. https://www.hhs.gov/about/leadership/rachel-levine.html.

Equality Forum. "LGBT History Month—October 22: Rachel Levine." QnotesCarolinas, October 22, 2018. Accessed May 28, 2022. https://qnotescarolinas.com/lgbt-history-month-october-22-rachel-levine/.

Huber, Craig. "Twitter Flags AG Paxton's Tweet about Rachel Levine as Hateful, Leaves It Accessible." *Spectrum News 1 (Texas)*, March 18, 2022. Accessed May 31, 2022. https://spectrumlocalnews.com/tx/south-texas-el-paso/news/2022/03/18/twitter-flags-ag-paxton-s-tweet-about-rachel-levine-as-hateful--leaves-it-accessible.

Kesslen, Ben. (2021, 24 October). "Rep. Jim Banks Suspended from Twitter for Misgendering Trans Government Official Rachel Levine." *NBC News*, October 24, 2021. Accessed May 31, 2022. https://www.nbcnews.com/nbc-out/out-news/rep-jim-banks-suspended-twitter-misgendering-trans-government-official-dr-n1282233.

Lange, Kaitlin. "Rep. Jim Banks Faces Criticism for Tweets about First Transgender Four-Star Officer." *Indianapolis Star*, October 19, 2021. Accessed May 31, 2022. https://www.indystar.com/story/news/politics/2021/10/19/rep-jim-banks-faces-criticism-tweets-dr-rachel-levine/8528034002/.

PennState. "Research Output: Rachel Levine." n.d. Accessed May 30, 2022. https://pennstate.pure.elsevier.com/en/searchAll/index/?search=rachel+levine&pageSize=25&showAdvanced=false&allConcepts=true&inferConcepts=true&searchBy=PartOfNameOrTitle.

Reynolds, Daniel. (2020, March 31). "Meet the Transgender Doctor Leading Pennsylvania's COVID-19 Response." *Advocate*, March 31, 2020. Accessed May 28, 2022. https://www.advocate.com/health/2020/3/30/meet-transgender-doctor-leading-pennsylvanias-covid-19-response.

Rubinkam, Michael. "Biden Picks Rachel Levine, Who Drew Credit and Criticism for Handling of PA's COVID-19 Crisis, as Assistant Health Secretary." *Associated Press*, January 19, 2021. Accessed May 31, 2022. https://www.mcall.com/news/breaking/mc-nws-dr-rachel-levine-chosen-as-assistant-health-secretary-20210119-pr6jvc6fsbhiljgzigcswr47eu-story.html.

Srikanth, Anagha. "Rachel Levine Could Be the First Transgender Official Confirmed by Congress. Who Is She?" *The Hill*, January 19, 202. Accessed May 28, 2022. https://thehill.com/changing-america/respect/diversity-inclusion/534777-rachel-levine-could-be-the-first-transgender/.

Tyson, Ann Scott. "Army Promotes its First Female Four-Star General." *Washington Post*, November 15, 2008. Accessed Oct 11, 2022. https://www.washingtonpost.com/wp-dyn/content/article/2008/11/14/AR2008111400259.html?hpid=sec-nation.

US Senate. "Question: On the Nomination (Confirmation: Rachel Leland Levine, of Pennsylvania, to be an Assistant Secretary of Health and Human Services." Roll Call Vote 117th Congress—1st Session, March 24, 2021. Accessed May 28, 2022. https://www.senate.gov/legislative/LIS/roll_call_votes/vote1171/vote_117_1_00134.htm.

Zezima, Katie. (2016, 1 June). "Meet Rachel Levine, One of the Very Few Transgender Public Officials in America." *Washington Post*, June 1, 2016. Accessed June 30, 2022. https://www.washingtonpost.com/politics/meet-rachel-levine-one-of-the-very-few-transgender-public-officials-in-america/2016/06/01/cf6e2332-2415-11e6-8690-f14ca9de2972_story.html.

Wolf, Tom. "Gov. Wolf Issues Statement on Hate Targeting Transgender Pennsylvanians." WJACTV. July 22, 2020. Accessed August 6, 2024. https://wjactv.com/news/local/gov-wolf-gives-statement-on-hate-targeting-transgender-pennsylvanians.

17

CHANGING THE BODY TO MATCH THE MIND
The Development of Gender-Affirming Surgery in the United States

Carolyn Wolf-Gould

So, why change one's body?[1] Possibly because the body is where we live and through it we communicate to others. The reactions our bodies receive from others affects how we interact. I wanted to change my body because I felt invisible. In a female body, I felt as if I couldn't fully exist, as if the masculine part of me was compressed inside me to a degree that was not just uncomfortable, but downright painful. We all have hidden components of our personality or selves that we either want to protect or yearn to have others see. We each have to find the balance for ourselves, bringing out those hidden attributes or somehow finding that place of comfort in our own skins, in our own lives. We all want to find fulfillment. For some people that means something as simple as changing hairstyles or driving a certain car, for others it means serious exercising and buying a new wardrobe. For still others it means giving up a boring job and attempting to change careers or going back to school to get that degree. For some people it means adopting a new religious practice or confirming the one in which we were raised. For others it means adopting an androgynous or overtly confrontational style of dress and grooming. For some of us it means changing our sex visibly, legally, internally, and externally—fundamentally and dramatically changing our bodies.

Surgery is not what transness is ultimately about. Transness is about life. It's about relationships, and not just intimate ones. Being a trans person is not something we do in the privacy of our own bedrooms; it affects every aspect of our lives, from our driver's licenses to our work histories, from our birth certificates to our school transcripts to our parents' wills, and every relationship represented by those paper trails. Still, for many of us, surgery is a crucial part of managing our gender incongruence.[2]

—Jamison Green, 2020

Human external genitalia are ambisexual (of indeterminate gender) until nine weeks gestational age, when the penis and clitoris form from the same genital tubercle, depending on the absence or presence of specific sex hormones.[3] Similarly, the scrotum and labia emerge from the same embryologic labioscrotal folds. During gender-affirming procedures, surgeons alter the form of these homologous structures to maintain function in the neogenitalia and create an aesthetic result. The glans of the penis, with its collection of sensitive nerve endings, becomes the similarly sensitive clitoris. The clitoris is either transformed into a small phallus (metoidioplasty) or placed at the base of a neophallus to preserve erotic sensation. Labial tissue is converted into a scrotum. We spring into this world as anatomical products of the same (miraculous) embryologic process—and for a gender surgeon, the penis and vagina are fundamentally more alike than different.

Transgender people wished to alter their bodies long before surgeons knew safe and effective techniques to assist them. Descriptions of eunuchs exist worldwide since ancient times, and castration (orchiectomy, penectomy, or some combination of both) was often a forced procedure to eliminate sexual/reproductive function or preserve a soprano voice.[4] In some cultures, transgender people, like the *hijra* of India, availed themselves of this procedure.[5]

The first documented account of an individual requesting gender surgery involved the Roman Emperor, Marcus Aurelius Antoninus (204–222 AD), posthumously named Elagabalus due to her devotion to the deity Elagabal.[6] Elagabalus assumed the throne at age fourteen.[7] Historians describe her four-year rule as notable for decadence, excess, zealotry, and transgressive sexual behaviors and gender presentations.[8] She allowed women into the Senate chambers.[9] She removed Jupiter from the head of the Roman Pantheon, replacing him with the alien Sun God, Elagabal—angering the Senate, the Praetorian

Guard, and the Roman people.[10] She exhibited feminine mannerisms and married four women and two men, one a chariot driver named Hierocles.[11] Elagabalus relished being called Hierocles's mistress, wife, and queen.[12] She wore makeup and wigs, preferred to be called a lady rather than a lord, and offered vast sums to any physician who could surgically alter her body and equip her with a vagina.[13]

The first known case of surgical gender reassignment dates back to first century BC.[14] Diodorus Siculus recorded the story of this individual, Callo, in *Bibliotheca Historica*:

> Callo [was] supposed to be a girl. Now the orifice with which women are provided, had in her case no opening. . . . She had from birth a perforation through which she excreted liquid residues . . . since she was incapable of intercourse as a woman, was obliged to submit to unnatural embraces. Later a tumor appeared on her genitals and . . . a doctor was called in. He cut into the swollen area, whereupon a man's privates protruded. He took steps to remedy the remaining deficiencies. First of all, cutting into the glans he made a passage into the urethra and using a silver catheter drew off the liquid residues. Then, by scarifying the perforated area he brought the parts together. Callo laid aside her loom-shuttles and all other instruments of women's work and taking in their stead the garb and status of a man changed her name to Callon.[15]

Contemporary clinicians attribute the findings in this case to a disorder of sexual development—specifically male pseudohermaphroditism, which led to ambiguous genitalia and a concealed penis.[16]

Gender-affirming surgical care in the United States commenced when American patients with a drive to transition approached doctors, specifically ones who listened, empathized, and agreed to attempt surgical procedures that theretofore were only offered overseas. The first gender surgeries took place in the 1920s at Magnus Hirschfeld's Institute for Sexual Science in Berlin. In 1952, after medically and surgically transitioning in Denmark, Christine Jorgensen returned to the United States, inspiring transgender Americans to request surgical transitions at home. Initially, US surgeons were reluctant to offer care for many reasons, but the country has moved beyond its turbulent beginnings; as of 2019, twenty-three major centers offered gender-affirming surgery,[17] and at this writing, a patient-focused website lists ninety-seven surgeons who perform vaginoplasty, seventy who perform phalloplasty, and hundreds who perform top (chest/breast), voice, facial, and body contouring procedures.[18] The history of chest/breast and body-affirming procedures would also offer important insights but is beyond the scope of this volume.[19] This chapter will review gender-affirming genital and facial surgical history from the early beginnings, to the present, and through to the evolving future—a process that has involved thousands of surgeons from multiple subspecialties across the globe.

THE EMERGENCE OF FEMINIZING SURGICAL PROCEDURES

Within increasingly tolerant pre-World War II Germany, Berlin became fertile ground for the first surgical change of sex. Hirschfeld opened the Institute for Sexual Science in Berlin in March 1919 and spent the next fourteen years describing and attempting to help patients who met his new diagnostic term *transsexual*. Dora "Dorchen" Richter (1891–1933), a patient who received hormone therapy from Hirschfeld, underwent orchiectomy in 1921 and, in 1931, became the first patient to request and submit to penectomy and vaginoplasty, under the care of Ludwig Levy-Lenz and Erwing Gohrbandt, respectively.[20] Felix Abraham, a psychiatrist who worked at the Institute, published an account of Richter's procedure as part of two case studies. The castration had the effect—albeit not extensive—of making her body fuller, restricting her beard growth, making visible the first signs of breast growth, and giving the fat pad a more feminine shape.[21] Abraham also described the new vaginoplasty procedure, which involved creating a space for the neovagina by separating the muscles of the perineum and lining the space with skin grafts from the upper leg. The surgeon stitched sponges in place to ensure the patency of the vaginal canal as it healed.[22] Abraham concluded this paper by stating, "It was not easy for us to decide on the described procedures, but the patients were not to be dismissed and were also in a mental state that made it probable that self-mutilation, with life-endangering complications, could be possible. . . . This surgery was . . . a kind of emergency surgery necessary to save patients from worse self-inflicted procedures."[23]

Niels Hoyer's widely published book *Man into Woman*[24] contains semi-autobiographical accounts of Lili Elbe's surgical transition in the early 1930s. Elbe too first underwent orchiectomy under the care of Gohrbandt in Berlin[25] and, later, a penectomy and implantation of an ovary by Kurt Warnekros at the Dresden Municipal Women's Clinic.[26] Hoyer's portrayal of Elbe's sudden and miraculous metamorphosis to female after removal of her testes was not physiologically accurate but caught the attention of both cis and transgender people. Accounts of her experience also inspired the trope of the gender surgeon as larger than life, even God-like. Hoyer described one of Elbe's experiences with her surgeon: "What power radiated from this strange person? Here in the Women's Clinic was a god whom all feared, whom all revered. In what did his power consist? . . . I was only one of the many who believed in this man through the mere force of belief, who believed in the helper in him through their belief in some kind of helper."[27] In 1931, Elbe returned to Dresden for her last operation—possibly a vaginoplasty, although popular mythology claims uterine transplant.[28] Elbe died of complications related to her surgery; historians have suggested heart attack, kidney disease, appendicitis, and cancer.[29] She was buried in the Trinitatis Cemetery, near her cherished Dresden women's clinic.

Upon Adolf Hitler's election as Germany's chancellor in 1933, nonbinary gender expression and homosexuality came under attack. Hitler's regime viewed the increasing LGBT visibility in Berlin under the Weimar Republic as particularly loathsome and evinced special hatred for Hirschfeld, an out gay man, a Jew, and a doctor who specialized in human sexuality. Just three months after Hitler's election, a mob looted and burned Hirschfeld's Sexual Institute and its records.[30] Widely published photographs of this conflagration illustrate Germany under Nazi rule, but few know that these images depict the historical erasure of Hirschfeld's defining work with transsexual people—and the lives of transsexual people who told their stories to Hirschfeld.[31] When this atrocity occurred, Hirschfeld was on a world tour; he realized he couldn't return to Germany. Sexologists Max Marcuse, Eugen Steinach, Ludwig Levy-Lenz, and other clinician-scholars of Jewish descent also fled the county.[32] Hirschfeld died on his sixty-seventh birthday in 1935, still in exile, in Nice. In contrast to the experience of their Jewish peers, physicians Gohrbandt and Warnekros connected with the National Socialist Party. Gorhbandt later joined the Luftwaffe as chief medical advisor and participated in the grisly medical experiments performed at Dachau.[33]

In the 1950s, several surgeons across the globe experimented with feminizing genital surgeries. Sir Archibald McIndoe (1900–1960),[34] a New Zealand surgeon who settled in Britain and became a mentee of Sir Harold Gillies, developed the McIndoe vaginoplasty for cisgender women with vaginal atresia or stenosis. His procedure involved suturing split-thickness skin grafts[35] around a tubular form, which he then inserted into a space dissected between the bladder and the rectum.[36] Some later gender surgeons briefly adapted this technique, using full-thickness grafts[37] to avoid postoperative constriction of the vaginal canal and prolonged use of internal forms.[38] In 1951, Gillies performed one of the earliest vaginoplasty operations on Roberta Cowell, employing his newly conceived foreskin and penile skin inversion method to create a rudimentary vagina. Georges Burou (1910–1987) independently developed the same anterior pedicle flap[39] prototype in 1956, a procedure referred to as the penile inversion vaginoplasty.[40] Burou, a gynecologist by training, achieved legendary status practicing genital surgery for trans women in Casablanca, Morocco, from the late 1950s until the mid-1970s.[41] Burou profited from increased demand for his services after European countries backed away from performing these procedures.

Jorgensen traveled to Denmark in 1950 where first she received hormone therapy and then underwent a series of demasculinizing operations that included orchiectomy in 1950 and penectomy in 1951.[42] In 1954, after her return to the United States, Jorgensen underwent vaginoplasty under the direction of Joseph Angelo (the husband of one of her classmates at the Manhattan Medical and Dental Assistant School) and Harry Benjamin.[43] After Jorgenson's publicized return to the United States in 1952, transgender Americans reached out to her Danish physicians for care, but the Copenhagen team was unable to meet the demand. During the 1950s and 1960s, transsexualism was considered a male condition, and surgical requests largely came from transgender women seeking vaginoplasty. Soon afterward, Danish authorities closed the country to transgender medical tourists.[44]

In the United States at this time, the mayhem statutes prohibited orchiectomy in all fifty states. While searching for surgical care for his patients, Benjamin reached out to psychiatrist Frederik Hartsuiker in Holland, an expert in prescribing castration for sex offenders.[45] A skeptic, Hartsuiker eventually engaged the services of Amsterdam surgeon H. C. Koch, Jr., but only for demasculinization (castration and penectomy), as feminizing surgeries were then prohibited in the Netherlands.[46] This connection ended in 1955 when Dutch clinicians and hospitals decided that care of foreign transsexuals was no longer their responsibility.[47] Stymied for options, those who could afford the expense traveled for surgery, usually to the "hush hush clinics" in Mexico or to Burou in Casablanca.[48]

In 1965, the Johns Hopkins Hospital in Baltimore opened the Moore Clinic, the first US university-affiliated institution for gender-affirming healthcare.[49]

Respect for Johns Hopkins as a hospital and academic center suddenly legitimized gender surgery and ended prohibition by the mayhem statutes. Soon, other academic centers opened gender programs across the nation. The clinicians intended to provide medical care, including sex reassignment surgery, and to study the scientific, ethical, religious, and legal ramifications of medical care for transsexuals.[50] The founding members of this program included Milton T. Edgerton and John Hoopes (both plastic surgeons), Howard Jones (gynecology), Horst Schirmer (urology), John Money (psychologist), Norman Knorr (psychiatry), and Claude Migeon (endocrinology).[51]

For vaginoplasty, the Hopkins surgeons employed a two-stage technique with a penile inversion pedicle flap, the glans penis simulating the cervix at the apex of the vagina, and scrotal strips fashioned into labia majora.[52] The description of their procedure included no effort to ensure clitoral sensation/sexual function or create aesthetic vulvar anatomy, improvements that came after the advent of microsurgical techniques. Maryland Blue Cross covered part of the surgical costs, but most insurance companies refused to pay for procedures.[53] Few who sought surgery could pay out of pocket. In 1970, a vaginoplasty cost approximately $1,200, a fee split by the plastic surgeon, gynecologist, and urologist. The hospital charged patients $125 per day for the typical twenty-five-day postoperative course.

Few patients received gender-affirming surgery. They faced a lengthy and complex evaluation process as they attempted to meet Hopkins' strict surgical requirements.[54] By 1972, only sixteen transgender women and seven transgender men had received primary gender-affirming procedures at Hopkins, despite evaluation of more than 2,400 transsexuals.[55] Modern Hopkins clinicians suggest that the clinic's main contribution to the field was in demonstrating the value of having a team approach to evaluation and care, including input from clinicians in medicine, mental health, and surgery.[56] In 1983, at his address as the incoming president of the Harry Benjamin International Gender Dysphoria Association, Edgerton recommended this interdisciplinary approach as the mainstay of care. He urged physicians to withhold judgment of transsexual patients until they have had experience with "these desperate and complex patients."[57] He reassured doubting colleagues by observing that very few patients regretted "sex-change surgery," even with complications.[58]

In 1979, Paul McHugh became the head of the psychiatry department with the expressed intention of ending the gender surgical program.[59] He cited a recently published paper by Jon Meyer and Donna Reter, which suggested that "sex reassignment surgery confers no objective advantage in terms of social rehabilitation" as one of the reasons to close the Hopkins gender program.[60] While the decision to close the clinic was heavily influenced by this paper (immediately viewed by many as biased and inaccurate), problems regarding the lack of stable funding, failure to reimburse physicians and staff for their time, trouble with administrative personnel, and difficulty in finding patients who could afford surgery also contributed.[61] Dozens of university centers across the country followed suit, closing their doors on an increasingly desperate trans community.[62]

It was in this setting, that John Ronald Brown (1922–2010) emerged to fill a surgical void. Brown, the son of a Mormon physician, graduated from the University of Utah Medical School in 1947 with a degree in general practice.[63] For the next twenty years he served as a general practitioner in California, Alaska, Hawaii, and the Marshall Islands and then elected to pursue surgical training. He attended a residency program in plastic surgery at New York's Columbia-Presbyterian Hospital but, to his disappointment, never achieved certification from the American Board of Plastic Surgery, a deficiency that prevented him from gaining hospital surgical privileges.

Brown set out to work in San Francisco in the early 1970s, operating in a few rooms off a busy street and assisted by an ex-con without medical training, referred to as Dr. James Spence.[64] Brown ignored the criteria for surgery imposed by the gender clinics and operated on anyone who requested care and had the money, regardless of their emotional or physical stability. He allowed unlicensed people (including other transsexual patients) to write prescriptions under his name, diagnose patients, and provide clinical care. He lied on insurance forms and failed to hospitalize patients with life-threatening complications. Most in the trans community acknowledged that Brown had significant faults—for example, he had no common sense; he walked into doors and could not balance his checkbook—but some patients praised his results, his accessibility, and his $2,500 charge for a vaginoplasty.[65] Brown distributed an advertising brochure, claiming: "John Brown pussies are the prettiest pussies . . . 99% orgasmic . . . natural appearance."[66] Most patients remained unaware of his incompetence. Contemporary surgeons, including Jack Fisher, a plastic surgeon with the University of California San Diego, who cared for Brown's failed cases, concluded: "He's a terrible, appalling, technical surgeon. . . . He doesn't know how to make a straight incision . . . hold a knife . . . no regard for limiting blood loss. [He has] been committing crimes against humanity for years."[67] In 1977, the California Board of Medical Quality Assurance revoked Brown's license for "gross negligence, incompetence and practicing unprofessional medicine in a manner which involved moral turpitude."[68]

Later that year, Brown claimed that God spoke to him one evening as he walked on his ranch. "You should know that the details of your life have been arranged so that you would be where you are now, doing what you are doing. . . . What you are doing is appreciated because these are my children, too."[69] Brown believed God was referring to his work with transsexuals and continued to perform gender surgeries underground, living in Southern California but operating in Mexico. Activist Dallas Denny warned the trans community of his dangerous practices for years, referring to him as Tabletop Brown because of his willingness to perform surgery in "motel rooms and on kitchen tables leaving his victim to wake up in the back seat of her car or on a couch in an abandoned house."[70] Patients complained of botched surgeries, and videos later found in Brown's home revealed his deadly practices.[71] Lin Fraser, a psychotherapist and international expert in gender dysphoria, witnessed Brown perform a surgery in a San Francisco garage.[72] After being convicted in 1991 for operating without a license,[73] Brown spent nineteen months in prison but emerged undeterred. He stopped practicing only after his conviction for the 1998 murder of Phillip Bondy, an elderly New Yorker who paid Brown ten thousand dollars to amputate his healthy leg to satisfy a sexual fetish.[74] Brown was extradited from Mexico to the United States, convicted of second-degree murder, and sentenced to fifteen years in prison, where he remained until his death in 2010.

During this time, Stanley Biber (1923–2006) emerged as the most popular gender surgeon in the world. Biber was born in Des Moines, Iowa, to Jewish parents who hoped he would become a rabbi. Instead, he followed his dream and became a general surgeon. He graduated from the University of Iowa Medical School in 1948, completed his residency in the Panama Canal Zone, and then joined the US Army, where he served as chief surgeon in a mobile army surgical hospital in the Korean conflict.[75] In 1956, Biber accepted a position as a staff physician at the United Mine Workers Clinic in the tiny town of Trinidad, Colorado (population nine thousand), an opportunity that allowed him to purchase a ranch and ride in cattle drives while working as a small-town general surgeon. There, Biber gained the trust of the citizenry as he set bones, replaced hips, removed gallbladders, and delivered babies at Mount Saint Rafael Hospital, a Catholic institution run by nuns. Biber latched on to Old West values, favoring blue jeans, bulky silver belt buckles, and pickup trucks.[76] Martin Smith described Biber as a "cowboy with a scalpel," a "short, avuncular surgeon, a former weightlifter, [who] looked a bit like a cannonball with glasses."[77] Biber cared for his patients in a humble office, accessed via a wheezy, rattletrap elevator, in the upper story of Trinidad's First Bank, a building described by Smith as tenement-like, with flaking paint.[78]

In 1969, a local social worker and friend came out to Biber—who had to ask her to explain what she meant by the term *transsexual*—and asked him to perform her vaginoplasty.[79] Although he listened with surprise, he was confident of his ability to learn new surgical techniques and tentatively agreed to take on this project.[80] He consulted Benjamin and requested references from John Hoopes at Johns Hopkins; these likely included Burou's sketches of his penile inversion procedure. (See Figure 4.1 in this volume.) One imagines Biber, scalpel in hand, shifting his gaze from his patient's perineum to the drawing at his side—Study. Cut. Cauterize. Study again. He denuded the penis, inverted the skin on an abdominal flap to create a vagina, pushed it into the space that he dissected between the bladder and rectum, and sutured the distal end of his tube to the prostatic pedicle.[81] He fashioned the surrounding tissue into a vulva. "It looked like hell," he reported to *Rocky Mountain News* in 2004. "It was terrible. But it functioned, and she was very happy with it because it functioned."[82]

Biber's early surgeries (and later Donald Laub's)[83] lacked the technical elegance of skilled surgeons today. In 1998, Biber and Laub described their penile inversion technique, which, like the Hopkin's method, placed the glans of the penis (which resembles the shape of the cervix) in the position of cervix uteri.[84] They made no mention of attempts to preserve orgasmic response and fashioned the clitoris, not from the glans (as is done today), but from the erectile tissue that previously surrounded the urethra.[85] Over time, as Biber treated more patients and refined his techniques, his reputation for compassionate care and good outcomes spread by word of mouth throughout the global trans community.

With the closure of the Johns Hopkins gender clinic and other university centers after 1979 and the retirement of Burou in Morocco, rural Trinidad became the primary location worldwide for transgender surgery. During his thirty-five-year career, Biber performed more than five thousand gender surgeries (vaginoplasty, phalloplasty, and facial feminization).[86] In the 1990s, newspaper articles estimated he had performed sixty percent of the world's sex-change surgeries.[87] At first, he saw only trans women but had a fifty–fifty mix of transfeminine and transmasculine patients by the end of his career.[88]

Biber kept his work hidden at first, concealing the files for his first few cases in a safe in the hospital administrator's office. But as his number of transsexual patients swelled, he realized he needed the support of his hospital and the town.[89] He offered a series of lectures describing the "transsexual phenomenon" as a medical condition that deserved compassion. Trinidad's population reacted with mixed feelings, but most welcomed the influx of medical tourists and their cash.[90] Although no documentation exists to support this claim, a popular story in Trinidad reported that in 1969, Biber received a special dispensation from Pope Paul VI to perform gender surgeries at his Catholic institution.[91] Whether true or not, this tale calmed the locals. Biber's work also helped keep the hospital solvent and local businesses raked in cash from his patients.[92] As Biber entered his eighties, patients complained that his age started to show.[93] Several gender surgeons trained with Biber, and he handpicked one of his protégés—gynecologist Marci Bowers—to take over his gender surgical practice.

Bowers graduated from the University of Minnesota in 1986, completed her residency in obstetrics and gynecology, and joined the Polyclinic and Swedish Medical Center in Seattle to begin a thriving practice, eventually rising to become the chief of her department.[94] She began her gender transition after 1996, while serving as chief, and received staggering scrutiny from colleagues.[95] Bowers first visited Biber's practice on May 25, 2000, a day the *Associated Press* proclaimed Trinidad "the Sex Change Capital."[96] She watched Bieber perform a vaginoplasty.

In 2003, Bowers moved to Trinidad to begin working with Biber, first to learn and then to improve upon his technique—particularly around genital sensitivity—by creating a homologous clitoris from available erectile tissue.[97] "'Some didn't have the hands. Some didn't have the courage. Some didn't have the heart.' When I finally came," said Bowers, "he said 'Marci is the only one to have all three.'"[98] In mid-2003, Biber's malpractice carrier suddenly closed, and Bowers became the first transgender surgeon to complete solo vaginoplasty.[99]

Bowers's status as a transgender woman was not explained to the local townspeople before her arrival and, as is typical for doctors who take over another's practice, most in Trinidad expected Bowers to replicate Biber's unconventional style. Although unconventional, Bowers was not a swashbuckling cowboy, driving cattle on her days off. She was sophisticated, a feminist with an immense personal investment in her work, and she began to employ her nimble hands, intelligence, lived experience, and new fame, not only to refine and innovate surgical techniques but also to change the hearts and minds of a nation that disregarded transgender people. Bowers not only advanced surgical outcomes in Trinidad but also worked with the media to bring trans healthcare into the spotlight. She operated on approximately 110–120 patients per year.[100] After Biber's death in 2006, Bowers struggled with administrators at Mount Saint Rafael Hospital, who objected to the increased publicity, among other concerns. In 2010, Bowers left Trinidad to open a practice in Burlingame, California, ending Trinidad's forty-one-year stint as the sex change capital of the world.

Like Biber and Brown, Laub also began offering gender-affirming surgical care during the 1970s. In 1968, he cofounded Stanford's early gender dysphoria program with psychiatrist Norman Fisk. Laub, a Marquette University Medical School graduate, specialized in plastic surgery, recognized the specific needs of transgender patients, and developed several important new surgical options for transfeminine and transmasculine people. For trans women, he pioneered the rectosigmoid vaginoplasty—which he dubbed the "Rolls Royce vagina"—by creating the vaginal vault with a section of the sigmoid colon. This allowed for a well-lubricated vagina with significantly increased girth as compared to the penile inversion technique that he dismissed as the "Volkswagen vagina."[101] But time exposed the pitfalls of this approach, namely greater invasiveness, higher complication rates, the requirement for postoperative colon screening, excessive mucous production, and less convincing visual appearance. Currently, most US gender surgeons consider rectosigmoid vaginoplasty a secondary or salvage procedure.

By the end of the twentieth century, transgender people found more options for gender-affirming surgical care. During this time, a still small but increasing number of surgeons offered care in North America. Eugene Schrang (Neenah, Wisconsin) and Toby Meltzer (Scottsdale, Arizona) developed sizable practices in the United States. Yvon Ménard and later Pierre Brassard provided surgery for US citizens (and those from other countries) in Montreal, Canada.[102] The World Professional Association for Transgender Health's *Standards of Care* recommended clear steps for psychological assessment before surgery. Transgender people created online forums to discuss their surgical results and experience with their surgeon, and trans activists began to establish expectations about quality and cultural competency. Transgender clinicians began to enter the field in greater numbers, with a focus on normalizing the trans experience and facilitating access to improved care.

The first who translated her transgender status into an opportunity to better the lives of other trans persons via education was Sheila Kirk (1930–2019). Kirk, a graduate of Boston University School of Medicine, specialized in gynecology. In 1996, she published several landmark health resource books on feminizing hormones, masculinizing hormones, and a guide for physicians.[103] She also coauthored a book on transgender HIV care.[104] She became the first transgender surgeon to serve on the board of the Harry Benjamin International Gender Dysphoria Association and coauthored the sixth edition of the World Professional Association for Transgender Health's *Standards of Care*.[105] She served as a founding member of the International Foundation for Gender Education and, in 1998 at age sixty-eight, opened the Transgender Surgical and Medical Center in Pittsburgh, Pennsylvania.[106] Although short-lived, the center was the first to be established by a transgender woman. In coordination with plastic surgeons J. William Furtrell and Ernest Manders, the center offered trans-affirming counseling, gynecological care, and a narrow repertoire of gender-affirming surgical procedures.[107] Kirk might have assisted with some of these surgeries but did not perform them herself.

Surgeons from around the globe continued to refine vaginoplasty techniques in the later twentieth and early twenty-first centuries. Differences in functional approaches tended to highlight aesthetic differences. Patients expected to be orgasmic, avoid urinary complications, attain a depth of at least ten centimeters, have an aesthetic appearance, and suffer only a narrow range of minor complications. S. Shan Ratnam performed the first vaginoplasty in Singapore in 1971 and later opened his Gender Identity Clinic at the National University Hospital.[108] In Thailand in 1975, Preecha Tiewtranon and Prakob Thongpeaw performed the first vaginoplasty at Chulalongkorn University Hospital.[109] Tiewtranon trained most of the one hundred existing vaginoplasty surgeons in Thailand. From 1975 to 2013, Tiewtranon and his team performed three thousand vaginoplasties, refining a technique over decades that achieved a result close to that of a cisgender woman in terms of cosmesis and functionality.[110] American plastic surgeon Bangalore Jayaram and colleagues published one of the case series on complications and undesirable results of vaginoplasty, problems they attributed to faulty surgical techniques and poor postoperative follow-up, due to the need to travel for surgeries.[111] At this time, no guidelines existed, and papers like this became the impetus for developing standards of care. In the early 1980s, Belgian surgeon Stan Monstrey joined the small gender team at the University of Ghent to become a leading clinician, researcher, and educator for feminizing and masculinizing surgeries.[112] Similarly, Dutch plastic surgeon, J. Joris Hage practiced and published numerous articles on improving gender surgical techniques.[113] In 1992, Chinese surgeon R. H. Fang introduced the concept of dorsal nerve preservation in male-to-female vaginoplasty, allowing homologous (same anatomical derivation as the cisgender clitoris) clitoral sensation.[114] In 2019, Suporn Watanyusakul, also from Thailand, described techniques that improve the vulvar aesthetic appearance.[115] Several teams developed techniques to create a mucosal lining for the neovagina, including the use of oral mucosal grafts or the use of cultured autologous oral epithelial cells.[116] More recently, Adam Jacoby and colleagues described the Davydov technique, a revolutionary robotic vaginoplasty that employs a peritoneal flap to effect an increase in vaginal depth in patients with insufficient genital skin.[117]

MASCULINIZING SURGICAL PROCEDURES

Physician Alan Hart underwent the first masculinizing surgery in the United States in 1910, a hysterectomy performed by Joshua Gilbert at the University of Oregon.[118] Gilbert's publication about Hart brought discussion of transmasculine healthcare to US physicians.

Most transgender men seek top surgery as part of gender transition, with fewer opting for bottom surgeries, including hysterectomy, metoidioplasty, and phalloplasty. Phalloplasty is one of the more challenging procedures in reconstructive surgery and has a higher complication rate than other gender-affirming procedures. Hage and colleagues defined the ideal goals of phalloplasty as:

> [T]he construction in a one-stage operation of an aesthetically pleasing neo-phallus with erogenous and tactile sensation, permitting the patient to void while standing and to engage in sexual intercourse like a natural man. The meatus should be at the top of the penis and a urine stream, not a spray, should break cleanly from it. The phallus should be in the midline just below the pubis and should be of appropriate size and shape.[119]

All should be done with few complications and minimal scarring. While surgeons continue to develop new techniques, none of the past or present procedures consistently meet these goals.[120] The techniques for phalloplasty developed in parallel to the advancement of new kinds of flaps for reconstructive surgery. The first surgeons used random pedicled tube flaps[121] that they periodically relocated until they reached the desired location. Subsequent surgeons employed pedicled island flaps[122] and myocutaneous flaps,[123] keeping the donor site adjacent to the neogenitalia. As microsurgical techniques improved in the latter half of the twentieth century, surgeons began using free flaps,[124] allowing the use of tissue from numerous places on the body.

In 1936, Russian surgeon Nikoalai A. Bogoraz (1874–1952) published the first report of phalloplasty; it involved a twenty-three-year-old man whose wife cut his penis off at the root in a fit of jealousy.[125] Bogoraz created the neophallus by crafting tube pedicle grafts from the abdominal skin around an eight-centimeter section of rib cartilage for stiffness. He recreated the urethra with scrotal skin. He reported that the phallus was erectile, that the young man's sexual sensations were preserved, and that his wife was satisfied with marital sexual relations.

The subspecialty field of plastic surgery developed during World War I, when surgeons began to treat soldiers with facial and body wounds from blast injuries. Gillies (later dubbed the father of the field of plastic surgery) was born in New Zealand. He moved to London first to receive surgical training in otolaryngology and then to practice.[126] His plan to become a successful ear, nose, and throat surgeon was derailed by World War I. Gillies volunteered for the Red Cross. In England, he met August Valadier and, in France, Hippolyte Morestin; both surgeons were pioneering techniques for facial reconstructive surgery.[127] Gillies opened Queen's Hospital in Sidcup, Kent, in 1917, with more than one thousand beds and dozens of surgeons from across the globe.[128]

In 1946, physician Michael Dillon reached out to Gillies with a completely new kind of request—phalloplasty for gender reassignment. Dillon underwent a series of thirteen surgeries over four years, laying the foundation for phalloplasty procedures for the next forty years.[129] Gilles created Dillon's neophallus by modifying the Maltz procedure described in 1946, the first penis surgically constructed with a functional urethra.[130] Gillies rolled "a tube of tissue on the abdominal wall to create a urethra. He surrounded this with another tube pedicle thereby, producing a composite homogeneous penis. The upper end of the tube pedicle was then divided, and the new urethra anastomosed to the natural urethral aperture . . . the end of the tube was then modeled to resemble the glans penis."[131] Surgeons relied on this technique for the next forty years, despite the disadvantages of the tubed flap method, which included multiple surgical stages, scarring of the abdomen, hematomas (a pool of clotted or partially clotted blood), lack of sensation, and a multitude of complications with the neourethra, including fistula, strictures, urinary incontinence, infections, and the presence of urethral hair, which caused stone formation and infections that led to fistulae.[132]

In the 1970s, several surgeons experimented with new phalloplasty techniques. In 1971, Israeli and American surgeons Isaac Kaplan and David Wesser, who served in a plastic surgery relief unit in Vietnam, noted a startling number of young men with amputation of the penis due to carcinoma.[133] They developed a rapid method to construct a functional (able to stand to pee) and sensate penis by creating a urethra from the delicate scrotal skin and then attaching a contiguous (attached) thigh flap that included branches of the genital femoral nerve to create the neophallus. These surgeons documented preserved sensation by stroking the penis to induce the cremasteric reflex. (When one stroked the inner thigh, the cremasteric muscle contracted to elevate the testes.) Kaplan later noted that this operation could be employed for "female transsexuals" using labial skin for the urethra. In 1972, the Columbian surgeon Miguel Orticochea developed a new method to reconstruct the amputated penis, a condition that resulted in loss of "normal . . . sexual activity . . . the characteristic male stance for micturition; [which caused] emotional disorders . . . [and loss] of the symbol of his manhood."[134] He created a compound pedicled musculocutaneous flap from the inner thigh, preserving both the contractile muscular elements and the obturator nerve. This enabled a patient to experience pain as well as erogenous, tactile, and thermal sensitivity. The addition of contractile muscle tissue from the thigh made it possible for his patients to contract their penis to diminish the length and enhance volume. Orticochea also embedded a flexible internal silastic rod within the neophallus for erectile function. His patients reported "practically normal sexual intercourse" and that both they and their wives achieved normal orgasms.[135] Laub also popularized the "post-modern penis,"[136] a rolled abdominal skin flap used to create a phallus. In the absence of a truly functional urethra, he recommended a removable silicone device to allow urination while standing.

In 1983, Chinese surgeons Ti-Shang Chang and Wen-Yi Hwang introduced the radial forearm free flap for use in phalloplasty procedures, a technique still preferred owing to the flap's skin quality, aesthetic look, and appropriate size.[137] The disadvantages include significant donor site scarring of the forearm and thus stigmata for being transmasculine and having had phalloplasty, lack of sensation, and the potential for strictures and fistulae involving the neourethra. To address strictures and fistulae, Singapore surgeon Colin Song and colleagues modified the radial forearm free flap in a two-stage procedure that involved prelamination of the neourethra on the donor arm before surgical transfer three months later.[138] American surgeon David Gilbert and colleagues demonstrated microsurgical reinnervation of the neophallus via the pudendal nerve to create return of tactile and erogenous sensation.[139] Serbian surgeon, Sava Perovic and colleagues developed a phalloplasty technique using a musculocutaneous latissimus dorsi flap that allowed for a phallus of good size and appearance and safe implantation of a penile prosthesis.[140]

Surgeons have attempted to enable rigidity of the neophallus with various inflatable or noninflatable implants of bone, cartilage, acrylic, and silicone.[141] Surgeons continue to refine phalloplasty techniques in search of an ideal procedure that affords cosmesis and function with fewer complications. Currently, microsurgical free flaps remain the standard of care.

In 1976, Laub introduced a new technique for trans men—metoidioplasty—performing the first case on Steve Dain, who helped him conceive this procedure.[142] Laub claimed that he and F. G. Bouman (Netherlands) created metoidioplasty virtually simultaneously (in the mid-1970s) and independently.[143] Laub and Bouman had different goals in mind: Bouman was looking for a way to facilitate standing micturition without the complications and costs of phalloplasty, and Laub was looking for a way to preserve and enhance sexual satisfaction without the complications and costs of phalloplasty.[144] This operation involved the creation of a small phallus from the clitoris, which often enlarges and elongates as a result of testosterone therapy. In a simple metoidioplasty, the clitoris is released from its attachments to the labia minora and from its tethering suspensory ligaments to the pubic bone.[145] The labial skin is freed and wrapped around to create a penile tube. In a metoidioplasty with urethral lengthening, the mucosal aspects of the labia minora are rearranged to extend the urethra to the glans penis. The ring metoidioplasty employs a ringed flap from inside the vagina to facilitate urethral lengthening.[146] The Serbian surgeons further modified this procedure by using grafts from the buccal mucosal (inside of the cheek) and genital flaps from the clitoral skin and labia minora to create a neourethra that ends at the tip of the glans.[147]

The metoidioplasty procedure creates a phallus with intact sensation, erectile rigidity (usually without a prosthesis), few scars, and requires short hospital stays. The downsides are the phallus is smaller and shorter than those of cisgender men, and all procedures accompanied by urethral lengthening to enable the patient to stand to pee are more likely to involve complications. The patient may also request scrotoplasty, with scrotal skin formed from the labia and filled with prosthetic testicular implants. Complications of metoidioplasty range from minor and self-limited, such as urinary tract infections, minor wound disruptions, and dribbling or spraying of urine, to significant complications including urethral strictures and/or fistula, and/or displacement or extrusion of the testicular implants.[148]

Despite the advances in penile construction, before the twenty-first century, researchers failed to systematically evaluate patient satisfaction with metoidioplasty and phalloplasty. In 2006, Dutch surgeon J. Joris Hage published an outcome study on metoidioplasty, detailing the complications seen in seventy patients.[149] American surgeon Jordan Frey et al. performed a meta-analysis of fifty-four patients with metoidioplasty and sixty with phalloplasty, asking "Is the 'ideal' neophallus an achievable goal?"[150] Their transmasculine subjects reported significantly higher rates of satisfaction with metoidioplasty compared to phalloplasty around penile aesthetics (eighty-seven vs. seventy percent), erogenous sensation (one hundred vs. sixty-nine percent), ability to have intercourse (fifty-one vs. forty-three percent), and similar results for standing micturition (eighty-nine percent). The authors concluded by bemoaning the scarcity of outcome studies for transgender men who underwent genital surgery.

FACIAL FEMINIZATION AND MASCULINIZATION SURGERIES

> If on a Saturday morning, someone knocks at the door and you wake up and get out of bed with messy hair, no makeup, no jewelry, and answer the door, the first words you'll hear from the person standing there are, "Excuse me, ma'am. . . ."
>
> —Douglas Ousterhout

The birth of craniofacial surgery dates to the 1960s and 1970s, with the work of the European surgeons, Paul Tessier[151] and Hugo Obwegeser,[152] plastic surgeons who trained with Sir Harold Gillies to develop a new and rapidly adopted subspecialty that involved manipulation of skeletal supports to the face, at first to repair war- or birth-related anomalies and later for aesthetic applications. Douglas Ousterhout, a US surgeon, trained with Tessier, and later established the field of facial feminization surgery.

In 1982, a colleague approached Ousterhout, who was at that time a prominent craniofacial reconstructive surgeon in San Francisco, asking him to feminize the face of his patient, a trans woman named Candice.[153] Candice had undergone feminizing genital surgery, an event that changed her life in profound ways, but the surgery had no impact on how others perceived her gender in everyday life. Dr. O (as he is affectionately called) realized that, while he had spent his career reconstructing the faces of patients with disfiguring facial injuries and congenital deformities, he had not the slightest notion "about the difference between a boy and girl's skull."[154] Rather than refuse Candice's request, he set about to research the difference between masculine and feminine craniofacial features.

Ousterhout graduated from the University of Michigan with a medical and dental degree, completed his plastic surgery residency at Stanford University in 1972, studied with Tessier, and later assisted with the opening of the Center for Craniofacial Anomalies at the University of California San Francisco in 1954.[155] To care for Candice, he first reviewed the literature of early twentieth-century anthropologists to determine the bony sites on skulls used to classify dry skulls as male or female. Then, he quantified these differences using measurements derived from a developmental orthodontic study based on X-rays of the head. Next, he evaluated a collection of 1,400 skulls to understand how to view skulls as distinctly masculine or feminine. Finally, he put his new skills to work by measuring and then surgically altering the shape of trans women's skulls to match his calculation of the "female mean."[156]

Ousterhout developed a set of procedures to feminize first the bony and then the soft tissue of the face.[157] He reshaped the square, masculine jaw by removing bone to create a pointy chin and softer angular jawline. He reduced the masculine brow prominence by bossing the bone above the eyes and repositioning the anterior wall of the frontal sinus and setting it back. He advanced the scalp onto the forehead, rounding the M-shaped masculine hairline, and shortened the upper lip to create the feminine "tooth show" that occurs with the mouth slightly open. He shaved the Adam's apple, augmented the lips, and in so doing, launched the field of facial feminization surgery. His 2009 book, *Facial Feminization Surgery*,[158] described the various techniques he perfected over his career and became the guide for the surgeons across the world, who continue to refine his procedures.

Critics of Ousterhout's work point out that studies to define femininity primarily involved Western concepts and white faces and failed to acknowledge racial differences.[159] The techniques erased ethnic characteristics like the Greek nose or the Asian jaw.[160] Some complained of a "cookie-cutter" effect and argued that Dr. O's work created faces with identical shapes and a family resemblance.[161] The procedures were originally designed to render trans women invisible and ensure they would pass as cisgender women, but as queer and feminist activists began to inform American culture, critics condemned these racial and cisheteronormative standards of femininity for reinforcing cultural binary expectations for acceptable gender presentation, assumptions that also reflected racial bias.[162]

Testosterone therapy adequately masculinizes the face and brow line for most transmasculine people, and the field of facial masculinization surgery has not received much attention until recently.[163] In 2011, Ousterhout pioneered masculinizing facial surgical techniques, with a description of procedures on the chin, forehead, and mandible.[164] Masculine facial characteristics include a square jaw, a wide and high forehead, a prominent supraorbital rim, a wider nose, and a projected chin. In 2021, American surgeon Jason Harris and colleagues published new plastic surgical techniques to achieve a masculine appearing face, using forehead lengthening, rhinoplasty, lip modification, chin implants, bone grafts, and thyroid cartilage enhancement.[165]

Historically, facial gender-affirming surgeries have been considered "cosmetic" and not covered by insurance, although this is beginning to change as studies document the improved quality of life and safety for those who are not visibly transgender.[166] More recent nonsurgical approaches to facial feminization and masculinization may add to or take the place of these techniques, including the use of neurotoxins (that is, Botox), fillers, and injectable products to alter facial lines.[167]

CONCLUSION

Prior to the twenty-first century, surgeons who desired training in gender-affirming procedures found few opportunities in the United States. Established surgeons were reluctant or unable to train others due to financial fears or limitations on training imposed by their hospitals; no American gender surgical training fellowships existed. In 2007, Stan Monstrey, then serving as president of the World Professional Association for Transgender Health, convened the first international meeting of gender surgeons in Chicago.[168] This surgeons-only event is now held biennially as part of the World Professional Association for Transgender Health's International Symposia, offering surgeons from across the globe the opportunity to meet and discuss surgical techniques and challenges.

In 2017, American surgeon Loren Schechter and colleagues published "Gender Confirmation Surgery: Guiding Principles,"[169] a framework for creating formal surgical training programs that employed a multidisciplinary treatment model and quality measures that was adopted by the board of the World Professional Association for Transgender Health. Concurrently, Schechter opened the first US gender surgical fellowship training program in Chicago. At present, gender surgical training programs also exist in New York City, Oregon, Maryland, Michigan, Utah, and California.

Few anticipated the tremendous surge in demand for services seen over the last decade.[170] During this time, a sea change began to occur around trans visibility, acceptance, and human rights. Legal advocates established the right to gender-affirming care based on new studies demonstrating that appropriate care reduced morbidity and mortality.[171] First, the World Professional Association for Transgender Health, and then multiple medical professional organizations, issued or endorsed statements affirming the *medical necessity* of trans-affirming care.[172] Insurance companies, including Medicare in 2014, began covering procedures.[173] New surgical centers have opened in numerous academic centers across the United States to meet the growing demand for care.

The increasing demand for services has also come with requests for new kinds of care. Nonbinary transitions move surgeons toward more creative, less binary surgical interventions.[174] For example, some individuals request metoidioplasty without removal of the vagina. Others request mastectomy with masculine chest reconstruction without nipple graft or tattoo. Some seek nullification surgery. The use of pubertal blockade for transgender youth necessitates new surgical protocols to address preservation of sexual function, fertility, and surgery with less tissue/underdeveloped organs. Surgeons are developing skeletal body modifications, including pelvic osteopathy to create an hourglass shape[175] and shoulder width reduction or widening surgery to align the skeletal chest width with one's gender identity.[176] The development of penile transplants for cisgender men and uterine transplants for cisgender women inspires hope that transgender people may eventually avail themselves of these options.[177] American surgeon Alireza Jahromi and colleagues described necessary steps for creating the first uterine transplant program for transgender women, including the possibility of harvests from transgender men who are also undergoing gender surgery.[178] As demand continues to drive care and surgeons strive to meet that demand, surgeons continue to refine and expand surgical techniques, furthering discussion around our increasingly nuanced understanding of gender identity, gender expression, and the provision of competent and affirming surgical care.

NOTES

1. Thank you to Dr. Loren Schechter for his assistance with this chapter.
2. Green, *Becoming a Visible Man*, 84.
3. Aatsha and Kewal, "Embryology, Sexual Development," 1.
4. Pemberton, "Castrati: Did the End Justify the Means?"
5. See chapter 1 in this volume.
6. Martjin Icks, "Cross-Dressers in Control." Although typically referred to in historical texts with masculine pronouns, Elagabalus' contemporary historian, Cassius Dio described her with feminine pronouns. Sources report that she wished to be addressed as a lady and due to this stated preference, I do the same.
7. Kamezis, "The Fall of Elagabalus," 350.
8. Kamezis, "The Fall of Elagabalus," 351–53.
9. Zanghellini, *The Sexual Constitution of Political Authority*, 60.
10. Kamezis, "The Fall of Elagabalus," 351–53.
11. *Encyclopedia Britannica*, "Vestal Virgins: Roman Religion." Including marriage to and defilement of the vestal virgin Aquilia Severa during a period when vestal virgins were punished with live burial for engaging in sexual intercourse.
12. Zanghellini, *The Sexual Constitution of Political Authority*, 59.
13. Icks, "Cross-Dressers in Control." No documentation exists to describe if anyone attempted this surgery.
14. Markantes et al., "Callo."
15. Markantes et al., "Callo."
16. Markantes et al., "Callo," 450. Some speculate that this was a 46, XY disorder due to 5a reductase type 2 or HSD17B3 deficiency.
17. Brooks, "Why the Growth of Transgender Surgery Centers in the U.S. Matters."
18. TransHealthCare, "Find a Surgeon for Gender Affirming Surgery."
19. I found references on techniques for these various surgeries but little on the history.
20. Elbe, Tonning, and Feldman, *Man Into Woman*, 8–10.
21. Abraham, "Genital Reassignment on Two Male Transvestites," 1.
22. Abraham, "Genital Reassignment on Two Male Transvestites," 2.
23. Abraham, "Genital Reassignment on Two Male Transvestites," 3.
24. Elbe, *Man Into Woman*, 138–39.
25. Elbe, Tonning, and Feldman, *Man Into Woman*, 8–10.
26. Elbe, Tonning, and Feldman, *Man Into Woman*, 8–10.
27. Elbe, *Man Into Woman*, 135, 156.
28. Elbe, Tonning, and Feldman, *Man Into Woman*, 8–10; Meyerowitz, *How Sex Changed*, 120.
29. Elbe, Tonning, and Feldman, *Man Into Woman*, 8–10.

30. Beachy, *Gay Berlin*, 241–43.
31. Schillace, "The Forgotten History."
32. Meyerowitz, *How Sex Changed*, 292; Schillace, "The Forgotten History."
33. Elbe, Tonning, and Feldman, *Man Into Woman*, 8–10.
34. Pinney and Metcalfe, "Sir Archibold McIndoe and the Guinea Pig Club."
35. ScienceDirect, "Split Thickness Skin Graft." A split thickness skin graft made from the epidermis and part of the dermis.
36. Wheeless and Roenneburg, "McIndoe Vaginoplasty for Neovagina."
37. Ray and Rao, "Full Thickness Skin Grafts." A full thickness skin graft is made from the dermis and epidermis.
38. Laub, Laub, and Riber "Vaginoplasty for Gender Confirmation"; Wheeless and Roenneburg, "McIndoe Vaginoplasty for Neovagina."
39. Medical Library, "Pedicle Flap." A pedicle flap consists of the full thickness skin and the subcutaneous tissue, attached by tissue containing its blood supply.
40. Hage, Karim, and Laub, "On the Origins of Pedicled Skin Inversion Vaginoplasty." Laub, *Second Lives*, 120. In 2019, Laub described the (modernized) penile inversion technique in layperson's terms: "It involves forming space between the rectum and the bladder and inverting the penis—essentially turning it inside out like a sock—and using the skin of the penis and sometimes skin grafts from the scrotum to line the vaginal vault. The testicles are removed, and scrotal skin is used to make the labia minora. The nerves and skin of the glans penis—the sensitive tip—are used to make the clitoris. The urethra is shortened, and sensitive urethral mucosa is placed in between the labia minora, the inner folds of the vagina."
41. See chapter 4 in this volume.
42. See chapter 6 in this volume.
43. Harrity, "#TBT: Christine Jorgensen." Her vaginoplasty was allowed in the United States despite the Mayhem statutes as she no longer had testes.
44. Bakker, "In the Shadows of Society," 148.
45. Bakker, "In the Shadows of Society," 148–58.
46. Bakker, "In the Shadows of Society," 152.
47. Bakker, "In the Shadows of Society," 153.
48. Skidmore, "Constructing the 'Good Transsexual,'" 284.
49. Siotos et al., "Origins of Gender Affirmation Surgery," 1.
50. Siotos et al., "Origins of Gender Affirmation Surgery," 2.
51. Harvard Library, John E. Hoopes Papers Collection; Edgerton, "The Role of Surgery in the Treatment of Transsexualism."
52. Edgerton and Bull, "Surgical Construction of the Vagina."
53. Siotos et al., "Origins of Gender Affirmation Surgery," 2–3.
54. See chapter 11 in this volume.
55. Siotos et al., "Origins of Gender Affirmation Surgery," 2–3.

56. Siotos et al., "Origins of Gender Affirmation Surgery," 2.
57. Edgerton, "The Role of Surgery in the Treatment of Transsexualism," 473.
58. Edgerton, "The Role of Surgery in the Treatment of Transsexualism," 474.
59. McHugh, "Psychiatric Misadventures," 501.
60. Meyer and Reter "Sex Reassignment: Follow-Up," 1015.
61. Siotos et al., "Origins of Gender Affirmation Surgery," 2–3.
62. See chapter 11 in this volume.
63. Ciotti, "Why Did He Cut That Man's Leg?"
64. Ciotti, "Why Did He Cut That Man's Leg?"
65. Brody, "Benefits of Transsexual Surgery." The gender clinics charged $5,000–$10,000.
66. Zagria Blogspot. "John Ronald Brown: Part II."
67. Ciotti, "Why Did He Cut That Man's Leg?"
68. Medical Quality State of California, "In the Matter of the Petition for Reinstatement of Revoked Certificate of: John Ronald Brown."
69. Ciotti, "Why Did He Cut That Man's Leg?"
70. Denny, "The Tijuana Experience" and "'Tabletop' John Brown Gets His."
71. Ciotti, "Why Did He Cut That Man's Leg?
72. Personal communication with Jamison Green, 2021.
73. People v. Brown.
74. Brang, McGeoch, and Ramachandran, "Apotemnophilia"; Ciotti, "Why Did He Cut That Man's Leg?"; Novais et al., "Apotemnophilia"; Sedda and Bottini, "Apotemnophilia, Body Integrity Identity Disorder or Xenomelia?"; Dotinga, "Out on a Limb." The name of this disorder is apotemnophilia, the uncontrollable desire to amputate healthy limbs, which may have a neurological basis. While referred to as a "sexual fetish" in reports on John Brown, it may or may not involve erotic fantasies. Some individuals state that that they seek amputation to feel complete.
75. Fox, "Stanley H. Biber"; Carnahan, "At 81, Sex-Change 'King' Just an Old Country."
76. Fox, "Stanley H. Biber"; Carnahan, "At 81, Sex-Change 'King' Just an Old Country."
77. Smith, *Going to Trinidad*, 14, 31.
78. Smith, *Going to Trinidad*, 43.
79. Carnahan, "At 81, Sex-Change 'King' Just an Old Country."
80. Smith, *Going to Trinidad*, 39–40.
81. Laub, Laub, and Riber "Vaginoplasty for Gender Confirmation," 464–65.
82. Carnahan, "At 81, Sex-Change 'King' Just an Old Country."
83. Laub, Laub, and Riber, "Vaginoplasty for Gender Confirmation."
84. Laub, Laub, and Riber, "Vaginoplasty for Gender Confirmation," 465.
85. Laub, Laub, and Riber, "Vaginoplasty for Gender Confirmation," 464.

86. Fritz and Mulkey, "The Rise and Fall of Gender Identity Clinics."
87. Carnahan, "At 81, Sex-Change 'King' Just an Old Country."
88. Brooks, "Why the Growth of Transgender Surgery Centers in the U.S. Matters."
89. Carnahan, "At 81, Sex-Change 'King' Just an Old Country."
90. Arrillaga, "Onetime Coal-Mining Town Bolstered by Changing Economy." Most, but not all, welcomed Biber's transsexual practice and patients. Monica Violante, owner of the Main Street Bakery said, "Nobody cares. It's just a part of Trididad." The Rev. Verlyn Hanson of the First Baptist Church disagreed: "The love of money is the root of all evil, and people will overlook a lot of evil to have a stronger economy."
91. Smith, *Going to Trinidad*, 74–75.
92. Carnahan, "At 81, Sex-Change 'King' Just an Old Country."
93. Smith, *Going to Trinidad*, 141–42.
94. Smith, *Going to Trinidad*, 143–45.
95. Lopez, "Burlingame Based Physician Makes History in Trans Medical Field." Bowers was the second physician practicing at Seattle's Swedish Medical Center to transition in less than three years. The first, Anne Lawrence (1950-), an anesthesiologist, had been under enormous scrutiny after her transition, was not well received by hospital staff and colleagues, and was forced to resign after examining the pelvis of an anesthetized patient without prior consent. James, "Lawrence Exposé." Lawrence went on to establish herself both as a hero and a villain for the transgender community. First, she built one of the early websites comparing postoperative photos of each surgeon. She collected these graphic surgical outcomes by soliciting impromptu photo sessions with patients she knew to be postop, then categorizing them according to surgeon. Although brazen in her technique, the posting of these photos did much to raise the bar for surgeons in terms of aesthetic and functional quality. She was one of the first to publish an outcome study based on the largest cohort of patients to date who reported on their experience with vaginoplasty. She concluded that that patient satisfaction was high, despite (rare) complications and regardless of the experience of the surgeon. Lawrence, "Factors Associated with Satisfaction or Regret." Personal communication with Dallas Denny and Jamison Green, 2021.
96. Arrillaga, "Colorado Town the 'Sex-Change Capital.'"
97. Smith, *Going to Trinidad*, 150–51.
98. Smith, *Going to Trinidad*, 149.
99. Carnahan, "At 81, Sex-Change 'King' Just an Old Country."
100. Mestas, "Trinidad Doctor Battled Hospital."; Smith, *Going to Trinidad*, 197–202.
101. Laub, *Second Lives, Second Chances*, 199–22.
102. Sherkin, Seidl, and Hagen, *When Gender Is in Question*, 69.
103. Kirk, *Feminizing Hormonal Therapy for the Transgendered*; *Masculinizing Hormonal Therapy for the Transgendered*; *Physician's Guide to Transgendered Medicine*.

104. Coleman, Kirk, and Bockting, *Transgender and HIV*.

105. Meyer et al., "The Harry Benjamin International Gender Dysphoria"; World Professional Association for Transgender Health, "WPATH Remembers Sheila Kirk."

106. Leach, "Pittsburgh Trans Doctor Opens Sex Reassignment Clinic."

107. Leach, "Pittsburgh Trans Doctor Opens Sex Reassignment Clinic."

108. Tan, "S Shan Ratnam."

109. Wangjiraniran et al. "Male-to-Female Vaginoplasty," 2.

110. Wangjiraniran et al. "Male-to-Female Vaginoplasty," 2, 7. Today, Thailand remains one of the foremost international destinations for gender affirming surgeries.

111. Jayaram, Stuteville, and Bush, "Complications and Undesirable Results."

112. Platel and Van Laeche, "Transformations Over Time"; Monstrey, Ceulemans, and Hoebeke," Sex Reassignment Surgery in the Female-to-Male Transsexual"; Monstrey et al., "Chest-Wall Contouring Surgery"; Ettner, Monstrey, and Coleman, *Principles of Transgender Medicine and Surgery*; Doornaert et al., "Penile Reconstruction with the Radial Forearm Flap."

113. Hage, "Chest-Wall Contouring"; Hage, Bloem, and Suliman, "Review of the Literature on Techniques for Phalloplasty"; Hage, "Metaidoioplasty"; Hage and van Turnhout, "Long-Term Outcome of Metaidoioplasty"; Hage et al., "Gender-Confirming Facial Surgery"; Hage et al., "Phalloplasty in Female-to-Male Transsexuals."

114. Fang, Chen, and Ma, "A New Method for Clitoroplasty."

115. Watanyusakul, "Vaginoplasty Modifications to Improve Vulvar Aesthetics."

116. Dessy et al., "The Use of Cultured Autologous Oral Epithelial Cells for Vaginoplasty in Male-to-Female Transsexuals"; Wei et al., "Autologous Buccal Micro-Mucosa Free Graft"; Lin et al., "Use of Autologous Buccal Mucosa for Vaginoplasty."

117. Jacoby et al., "Robotic Davydov Peritoneal Flap Vaginoplasty."

118. Gilbert, "Homo-Sexuality and Its Treatment."

119. Hage, Bloem, and Suliman, "Review of the Literature on Techniques for Phalloplasty," 1095.

120. Frey et al., "A Systematic Review of Metoidioplasty and Radial Forearm Flap."

121. Medical Dictionary, "Tubed Pedicle Flap." A bipedicle flap made by elevating a long strip of tissue from its bed except at the two extremities, the cut edges then being sutured together to form a tube.

122. Kimyai-Asadi and Goldberg, "Island Pedicle Flap."

An island of skin that is detached from its epidermal and dermal attachments while retaining its vascular supply from an underlying pedicle.

123. Free Dictionary by Farlex. A compound flap of skin and muscle with adequate vascularity to permit sufficient tissue to be transferred to the recipient site.

124. Free Dictionary by Farlex. An island flap detached from the body and reattached at the distant recipient site by microvascular anastomosis.

125. Schultheiss, Gabouev, and Jonas, "Nikolaj A. Bogoraz (1874–1952)."

126. See chapter 4 in this volume.
127. Bamji, "Sir Harold Gillies: Surgical Pioneer," 144.
128. Bamji, "Sir Harold Gillies: Surgical Pioneer," 144.
129. Nair, "Sir Harold Gillies."
130. Hoopes, "Operative Treatment of the Female Transsexual," 342–43.
131. Nair, "Sir Harold Gillies."
132. Noe et al., "Construction of Male Genitalia," 301.
133. Kaplan and Wesser, "A Rapid Method of Constructing a Sensitive Functional Penis."
134. Orticochea, "A New Method of Total Reconstruction of the Penis," 347.
135. Orticochea, "A New Method of Total Reconstruction of the Penis," 366.
136. Laub, *Second Lives, Second Chances*, 123–25.
137. Chang and Hwang, "Forearm Flap in One-Stage Reconstruction of the Penis."
138. Song et al., "Modifications of the Radial Forearm Flap Phalloplasty."
139. Gilbert et al., "Phallic Reinnervation via the Pudendal Nerve."
140. Perovic et al., "Total Phalloplasty Using a Musculocutaneous Latissimus Dorsi Flap."
141. Rooker et al., "The Rise of the Neophallus"; Noe et al., "Construction of Male Genitalia."
142. Hage, "Metaidoioplasty," 161; Laub, *Second Lives, Second Chances*, 125.
143. Green, *Becoming a Visible Man*, 2nd ed., 107.
144. Personal communication with Jamison Green, 2021.
145. Green, *Becoming a Visible Man*, 110.
146. Djordjevic, Stojanovic, and Bizic, "Metoidioplasty: Techniques and Outcomes."
147. Djordjevic et al., "Metoidioplasty as a Single Stage Sex Reassignment Surgery"; Djordjevic, Stojanovic, and Bizic, "Metoidioplasty: Techniques and Outcomes."
148. Djordjevic, Stojanovic, and Bizic, "Metoidioplasty: Techniques and Outcomes."
149. Hage and van Turnhout, "Long-Term Outcome of Metaidoioplasty."
150. Frey et al., "A Systematic Review of Metoidioplasty and Radial Forearm Flap."
151. Tessier was from France. Bhattacharya, "Dr. Paul Tessier"; David, "Obituary—Dr. Paul Tessier."
152. Naini, "Hugo L. Obwegeser." Obwegeser was born in Austria, moved to Switzerland due to threat of Nazi persecution.
153. Plemons, "Description of Sex Difference as Prescription for Sex Change," 658.
154. Plemons, "Description of Sex Difference as Prescription for Sex Change," 658.
155. Deschamps-Braly Clinic, "Dr. Douglas K. Osterhout [Retired]."
156. Plemons, "Description of Sex Difference as Prescription for Sex Change," 666.
157. Ousterhout, *Facial Feminization Surgery* and "Dr. Paul Tessier and Facial Skeletal Masculinization."
158. Ousterhout, *Facial Feminization Surgery*.

159. Cho, Massie, and Morrison, "Ethnic Considerations for Rhinoplasty in Facial Feminization."

160. Plemons, "Making the Gendered Face," 125–45.

161. Plemons, "Making the Gendered Face," 141.

162. Richie, "A Queer, Feminist Bioethics Critique."

163. Deschamps-Braly, "Approach to Feminization Surgery"; Sayegh et al., "Facial Masculinization Surgery"; Harris, Premaratne, and Spector, "Facial Masculinization from Procedures to Payment."

164. Ousterhout, "Dr. Paul Tessier and Facial Skeletal Masculinization."

165. Harris, Premaratne, and Spector, "Facial Masculinization from Procedures to Payment."

166. Harris, Premaratne, and Spector, "Facial Masculinization from Procedures to Payment."

167. Ascha et al., "Nonsurgical Management of Facial Masculinization and Feminization."

168. Personal communication with Dr. Loren Schecter, 2021.

169. Schechter et al., "Gender Confirmation Surgery."

170. Personal communication with Loren Schecter, 2021.

171. Fields v. Smith; see also chapter 15 in this volume.

172. Green, "Unbending the Light," 515.

173. Green, "Unbending the Light," 511–12.

174. Berli et al., "Patient Responsive Care."

175. Jones, "A New Plastic Surgery Technique for Hip Widening"; Williams, "Pelvic Beauty' Becomes Achievable."

176. Eppley, "Shoulder Narrowing & Widening Surgery."

177. Jones et al., "Perceptions and Motivations for Uterus Transplant"; Preto et al., "The Frontier of Penile Implants in Phalloplasty."

178. Jahromi et al., "Uterine Transplantation and Donation in Transgender Individuals."

WORKS CITED

Aatsha, P. A., and Krishan Kewal. "Embryology, Sexual Development." In *StatPearls* [Internet]. Updated August 28, 2023. Treasure Island, FL: StatPearls Publishing, 2021. Accessed September 29, 2022. http://www.ncbi.nlm.nih.gov/books/NBK557601/.

Abraham, Felix. "Genital Reassignment on Two Male Transvestites." *Genitalumwandlungen an Zwei Männlichen Transvestiten. Zeitschrift Für Sexualwissenschaft Und Sexualpolitik* 18 (1931): 223–26. Reprint in *International Journal of Transgenderism*, 2, no. 1 (1998): 1–4.

Arrillaga, Pauline. "Onetime Coal-Mining Town Bolstered by Changing Economy." *Los Angeles Times*, June 4, 2000. Accessed August 14, 2024. https://www.latimes.com/archives/la-xpm-2000-jun-04-me-37512-story.html

Ascha, Mona, Marco Swanson, Jonathan Massie, et al. "Nonsurgical Management of Facial Masculinization and Feminization." *Aesthetic Surgery Journal* 39, no. 5 (2018): NP123–37. https://doi.org/10.1093/asj/sjy253.

Bakker, Alex. "In the Shadows of Society: Trans People in the Netherlands in the 1950s." In *Others of My Kind: Transatlantic Transgender Histories*, 133–75. Calgary, Alberta: University of Calgary Press, 2020.

Bamji, Andrew. "Sir Harold Gillies: Surgical Pioneer." *Trauma* 8, no. 3 (2006): 143–56. https://doi.org/10.1177/1460408606072329.

Beachy, Robert. *Gay Berlin: Birthplace of a Modern Identity*. New York: Vintage Books, 2014.

Berli, Jens U., Daniel Dugi, Mary Marsiglio, Christina Milano, and Amy Penkin. "Patient Responsive Care: Engaging the Multi-Disciplinary Team to Deconstruct Binary Models of Gender Affirming Surgical Care." Virtual presentation, Seeking Equity in a Time of Hope and Challenge: USPATH, November 6, 2021. Accessed November 10, 2021. https://www.wpath.org/media/cms/Documents/USPATH/2021/3275-USPATH2021-Full%20Schedule-FINAL.pdf.

Bhattacharya, Surajit. "Dr. Paul Tessier." *Indian Journal of Plastic Surgery* 41, no. 2 (2008): 244–45. Accessed September 29, 2022. https://www.ncbi.nlm.nih.gov/pmc/articles/PMC2740534/.

Brang, David, Paul D. McGeoch, and Vilayanur S. Ramachandran. "Apotemnophilia: A Neurological Disorder." *NeuroReport* 19, no. 13 (2008): 1305–06.

Brody, Jane. "Benefits of Transsexual Surgery Disputed as Leading Hospital Halts the Procedure." *New York Times*, October 2, 1979. Accessed September 29/2022. https://www.nytimes.com/1979/10/02/archives/benefits-of-transsexual-surgery-disputed-as-leading-hospital-halts.html.

Brooks, Arnold Thomas. "Why the Growth of Transgender Surgery Centers in the U.S. Matters." TransHealthCare. November 11, 2019. Accessed September 29, 2022. https://transhealthcare.org/news/transgender-surgery-centers/.

Carnahan, Ann. "At 81, Sex-Change 'King' Just an Old Country." *Rocky Mountain News*, August 16, 2004.

Caughie, Pamela, and Sabine Meyer. "Introduction." In *Man Into Woman: A Comparative Scholarly Edition*, 8–10. London: Bloomsbury Academic, 2020.

Chang, Ti-Shang, and Wen-Yi Hwang. "Forearm Flap in One-Stage Reconstruction of the Penis." *Plastic and Reconstructive Surgery* 74, no. 2 (1983): 251–58.

Cho, Daniel Y., Jonathan P. Massie, and Shane D. Morrison. "Ethnic Considerations for Rhinoplasty in Facial Feminization." *JAMA Facial Plastic Surgery* 19, no. 3 (2017): 243. https://doi.org/10.1001/jamafacial.2017.0223.

Ciotti, Paul. "Why Did He Cut That Man's Leg? The Peculiar Practice of Dr. John Ronald Brown." *LA Weekly*, December 15, 1999. Accessed September 29, 2022. https://web.archive.org/web/20070930154730/http://www.laweekly.com/index3.php?option=com_content&task=view&id=6108&Itemid=9&pop=1&page=0.

Coleman, Edmond J., Sheila Kirk, and Walter O. Bockting. *Transgender and HIV: Risks, Prevention, and Care*. New York: Routledge, 2014.

David, David. "Obituary—Dr. Paul Tessier." *Journal of Plastic, Reconstructive & Aesthetic Surgery* 61, no. 9 (2008): 1008. https://doi.org/10.1016/j.bjps.2008.07.005.

Denny, Dallas. "'Tabletop' John Brown Gets His." *Transgender Forum* (blog), 1999. Accessed September 29, 2022. http://dallasdenny.com/Writing/2013/04/24/tabletop-brown-gets-his-1999/.

———. "The Tijuana Experience." *Alicia's TV Girl Talk* 4, no. 9 (1992): 18. Accessed September 29, 2022. http://dallasdenny.com/Writing/2011/10/22/the-tijuana-experience/.

Deschamps-Braly Clinic (website). "Dr. Douglas K. Osterhout [Retired] R." n.d. Accessed March 27, 2021. https://deschamps-braly.com/dr-ousterhout-facial-feminization-surgeon-ffs/.

Deschamps-Braly, Jordan C. "Approach to Feminization Surgery and Facial Masculinization Surgery: Aesthetic Goals and Principles of Management." *Journal of Craniofacial Surgery* 30, no. 5 (2019): 1352–58. https://doi.org/10.1097/SCS.0000000000005391.

Dessy, Luca A., Marco Mazzocchi, Federico Corrias, Simona Ceccarelli, Cinzia Marchese, and Nicolò Scuderi. "The Use of Cultured Autologous Oral Epithelial Cells for Vaginoplasty in Male-to-Female Transsexuals: A Feasibility, Safety, and Advantageousness Clinical Pilot Study." *Plastic and Reconstructive Surgery* 133, no. 1 (2014): 158–61. https://doi.org/10.1097/01.prs.0000435844.95551.35.

Djordjevic, Miroslav L., Borko Stojanovic, and Marta Bizic. "Metoidioplasty: Techniques and Outcomes." *Translational Andrology and Urology* 8, no. 3 (2019): 248–53. https://doi.org/10.21037/tau.2019.06.12.

Djordjevic, Miroslav L., Dusan Stanojevic, Marta Bizic, et al. "Metoidioplasty as a Single Stage Sex Reassignment Surgery in Female Transsexuals: Belgrade Experience." *Journal of Sexual Medicine* 6, no. 5 (2009): 1306–13. https://doi.org/10.1111/j.1743-6109.2008.01065.x.

Doornaert, M., P. Hoebeke, P. Ceulemans, G. T'Sjoen, G. Heylens, and S. Monstrey. "Penile Reconstruction with the Radial Forearm Flap: An Update." *Handchirurgie · Mikrochirurgie · Plastische Chirurgie* 43, no. 4 (2011): 208–14. https://doi.org/10.1055/s-0030-1267215.

Dotinga, Randy. "Out on a Limb." *Salon*, 2000. Accessed September 29, 2022. https://www.salon.com/2000/08/29/amputation/.

Edgerton, M. T. "The Role of Surgery in the Treatment of Transsexualism." *Annals of Plastic Surgery* 13, no. 6 (1984): 473–81. https://doi.org/10.1097/00000637-198412000-00003.

Edgerton, M. T., and John Bull "Surgical Construction of the Vagina and Labia in Male Transsexuals." *Plastic and Reconstructive Surgery* 46, no. 6 (1970): 529–39.

Elbe, Lili. *Man Into Woman*, 3rd ed., edited by Neils Hoyer. New York, NY: Popular Library, 1933.

Elbe, Lili, Erik Tonning, and Matthew Feldman. *Man Into Woman: A Comparative Scholarly Edition*, edited by Pamela L. Caughie and Sabine Meyer. London: Bloomsbury Academic, 2020.

Encyclopedia Britannica. "Vestal Virgins: Roman Religion." Accessed September 3, 2021. https://www.britannica.com/topic/Vestal-Virgins.

Eppley, Barry. "Shoulder Narrowing & Widening Surgery." Dr. Barry L. Eppley, MD (website). n.d. Accessed November 7, 2021. https://www.eppleyplasticsurgery.com/shoulder-narrowing-widening/.

Ettner, Randi, Stan Monstrey, and Eli Coleman. *Principles of Transgender Medicine and Surgery*. New York: Routledge, 2016. Accessed September 29, 2022. https://books.google.com/books?hl=en&lr=&id=LwszDAAAQBAJ&oi=fnd&pg=PP1&dq=Principles+of+Transgender+Medicine+and+Surgery&ots=cvuWhSnPjJ&sig=kgm7vVHi6HO4OiOlpPDwtG5bClk.

Fang, R. H., C. F. Chen, and S. Ma. "A New Method for Clitoroplasty in Male-to-Female Sex Reassignment Surgery." *Plastic and Reconstructive Surgery* 89, no. 4 (1992): 679–82; discussion 683.

Fields v. Smith, 653 F.3d 550. 7th Circuit, 2011.

Fox, Margalit. "Stanley H. Biber, 82, Surgeon Among First to Do Sex Changes, Dies." *New York Times*, sec. Obituaries, January 21, 2006. Accessed September 29, 2022. https://www.nytimes.com/2006/01/21/us/stanley-h-biber-82-surgeon-among-first-to-do-sex-changes-dies.html.

Free Dictionary by Farlex. "Free Flap." Accessed March 24, 2021. https://medical-dictionary.thefreedictionary.com/free+flap.

———. "Myocutaneous Flap." Accessed March 24, 2021. https://medical-dictionary.thefreedictionary.com/myocutaneous+flap.

———. "Tubed Pedicle Flap." Accessed March 24, 2021. https://medical-dictionary.thefreedictionary.com/tubed+pedicle+flap.

Frey, Jordan D., Grace Poudrier, Michael V. Chiodo, and Alexes Hazen. "A Systematic Review of Metoidioplasty and Radial Forearm Flap Phalloplasty in Female-to-Male Transgender Genital Reconstruction: Is the 'Ideal' Neophallus an Achievable Goal?" *Plastic and Reconstructive Surgery. Global Open* 4, no. 12 (2016): e1131. https://doi.org/10.1097/GOX.0000000000001131.

Fritz, Melanie, and Nat Mulkey. "The Rise and Fall of Gender Identity Clinics in the 1960s and 1970s." *Bulletin of the American College of Surgeons*, April 2, 2021. Accessed October 1, 2022. https://bulletin.facs.org/2021/04/the-rise-and-fall-of-gender-identity-clinics-in-the-1960s-and-1970s/.

Gilbert, D. A., M. W. Williams, C. E. Horton, et al. "Phallic Reinnervation via the Pudendal Nerve." *Journal of Urology* 140, no. 2 (1988): 295–99. https://doi.org/10.1016/s0022-5347(17)41587-4.

Gilbert, J. Allen. "Homo-Sexuality and Its Treatment." *Journal of Nervous and Mental Disease* 52, no. 4 (1920): 297–322.

Green, Jamison. *Becoming a Visible Man*. Nashville, TN: Vanderbilt University Press, 2004.

———. *Becoming a Visible Man*. 2nd ed. Nashville, TN: Vanderbilt University Press, 2020.

———. "Unbending the Light: Changing Laws and Policies to Make Transgender Health Visible; Reflections of an Advocate." *Journal of Law, Medicine & Ethics* 50, no. 3 (2022): 509–18.

Hage, J. Joris. "Chest-Wall Contouring in Female-to-Male Transsexuals: Basic Considerations and Review of the Literature." *Plastic and Reconstructive Surgery* 96, no. 2 (1995): 386–91.

———. "Metaidoioplasty: An Alternative Phalloplasty Technique in Transsexuals." *Plastic and Reconstructive Surgery* 97, no. 1 (1996): 161–67. https://doi.org/10.1097/00006534-199601000-00026.

Hage, J. Joris, Alfred G. Becking, Floris H. de Graaf, and D. Bram Tuinzing. "Gender-Confirming Facial Surgery: Considerations on the Masculinity and Femininity of Faces." *Plastic and Reconstructive Surgery* 99, no. 7 (1997): 1799–807.

Hage, J. J., Joannes Bloem, and H. M. Suliman. "Review of the Literature on Techniques for Phalloplasty with Emphasis on the Applicability in Female-to-Male Transsexuals." *Journal of Urology* 150, no. 4 (1993): 1093–98.

Hage, J. J., C. A. Bout, J. J. Bloem, and J. A. Megens. "Phalloplasty in Female-to-Male Transsexuals: What Do Our Patients Ask For." *Annals of Plastic Surgery* 30, no. 4 (1993): 323–26. https://doi.org/10.1097/00000637-199304000-00006.

Hage, J. Joris, Refaat B. Karim, and Donald R. Laub Sr. "On the Origin of Pedicled Skin Inversion Vaginoplasty: Life and Work of Dr Georges Burou of Casablanca." *Annals of Plastic Surgery* 59, no. 6 (2007): 723–29.

Hage, J. Joris, and Arjen A. W. M. van Turnhout. "Long-Term Outcome of Metaidoioplasty in 70 Female-to-Male Transsexuals." *Annals of Plastic Surgery* 57, no. 3 (2006): 312–16. https://doi.org/10.1097/01.sap.0000221625.38212.2e.

Harris, Jason, Ishani D. Premaratne, and Jason A. Spector. "Facial Masculinization from Procedures to Payment: A Review." *LGBT Health* 8, no. 7 (August 2021). https://doi.org/10.1089/lgbt.2020.0128.

Harrity, Christopher. "#TBT: Christine Jorgensen." Advocate, November 20, 2014. Accessed September 29, 2022. http://www.advocate.com/politics/transgender/2014/11/20/tbt-christine-jorgensen.

Harvard Library. John E. Hoopes Papers Collection. Accessed October 20, 2021. https://hollisarchives.lib.harvard.edu/repositories/14/resources/7679/collection_organization.

Hoopes, John E. "Operative Treatment of the Female Transsexual." In *Transsexualism and Sex Reassignment*, 331–23. Baltimore, MD: Johns Hopkins Press, 1969.

Icks, Martijin. "Cross-Dressers in Control: Transvesticism, Power and the Balance Between the Sexes in the Literary Discourse of the Roman Empire." In *TransAntiquity: Cross-Dressing and Transgender Dynamics in the Ancient World*, edited by Domitilla Campanile, Filippo Carlà-Uhink, and Margherita Facella, 65–82. Abingdon, Oxon: Routledge, 2017. Accessed August 22, 2022. https://www.google.com/books/edition/TransAntiquity/39ENDgAAQBAJ?hl=en&gbpv=1&dq=Icks,+Martijin.+Cross-Dressers+in+Control:+Transvesticism,+Power+and+the+Balance+between+the+Sexes+in+the+Literary+Discourse+of+the+Roman+Empire.+In&pg=PT94&printsec=frontcover.

Jacoby, Adam, Samantha Maliha, Michael A. Granieri, et al. "Robotic Davydov Peritoneal Flap Vaginoplasty for Augmentation of Vaginal Depth in Feminizing Vaginoplasty." *Journal of Urology* 201, no. 6 (2019): 1171–76. https://doi.org/10.1097/JU.0000000000000107.

Jahromi, Alireza, Sydney Horen, Amir Dorafshar, et al. "Uterine Transplantation and Donation in Transgender Individuals; Proof of Concept." *International Journal of Transgender Health* 22, no. 4 (May 2021): 349–59. https://doi.org/10.1080/26895269.2021.1915635.

James, Andrea. "Lawrence Exposé," *Transgender Map* (blog), October 6, 2019. Accessed September 29, 2022. https://www.transgendermap.com/community/roberta-angela-dee/.

Jayaram, B. N., O. H. Stuteville, and I. M. Bush. "Complications and Undesirable Results of Sex-Reassignment Surgery in Male-to-Female Transsexuals." *Archives of Sexual Behavior* 7, no. 4 (1978): 337–45. https://doi.org/10.1007/BF01542042.

Jones, Benjamin P., Abirami Rajamanoharan, Saaliha Vali, et al. "Perceptions and Motivations for Uterus Transplant in Transgender Women." *JAMA Network Open* 4, no. 1 (2021): e2034561. https://doi.org/10.1001/jamanetworkopen.2020.34561.

Jones, Zinnia. "A New Plastic Surgery Technique for Hip Widening." *Gender Analysis* (blog), February 1, 2018. Accessed September 29, 2022. https://genderanalysis.net/2018/02/a-new-plastic-surgery-technique-for-hip-widening/.

Kamezis, Adam. "The Fall of Elagabalus as Literary Narrative and Political Reality." *Historia* 65 (2016): 348–90.

Kaplan, I., and D. Wesser. "A Rapid Method of Constructing a Sensitive Functional Penis." *Harefuah* 79, no. 1 (1970): 19–20.

Kimyai-Asadi, Arash, and Leonard H. Goldberg. "Island Pedicle Flap." *Dermatologic Clinics* 23, no. 1 (2005): 113–27.

Kirk, Sheila. *Feminizing Hormonal Therapy for the Transgendered*. Watertown, MA: Together Lifeworks, 1996.

———. *Masculinizing Hormonal Therapy for the Transgendered*. Watertown, MA: Together Lifeworks, 1996.

———. *Physician's Guide to Transgendered Medicine*. Watertown, MA: Together Lifeworks, 1996.

Laub, Donald. *Second Lives, Second Chances*. Toronto, Ontario: ECW Press, 2019.

Laub, Donald R., Donald Laub, and Stanley Riber. "Vaginoplasty for Gender Confirmation." *Clinics in Plastic Surgery* 15, no. 3 (1988): 463–70.

Lawrence, Anne A. "Factors Associated with Satisfaction or Regret Following Male-to-Female Sex Reassignment Surgery." *Archives of Sexual Behavior* 32, no. 4 (2003): 299–315.

Leach, Dawn. "Pittsburgh Trans Doctor Opens Sex Reassignment Clinic." *Gay People's Chronicle*, June 5, 1998. Accessed September 29, 2022. http://www.ifge.org/news/1998/july/nws7128a.htm.

Lin, W. C., Cherry Y. Y. Chang, Y. Y. Shen, and H. D. Tsai. "Use of Autologous Buccal Mucosa for Vaginoplasty: A Study of Eight Cases." *Human Reproduction* 18, no. 3 (2003): 604–07. https://doi.org/10.1093/humrep/deg095.

Lopez, Sierra. "Burlingame Based Physician Makes History in Trans Medical Field." *San Mateo Daily Journal*, July 18, 2020. Accessed September 29, 2022. https://www.smdailyjournal.com/news/local/burlingame-based-physician-makes-history-in-trans-medical-field/article_ebe14c50-c8a9-11ea-80bc-070a4504e437.html.

Markantes, Georgios, Efthimios Deligeoroglou, Anastasia Armeni, et al. "Callo: The First Known Case of Ambiguous Genitalia to Be Surgically Repaired in the History of Medicine, Described by Diodorus Siculus." *Hormones*, 14, no. 3 (2015): 459–61. https://doi.org/10.14310/horm.2002.1608.

Medical Quality State of California. In the Matter of the Petition for Reinstatement of Revoked Certificate of: John Ronald Brown, 1983. Accessed September 29, 2022. https://www2.mbc.ca.gov/BreezePDL/document.aspx?path=%5CDIDOCS%5C20151015%5CDMRAAAFC4%5C&did=AAAFC151015180442278.DID.

McHugh, Paul R. "Psychiatric Misadventures." *American Scholar* 61, no. 4 (1992): 497–510.

Mestas, Anthony A. "Trinidad Doctor Battled Hospital." *Pueblo Chieftain*, August 1, 2010. Accessed September 29, 2022. https://www.chieftain.com/story/news/2010/08/01/trinidad-doctor-battled-hospital/8416043007/.

Meyer, Jon K., and Donna J. Reter. "Sex Reassignment: Follow-Up." *Archives of General Psychiatry* 36, no. 9 (1979): 1010–15.

Meyer, Walter, Walter O. Bockting, Peggy Cohen-Kettenis, et al. "The Harry Benjamin International Gender Dysphoria Association's Standards of Care for Gender Identity

Disorders, Sixth Version." *Journal of Psychology & Human Sexuality* 13, no. 1 (2002): 1–30. https://doi.org/10.1300/J056v13n01_01.

Meyerowitz, Joan. *How Sex Changed*. Cambridge: Harvard University Press, 2009.

Monstrey, Stan J., Peter Ceulemans, and Piet Hoebeke. "Sex Reassignment Surgery in the Female-to-Male Transsexual." *Seminars in Plastic Surgery* 25, no. 3 (2011): 229–44. https://doi.org/10.1055/s-0031-1281493.

Monstrey, Stan, Gennaro Selvaggi, Peter Ceulemans, et al. "Chest-Wall Contouring Surgery in Female-to-Male Transsexuals: A New Algorithm." *Plastic and Reconstructive Surgery* 121, no. 3 (2008): 849–59. https://doi.org/10.1097/01.prs.0000299921.15447.b2.

Naini, Farhad B. "Hugo L. Obwegeser (1920–2017)—The Father of Modern Orthognathic Surgery." *Journal of Orthodontics* 44, no. 4 (2017): 317–19. https://doi.org/10.1080/14653125.2017.1392064.

Nair, Rajesh. "Sir Harold Gillies: Pioneer of Phalloplasty and the Birth of Uroplastic Surgery." *Journal of Urology* 183, no. 4 (2010): e437.

Noe, Joel M., Ronald Sato, Clifford Coleman, and Donald R. Laub. "Construction of Male Genitalia: The Stanford Experience." *Archives of Sexual Behavior* 7, no. 4 (1978): 297–303.

Novais, C., M. J. Peixoto, M. Mota Oliveira, and A. Côrte-Real. "Apotemnophilia: Psychiatric Disorder, Neurological Disorder or Not a Disease at All?" *European Psychiatry*, Abstracts of the 24th European Congress of Psychiatry, 33, S1 (March 2016): S155. https://doi.org/10.1016/j.eurpsy.2016.01.286.

Orticochea, M. "A New Method of Total Reconstruction of the Penis." *British Journal of Plastic Surgery* 25, no. 4 (1972): 347–66. https://doi.org/10.1016/s0007-1226(72)80077-8.

Ousterhout, Douglas K. *Facial Feminization Surgery: A Guide for the Transgendered Woman*. Omaha, NE: Addicus Books, 2009.

———. "Dr. Paul Tessier and Facial Skeletal Masculinization." *Annals of Plastic Surgery* 67, no. 6 (2011): S10. https://doi.org/10.1097/SAP.0b013e31821835cb.

Pemberton, Marilyn. "Castrati: Did the End Justify the Means?" *Historia: Magazine of the Historical Writers' Association*, January 17, 2020. Accessed September 29, 2022. http://www.historiamag.com/castrati-end-justify-means/.

People v. Brown, 91 Cal.App.4th 256, 109 Cal. Rptr. 2d 879, Cal. Ct. App., 2001.

Perovic, Sava V., Rados Djinovic, Marko Bumbasirevic, Miroslav Djordjevic, and Petar Vukovic. "Total Phalloplasty Using a Musculocutaneous Latissimus Dorsi Flap." *BJU International* 100, no. 4 (2007): 899–905; discussion 905. https://doi.org/10.1111/j.1464-410X.2007.07084.x.

Pinney, Jacquie, and Anthony Metcalfe. "Sir Archibald McIndoe and the Guinea Pig Club." *PMFA Journal* 1, no. 2 (2014). Accessed September 29, 2022. https://www.thepmfajournal.com/features/post/sir-archibald-mcindoe-and-the-guinea-pig-club.

Platel, Alain, and Frank Van Laeche. "Transformations over Time: Interview with Plastic Surgeon Stan Mosnstrey." *LaGeste Newsletter*, 2024. Accessed August 13,2024. https://www.lageste.be/en/interview-with-plastic-surgeon-stan-monstrey

Plemons, Eric. *The Look of a Woman: Facial Feminization Surgery and the Aims of Trans-Medicine*. Durham, NC: Duke University Press, 2017. Accessed September 29, 2022. https://www.google.com/books/edition/The_Look_of_a_Woman/L3MtDwAAQBAJ?hl=en&gbpv=0.

Plemons, Eric D. "Description of Sex Difference as Prescription for Sex Change: On the Origins of Facial Feminization Surgery." *Social Studies of Science* 44, no. 5 (2014): 657–79.

Plemons, Eric Douglas. "Making the Gendered Face: The Art and Science of Facial Feminization Surgery." PhD diss., University of California, Berkeley, 2012. Accessed September 29, 2022. https://escholarship.org/uc/item/6gw4b97x

Preto, Mirko, Gideon Blecher, Massimiliano Timpano, Paolo Gontero, and Marco Falcone. "The Frontier of Penile Implants in Phalloplasty: Is the ZSI 475 FTM What We Have Been Waiting For?" *International Journal of Impotence Research* 33 (January 2021): 1–5. https://doi.org/10.1038/s41443-020-00396-2.

Ray, Saikat, and Krishna Rao. "Full Thickness Skin Grafts. Skin Grafts—Indications, Applications and Current Research." IntechOpen, 2011. https://doi.org/10.5772/22385.

Richie, Cristina. "A Queer, Feminist Bioethics Critique of Facial Feminization Surgery." *American Journal of Bioethics* 18, no. 12 (2018): 33–35.

Rooker, Steven, Krishna Vyaas, Emily DiFilippo, Ian Nolan, Shane Morrison, and Richard Santucci. "The Rise of the Neophallus: A Systematic Review of Penile Prosthetic Outcomes and Complications in Gender-Affirming Surgery." *J Sex Med* (2019): 1–12. Accessed August 13, 2024. https://cranects.com/wp-content/uploads/sites/307/2019/10/Penile-Implant.pdf.

Sayegh, Farah, David Ludwig, Mona Ascha, et al. "Facial Masculinization Surgery and Its Role in the Treatment of Gender Dysphoria." *Journal of Craniofacial Surgery* 20, no. 5 (2019): 1339–46. https://doi.org/10.1097/SCS.0000000000005101.

Schechter, Loren S., Salvatore D'Arpa, Mimis N. Cohen, Ervin Kocjancic, Karel E. Y. Claes, and Stan Monstrey. "Gender Confirmation Surgery: Guiding Principles." *Journal of Sexual Medicine* 14, no. 6 (2017): 852–56. https://doi.org/10.1016/j.jsxm.2017.04.001.

Schillace, Brandy. "The Forgotten History of the World's First Trans Clinic." *Scientific American*, May 10, 2021. Accessed August 24, 2022. https://www.scientificamerican.com/article/the-forgotten-history-of-the-worlds-first-trans-clinic/.

Schultheiss, Dirk, Alexander Gabouev, and Udo Jonas. "Nikolaj A. Bogoraz (1874–1952): Pioneer of Phalloplasty and Penile Implant Surgery." *Journal of Sexual Medicine* 2, no. 1 (2005): 139–46. https://onlinelibrary.wiley.com/doi/abs/10.1111/j.1743-6109.2005.20114.x.

Science Direct. "Split Thickness Skin Graft—an Overview." n.d. Accessed September 21, 2021. https://www.sciencedirect.com/topics/medicine-and-dentistry/split-thickness-skin-graft.

Sedda, Anna, and Gabriella Bottini. "Apotemnophilia, Body Integrity Identity Disorder or Xenomelia? Psychiatric and Neurologic Etiologies Face Each Other." *Neuropsychiatric Disease and Treatment* 10 (July 2014): 1255–65. https://doi.org/10.2147/NDT.S53385.

Sherkin, Suzanne, Helma Seidl, and Skyler Hagen. *When Gender Is in Question: A Guide to Understanding*. Victoria, BC, Canada: Friesen Press, 2021.

Siculus, Diodorus. *Library of History, Volume XI: Fragments of Books 21–32*. Loeb Classical Library 409. Translated by Francis R. Walton. Cambridge: Harvard University Press, 1957. Quoted in Markantes et al., "Callo." https://doi.org/10.14310/horm.2002.1608.

Siotos, Charalampos, Paula M. Neira, Brandyn D. Lau, et al. "Origins of Gender Affirmation Surgery: The History of the First Gender Identity Clinic in the United States at Johns Hopkins." *Annals of Plastic Surgery* 83, no. 2 (2019): 132–36. https://doi.org/10.1097/SAP.0000000000001684.

Skidmore, Emily. "Constructing the 'Good Transsexual': Christine Jorgensen, Whiteness, and Heteronormativity in the Mid-Twentieth-Century Press." *Feminist Studies* 37, no. 2 (2011): 270–300.

Smith, Martin. *Going to Trinidad: A Doctor, a Colorado Town, and Stories from an Unlikely Gender Crossroads*. Denver, CO: Bower House, 2021.

Song, Colin, Manzhi Wong, Chin-Ho Wong, and Yee-Siang Ong. "Modifications of the Radial Forearm Flap Phalloplasty for Female-to-Male Gender Reassignment." *Journal of Reconstructive Microsurgery* 27, no. 2 (2011): 115–20. https://doi.org/10.1055/s-0030-1268210.

Tan, Roy. "S Shan Ratnam." Singapore LGBT Encyclopaedia Wiki. n.d. Accessed October 20, 2021. https://the-singapore-lgbt-encyclopaedia.wikia.org/wiki/S_Shan_Ratnam.

TransHealthCare, "Find a Surgeon for Gender Affirming Surgery." TransHealthCare, n.d. Accessed September 23, 2021. https://www.transhealthcare.org/.

Wangjiraniran, Burin, Gennaro Selvaggi, Prayuth Chokrungvaranont, Sirachai Jindarak, Sutin Khobunsongserm, and Preecha Tiewtranon. "Male-to-Female Vaginoplasty: Preecha's Surgical Technique." *Journal of Plastic Surgery and Hand Surgery* 49, no. 3 (2015): 153–59. https://doi.org/10.3109/2000656X.2014.967253.

Watanyusakul, Suporn. "Vaginoplasty Modifications to Improve Vulvar Aesthetics." *Urologic Clinics of North America* 46, no. 4 (2019): 541–54. https://doi.org/10.1016/j.ucl.2019.07.008.

Wei, Shu-Yi, Feng-Yong Li, Qiang Li, et al. "Autologous Buccal Micro-Mucosa Free Graft Combined with Posterior Scrotal Flap Transfer for Vaginoplasty in Male-To-Female Transsexuals: A Pilot Study." *Aesthetic Plastic Surgery* 42, no. 1 (2018): 188–96. https://doi.org/10.1007/s00266-017-0977-x.

Wheeless, Clifford and Marcella Roenneburg. "McIndoe Vaginoplasty for Neovagina." *Atlas of Pelvic Surgery*, n.d. Accessed September 5, 2021. https://atlasofpelvicsurgery.org/2VaginalandUrethra/13McIndoeVaginoplastyforNeovagina/chap2sec13.html.

Williams, Constance. "'Pelvic Beauty' Becomes Achievable, Harvard Professor Says." *Korea Biomedical Review*, October 20, 2017. Accessed September 29, 2022. http://www.koreabiomed.com/news/articleView.html?idxno=1649.

World Professional Association for Transgender Health Bulletin. "WPATH Remembers Sheila Kirk, MD, 1930–2019." May 6, 2020. Accessed September 29, 2022. https://listloop.com/wpath/mail.cgi/archive/adhoc/20200526073422/.

Zagria Blogspot. "John Ronald Brown: Part II." A Gender Variance Who's Who (blog), May 20, 2017. Accessed September 29, 2022. https://zagria.blogspot.com/2017/05/john-ronald-brown-part-ii.html.

Zanghellini, Aleardo. *The Sexual Constitution of Political Authority: The "Trials" of Same-Sex Desire*. Abingdon, Oxon: Routledge, 2015.

17.1. PROFILE: ALAN HART (1890–1962)

Carolyn Wolf-Gould

In 1918, Alan Hart was the first transgender individual in the United States to receive supportive care from a physician, J. Allen Gilbert, who eventually provided the first gender-affirming hysterectomy. Gilbert's publication of Hart's medical history and Hart's subsequent distinguished career paved the way for people like Reed Erickson, who promoted access to medical and surgical transitions for those seeking relief from gender dysphoria.

Assigned female at birth in 1890 and christened Alberta Lucille, Hart grew up in a rural community in Oregon. From a young age he identified as male, assuring his mother he would "grow up to be a man and take care of [her]."[1] As a child, he gravitated toward traditionally masculine activities such as farm chores, collecting pocket knives, and chopping wood. He preferred boy's clothing and begged his parents to let him cut his hair and wear trousers, believing this would allow him to be a boy in the world. As Hart grew older, he excelled in all aspects of school; took up hunting, rowing, and football; and fantasized about being married to and making love to a woman as a man, although "the exact nature of the sex act was not yet clear in her [sic] mind."[2] He observed the anatomy of farm animals and peeked through holes in the outhouse to study the boys. He developed crushes on his female classmates, teachers, and the family servants, eventually entering into a series of passionate relationships with different women.

Hart graduated from Albany College (now Lewis and Clark College) in 1912,[3] developed a romantic relationship with a female classmate, and supported them both by rapidly depleting his newly acquired inheritance. He struggled with love affairs, began to drink and smoke, and frequented the theaters and cabarets in nearby cities.[4] Hart often passed as a man. In 1913, he entered the University of Oregon Medical College and once again proved himself an excellent student. He graduated in 1917; "[she] was the only woman in the class and took with top academic honors."[5]

In medical school, Hart grappled with his "condition" by reading medical literature and books. "At first, [she] was plunged into self-condemnation and misery, but very soon came to take a saner view and face [her] problem as best she could."[6] In 1918, at age twenty-six, he sought medical care from the progressive physician J. Allen Gilbert. After psychotherapy and hypnosis proved unsuccessful in altering his masculine identity, Hart told Gilbert he possessed an "utter loathing of the female type of mind" and wanted no treatment that would "deprive [her] of [her] masculine ambitions and tastes."[7] Gilbert acknowledged his own confusion around "such a psychological muddle," noting that Hart "knew nothing of psychopathy and did not realize that [her] own condition was abnormal; it always seemed perfectly right to [her]."[8] He eventually agreed to help Hart "prepare definitively and permanently for the role of the male in conformity with [her] real nature all these years."[9]

What is perhaps most remarkable about Hart's story is that he justified his need for a hysterectomy with an argument in favor of eugenics: "[She] realized and urged the advisability of sterilization of [herself], as well as of any individual afflicted as [she] was."[10] Gilbert, after long hesitation and deliberation, performed the operation, after which his patient renamed himself Alan, cut his hair, donned masculine clothing, eloped with Inez Stark, and "started as a male with a new hold on life and ambitions worthy of [her] high degree of intellectuality."[11]

After graduation, Hart was appointed to a hospital as an intern, but post-transition life proved difficult. Hart was outed by a colleague—and ultimately hounded out of the workplace.[12] With similar gender-related harassment over the next few years, he repeatedly "resigned" from multiple positions in Western and Midwestern hospitals. Unable to cope with these frequent disruptions, Stark left him in 1923.

Eventually Hart earned a master of medical science degree in radiology from the University of Pennsylvania and a master of public health from Yale.[13] In 1925 he settled into marriage with Edna Ruddick, who remained with him until his death.[14] He developed expertise on tuberculosis and the use of X-rays for its detection, serving in antituberculosis programs in New Mexico, Illinois, Washington, Idaho, and finally, Connecticut, where he worked in the state's Department of Health's tuberculosis office from 1945 until 1962.[15] He also published short stories, four novels (some loosely based on his own history), and a nonfiction book on the use of X-rays and radium.[16]

Hart's singular experience and the attendant publicity contributed to the idea that gender identity existed only as a binary, a belief that persisted for decades. In 1918, he spoke to a reporter for the *Daily Democrat* newspaper, stating "I had to do it. . . . For years I had been unhappy. . . . There can be no dual sex in a person. It is either one or the other."[17]

After World War II, hormone therapy became available, and Hart used testosterone to masculinize his body.[18] He believed his transition was a process that *affirmed*, rather than *changed* his gender. Hart proclaimed, "Each of us must take into account the raw material which heredity dealt us at birth and the opportunities we have had along the way, and then work out for ourselves a sensible evaluation of our personalities and accomplishments."[19]

NOTES

1. Gilbert, "Homo-Sexuality and Its Treatment," 300.
2. Gilbert, "Homo-Sexuality and Its Treatment," 302. All references to Alan Hart in Gilbert's paper refer to him with feminine pronouns.
3. Booth and Lauderdale, "Life and Career," 5.
4. Gilbert, "Homo-Sexuality and Its Treatment," 310.
5. Booth and Lauderdale, "Life and Career," 5.
6. Gilbert, "Homo-Sexuality and Its Treatment," 317.
7. Gilbert, "Homo-Sexuality and Its Treatment," 319.
8. Gilbert, "Homo-Sexuality and Its Treatment," 309.
9. Gilbert, "Homo-Sexuality and Its Treatment," 320.
10. Gilbert, "Homo-Sexuality and Its Treatment," 321.
11. Gilbert, "Homo-Sexuality and Its Treatment," 321; Young, "Alan Hart (1890–1962)."
12. *Morning Register*, "Posed as Dr. 'Alan' Hart"; *Eugene Guard*, "Women's Hospital Intern"; *Hartford Courant*, "Dr. Hart Dies"; Booth and Lauderdale, "Life and Career," 5; Gilbert, "Homo-Sexuality and Its Treatment," 321.
13. *Hartford Courant*, "Dr. Hart Dies."
14. Booth and Lauderdale, "Life and Career," 6.
15. *Hartford Courant*, "Dr. Hart Dies"; *Morning Register*, "Posed as Dr. 'Alan' Hart"; *Spokesman-Review*, "32 Reactors"; *Herald-Bulletin*, "Dr. Alan Hart"; *Record-Journal*,

"350 Volunteers"; Boag, *Re-Dressing America,* 14; Booth and Lauderdale, "Life and Career," 6; *Idaho Evening Times,* "Specialist Will Assist Doctors."
   16. Booth and Lauderdale, "Life and Career," 6; Hart, *These Mysterious Rays.*
   17. *Albany Daily Democrat,* "Dr. Hart Explains Change."
   18. Young, "Alan Hart (1890–1962)."
   19. Booth and Lauderdale, "Life and Career," 8.

WORKS CITED

Albany Daily Democrat. "Dr. Hart Explains Change to Male Attire." March 26, 1918, 1.
Boag, Peter. *Re-Dressing America's Frontier Past.* Berkeley, CA: University of California Press, 2011.
Booth, Brian, and Thomas Lauderdale. "The Life and Career of Alberta Lucille/Dr. Alan Hart with Collected Early Writings." Lewis & Clark Digital Collection. 1999. Archival materials printed by the Aubrey Watzek Library. Portland, OR: Lewis & Clark College, 2003. Accessed January 9, 2021. https://specialcollections.lclark.edu/items/show/36925.
Eugene Guard. "Woman's Hospital Intern Masquerades as a Man." February 5, 1918, 1.
Gilbert, J. Allen. "Homo-Sexuality and Its Treatment." *Journal of Nervous and Mental Disease* 52, no. 4 (1920): 297–322.
Hart, Alan. *These Mysterious Rays: A Nontechnical Discussion of the Uses of X Rays and Radium.* New York: Harper & Brothers, 1943.
Hartford Courant. "Dr. Hart Dies at 71, State X-Ray Director." July 3, 1962, 7.
Herald-Bulletin. "Dr. Alan Hart to Be In Twins Falls Soon." February 27, 1936, 7.
Idaho Evening Times. "Specialist Will Assist Doctors; Anti-Tuberculosis Association Brings Dr. Alan Hart Here as Consultant." March 6, 1936, 3.
Morning Register. "Posed as Dr. 'Alan' Hart." February 6, 1918, 1.
Record-Journal. "350 Volunteers to Conduct Chest X-Ray Canvass Locally." October 6, 1955, 14.
Spokesman-Review. "32 Reactors are Found by Tuberculosis Tests." June 9, 1935, 13.
Young, Morgen. "Alan Hart (1890–1962)." *Oregon Encyclopedia,* October 4, 2019. Accessed January 10, 2021. https://www.oregonencyclopedia.org/articles/hart_alan_1890_1962_/#.X_tlGulKjt1.

17.2. PROFILE: ELMER BELT (1893–1980)

Amy Block

Arthur Elmer Belt, the son of a postmaster, was born in 1893 and grew up in southern California. He rode a horse daily to his Los Angeles high school, where he completed science projects on the inner workings of the kidney.[1] Belt attended medical school at the University of California Berkeley, pursued further training in urology at the University of California San Francisco and the Brigham Hospital in Boston, and was later instrumental in establishing the University of California Los Angeles medical campus.[2] His friends included novelist Upton Sinclair and Earl Warren, the governor of California and eventual chief justice of the US Supreme Court.[3] By all accounts, he enjoyed a loving marriage to his wife Mary Ruth and raised two sons. He even gained some notoriety as a lifelong collector of Leonardo da Vinci's books and drawings.[4]

Without much fanfare, Belt also performed some of the earliest recorded gender-affirming surgeries in the United States. Postwar California was home to Robert Stoller, a Los Angeles psychoanalyst who was sympathetic to trans patients, as well as Harry Benjamin, the pioneering endocrinologist who had offices in San Francisco and New York.[5] Benjamin consulted Belt about surgical possibilities for his male-to-female patients in the early 1950s.[6] Belt's training in urology had familiarized him with a range of genital reconstruction procedures necessitated by physical trauma, sterility, and cancers.[7] When he began to treat transgender patients, Belt described himself as a "softie" who had "a strong sense of compassion for these poor devils."[8]

During this time, surgeons offering gender-affirming surgery in the United States faced legal challenges due to Mayhem statutes. Dating back to medieval England, the concept of mayhem—or maim—made it a felony to injure a man in such a way that he was unable to fight for his country.[9] In 1949, the attorney general of California advised Benjamin that surgical disturbance of the male genitals would constitute mayhem. No doctor was ever prosecuted for trans care under these statutes, but they had the intended effect of intimidating surgeons.[10]

To sidestep the Mayhem statutes, Belt devised a legal feminizing method that recessed the testes through the inguinal canals and preserved them whole in the abdomen.[11] Estrogen therapy then offset the hormonal effects of the gonads. Belt performed vaginoplasties on patients after these procedures, including on patients like Anette Dolan, who, in 1953, removed her own testes at home.[12] By the late 1960s, sufficient court cases had been decided in favor of gender-affirming surgeries, including those affecting the gonads, that the threat of mayhem receded.[13]

Transgender women's accounts of Belt run the gamut. Carla Sawyer complained about the roughness Belt used at a postop dilating appointment, and Aleshia Brevard reported that he was "condescending and rude."[14] The doctor himself complained in a letter to his nephew Willard Goodwin, a urologist, that his trans patients "lie when there is no need for it whatever."[15] In one case, Belt wrote that "the patient came in after all was done expressing dissatisfaction because there was not a uterus with tubes and ovaries" for having a baby.[16] Still, patients sought him out during those years as one of the few practitioners offering "sex changes" in the United States. Belt also wrote certified letters recommending that his patients' legal sex be changed to reflect their experienced gender and new parts.[17]

In late 1954, a committee of doctors at the University of California Los Angeles, including staff psychiatrists and his nephew Goodwin, advised Belt to stop performing gender-affirming procedures.[18] Belt nevertheless continued to operate at Good Samaritan, a different Los Angeles hospital where he had privileges, before finally ceasing gender-affirming surgery altogether in 1962 at the request of his wife and son.

An office fire in 1958 destroyed Belt's records, making it impossible to know the true extent of his trans surgical career.[19] He avoided publicity around this aspect of his work and resumed a quiet life until his death in 1980.

Belt may have quietly introduced feminizing genital surgery to the United States, but other surgeons did not generally accept or perform these procedures until Johns Hopkins opened the first medical gender center in 1965. Numerous other academic institutions followed suit. In a twist, Belt's nephew Goodwin upheld the family legacy when he himself performed a gender-affirming surgery for a trans woman named Barbara at the University of California Los Angeles in 1968.[20] A lawyer representing California's university system assured him that the state would pay for any legal bills in the unlikely event of Mayhem charges.[21] Goodwin later joined the ranks of Stoller and Richard Green at the University of California's interdisciplinary Gender Identity Clinic,[22] which provided vital services but also pressured some of its young patients to conform to gender norms rather than explore their true identities.[23]

NOTES

1. Marmor, "In Obscure Rebellion," 413.
2. Dibner, "Elmer Belt," 837.
3. Dibner, "Elmer Belt," 837.
4. Marmor, "In Obscure Rebellion," 414.
5. Reay, "The Transsexual Phenomenon," 1043.

6. Meyerowitz, "A 'Fierce and Demanding' Drive," 371.
7. Belt, "A Chat with Elmer Belt," 399.
8. Meyerowitz, "A 'Fierce and Demanding' Drive," 371.
9. Lewis, "The Lawfulness of Gender Reassignment Surgery," 62.
10. Lewis, "The Lawfulness of Gender Reassignment Surgery," 69.
11. Lewis, "The Lawfulness of Gender Reassignment Surgery," 71.
12. Meyerowitz, "A 'Fierce and Demanding' Drive," 371.
13. Lewis, "The Lawfulness of Gender Reassignment Surgery," 82.
14. Meyerowitz, "A 'Fierce and Demanding' Drive," 380.
15. Meyerowitz, "A 'Fierce and Demanding' Drive," 381.
16. Meyerowitz, "A 'Fierce and Demanding' Drive," 372.
17. Meyerowitz, "A 'Fierce and Demanding' Drive," 381.
18. Meyerowitz, "A 'Fierce and Demanding' Drive," 371.
19. Louise M. Darling Biomedical Library, Elmer Belt Papers.
20. Green, "Robert Stoller's Sex and Gender," 1459.
21. Green, "Robert Stoller's Sex and Gender," 1460.
22. Herdt, "Robert J. Stoller in the Clinic and the Village," 19.
23. Goulding, "UCLA Study Tried to Change Children's Gender Identity."

WORKS CITED

Belt, Elmer. "A Chat With Elmer Belt." *Urology* 10, no. 4 (1977): 398–402.

Dibner, Bern. "Elmer Belt (1893–1980)." *Technology and Culture* 22, no. 4 (1981): 837–38.

Goulding, Susan. "UCLA Study Tried to Change Children's Gender Identity in the 1960s, Say Two Educators." *Orange County Register*, November 18, 2019.

Green, Richard. "Robert Stoller's Sex and Gender: 40 Years On." *Archives of Sexual Behavior* 39, no. 6 (2010): 1457–65.

Herdt, Gilbert. "Robert J. Stoller in the Clinic and the Village." *Psychoanalysis and History* 22, no. 1 (2020): 15–34.

Lewis, Penney. "The Lawfulness of Gender Reassignment Surgery." *American Journal of Legal History* 58, no. 1 (2018): 56–85.

Louise M. Darling Biomedical Library, Special Collections. Elmer Belt Papers: Descriptive Summary. 2010. Accessed October 5, 2021. https://oac.cdlib.org/findaid/ark:/13030/kt2199r6k1/entire_text/.

Marmor, Max C. "In Obscure Rebellion: The Collector Elmer Belt." *Journal of Library History (1974–1987)* 22, no. 4 (1987): 409–24.

Meyerowitz, Joanne. "A 'Fierce and Demanding' Drive." In *The Transgender Studies Reader*, edited by Susan Stryker and Stephen Whittle, 362–82. New York: Routledge, 2006.

Reay, Barry. "The Transsexual Phenomenon: A Counter-History." *Journal of Social History* 47, no. 4 (2014): 1042–70.

17.3. PROFILE: CHRISTINE McGINN (1969–)

Yongha Kim

Christine McGinn was the first trans-identified, board-certified plastic surgeon to perform gender-affirming surgeries. She is the founder and acting director of the Papillon Gender Wellness Center, a clinic established in 2007 in New Hope, Pennsylvania, that provides holistic and affirming care for transgender and gender-diverse (TGD) patients.

McGinn attributes her approach in medicine to the holistic medical education she received at Philadelphia College of Osteopathic Medicine.[1] She graduated in 1995 on the US Navy's Health Professions Scholarship and served as a naval flight surgeon from 1995 to 2000, as well as in the Inactive Ready Reserves until 2004.[2] Her career as a flight surgeon was a distinguished one—she was invited by National Aeronautics and Space Administration (NASA) to participate in two space missions and was nominated as a Flight Surgeon of the Year for the US Navy in the last year of her service.[3] She was honorably discharged after being passed over for promotion to lieutenant commander for publicly stating she was a lesbian in an interview with Lester Holt on MSNBC, thus violating the Don't Ask Don't Tell policy.[4] The day before her discharge, she changed her legal name, requiring the Navy to discharge her under her new name, Christine McGinn.[5] In 2021, NASA's chief health and medical officer invited her to return and help develop medical guidelines for TGD astronaut candidates.

In 2005, while McGinn was in surgical training, former Surgeon General David Satcher invited her to serve as a member of the National Advisory Council at the Center of Excellence in Sexual Health at Morehouse School of Medicine.[6] As a physician, veteran, and transgender person, McGinn helped build consensus on sexual health policy with other sexual health leaders. In 2006, with the connections she formed while serving in this role, she contributed functional information on transgender orgasm and collaborated on the book *The Science of Orgasm*.

In 2007, McGinn established the Papillon Gender Wellness Center and dedicated herself to providing care for TGD people. She understood the importance of a holistic approach in gender care and pioneered a clinic that incorporated various aspects of transition, including surgery, endocrinology, hair removal, mental health therapy, community outreach, and fertility.[7] Many clinics across the United States have replicated this model of care.

As a national, public-facing figure, McGinn is a vocal advocate for transgender communities and has raised awareness of TGD rights. She spoke out for the inclusion of TGD people in organized athletics in the *New York Times* in 2008 and again in the documentary *Game Face* (2015).[8] She appeared on the *Oprah Winfrey Show* to share her experience being the first woman to have "fathered her child and also breastfed"; she had used her previously cryogenic sperm for in vitro fertilization with her wife.[9] She was featured in the award-winning documentary *Trans* and served as a surgical advisor for the Academy Award–winning feature film *The Danish Girl* (2015).[10] In 2016, when the Trump administration issued a ban on trans military personnel, she publicly announced she would provide free gender-affirming surgery to TGD service members who were denied treatment by government insurance programs.[11]

Today, McGinn remains dedicated to the day-to-day operation of the Papillon Center and continues to provide holistic TGD healthcare to those in need.

NOTES

1. McGinn, interview with the author.
2. Bondy, "I Just Had to Suppress Everything."
3. *Trans.*
4. McGinn, interview with the author.
5. *Trans.*
6. McGinn, interview with the author.
7. Papillon Gender Wellness Center, "About Us."
8. McGinn, interview with the author.
9. *Trans.*
10. McGinn, interview with the author.
11. Perez, "Ex-Navy Surgeon Promises Free Surgery."

WORKS CITED

Bondy, Haley. "'I Just Had to Suppress Everything': What It's Like to be Transgender in a Male-Dominated Field." *MSNBC: Know Your Value*, June 21, 2019.

Accessed June 2021. https://www.nbcnews.com/know-your-value/feature/i-just-had-suppress-everything-what-it-s-be-transgender-ncna1019636.

McGinn, Christine. Interview with author. February 2022.

Papillon Gender Wellness Center. "About Us." 2015. Accessed June 2021. https://www.drchristinemcginn.com/aboutus/.

Perez, Medardo. "Ex-Navy Surgeon Promises Free Surgery for Transgender Troops." *NBC News*, July 13, 2017. Accessed June 2021. https://www.nbcnews.com/feature/nbc-out/ex-navy-surgeon-promises-free-surgery-transgender-troops-n788126.

Trans. Directed by Chris Arnold. Produced by Mark Schoen. Performed by Christine McGinn, Masen Davis, Jamison Green, and Tiffany Woods. 2012.

18

THE TREATMENT OF TRANSGENDER AND GENDER-DIVERSE CHILDREN AND ADOLESCENTS

Diane Ehrensaft

In this chapter, I trace the historical trajectory from curative to supportive models of care for transgender and gender-diverse (TGD) children. I discuss children and adolescents whose gender identities are distinct from their assigned sex at birth. Developmentally, they are prepubertal or in puberty. Their identity challenges the genders others assume them to be based on social norms in their cultures. Their visibility has increased in the first part of the twenty-first century, as evidenced by the growing numbers of children brought to gender clinics for support,[1] the growth in the number of those clinics,[2] and the attention given to gender-diverse children in the social and public media, as well as in the political arena. Nevertheless, they have existed since time immemorial.[3]

When it comes to the care of these young people, history has shown the mental health field to have been paradoxically problematic and enlightened as knowledge and treatment protocols evolved. Mental health practitioners have attempted either to cure or to support children and youths' diverse gender identities and expressions. As we moved into the third decade of the twenty-first century, the ascendance of the gender affirmative model[4] as the prevailing model of care for TGD children has been met with an alarming backlash internationally, with judicial and legislative actions intent on squashing supportive mental health and medical treatments for these youth. International, national, and state health and advocacy organizations have responded by signing joint statements and providing expert testimony, thus highlighting the scientific evidence for gender-affirming care for trans children and youth.

PSYCHOANALYSIS PLAYS ITS HAND

Following the footprint of psychosexual stages of development outlined by the Freuds (Sigmund and Anna) in the early to mid-twentieth century, a trope of gender development coalesced, first in Vienna and then later in Hampstead, England.[5] In this model, an infant was assigned a sex at birth based on genitalia: male or female. Within the first two years of life, the child learned their core gender identity based on their sex designation (that is, I am a girl; I am a boy). From two to six years of age, the child learned what it meant to be a boy or a girl and was socialized into appropriate gender roles based on sociocultural expectations. In this same age range, they fell in love with their opposite-sex parent (with the assumption that all children had only two parents and those two parents were of the opposite sex); discovered the dangers of that fantasized love affair; and rejected that desire in place of identification with their same-sex parent. If all went well, by age six the child was clear in their core gender identity, accepted this status as permanent and irreversible, and solidified a heterosexual/straight orientation.[6] According to this psychoanalytic model, if a child had not reached these milestones by age six, there was cause for concern, and the child, along with their parents, was referred for psychiatric help to analyze and address the source of this developmental failure. This model prevailed and underlay much of psychiatry throughout the twentieth century, and sometimes it still persists.

Dr. Robert Stoller, working at the University of California Los Angeles from the 1950s until his tragic death in a car accident in 1991, was a psychiatrist and psychoanalyst who translated this trope into an intervention model. The main targets in his approach were "effeminate" boys who did not abide by the gender norms of the time. His psychoanalytic approach to these youth was predicated on two hypotheses: (1) their gender expressions and gender identities emerged from a specific set of dynamics; (2) their femininity was a result of too much gratification (on the part of the mother), rather than a defense against primitive, overwhelming anxiety. Stoller's treatment of choice was individual psychoanalysis with the child, the mother, and the father. The description of the pool of children treated is anatomically normal, graceful, charming, feminine in appearance, liked to dress in girls' clothes, played exclusively with girls in girls' activities, wanted their body changed to female. In regard to the children's gender history, parents reported these behaviors were evident since approximately one year of age.[7] By contemporary gender-affirming standards, these youth would likely be considered transgender or gender-diverse, perhaps wanting to explore social transitions. By Stoller's standards, these children were suffering from a gender disorder caused by parental foibles (overinvolved mother, distant or ineffectual father) and in need of a cure.[8]

Colette Chiland later adopted Stoller's model in France in the early twenty-first century, recommending intensive psychotherapy for the child, individual treatment for each parent, and an occasional joint parent session. If there was a question at the initial evaluation that the child was presenting with an apparent transgender identity, clinicians sent the child to an endocrinologist to rule out a disorder of sex development before any psychological treatment could begin. This was to make sure the child was normal anatomically, that is, endosex (not intersex). Chiland, as did Stoller, recommended a therapist of the same birth-assigned sex as the child because "in our view, it is good for the child to interact with a same-sex adult who is at ease with his sex, as his same-sex parent is not—nor indeed is his other-sex parent."[9] Regarding treatment outcome, the goal was to cure the gender anomalies and ward off a transsexual adulthood: "It is evident to all concerned with transsexualism that the treatment prognosis is better in childhood than in adolescence and adulthood, and that the parents must also receive attention."[10]

Calling on a different set of psychoanalytic postulates, Susan Coates (director of the Childhood Gender Identity Service at St. Luke's-Roosevelt Hospital Center in New York City from 1980 until 1997) and her associates developed a model of treatment based on the assumption that trauma or early attachment disruptions underlay gender dysphoria in young children and that treatment of the trauma or attachment disorders would alleviate or remove the gender anomalies.[11] For example, a little boy who was the victim of a car accident in which he lost his mother soon after adopted the accouterments of a female and announced having a gender identity as female. Clinicians interpreted this gender crossing as the child holding onto the dead mother by becoming the mother. Treatment involved psychotherapy to enable the child to work through the trauma of the accident and loss of the mother, with the assumption that the feminine expression and female gender identity would remit following treatment. Coates failed to publish information regarding the long-term outcomes for this child regarding gender identity and/or expression. While the trauma/attachment disruption theory may have applied to this particular child, no evidence exists documenting the evidence of trauma and/or attachment disruptions as a causative factor or even appearing at all in the vast majority of children who articulate a transgender identity.

In sum, psychoanalysis set the stage for reparative practices, defined as therapy attempting to change the gender behaviors, ideations, and identifications of young children to ward off a gay or transgender outcome. Then, social engineering and behavior modification programs took over, a phenomenon to which we now turn.

RICHARD GREEN AND THE SISSY BOY MODEL

There was no ambiguity in the treatment program set up by Richard Green at the University of California Los Angeles in the 1980s. He dedicated his book *Sissy Boy Syndrome and the Development of Homosexuality* to Stoller, "who sustained me."[12] He recommended that effeminate boys receive treatment to eliminate their feminine behaviors and redirect them to cisnormative and heteronormative standards. The psychoanalytic principles of parents' influence on their sons' behaviors stood firmly within his theoretical understanding of gender development, yet the actual parameters of treatment followed social engineering and behavior modification rubrics. As described in *Sexual Identity Conflict in Children and Adults*, Green recommended that (1) fathers augment contact with their boys by finding activities within their mutual interests and competencies; (2) parents engineer playdates with nonaggressive male peers; (3) parents discourage feminine physical gestures to avoid negative social feedback and isolation from other boys; and (4) therapeutic goals should include reducing current psychic pain to allow for a wider range of social options in the future. Green's approach also involved direct shaming, as revealed in his report to a mother about her six-year-old child Nick, who was enrolled in Green's longitudinal research project. Green described Nick as a boy who liked girl things and did not want to play ball—and went on to confront these behaviors: "I told him that as he grows up, and if he continues to do sissy things, that he won't have many friends, and people will make fun of him, and that he'll be very unhappy."[13] Green instructed Nick's mother to offer praise for any masculine behaviors. He encouraged Nick's father to take over regarding activities, asking the mother to step aside: "You've got to get these mothers out of the way. Feminine [boys] don't need their mothers around."[14]

The effects of this modality of treatment are best reflected in Green's treatment notes about Nick: "Today he had a fantasy about another 'feminine' boy whom he knows I see here. He said, 'He should be spanked. Or at least reminded. He probably wants to be a girl because he can wear girls' dresses and have long hair. But he shouldn't do this because children will make fun of him. Boys burn up dresses of boys. Boys can go places and have more fun.'"[15] From a psychoanalytic perspective, this progress note suggests evidence of a child who was socially induced to turn passive into active by attacking a child similar to himself and dissociating from his authentic gender self through reaction formation. In other words, after Nick was instructed and socially engineered to repudiate all he once experienced as good, he now deemed the behavior bad and deserving of punishment (as might very well have happened to Nick if his parents followed Green's directive to negatively reinforce or punish "gender inappropriate" behaviors). Situating Green's work within a more recent study of shame and depression in treatment modalities for gender-diverse children,[16] the case of Nick (and other of Green's reported cases) would be evaluated not as facilitating confidence and well-being but rather as inducing shame and repudiation, the perhaps unintended but inevitable outcome of the "sissy boy" approach.

The form of treatment practiced by Green and associates at the University of California Los Angeles is now illegal in several US states and municipalities and all of Canada. California, the state in which Green conducted his clinic, was the first of many, in 2012, to pass legislation (Senate Bill 1172) banning mental health professionals from engaging in reparative forms of therapy with minors who are gender-diverse or potentially members of a sexual minority. More specifically, these state laws declared that no mental health professional should attempt to change a child's gender behaviors, roles, or identity. The growing body of evidence documenting the harm (sometimes fatal) done to sexual and gender minorities when professionals attempt to redirect a child's sexuality and/or gender identity informed these statutes. This harm includes anxiety, depression, self-harm, substance abuse, eating disorders, unsafe sexual practices, and suicidality.[17] The statutes also coincided with policy statements from major international and national organizations involved in the psychological care of children and youth, all of which articulated reparative forms of therapy as ineffective, harmful, and unethical.[18]

A report from a man who was once Green's patient speaks poignantly to the harm done. The parents of Karl Bryant, now a gay sociologist who studies the history of the treatment of gender-expansive children, brought Byrant to Green in 1967 to cure his sissy behaviors. Bryant reports that between the ages of five and eight, Green provided treatment to ensure he learned to act more like a boy. He recalls that Green stressed the benefits of being a boy in contrast to the challenges faced by a girl. Green encouraged Bryant's father to develop a closer relationship with him and trained his parents to establish more conventional gender role behaviors at home. Bryant's take-away message was that you can *want* to be someone you're not, but it's never going to happen. Only in adulthood did Bryant come to realize that this therapy did more harm than good, particularly the directives given to his parents: "I was told that the way I felt about that aspect of myself [his gender expressions and his attraction to boys] was wrong, was sick, needed to be changed. It was a little different than a kid on the playground threatening to beat you up—you know they're the enemy. This was my parents, people I trusted." [19]

LIVING-IN-YOUR-OWN-SKIN MODEL

Kenneth Zucker, an American psychologist, worked as the clinical lead of the Gender Identity Clinic for Children at the Centre for Addiction and Mental Health (CAMH) in Toronto, Canada, from 1981 to 2015, when his gender clinic was closed by the hospital for alleged unethical practices. Zucker followed the directives of Green's program, with one additional objective: to ward off a transgender future. Although Zucker and his colleagues consistently denied that their interventions equated with reparative therapy, it is difficult to discern how it was different. Susan Bradley, Zucker, and their colleagues at CAMH adapted Green's methods and set as the treatment goal for young children acceptance of the gender that matched their assigned sex at birth.[20] Their underlying premise was that young children have a malleable gender identity and could be influenced to achieve psychological congruence between their sexed body and the gender identity that matched that body or, metaphorically, "live in their own skin."[21] The rationale for implementing this treatment was that going through life as a cisgender rather than transgender individual relieved the child of the stigma of being transgender and the added burden of medical interventions (hormones, surgeries) that might accompany a transgender identity. As quoted in a *Metro* article, Zucker stated "You are lowering the odds that as such a kid [that is, a gender-expansive child] gets older, he or she will move into adolescence feeling so uncomfortable about their gender identity that they think that it would be better to live as the other gender and require treatment with hormones and sex-reassignment surgery."[22] This model gained ascendance during the era in which expanded medical services became available to transgender adolescents and adults, including puberty blockers to pause pubertal development for youth exploring their gender, gender-affirming hormones, and gender-affirming surgical interventions. The assumption was that no parent would want this fate for their child if it could be prevented. Zucker attained a position of authority by publishing many articles and attaining the position of editor at the prestigious journal *Archives of Sexual Behavior*, where he exercised his editorial prerogative to ensure his own theories were propagated and extensively cited.

Implementing this model of treatment required that the child and family first undergo an extensive evaluation and that the parents agree to implement the treatment plan. The plan involved removing toys and activities considered nonnormative and replacing them with toys and activities typically associated with a child's birth-assigned sex; introducing same-sex playmates to replace opposite-sex playmates; encouraging the same-sex parent to become more active in the child's life while asking the opposite-sex parent to step back; and involving both parents and the child in ongoing psychotherapy to address their psychodynamic issues. Parents who could not agree to these methods of treatment (many expressed that they could not bear doing this to their child) were typically labeled as resistant or in denial rather than as exercising their rights as informed consumers.[23]

If the above-mentioned efforts were not implemented, or if a child still expressed a desire to live as another gender by adolescence, the treatment team advised that the sensitive period for gender malleability was over; and it was too late for the living-in-your-own-skin methods to be effective. At that point, they supported the youth socially transitioning and later receiving medical interventions (hormones, surgery) to achieve gender congruence. In sum, Zucker's living-in-your-own-skin model integrated a form of behavior modification, social engineering, and psychodynamic psychotherapy to achieve the set goals of gender congruence between assigned sex at birth and the child's gender identity, until it was too late to do so.[24] I refer to this model as the "bending the twig" approach. The treatment team (primarily the parents) bent the child's natural growth to suit societal expectations of the child's gender identity while these youth were still thought to be tender and malleable.

The living-in-your-own-skin model is no longer legal in the province of Ontario. In 2015, the Legislative Assembly of Ontario passed Bill 77, the *Affirming Sexual Orientation and Gender Identity Act*, which banned mental health practices that attempted to change a child's gender identity, expressions, or sexual identity. Later that year, Zucker's gender program at CAMH closed. Following complaints from the community that the service caused harm to children and after an internal review of the clinic's practices, the Center let Zucker go. He sued and, in October 2018, received a settlement from CAMH consisting of more than half a million dollars in damages, legal fees, and interest, plus a public apology.[25] Zucker remains in private practice.

THE WATCHFUL WAITING MODEL

At the same time the gender program at the CAMH was in operation, a group of professionals in the Netherlands developed their own treatment center, housed at the Vrije Universiteit Medical Center in Amsterdam. Their care model, developed within their pediatric gender clinic (opened in 1987), became known as the watchful waiting model.[26] This clinic was the first program to offer GnRH analogs (puberty blockers) to youth who were exploring their gender identity. Such treatment provided young people an opportunity to pause puberty before they confirmed a transgender pathway with social and medical transitions.

Their treatment protocols started well before the stage of puberty. Parents brought children to the clinic at a young age, typically because they observed that their child was either not developing in a gender-conforming fashion or showed stress related to gender expectations. Many of their preliminary evaluative procedures were similar to those used at Zucker's program in Toronto; in fact, Zucker worked closely with the Dutch program, adapting their assessment instruments in his own clinic. They first submitted children to a battery of tests to determine whether they exhibited gender dysphoria and to identify co-occurring psychological issues. They offered ongoing psychotherapy to the prepubertal children diagnosed with gender dysphoria (or previously, the *Diagnostic Statistical Manual of Mental Disorders, Fourth Edition*, diagnosis of gender identity disorder) and psychological supports for their parents.

The clinicians encouraged parents to allow their children to explore and express gender naturally at home or in specific protected environments. However, for young children who articulated a gender identity that did not match their assigned sex at birth, they recommended a watchful waiting approach. They suggested postponing some social transition interventions, such as name/pronoun change and gender marker change, until adolescence. They rationalized this waiting period as follows: (1) their research demonstrated that only a small percentage of the children who received a diagnosis in early childhood maintained that diagnosis into adolescence, so they felt it was best to wait until adolescence and the beginning stages of puberty to better discern if this child was transgender;[27] (2) although a child might appear clear in their affirmed gender identity at a young age, allowing them to transition early in life might cognitively pigeonhole them prematurely, depriving them of the opportunity for further exploration of their gender identity; and (3) premature social transition might prevent a child from being realistic about the biological features of their body based on their sex.

If by adolescence the youth still qualified for a gender dysphoria diagnosis and articulated a transgender identity, the clinicians and family helped the child socially transition without restrictions and offered medical interventions to allow greater gender congruence, with age requirements set for puberty blockers, gender-affirming hormone therapy, and surgeries. In sum, this approach supported a child as they evolved into their authentic gender identity (without attempts to persuade them to live in their own skin); however, it also recommended caution for prepubertal children regarding changes in their gender expression, postponing social transitions until adolescence. In its original iteration, the model also endorsed waiting to start hormone therapy until age sixteen, the legal age of majority in the Netherlands.

The main change effort evidenced in the Dutch protocol involved asking the prepubertal gender dysphoric child who desired social transition to wait until later. I consider this approach "the hold back model." Although the proponents of the Dutch model reported no untoward effects of asking a child to wait until puberty before socially transitioning, they lacked evidence that compared the outcomes for these children with those afforded the opportunity to socially transition before puberty. More recently, Kristina Olson and her associates at the TransYouth Project at the University of Washington published data that challenged the need for watchful waiting. They matched prepubertal transgender children with a cisgender control group and demonstrated that children who underwent an early social transition were equal to their peers in social-emotional and cognitive development and showed no increase in psychological problems.[28]

Those of us who developed the gender affirmative model of care are indebted to the team in the Netherlands, as they set the stage for health-generating and innovative care of gender-diverse children and youth. However, the holding back component is a fault line in their approach. A few years ago, I received an email from a parent from the Netherlands that spoke to the problem:

Dear Mrs. Ehrensaft,

You do not know me at all, and your time is precious, but as a mother of 3 wonderful children of which our B, born as a boy, with twin brother S, 6 years old, I cannot do otherwise than reach out even across the borders of our country. . . . all for B's well-being.
  Last month she told me: "Mummy until I was 3 years old, I really thought I WAS a girl . . . now I know I am not." And then I explain that how you feel inside is just as real as my oldest daughter knows she is a girl, beyond doubt. In our opinion, B is not confused. But the specialist team we consulted tells all parents of children with gender dysphoria: "Do not give too much room; he or she will probably outgrow it. . . . It is not so hard to dress neutrally." But after a year of struggling, crying of B "Why can't I dress the way I want to, Mom?" We felt we had to give more space.
  What do you think of our way of responding?
  Thank you so much for your time
  A mother with tears in her heart.

This mother saw that her transgender daughter was guided to hide her true gender in a neutral gender expression and knew that her daughter had been coaxed, even if gently, to accept that her body was male. The mother felt her child's pain in being unable to live authentically, and in writing to me, she pushed back against the clinic's instruction to limit her child's freedom of gender expression.

THE GENDER AFFIRMATIVE MODEL

If the live-in-your-own-skin model is the bend the twig approach and the Dutch protocol the hold back model, the gender affirmative model (GAM) serves in contrast as the "listen and act" model. The GAM, the newest approach for addressing the needs of transgender young people, evolved from the Dutch protocol and stands as an antidote to reparative models of care. The move toward this model of care occurred organically around the globe as practitioners, community members, families, and theorists in the first decade of the twenty-first century began to coalesce around an understanding of gender-diverse children, including that gender expressions and identity exist across a spectrum (rather than within two boxes) and that a child of any age had a right to live in their authentic gender. The development of the model coincided with the establishment of new pediatric gender clinics, with the first in the United States, the Gender Management Services Clinic at Boston Children's Hospital under the leadership of Norman Spack, opening in 2007. The basic building blocks of this model were established by the second decade of the twenty-first century.

In 2013, an interdisciplinary group of professionals from the first four major US sites for pediatric gender care launched a multisite National Institutes of Health study on the effects of puberty blockers and hormone therapy in youth, and they published a paper outlining the major tenets of the gender affirmative model as understood at that time.[29] The authors came from the University of California San Francisco, Boston Children's Hospital, Lurie's Children's Hospital in Chicago, and Children's Hospital Los Angeles. Following is the comprehensive list of those tenets, as delineated in the 2013 article, amended for explication:

- Gender variations are not disorders, nor are they pathological.

- Gender variations are healthy expressions of infinite possibilities of human gender.

- Gender presentations are diverse and varied across cultures, requiring cultural sensitivity to those variations.

- Gender involves an interweaving of nature, nurture, and culture—no one of these stands alone in shaping gender.

- A person's gender may be binary; a person's gender may be fluid or multiple.

- If a person is suffering from any emotional or psychiatric problem connected to their gender, this is likely because of negative reactions to the child from the outside world.

- If there is gender pathology, we will find it not in the child but in the culture (otherwise known as transphobia).[30]

The conclusion from these premises is that striving toward an authentic gender identity is the cure rather than a disease in need of cure and that efforts for "cure" should be directed toward changing the environmental factors that impede a person's gender health.

The underlying premise of the GAM is that an individual is capable of articulating their authentic gender identity at any age. The role of the clinician is to listen to the child, assess what the child is saying about their gender, and help the child live in that gender, whatever form that might take.[31] Unlike the living-in-your-own-skin model, the clinician does not attempt to change a child's gender behaviors, nor are the parents recommended to do so. In contrast to the watchful waiting model, the GAM is based on stages, not ages, meaning there is no set age for gender affirmation, only the child's stage of readiness for steps in gender congruence, including social transitions for prepubertal children.

Practitioners who adopt this model vary in their evaluative procedures. Some, like practitioners using the live-in-your-own-skin and watchful waiting models, administer formal evaluations to determine a child's gender status and any co-occurring psychological issues.[32] Others, following the tenet that gender expansiveness is a healthy variation of development and is not necessarily subject to a mental health diagnosis, forego formal psychological assessments and replace them with patient consultations. Practitioners recommend psychotherapy only if the child (or parent) demonstrates signs of stress or distress or needs a "room of their own" to further explore their gender.[33] They emphasize an ecological process, evaluating the systems in which the child is growing, including family, daycare, school, and religious institutions, ultimately striving to institute plans in each of those domains to assure support and acceptance.[34] This model promotes interdisciplinary teams of mental health and medical providers; the child, parents, and allied professionals are critical members of the care team.[35] Clinicians pay attention to siblings, grandparents, and other extended family members under the principle that family acceptance is crucial to a child's gender health[36] and that anyone intimately related to the child may need support as they adjust to the child's newly articulated gender self.[37]

The main arena in which the GAM pushes beyond the watchful waiting model is around the issue of social transitions. Following the dictum that gender health is defined as the opportunity for a child to explore and live in the gender that feels most authentic to them with no rejection or aspersion, the GAM asserts that preventing a child from doing so is unnecessary and possibly harm inducing, rather than risk aversive.[38] Further, since the GAM contends that knowing one's gender is a lifelong developmental process, GAM practitioners are less concerned that an early social transition might lock a child into a fixed gender identity. Instead, GAM practitioners make every effort to leave all gender pathways open, with opportunities for the child to evolve into a different gender, either in expressions or identity—or both—over time.

The GAM is opposed to the underlying premises of the living-in-your-own-skin model, that is, that a young child's gender identity is malleable, that a cisgender outcome is superior to a transgender outcome, and that parents should engage in social engineering practices to contort the natural unfolding of their child's authentic gender self. The GAM is critical of both the living-in-your-own-skin and watchful waiting models for conflating gender identity with gender expression and relying on data from their own clinics to argue that most children outgrow their gender dysphoria by adolescence. In reality, young children who are transgender do not outgrow their transgender identity; young children who are expansive in their gender expressions may not be dealing with gender identity issues. The GAM recognizes that children will follow different developmental pathways that should be consistently left open to them, and this includes the pathway to a social transition from one gender to another if their identity warrants this change.[39]

As the newest kid on the block, the GAM is criticized for lacking empirical scientific evidence to demonstrate its effectiveness, including its claims that early social transitions are in a child's best interest and cause no harm.[40] The aforementioned research of Olson and associates at the University of Washington does provide evidence to support one aspect of the GAM: children who socially transitioned at an early age did as well mental health–wise as a matched group of cisgender children. Nonetheless, more evidence is warranted, particularly regarding children who have transitioned at an early age, to assess whether early social transitions facilitate optimal outcomes for gender resilience and confidence. Some claim that the GAM rubber stamps whatever a child articulates about their gender based on the major premise: "If you want to know a child's gender, it is not for us to say, but for the child to tell." This assertion is a misperception of the approach, which instead employs an exploratory, collaborative treatment model with the child at the center, joined by the family and interdisciplinary team of gender specialists who listen over time to what the child is communicating about their gender.

In the GAM, the change effort helps a child move from gender stress to gender health, defined as the opportunity to live in one's authentic gender with acceptance and support, free of aspersion, rejection, or prohibition.[41] This process enables a shift from gender dysphoria to gender euphoria, defined as the opportunity to live in one's authentic gender and the feelings of happiness that accompany that effort. Its methods follow the *Standards of Care* of the World Professional Association for Transgender Health and the guidelines of each of the major organizations that provide directives for gender care involving children and youth. The efficacy of this model might best be expressed in the words of a nine-year-old patient at the Child and Adolescent Gender Center clinic at the University of California San Francisco who socially transitioned from boy to girl at age eight. When asked, "What would you do if someone said you had to go back to living as a boy?" The child quickly answered: "I'd take 'em to court." Then, after a pause: "Or they could take me to court." Legislation in the United States is not yet fully informed by this model, but clearly this child was willing to fight for their identity.

CONCLUSION

While exploring the history of treatment for transgender children under the age of puberty, we follow an emerging trajectory of change efforts. These efforts originally centered around moving a child from gender expansiveness to confirmed heterosexuality and gender normativity. This reparative model morphed into a related change effort to move a child from a transgender to a cisgender outcome—the living-in-your-own skin model. This grew into the watchful waiting model, an approach that supported transgender outcomes but postponed change in case a child should grow out of their gender-expansive/transgender self. Most recently, a change effort emerged, one that helps move a child from gender stress to gender authenticity and the consolidation of a true gender self.[42] This latest is the GAM.

With clear evidence of harm, those drawn to reparative methods would do well to change their attitudes toward gender-expansive children. Those drawn to the watchful waiting and gender affirmative methods need to promote change in the world to allow all children to be recognized and supported in the gender most authentic to them, regardless of whether it matches the assigned sex at birth or the gender norms of the culture.

NOTES

1. Chen, Fuqua, and Eugster, "Referrals for Gender Dysphoria."
2. Hsieh and Leininger, "Resource List."

3. Gill-Peterson, *Histories of the Transgender Child*.
4. Keo-Meier and Ehrensaft, *The Gender Affirmative Model*.
5. Freud, "Three Essays on the Theory of Sexuality"; Freud, "Analysis of a Phobia in a Five-Year-Old-Boy"; Freud, "Femininity"; Freud, *"Normality and Pathology in Childhood*.
6. Tyson, "Developmental Line of Gender Identity"; Fast, "Aspects of Core Gender Identity"; Ehrensaft, *Gender Born, Gender Made*.
7. Stoller, *Presentations of Gender*.
8. Stoller, *Presentations of Gender*.
9. Chiland, *Transsexualism*, 66.
10. Chiland, *Transsexualism*, 65.
11. Coates et al., "The Etiology of Boyhood"; Marantz and Coates, "Mothers of Boys."
12. Green, *"Sissy Boy Syndrome,"* dedication page.
13. Green, *"Sissy Boy Syndrome,"* 274.
14. Green, *"Sissy Boy Syndrome,"* 275.
15. Green, *"Sissy Boy Syndrome,"* 271.
16. Wallace and Russell, "Attachment and Shame."
17. Bryant, "Making Gender Identity Disorder"; Kohli, "Gender Behavior Therapy"; Wallace and Russell, "Attachment and Shame"; Byne et al., "Report of the American Psychiatric Association"; Byne, "Regulations Restrict Practice"; Turban and Ehrensaft, "Gender Identity in Youth."
18. Coleman et al., *Standards of Care*; Telfer et al., *Australian Standards of Care*.
19. Kohli, "Gender Behavior Therapy."
20. Zucker and Bradley, *Gender Identity Disorder*.
21. Zucker et al., "Developmental, Biopsychosocial Model."
22. Cross, "Outcry Prompts CAMH."
23. Zucker and Bradley, *Gender Identity Disorder*.
24. Zucker et al., "Developmental, Biopsychosocial Model."
25. Hayes, "Doctor Fired from Gender Identity Clinic."
26. Cohen-Kettenis and Pfäfflin, *Transgenderism*; de Vries and Cohen-Kettenis, "Clinical Management of Gender Dysphoria."
27. Steensma and Cohen-Kettenis, "Gender Transitioning before Puberty?," 649–50; Steensma et al., "Factors Associated with Childhood Gender Dysphoria."
28. Durwood et al., "Mental Health and Self Worth"; Olson, "Prepubescent Transgender Children"; Olson, Key, and Eaton, "Gender Cognition"; Olson, Durwood et al., "Mental Health of Transgender Children."
29. Hidalgo et al., "The Gender Affirmative Model."
30. Ehrensaft, *The Gender Creative Child*, 15.
31. Hidalgo et al., "The Gender Affirmative Model."
32. Berg and Edwards-Leeper, "Child and Family Assessment."

33. Ehrensaft, *The Gender Creative Child.*
34. Kaufman and Tishelman, "Creating a Network of Professionals."
35. Sherer et al., "Child and Adolescent Gender Center."
36. Travers et al., *Impact of Strong Parental Support.*
37. Malpas et al., "Resilience in Trangender and Gender Expansive Children."
38. Ehrensaft et al., "Prepubertal Social Gender Transitions"; Keo-Meier and Ehrensaft, *The Gender Affirmative Model.*
39. Ehrensaft et al., "Prepubertal Social Gender Transitions."
40. Turban and Ehrensaft, "Gender Identity in Youth."
41. Hidalgo et al., "The Gender Affirmative Model"; Ehrensaft, *The Gender Creative Child.*
42. Ehrensaft, "From Gender Identity Disorder."

WORKS CITED

Beemyn, Genny, and Susan Rankin. *The Lives of Transgender People.* New York: Columbia University Press, 2011.
Berg, Dianne, and Laura Edwards-Leeper. "Child and Family Assessment." In *The Gender Affirmative Model: An Interdisciplinary Approach to Supporting Transgender and Gender Expansive Children*, edited by Colt Keo-Meier and Diane Ehrensaft, 101–24. Washington, DC: American Psychological Association Publications, 2018.
Bryant, Karl. "Making Gender Identity Disorder of Childhood: Historical Lessons for Contemporary Debates." *Sexuality Research and Social Policy* 3, no. 3 (2006): 23–39. https://doi.org/10.1525/srsp.2006.3.3.23.
Byne, William. "Regulations Restrict Practice of Conversion Therapy." *LGBT Health* 3, no. 2 (2016): 97–99. https://doi.org/10.1089/lgbt.2016.0015.
Byne, William, Susan J. Bradley, Eli Coleman, et al. "Report of the American Psychiatric Association Task Force on Treatment of Gender Identity Disorder." *Archives of Sexual Behavior* 41 (2012): 759–96. https://doi.org/10.1007/s10508-012-9975-x.
Chen, Melinda, John Fuqua, Erica A. Eugster. "Characteristics of Referrals for Gender Dysphoria over a 13-Year Period." *Journal of Adolescent Health* 58, no. 3 (2016): 369–71. https://doi.org/10.1016/j.jadohealth.2015.11.
Chiland, Colette. *Transsexualism: Illusion and Reality.* Middletown, CT: Wesleyan University Press, 2003.
Coates, Susan, Richard C. Friedman, and Sabrina Wolfe. "The Etiology of Boyhood Gender Identity Disorder: A Model for Integrating Temperament, Development, and Psychodynamics." *Psychoanalytic Dialogues* 1, no. 4 (1991): 481–523. https://doi.org/10.1080/10481889109538916.
Cohen-Kettenis, Peggy T., and Friedemann Pfäfflin. *Transgenderism and Intersexuality in Childhood and Adolescence: Making Choices.* Thousand Oaks, CA: Sage, 2003.

Coleman, Eli, Walter Bockting, Marsha Botzer, et al. "Standards of Care for the Health of Transsexual, Transgender, and Gender-Nonconforming People, Version 7." *International Journal of Transgenderism* 13, no. 4 (2012): 165–232. https://doi.org/10.1080/15532739.2011.700873.

Cross, J. S. "Outcry Prompts CAMH to Review Its Controversial Treatment of Trans Youth." *Metro*, 2015. Accessed August 21, 2024. https://web.archive.org/web/20150320203815/http://metronews.ca/news/toronto/1315743/outcry-prompts-camh-to-review-its-controversial-treatment-of-trans-youth/.

de Vries, Annelou L. C. and Peggy T. Cohen-Kettenis. "Clinical Management of Gender Dysphoria in Children and Adolescents: The Dutch Approach." *Journal of Homosexuality* 59, no. 3 (2012): 301–20. https://doi.org/10.1080/00918369.2012.653300.

Durwood, Lily, Katie A. McLaughlin, and Kristina R. Olson. "Mental Health and Self-Worth in Socially Transitioned Transgender Youth." *Journal of the American Academy of Child and Adolescent Psychiatry* 56, no. 2 (2017): 116–123.e2. Accessed August 21, 2024. https://www.sciencedirect.com/science/article/abs/pii/S0890856716319414.

Ehrensaft, Diane. "From Gender Identity Disorder to Gender Identity Creativity: True Gender Self Child Therapy." *Journal of Homosexuality* 59, no. 3 (2012): 337–56. https://doi.org/10.1080/00918369.2012.653303.

———. *Gender Born, Gender Made*. New York: The Experiment, 2011.

———. *The Gender Creative Child: Pathways for Nurturing and Supporting Children Who Live Outside Gender Boxes*. New York: The Experiment, 2016.

Ehrensaft, Diane, Shawn V. Giammattei, Kelly Storck, Amy C. Tishelman, and Colt St. Amand. "Prepubertal Social Gender Transitions: What We Know; What We Can Learn—A View from a Gender Affirmative Lens." *International Journal of Transgenderism* 19, no. 2 (2018): 251–68. https://doi.org/10.1080/15532739.2017.1414649.

Fast, Irene. "Aspects of Core Gender Identity." *Psychoanalytic Dialogues* 9, no. 5 (1999): 633–61. https://doi.org/10.1080/10481889909539349.

Freud, Anna. *Normality and Pathology in Childhood: Assessments of Development*. New York: International Universities Press, 1965.

Freud, Sigmund. "Analysis of a Phobia in a Five-Year-Old-Boy." In *The Standard Edition of the Complete Psychological Works of Sigmund Freud, Volume X (1909): Two Case Histories*, 5–149. London: Hogarth Press, 1909.

———. "Femininity." In *The Standard Edition of the Complete Psychological Works of Sigmund Freud, Volume 22 (1932–1936): New Introductory Lectures on Psycho-Analysis and Other Works*, 112–35. London: Hogarth Press and the Institute of Psycho-analysis, 1933.

———. "Three Essays on the Theory of Sexuality." In *The Standard Edition of the Complete Psychological Works of Sigmund Freud, Volume VII (1901–1905): A*

Case of Hysteria, Three Essays on Sexuality and Other Works, 135–243. London: Hogarth Press, 1905.

Gill-Peterson, J. *Histories of the Transgender Child.* Minneapolis: University of Minnesota Press, 2018.

Green, Richard. *Sexual Identity Conflict in Children and Adults*. New York: Basic Books, 1974.

———. *The "Sissy Boy Syndrome" and the Development of Homosexuality*. Hartford, CT: Yale University Press, 1987.

Hayes, Molly. "Doctor Fired from Gender Identity Clinic Says He Feels Vindicated after CAMH Apology, Settlement." *Globe and Mail*, October 7, 2018. Accessed June 9, 2021. https://www.theglobeandmail.com/canada/toronto/article-doctor-fired-from-gender-identity-clinic-says-he-feels-vindicated/.

Hidalgo, Marco A., Diane Ehrensaft, Amy C. Tischelman, et al. "The Gender Affirmative Model: What We Know and What We Aim to Learn." *Human Development* 56, no. 5 (2013): 285–90. https://doi.org/10.1159/000355235.

Hsieh, Sam, and Jennifer Leininger. "Resource List: Clinical Care Programs for Gender-Nonconforming Children and Adolescents." *Pediatric Annals* 43, no. 6 (2014): 238–44. https://doi.org/10.3928/00904481-20140522-11.

Kaufman, Randi, and Amy Tishelman. "Creating a Network of Professionals." In *The Gender Affirmative Model: An Interdisciplinary Approach to Supporting Transgender and Gender Expansive Children*, edited by Colt Keo-Meier and Diane Ehrensaft, 173–88. Washington, DC: American Psychological Association, 2018. https://doi.org/10.1037/0000095-011.

Keo-Meier, Colt, and Diane Ehrensaft, eds. *The Gender Affirmative Model: An Interdisciplinary Approach to Supporting Transgender and Gender Expansive Children*. Washington, DC: American Psychological Association, 2018.

Kohli, Sonaki. "Gender Behavior Therapy and Gay Conversion: UCLA's Past, California's Future." *Daily Bruin*, 2012. Accessed August 21, 2024. https://dailybruin.com/2012/11/15/gender-behavior-therapy-and-gay-conversion-uclas-past-californias-future.

Lev, Arlene Istar. "Disordering Gender Identity: Gender Identity Disorder in the DSM-IV-TR." *Journal of Psychology and Human Sexuality* 17, no. 3–4 (2005): 35–69.

Malpas, Jean, Elizabeth Glaeser, and Shawn V. Giammattei. "Building Resilience in Transgender and Gender Expansive Children, Families, and Communities: A Multidimensional Family Approach." In *The Gender Affirmative Model: An Interdisciplinary Approach to Supporting Transgender and Gender Expansive Children*, edited by Colt Keo-Meier and Diane Ehrensaft, 141–56. Washington, DC: American Psychological Association, 2018. https://doi.org/10.1037/0000095-009.

Marantz, Sonia, and Susan Coates. "Mothers of Boys with Gender Identity Disorder: A Comparison of Matched Controls." *Journal of the American Academy of Child and Adolescent Psychiatry* 30, no. 2 (1991): 310–15. https://doi.org/10.1097/00004583-199103000-00022.

Olson, Kristina R. "Prepubescent Transgender Children: What We Do and Do Not Know." *Journal of the American Academy of Child and Adolescent Psychiatry* 55, no. 3 (2016): 155–56.e3. https://doi.org/10.1016/j.jaac.2015.11.015.

Olson, Kristina R., Lily Durwood, Madeleine DeMeules, and Katie A. McLaughlin. "Mental Health of Transgender Children Who Are Supported in Their Identities." *Pediatrics* 137, no. 3 (2016): e20153223. https://doi.org/10.1542/peds.2015-3223.

Olson, Kristina R., Aidan C. Key, and Nicholas R. Eaton. "Gender Cognition in Transgender Children." *Psychological Science* 26, no. 4 (2015): 467–74. https://doi.org/10.1177/0956797614568156.

Pfäfflin, Friedemann, and Astrid Junge. *Sex Reassignment: Thirty Years of International Follow-up Studies after Sex Reassignment Surgery: A Comprehensive Review, 1961–1991*. Dusseldorf, Germany: Symposion Publishing, 1998. Accessed August 21, 2024. http://web.archive.org/web/20070503090247/http:/www.symposion.com/ijt/pfaefflin/1000.htm.

Sherer, Ilana, Stephen M. Rosenthal, Diane Ehrensaft, and Joel Baum. "Child and Adolescent Gender Center: A Multidisciplinary Collaboration to Improve the Lives of Gender Nonconforming Children and Teens." *Pediatrics in Review* 33, no. 6 (2012): 273–75. https://doi.org/10.1542/pir.33-6-273.

Steensma, Thomas D., Jenifer K. McGuire, Baudewijntje P. C. Kreukels, Anneke J. Beekman, and Peggy T. Cohen-Kettenis. "Factors Associated with Desistence and Persistence of Childhood Gender Dysphoria: A Quantitative Follow-up Study." *Journal of the American Academy of Child and Adolescent Psychiatry* 52, no. 6 (2013): 582–90. https://doi.org/10.1016/j.jaac.2013.03.016.

Steensma, Thomas D., and Peggy T. Cohen-Kettenis. "Gender Transitioning before Puberty?" *Archives of Sexual Behavior* 40 (2011): 649–50. https://doi.org/10.1007/s10508-011-9752-2.

Stoller, Robert J. *Presentations of Gender*. Hartford, CT: Yale University Press, 1985.

Telfer, Michelle M., Michelle A. Tollit, Carmen C. Pace, and Ken C. Pang. *Australian Standards of Care and Treatment Guidelines for Trans and Gender Diverse Children and Adolescents Version 1.1*. Vol. 1.1. Melbourne: Royal Children's Hospital, 2018. https://onlinelibrary.wiley.com/doi/full/10.5694/mja17.01044. Accessed August 21, 2024.

Travers, Robb, Greta Bauer, Jake Pyne, Kaitlin Bradley, Lorraine Gale, and Maria Papadimitriou. *Impacts of Strong Parental Support for Trans Youth: A Report Prepared for Children's Aid Society of Toronto and Delisle Youth Services*. Trans Pulse, 2012. Accessed August 21, 2024. http://transpulseproject.ca/wp-content/uploads/2012/10/Impacts-of-Strong-Parental-Support-for-Trans-Youth-vFINAL.pdf.

Turban, Jack. "Connecticut Bans Conversion Therapy for LGBT Youth." *Psychology Today*, 2017. Accessed August 21, 2024. https://www.psychologytoday.com/us/blog/political-minds/201705/connecticut-bans-conversion-therapy-lgbt-youth.

Turban, Jack L., and Diane Ehrensaft. "Research Review: Gender Identity in Youth: Treatment Paradigms and Controversies." *Journal of Child Psychology and Psychiatry* 59, no. 12 (2018): 1228–43. https://doi.org/10.1111/jcpp.12833. Accessed August 21, 2024.

Tyson, Phyllis. "A Developmental Line of Gender Identity, Gender Role, and Choice of Love Object." *Journal of the American Psychoanalytic Association* 30, no. 1 (1982): 61–86. https://doi.org/10.1177/000306518203000103.

Wallace, Robert, and Hershel Russell. "Attachment and Shame in Gender-Nonconforming Children and Their Families: Toward a Theoretical Framework for Evaluating Clinical Interventions." *International Journal of Transgenderism* 14, no. 3 (2013): 113–26. https://doi.org/10.1080/15532739.2013.824845.

Zucker, Kenneth J., Hayley Wood, Devita Singh, and Susan J. Bradley. "A Developmental, Biopsychosocial Model for the Treatment of Children with Gender Identity Disorder." *Journal of Homosexuality* 59, no. 3 (2012): 369–97.

Zucker, Kenneth J., and Susan J. Bradley. *Gender Identity Disorder and Psychosexual Problems in Children and Adolescents*. New York: Guilford Press, 1995.

18.1. THE PEDIATRIC GENDER MANAGEMENT SERVICE AND GENDER SURGERY CENTER AT BOSTON CHILDREN'S HOSPITAL

David A. Diamond

In 2006, an international consensus conference on the management of intersex disorders[1] convened in Chicago with the following objectives: discuss the more controversial issues in intersex management, provide management guidelines for intersex patients, and prioritize research questions.[2] Conference participants recommended that multidisciplinary teams be tasked with managing these complex patients at major referral centers. Norman Spack, a senior endocrinologist represented Boston Children's Hospital, and soon after the conference, he and I (author and pediatric urologist) agreed to create an interdisciplinary center for patients with disorders of sexual development at Boston Children's Hospital, with medical, surgical, mental health, and nursing support. They recruited Laura Edwards-Leeper from psychology, Francie Mandel from social work, and Rosemary Grant from urology nursing to support the Gender Management Service (GeMS; currently known as the Gender Multispecialty Service). The departments of medicine and urology jointly provided financial support for the mental health team. The half-day monthly clinic launched in

2007. At that time, Spack also managed a modest transgender endocrinology practice.

As the referrals for patients with disorders of sexual development increased, a surprising number of transgender youths also began to present to the clinic. After the first year, the transgender patients, who traveled from throughout the northeast, outnumbered the patients with disorders of sexual developments by three to one. Spack recognized the challenge of providing affirming care for gender dysphoric youth; his team needed more training. He knew of the groundbreaking work of the Dutch group led by Peggy T. Cohen-Kettenis and organized a visit to the Netherlands for Edwards-Leeper and himself to learn their approach.[3] The team learned to perform gender assessments for gender dysphoric youth and determine their appropriateness for medical interventions, including the use of puberty blockers—medications that halt puberty—in part to allow time for patients and their families to participate in counseling and assess a child's gender identity over time. Internally, the Boston Children's Hospital made the crucial decision to provide financial support for the program.[4]

The GeMS program rapidly gained national recognition for adopting the Dutch protocols, a step that revolutionized the treatment of transgender youth in the United States. Physicians who trained within GeMS brought these skills to other centers, including the University of Michigan (Child and Adolescent Gender Services), Chicago (Gender Identity and Sex Development), and Dallas, Texas (GENECIS-Gender Education and Care Interdisciplinary Support), and other hospitals (for example, in Seattle [Gender Clinic] and Philadelphia [Gender and Sexuality Development Clinic]) that went on to adopt the Boston model on their own. Currently, a modified version of these protocols, the Gender Affirmative Model,[5] is the standard of care for trans youth throughout most of the United States. Despite the proliferation of this model, the Arkansas legislature outlawed treatment of minors in 2021 for political reasons, enacting the "single most extreme anti-trans law to ever pass through a state legislature."[6] Numerous state legislatures were considering similar measures at the time of this writing.[7]

In 2017, gender-affirming surgical options were limited in Boston. The urologists at Boston Children's Hospital only assumed responsibility for the insertion and removal of the puberty blocking implant. That year, plastic surgeons at the hospital approached the urology department to discuss the increasing numbers of transmasculine individuals requesting phalloplasty and metoidioplasty, procedures that were unavailable at all Boston hospitals. The plastic surgeons had performed numerous chest (top) surgeries for the trans community and had developed a relationship with Fenway Health, the largest program for transgender medical care in the area. Boston Medical Center offered vaginoplasty and had a waiting list of more than two hundred adults. Graduates from the pediatric GeMS clinic wished to start college or enter the workplace in their affirmed gender and wanted to receive their surgical care at the same medical center before setting off.

The national climate for transgender surgical care had evolved by this time. Social media, television, film, and the lay press had brought prominent individuals and compelling stories on gender transition to national attention. Some college health plans, as well as public and private insurance, covered gender-affirming surgery. The team believed the time was ripe to garner institutional support for a surgical program at Boston Children's Hospital. As a team, the urologists and plastic surgeons approached the departments of surgery, nursing, anesthesia, and ethics, as well as hospital administrators and legal consultants to assess interest. Remarkably, they encountered overwhelming support for this program.

The new gender surgical team traveled to San Francisco, California, for training on transmasculine surgical procedures, particularly phalloplasty, and partnered with colleagues at Boston Medical Center to learn how to perform vaginoplasties. Within a few months, the hospital administration approved the creation of a Gender Surgical Center of Excellence and provided resources to assemble a team that included a registered nurse, a social worker, a researcher, and a program coordinator.[8] The finance division developed a business model with marketing to promote the new program.

The team performed the first radial forearm flap phalloplasty in January 2018. As of March 2021, the program has provided more than 650 consultations for masculinizing and feminizing top and bottom surgery. They completed fourteen phalloplasties, three metoidioplasties, and eight vaginoplasties despite the COVID-induced slowdown of the previous year. As reconstructive bottom surgeries are sterilizing procedures, the clinic offers these exclusively to adult patients but does provide top or chest surgery for transgender adolescents.

At the time of this publication, the GeMS program focuses solely on transgender youth, with a parallel clinic for children with disorders/differences of sexual development. The clinicians at the GeMS see 350 new patients per year, and the center is staffed with four psychologists, six endocrinologists, one nurse practitioner, one adolescent medicine physician, and two social workers.

The development and evolution of this program, responding to an unmet social and medical need, has been a remarkable success story for Boston Children's Hospital and the patients that it serves.

NOTES

1. The diagnostic term *intersex* later changed to *disorders of sexual development*. The field is now moving toward the less pathologizing term *differences of sexual development*, in parallel to diagnosis of *gender identity disorder*, which changed to the less pathologizing diagnosis, *gender dysphoria*.
2. Lee et al., "Consensus Statement."
3. de Vries and Cohen-Kettenis, "Clinical Management of Gender Dysphoria."
4. Spack et al., "Characteristics of Children and Adolescents," 419.
5. Keo-Meier and Ehrensaft, "Introduction," 14–15.
6. Yurcba, "Arkansas Passes Bill to Ban Gender-Affirming Care."
7. Lewis, "Alabama Senate Votes"; Movement Advancement Project, "LGBTQ Policy Spotlight."
8. Boskey et al., "Ethical Issues," 2.

WORKS CITED

Boskey, Elizabeth, Judith Johnson, Charlotte Harrison, et al. "Ethical Issues When Establishing a Pediatrics Gender Surgery Center." *Pediatrics* 143, no. 6 (2019): 1–12e.

de Vries, A. L. C., and P. T. J. Cohen-Kettenis. "Clinical Management of Gender Dysphoria in Children and Adolescents: The Dutch Approach." *Homosexuality* 59, no. 3 (2012): 301–20.

Keo-Meier, Colt, and Diane Ehrensaft, eds. "Introduction to the Gender Affirmative Model." In *The Gender Affirmative Model: An Interdisciplinary Approach to Supporting Transgender and Gender Expansive Children*, 3–19. Washington, DC: American Psychological Association, 2018.

Lee, P. A., C. P. Ahmed, S. F. Houk, and I. A. Hughes. "Consensus Statement on Management of Intersex Disorders Organized by the Lawson Wilkins Pediatric Endocrine Society and the European Society for Pediatric Endocrinology." *Pediatrics* 3 (2006): 301–20.

Lewis, Sophie. "Alabama Senate Votes to Make Hormone Therapy and Surgery for Trans Youth a Felony." *CBS News*, March 3, 2021. Accessed May 13, 2021. https://www.cbsnews.com/news/alabama-senate-bans-hormone-therapy-surgery-felony-transgender-youth/.

Movement Advancement Project. "LGBTQ Policy Spotlight: Efforts to Ban Health Care for Transgender Youth." April 2021. Accessed August 24, 2021. https://www.lgbtmap.org/2021-spotlight-health-care-bans.

Spack, N., L. Edwards-Leeper, H. Feldman, et al. "Characteristics of Children and Adolescents with Gender Identity Disorder Referred to a Pediatric Medical Center." *Pediatrics* 129, no. 3 (2012): 418–25.

Yurcba, Jo. "Arkansas Passes Bill to Ban Gender-Affirming Care for Trans Youth." *NBC News*, March 29, 2021. Accessed September 18, 2021. https://www.nbcnews.com/feature/nbc-out/arkansas-passes-bill-ban-gender-affirming-care-trans-youth-n1262412.

18.2. ADOLESCENT MEDICAL CARE

Tresne Hernandez and Katherine Blumoff Greenberg

While early sexologists, including Magnus Hirschfeld, Alfred Kinsey, and Harry Benjamin, recognized that many transgender adults first experienced gender dysphoria in early childhood,[1] clinicians did not begin to treat transgender youth with hormonal therapies until the mid-1990s and, then, only in the Netherlands.

Peggy T. Cohen-Kettenis and Annelou C. V. de Vries pioneered new medical interventions for transgender youth at the Utrecht University Hospital in the Netherlands. In the early Dutch model, clinicians recommended waiting until late adolescence for social and medical transition. They believed youth must experience early puberty to "know" their gender identity and that early transitions would preclude essential gender exploration.[2] In 1997, the Dutch group published their first paper on the treatment of youth as young as sixteen with hormonal therapies.[3] In 1998, they reported on their first patient treated with gonadotropin-releasing hormone analogs to halt puberty at an early stage to prevent the development of secondary sex characteristics, a revolutionary approach that enabled youth to experience puberty in their experienced gender.[4] Over the next several decades, the Dutch team published their evolving treatment protocols.[5] The 2009 Endocrine Society Guidelines included the Dutch recommendations to suppress puberty in youth who met certain criteria until age sixteen[6] and that the induction of puberty in the experienced gender with estrogen or testosterone therapy begin at age sixteen or older.[7]

In 2007, Norman Spack and his team at Boston Children's Hospital founded the first comprehensive academic gender clinic for youth in the United States—the Gender Management Service (now the Gender Multispecialty Service). This team followed the Dutch protocols and the newly published Endocrine Society Guidelines.[8] In the early 2010s, pediatric and adolescent gender health clinics proliferated throughout the United States. In 2014, Sam Hsieh and Jennifer Lieninger compiled and published a list of thirty-three centers that offered gender-affirming care for youth,[9] all following some version of the Dutch protocol.

In 2014, the Dutch group published the first outcome study for their evolved protocol, which involved the use of puberty blockers at Tanner stages two to three, hormone therapy after age sixteen, and referral to gender-affirming surgeries after age eighteen, when desired.[10] They demonstrated that the fifty-five youth with access to timely, gender-affirming care possessed improved psychological outcomes compared to nontransgender young adults in the general Dutch population. Publication of these outcome data enabled the further proliferation of programs treating adolescents and young adults; as of this writing, approximately sixty centers nationwide offer children and adolescents access to gender healthcare, with an estimated three hundred clinics or medical offices providing hormonal therapies for adolescents.[11] Most centers in the United States now base treatment on the gender affirmative model,[12] which allows children "to speak for themselves about their self-experienced gender identity and expressions and provid[es] support for them to evolve into their authentic gender selves, no matter at what age."[13] This model further encourages clinicians to listen carefully to youth and recognize that the exploration of their gender identity may be a fluid process that evolves over time.[14]

While the publication of the Dutch outcomes represented important data for US-based providers to use to guide care and counseling for transgender adolescents and their parents, many unanswered questions remained. For example, how should clinicians counsel youth and families about the potential loss of fertility and the physiological effects of prolonged use of puberty blockers (for instance, on bone health)? What are the medium- and long-term impacts of gender-affirming hormones on cardiometabolic health?[15]

In 2012, the National Institutes of Health funded the first significant study of transgender and gender-diverse (TGD) youth in the United States. Titled the Trans Youth Study, this important undertaking began enrolling subjects in 2015; it was a collaborative effort linking four academic pediatric gender centers that planned to follow youth for five years. The study addressed the safety and efficacy of early treatment, including the use of pubertal blockers and gender-affirming hormonal treatment, by examining physiologic parameters and physiological well-being, among other outcomes.[16] Other studies provided foundational data on the impact of chest binding on wellness,[17] the impact of various puberty-blocking medication formulations,[18] and the short-term cardiometabolic impacts of hormone therapies.[19]

Despite the proliferation of clinical services and research data, transgender youth and their families still face significant barriers to care. Increasing societal visibility and acceptance of trans identities has decreased stigma about coming out; a recent study found that nearly ten percent of the high school students surveyed reported a TGD identity.[20] Pediatric and adolescent gender health clinics report a recent significant uptick in the number of referrals for care.[21]

While the medical literature demonstrates improved mental health outcomes with early social[22] and medical transition,[23] these treatment decisions are now debated and decided within state governmental bodies. In recent years, we have seen landmark anti-LGBTQ state legislation. Only five months into 2021, the Human Rights Campaign was already able to report the most anti-LGBTQ bills ever introduced into state legislatures. Bills enacted into law included those limiting transgender youths' ability to participate in sports, as well as a bill in Arkansas preventing doctors from providing or referring for gender-affirming hormonal therapy for people younger than eighteen.[24] The lawmakers enacting these laws do not have experience or expertise in the needs of gender dysphoric youth, and their claims often fly in the face of published data and national and international best practices.

Our clinicians at Golisano Children's Hospital–University of Rochester Medical Center in Rochester, New York, strive to meet the needs of TGD youth for the nine-county Finger Lakes region, as well as large areas of Central and Western New York. Like many youth centers, we draw from a large catchment area; ours spans New York from the Pennsylvania borders to our borders with Canada and Vermont.

We began offering care for TGD youth in 2012. At that time, we cared for ten to fifteen patients, and our business plan anticipated five new patient referrals a year. A decade later, our practice now serves serve more than five hundred adolescents, young adults, and their families annually. We care for youth and young adults through age twenty-five. We employ a mental health collaborative model for youth under the age of eighteen and the informed consent model for young adults eighteen and older. We prescribe and manage puberty-blocking medications and hormone therapy, refer for gender-affirming surgical care, and support patients during their planning and recovery.

While our clinic is unique to our geographic location, it also represents the quality and variety of care currently available to TGD youth and families in many parts of the United States. In contrast, while some clinics struggle to meet the rising demand for services, many youths still live in areas without access to care. In many states, there is political movement to ban or lessen gender-affirming care for youth, despite medical evidence of its benefits, and clinicians and patients alike are in more precarious positions due to discriminatory and divisive political climates.

NOTES

1. Gill-Peterson, *Histories of the Transgender Child*, 61.
2. Ehrensaft, "Gender Nonconforming Youth," 62.
3. Cohen-Kettenis and van Goozen, "Sex Reassignment."
4. Cohen-Kettenis and van Goozen, "Pubertal Delay," 46–48.
5. Delemarre-van de Waal and Cohen-Kettenis, "Clinical Management of Gender Identity Disorder"; Rosenthal, "Challenges in the Care," 586.
6. Tanner, "Growth and Maturation during Adolescence." Including, but not limited to, fulfilling specific *Diagnostic and Statistical Manual of Mental Disorders* criteria and having experienced puberty to at least sexual maturity rating (SMR; formerly known as Tanner Stages) stage two. SMR staging is a system used to track the physical development of people during puberty.
7. Hembree et al., "Endocrine Treatment," 3132.
8. Spack et al., "Children and Adolescents."
9. Hsieh and Leininger, "Resource List."
10. de Vries et al., "Young Adult Psychological Outcome."
11. Society for Evidence Based Gender Medicine, "Gender-Affirming Hormones."
12. Keo-Meier and Ehrensaft, "Introduction."
13. Ehrensaft, "Gender Nonconforming Youth," 62.
14. Keo-Meier and Ehrensaft, "Introduction," 14.
15. Geist et al., "Pediatric Research and Health Care," 38.
16. Olson-Kennedy et al., "Creating the Trans Youth Research Network"; Bunim, "First U.S. Study of Transgender Youth"; NIH Reporter, "The Impact of Early Medical Treatment."
17. Julian et al., "The Impact of Chest Binding."
18. Olson-Kennedy et al., "Histrelin Implants."
19. Millington et al., "Association of High-Density Lipoprotein."
20. Kidd et al., "Prevalence of Gender-Diverse Youth."
21. Handler et al., "Trends in Referrals."
22. Olson et al., "Mental Health of Transgender Children."
23. Sorbara et al., "Mental Health and Timing."

24. Ronan, "2021 Officially Becomes Worst Year"; Walch et al., "Proper Care of Transgender and Gender Diverse Persons," 306–07; Carlisle, "Federal Judge Temporarily Halts Arkansas Transgender Health Care Ban."

WORKS CITED

Bunim, Juliana. "First U.S. Study of Transgender Youth Funded by NIH: Four Sites with Dedicated Transgender Youth Clinics to Examine Long-Term Treatment Effects." University of California San Francisco, August 17, 2015 2015. Accessed February 3, 2022. https://www.ucsf.edu/news/2015/08/131301/first-us-study-transgender-youth-funded-nih.

Carlisle, Madeleine. "Federal Judge Temporarily Halts Arkansas Transgender Health Care Ban, Arguing It Causes 'Irreparable Harm.'" *Time*, July 21, 2021. Accessed February 3, 2022. https://time.com/6082411/arkansas-trans-health-care-ban/.

Cohen-Kettenis, Peggy T., and Stephanie H. M. van Goozen. "Pubertal Delay as an Aid in Diagnosis and Treatment of a Transsexual Adolescent." *European Child & Adolescent Psychiatry* 7, no. 4 (1998): 246–48. https://doi.org/10.1007/s007870050073.

———. "Sex Reassignment of Adolescent Transsexuals." *Journal of the American Academy of Child & Adolescent Psychiatry* 36, no. 2 (1997): 263–71. https://doi.org/10.1097/00004583-199702000-00017.

de Vries, Annelou L. C., Jenifer K. McGuire, Thomas D. Steensma, et al. "Young Adult Psychological Outcome after Puberty Suppression and Gender Reassignment." *Pediatrics* 134, no. 4 (2014): 696–704. https://doi.org/10.1542/peds.2013-2958.

Delemarre-van de Waal, Henriette A., and Peggy T. Cohen-Kettenis. "Clinical Management of Gender Identity Disorder in Adolescents: A Protocol on Psychological and Paediatric Endocrinology Aspects." *European Journal of Endocrinology* 155, no. S1 (2006): S131–37. https://doi.org/10.1530/eje.1.02231.

Ehrensaft, Diane. "Gender Nonconforming Youth: Current Perspectives." *Adolescent Health, Medicine and Therapeutics* 8 (2017): 57–67. https://doi.org/10.2147/ahmt.s110859.

Geist, Claudia, Katherine B. Greenberg, Rixt A. C. Luikenaar, and Nicole L. Mihalopoulos. "Pediatric Research and Health Care for Transgender and Gender Diverse Adolescents and Young Adults: Improving (Biopsychosocial) Health Outcomes." *Academic Pediatrics* 21, no. 1 (2020): 32–42. https://doi.org/10.1016/j.acap.2020.09.010.

Gill-Peterson, Jules. *Histories of the Transgender Child*. Minneapolis, MN: University of Minnesota Press, 2018. http://www.jstor.org/stable/10.5749/j.ctv75d87g.

Handler, Ted, J. Carlo Hojilla, Reshma Varghese, Whitney Wellenstein, Derek D. Satre, and Eve Zaritsky. "Trends in Referrals to a Pediatric Transgender Clinic." *Pediatrics* 144, no. 5 (2019): e20191368. https://doi.org/10.1542/peds.2019-1368.

Hembree, Wylie C., Peggy Cohen-Kettenis, Henriette A. Delemarre-van de Waal, et al. "Endocrine Treatment of Transsexual Persons: An Endocrine Society Clinical Practice Guideline." *Journal of Clinical Endocrinology & Metabolism* 94, no. 9 (2009): 3132–54. https://doi.org/10.1210/jc.2009-0345.

Hsieh, Sam, and Jennifer Leininger. "Resource List: Clinical Care Programs for Gender-Nonconforming Children and Adolescents." *Pediatric Annals* 43, no. 6 (2014): 238–44. https://doi.org/10.3928/00904481-20140522-11.

Julian, Jamie M., Bianca Salvetti, Jordan I. Held, Paula M. Murray, Lucas Lara-Rojas, and Johanna Olson-Kennedy. "The Impact of Chest Binding in Transgender and Gender Diverse Youth and Young Adults." *Journal of Adolescent Health* 68, no. 6 (2021): 1129–34. https://doi.org/10.1016/j.jadohealth.2020.09.029.

Keo-Meier, Colt, and Diane Ehrensaft, eds. "Introduction." In *The Gender Affirmative Model: An Interdisciplinary Approach to Supporting Transgender and Gender Expansive Children*, 3–19. Washington, DC: American Psychological Association Publications, 2018. https://doi.org/10.1037/0000095-001.

Kidd, Kacie M., Gina M. Sequeira, Claudia Douglas, et al. "Prevalence of Gender-Diverse Youth in an Urban School District." *Pediatrics* 147, no. 6 (2021): e2020049823. https://doi.org/10.1542/peds.2020-049823.

Millington, Kate, Courtney Finlayson, Johanna Olson-Kennedy, Robert Garofalo, Stephen M. Rosenthal, and Yee-Ming Chan. "Association of High-Density Lipoprotein Cholesterol with Sex Steroid Treatment in Transgender and Gender-Diverse Youth." *JAMA Pediatrics* 175, no. 5 (2021): 520–21. https://doi.org/10.1001/jamapediatrics.2020.5620.

NIH Reporter. "The Impact of Early Medical Treatment in Transgender Youth." 2021. Accessed August 21, 2024. https://reporter.nih.gov/search/Toxa9FxgiESqgnX5B8cfCw/project-details/10122677#history.

Olson, Kristina R., Lily Durwood, Madeleine DeMeules, and Katie A. McLaughlin. "Mental Health of Transgender Children Who Are Supported in Their Identities." *Pediatrics* 137, no. 3 (2016): e20153223. https://doi.org/10.1542/peds.2015-3223.

Olson-Kennedy, Johanna, Yee-Ming Chan, Stephen Rosenthal, et al. "Creating the Trans Youth Research Network: A Collaborative Research Endeavor." *Transgender Health* 4, no. 1 (2019): 304–12. https://doi.org/10.1089/trgh.2019.0024.

Olson-Kennedy, Johanna, Laer H. Streeter, Robert Garofalo, Yee-Ming Chan, and Stephen M. Rosenthal. "Histrelin Implants for Suppression of Puberty in Youth with Gender Dysphoria: A Comparison of 50 Mcg/Day (Vantas) and 65 Mcg/Day (Supprelinla)." *Transgender Health* 6, no. 1 (2021): 36–42. https://doi.org/10.1089/trgh.2020.0055.

Ronan, Wyatt. "2021 Officially Becomes Worst Year in Recent History for LGBTQ State Legislative Attacks as Unprecedented Number of States Enact Record-Shattering Number of Anti-LGBTQ Measures into Law." Human Rights Campaign, news release, May 7, 2021. Accessed February 3, 2022. https://www.hrc.org/press-releases/2021-officially-becomes-worst-year-in-recent-history-for-lgbtq-state-legislative-attacks-as-unprecedented-number-of-states-enact-record-shattering-number-of-anti-lgbtq-measures-into-law.

Rosenthal, Stephen M. "Challenges in the Care of Transgender and Gender-Diverse Youth: An Endocrinologist's View." *Nature Reviews Endocrinology* 17, no. 10 (2021): 581–91. https://doi.org/10.1038/s41574-021-00535-9.

Society for Evidence Based Gender Medicine. "'Gender-Affirming Hormones and Surgeries for Gender-Dysphoric US Youth." May 28, 2021. Accessed February 3, 2022. https://segm.org/ease_of_obtaining_hormones_surgeries_GD_US.

Sorbara, Julia C., Lyne N. Chiniara, Shelby Thompson, and Mark R. Palmert. "Mental Health and Timing of Gender-Affirming Care." *Pediatrics* 146, no. 4 (2020): e20193600. https://doi.org/10.1542/peds.2019-3600.

Spack, Norman P., Laura Edwards-Leeper, Henry A. Feldman, et al. "Children and Adolescents with Gender Identity Disorder Referred to a Pediatric Medical Center." *Pediatrics* 129, no. 3 (2012): 418–25. https://doi.org/10.1542/peds.2011-0907.

Tanner, J. M. Growth and Maturation during Adolescence. *Nutrition Reviews* 39, no. 2 (1981): 43–55. https://doi.org/10.1111/j.1753-4887.1981.tb06734.x.

Walch, Abby, Caroline Davidge-Pitts, Joshua D. Safer, Ximena Lopez, Vin Tangpricha, and Sean J. Iwamoto. "Proper Care of Transgender and Gender Diverse Persons in the Setting of Proposed Discrimination: A Policy Perspective." *Journal of Clinical Endocrinology & Metabolism* 106, no. 2 (2020): dgaa816. https://doi.org/10.1210/clinem/dgaa816.

19

A HISTORY OF GENDER-AFFIRMING VOICE AND COMMUNICATION INTERVENTIONS

Jack Pickering and Terren Lansdaal

In September 2011, a small group of speech-language pathologists from around the world attended the 22nd Biennial Symposium of the World Professional Association of Transgender Health (WPATH) in Atlanta, Georgia. Among the symposium's activities was the introduction to the seventh version of the WPATH *Standards of Care (SOC)*, which for the first time included discussion of gender-affirming voice and communication intervention. The group of speech-language pathologists in attendance cheered this announcement—it had been far too long in coming. While this moment ushered the formal inclusion of gender-affirming voice and communication intervention into WPATH's standards, the history of voice and communication modification for the treatment of gender dysphoria had begun more than four decades earlier.

Most of the early work focused on transgender women, as feminizing hormone therapy does not impact the vocal instrument (the vocal folds, the throat, the mouth) of those who have already completed masculine puberty. In contrast, androgen treatments directly change the vocal instrument, which initially had a deprioritizing effect on the development of gender-affirming voice and communication intervention for transgender men. As such, protocols targeting transgender women have long driven clinical advancements for speech-language pathology. Treatment for transgender men and nonbinary people is no less urgent, though. Today, speech-language pathologists provide gender-affirming voice and communication intervention to transgender men, singers, youth, and those who identify outside the gender binary.

Why is gender-affirming voice and communication intervention important in transgender healthcare? In day-to-day interactions, a person's voice makes as strong an impression on others as one's outward appearance. Voice serves as a social cue in the complex process of perceiving gender, and based on the sound of their voice, transgender people may be perceived by others as their assigned, rather than experienced, gender. For many transgender people, voice is a trigger for dysphoria and a source of fear about judgment or violence. Others face actual judgment or violence when outed by a voice that is incongruent with their gender expression.

This chapter takes a historical perspective on gender-affirming voice and communication interventions for transgender and gender-diverse (TGD) people. The first author is a cisgender male speech-language pathologist who has provided voice and communication training at the College of Saint Rose in Albany, New York since 2007. The second is a nonbinary speech-language pathologist who entered the field with the specific intention of supporting TGD people. We focus on behavioral methods for modifying voice and communication, and we also briefly discuss the surgical procedures that increase vocal pitch.

THE EARLY YEARS IN VOICE INTERVENTION FOR TRANSGENDER WOMEN: 1970S–1990S

In 1985, Richard Adler, a speech-language pathologist in Atlanta, Georgia, opened a private practice after his academic program at Emory University closed. Within months, Emory's Department of Rehabilitation began to send him clients. Among those referred were transgender clients who wished to modify their voice. According to Adler, the referring speech pathologist assumed that as an out gay man, Adler would know how to work with transgender patients.[1]

Adler's intervention was influenced by his clinical expertise in voice, collaboration with his initial clients, the increasing sociolinguistic research in gender and communication, and a consultation with Carol Friedenberg, a speech-language pathologist in San Francisco, California, and one of the first in private practice working on transgender voice. He also read a 1983 article on transgender voice and communication by speech-language pathologist Jennifer Oates and Georgia Dacakis, both of Melbourne, Australia. From this initial experience, Adler created an intervention program that included eleven components of voice, speech, language, and nonverbal communication. The development of his practice led to a rapid influx of referrals and two to three new clients each week. As Adler tells it, the growth overwhelmed him. Thus began his illustrious career in gender-affirming voice and communication training.

In 1979, five years before Adler started his private practice, Oates also received a referral of a transgender client who wished to feminize her voice, this time from the Gender Dysphoria Clinic at Queen Victoria Hospital in Melbourne. Oates faced a similar conundrum to Adler's: they worked in a vacuum.[2] While new sociolinguistic literature described the differences between masculine and feminine communication styles (that is, pitch, vocal inflection, and nonverbal communication), little information existed on gender-affirming voice therapy. Oates's literature search revealed only two papers, both case studies that described behavioral techniques to train transgender women to feminize their voices: Meryle Kalra from Canada presented a case at the American Speech-Language-Hearing Association Convention in Chicago in 1977,[3] and Ralph Bralley and colleagues from the University of Virginia wrote a case study in 1978.[4] These papers described women who successfully changed their vocal pitch with voice training, but neither paper presented a comprehensive approach to voice and communication intervention.

Oates' early experiences led to an ongoing, long-standing collaboration with Georgia Dacakis, including the 1983 publication (mentioned above) that Adler used to develop his program. This paper offered the first description of a holistic voice and communication protocol for trans women.[5] Given the relative absence of research on transgender voice and communication, they described existing research from linguistics on gender-based differences in communication. They recommended that voice modification training involves attention to vocal characteristics that influence a listener's perception of gender (see table 19.1). They also described vocal health, or methods to care for the voice, and nonverbal communication skills to feminize communication styles for transgender women.

In their 1983 paper, Oates and Dacakis also reported on two experimental laryngeal surgeries designed to increase vocal pitch. Although surgeons began

Table 19.1. Vocal Characteristics that Influence a Listener's Perception of Gender

Pitch	The perceived highness or lowness of the voice. Female speakers have a higher pitch than males.
Fundamental frequency	The acoustic correlate of pitch, corresponding to the rate of vocal cord vibration when producing voice. Female speakers have higher fundamental frequency than males.
Prosody	The inflection, intonation, and stress of the voice. Females produce more varied prosody (particularly increased inflection) when speaking.
Voice quality	The overall nature of the sound produced by vocal cord vibration. Female speakers may be perceived as breathier than males.
Intensity	The acoustic correlate of loudness. Females may be perceived to produce a softer, less intense voice than males.
Resonance	The tone or timbre of speech created by modifications to voice in the throat, mouth, and nasal cavities. Female resonance is higher in frequency and perceived to be more forward in the vocal tract.
Articulation	The production of speech sounds. Females are perceived to be more precise than male speakers.

to develop pitch-altering surgical procedures around the same time speech-language pathologists developed behavioral voice and communication modification, speech-language pathologists and laryngeal surgeons did not routinely collaborate; such partnerships have become more common in recent times.

Adler, Oates, Dacakis, and Friedenberg are speech-language pathologists whose specialty is voice: vocal anatomy and physiology, normal voice production, and vocal health, as well as the assessment and treatment of physical or functional problems with the vocal mechanism (voice disorders). These pioneering clinicians understood that gender-affirming voice and communication intervention did not address a disordered voice; however, their knowledge and skill working with the human voice benefitted their transgender clients. They applied systematic behavioral methods to facilitate a safe change in the vocal characteristics of transgender women, described in table 19.1. Professional colleagues in the United States and around the world began to use these methods as the number of TGD people seeking gender-affirming voice and communication intervention increased during the 1980s and 1990s.

Shortly after Adler began his private practice in the mid-1980s, other speech-language pathologists across the United States began to work with transgender women on voice modification. These clinicians, often private practitioners or faculty members in university-based speech-language pathology programs, most often specialized in voice. University programs began to expose students to gender-affirming voice and communication training, the first at George Washington University, under the leadership of Joan Regnell in the early 1970s. Increasingly, textbooks in speech-language pathology began to mention intervention for transgender women as a potential path for practitioners.

The University of Washington was among the first university-based centers to develop a voice and communication program to serve transgender women. This program provided students with hands-on experience in gender-affirming voice and communication intervention. One beneficiary of this development was Sandy Hirsch, who saw her first client in 1988 as a graduate student and went on to become a national leader in the development and provision of TGD voice services.[6] The University of Washington continued to provide services to transgender women through the 1990s and into the new millennium, including the first group intervention program, developed by speech-language pathologist Michelle Mordaunt in 1995.[7] Mordaunt's structured group intervention program, which included important peer support unavailable during individual intervention, became a model for other universities and colleges, including my (Jack Pickering) institution, the College of Saint Rose. As Mordaunt directed her voice and communication training program, Hirsch began her thriving Seattle-based private practice Give Voice in 1996, serving TGD people.[8] Other speech-language pathologists across the United States began similar evolutionary steps.

As intervention and educational opportunities in gender-affirming voice and communication increased in the late 1980s and early 1990s, research emerged to provide insight into the effectiveness of training. For example, Dacakis demonstrated that the pitch of a transgender woman could be increased safely with behavioral intervention and described the correlation between the number of intervention sessions and change over time.[9] Speech-language pathologists Kay Mount and Shirley Salmon established that change in pitch and resonance improved a listener's perception of a feminine voice; changing both characteristics was more effective than changing one or the other.[10] These early studies provided clinicians with confidence and a clearer direction for intervention.

TRANSGENDER VOICE AND COMMUNICATION INTERVENTION: INTO THE NEW MILLENNIUM

In the period between 1997 and 2002, three new publications described gender-affirming voice and communication intervention for transgender women; the respective authors evaluated techniques employed during their own work with patients. Oates and Dacakis wrote the first article in 1997,[11] recommending that voice services for trans women focus on increasing pitch and fundamental frequency, increasing resonance frequencies, decreasing intensity, increasing breathy voice quality, and modifying intonation. They considered other aspects of communication, including articulation, rate of speech, vocabulary, style, and content, as well as nonverbal vocalizations such as coughing and laughing. Oates and Dacakis concluded that behavioral voice training required attention to more than the pitch of the voice, representing an important expansion of earlier protocols. Their systematic, multidimensional approach to voice and communication intervention led them to perform extensive research in transgender voice—work that continues to inform their present-day clinical program at LaTrobe University in Melbourne, Australia.[12]

After the publication of Oates and Dacakis's 1997 paper, two speech-language pathologists in the United States described behavioral voice and communication interventions. Marylou Gelfer, a university professor from Milwaukee, outlined a hierarchical approach to voice services that began with establishing a target pitch, effective use of inflection, and production of a vocal quality that was "light and clear."[13] She suggested the use of biofeedback to habituate the target pitch (voice apps serve this purpose today). In later stages of the program, she recommended the inclusion of language and nonverbal communication. The client and clinician needed to express satisfaction with results prior to ending treatment. Gelfer's later intervention research focused on treatment efficacy, significantly advancing the delivery of services for gender-affirming voice and communication.

Friedenberg, mentioned earlier, was the second American speech-language pathologist to add to the medical literature. She summarized Gelfer's approach and recommended that interventions also include consideration of a client's life experience, their transition process, and WPATH's (referred to at the time as Harry Benjamin International Gender Dysphoria Association) *SOC*. To insure appropriate holistic care for transgender individuals, she endorsed interdisciplinary collaboration with other helping professionals, such as medical and mental health clinicians. She urged clinicians to seek training in cultural competency and to center voice and communication intervention as an integral part of the broader transition process. She also addressed how gender, racial, and ethnic stereotypes, as well as cultural gender differences impact voice intervention.[14] Friedenberg's 2002 paper was the first to address the intersection of gender with race, ethnicity, and culture in regard to gender-affirming voice and communication intervention; significant gaps in research and care for voice interventions persist for transgender people of color.

In the 1990s, several transgender women also produced works intended to help others to feminize their voices. Two efforts of note are Alison Laing's 1987 *Speaking as a Woman*[15] and Melanie Phillips' VHS videotape "Melanie Speaks."[16] Laing emphasized feminine speech patterns such as a rise in pitch at the end of sentences. Phillips described her work to feminize her own voice and offered instructions for others like herself. "Melanie's tape gave trans women of her generation permission to speak on their own terms. And it showed them how to do it in a fun, inviting way. This wasn't a doctor or a psychologist ordering you to conform. It was another trans woman showing you how she did it. Melanie Speaks is also, in many ways, a relic of its time."[17]

By the turn of the century, speech-language pathologists possessed evidence-based research and resources on interventions for transgender women that they could use in their clinical work. And another resource surfaced at this time: the Internet. In the mid-1990s, the World Wide Web provided a platform for transgender women to share information with interested peers. Resources previously difficult to access became available through community-created websites and search engines. In early 2000, the owner of the website Transsexual Voice for the Tone Deaf wrote, "There is practically no help out there for people when it comes to getting a new voice."[18] After unsatisfactory experiences with three speech-language pathologists, she learned to feminize her voice on her own and then shared what she learned to help other trans women who struggled to find resources. Others wrote about their experiences on trans community forums and crafted their own guides. Now, entire online communities exist—most created and moderated by trans women—dedicated to sharing experiences and providing guidance for all aspects of gender-affirming voice and communication training.[19]

RESOURCES AND SERVICES EXPAND: 2006 TO THE PRESENT

In 2006, Adler, Hirsch, and Mordaunt published the seminal work in gender-affirming voice and communications efforts, a book entitled *Voice and Communication Therapy for the Transgender/Transsexual Client: A Comprehensive Clinical Guide*.[20] For more than a decade and through two revisions (2012 and 2019), this book served as the only comprehensive text describing behavioral intervention for voice and communication. Chapters focused on each of the primary characteristics of voice and communication (listed in table 19.1); integrated psychosocial and endocrinologic considerations; offered information on voice and communication services for trans men, trans actors, and singers; and advanced a more holistic perspective on gender transition for practicing clinicians.

The publication of Adler, Hirsch, and Mordaunt's book ushered in a period of increased interest in voice and communication services for trans women that continues today. Research surged in the field, leading to numerous publications supporting gender-affirming voice and communication intervention, as well as resources for clinicians and clients. In increasingly systematic ways, clinicians and TGD people discussed ongoing assessment of voice and intervention beyond increasing pitch. Evidence allowed clinicians to fine-tune their techniques for voice, resonance, and communication for TGD voices, including trans men.

Clinicians recently began to explore quality of life and voice satisfaction with transgender patients, providing important patient self-reported perception of their voice for the first time. In 2013, Dacakis and colleagues developed the Transsexual Voice Questionnaire to specifically address trans women's voice-related satisfaction.[21] Similar to other client self-perception measures, the questionnaire required an individual to rate the frequency (1 = never or rarely; 4 = usually or always) with which one of thirty situations occur (for example, "I am less outgoing because of my voice" and "When I laugh I sound like a man"). They determined that validity and reliability were strong in the original English version, as well as in other language versions of the tool. In 2017, Adrienne Hancock from George Washington University reported on TGD voice and communication from the perspective of the World Health Organization's *International Classification of Functioning*, emphasizing that measures of client self-perception are important and provide insight on the impact of voice on a trans women's functioning in the world.[22]

Shortly after publication of the first edition of *A Comprehensive Clinical Guide* in 2006, Adler began to lobby WPATH to include voice and communication in their *SOC*. Ultimately, he joined the WPATH Standards of Care Revision Committee for the seventh version (2011); consequently, this edition includes a section on gender-affirming voice and communication intervention. Adler's leadership created an important connection between the discipline of speech-language pathology and WPATH. Including information on voice and communication firmly established the critical role voice plays in someone's transition—and why voice intervention is an integral component of trans healthcare. The next version of the standards, the eighth version, once again includes voice and communication intervention and, for the first time, the revision committee includes a gender-diverse consumer of voice and communication services.

As the connection with WPATH was evolving, other US clinicians began to present on gender-affirming voice and communication at international, national, and regional conferences for speech-language pathologists and transgender health professionals, further expanding the field's footprint. Presentations on voice and communication were featured at transgender networking conferences like Fantasia Fair, Southern Comfort, and Gender Odyssey. At the 2015 American Speech-Language-Hearing Association national convention in Denver, Adler and Jack Pickering presented to an audience of close to five hundred speech-language pathologists, a testament to the professional interest that has been growing since the 1980s.[23]

GENDER-AFFIRMING VOICE INTERVENTION: MOVING FORWARD

Today, gender-affirming voice and communication training for trans women is well described, and ample evidence exists to support its use for people who can access the services. Even with increased provision of gender-affirming voice and communication interventions, barriers exist that may prevent TGD individuals from seeking care and affect clinicians' ability to offer comprehensive care.

For example, insurance often does not cover speech-language pathologist services, a matter that requires us to lobby for policy change. While the Affordable Care Act prohibits providers from withholding services based on gender identity, it does not require coverage for transition-related services. As of 2021, twenty-one states, along with the District of Columbia, provided coverage for gender-affirming care.[24] Private insurers vary around coverage of gender-affirming voice training services. One can appeal if coverage for voice intervention is denied, but systemic change will come only from advocating at the state level.

Apart from the need for increasing access to care, comprehensive, compassionate service provision is also necessary. The American Speech-Language-Hearing Association's 2017 ethics statement maintains that clinicians are expected to competently provide all clinical services in the field; if they feel unable to do so, they must refer patients to another professional who can provide the required services.[25] The document further states that individual speech-language pathologists are responsible for accessing continuing professional education to address knowledge gaps, learn new skills, and attend training on cultural and linguistic competency.

Under the umbrella of clinical services, gender-affirming voice and communication therapy falls within the speech-language pathologist's scope of practice. Speech-language pathologists in gender clinics, mental health counselors, doctors, and surgeons increasingly offer education to patients regarding vocal interventions. Nonetheless, there may be a misconception of the role of speech-language pathologists in supporting voice change in TGD individuals. In a 2014 survey by Jean Sawyer and colleagues, one respondent stated it would be offensive if a health care provider referred them to a speech-language pathologist, as it implied their speech was disordered due to their gender identity.[26]

If a TGD client does seek voice modification, they should be able to access competent and affirming care from a trained speech-language pathologist. Unfortunately, a 2015 survey regarding cultural competency of speech-language pathologists indicates another barrier.[27] While most of the speech-language pathologists surveyed reported feeling comfortable working with TGD clients, they did not perceive that they had adequate knowledge or experience in the provision of gender-affirming voice services. Half of the respondents could not describe transgender communication therapy and reported minimal knowledge regarding LGBT cultural competency. Approximately half of the respondents indicated that their master's in speech-language training curriculum did not include transgender communication therapy.[28] Fortunately, training opportunities have become more numerous in recent years, via courses and workshops. There are also resources and networking opportunities available for speech-language pathologists who are interested in TGD voice and communication.

Speech-language pathologists are not the only professionals who lack knowledge and experience in gender-affirming voice intervention. Students studying otolaryngology report less exposure to trans patient care compared to their peers in urology and plastic surgery. In a 2018 survey of 285 otolaryngology trainees, only thirty percent reported exposure to transgender care in their residency compared to sixty-four percent and fifty-three percent of urology and plastic surgery residents, respectively.[29] This educational gap would appear to create a barrier to pitch altering surgery for TGD people.

Even with these barriers, gender-affirming voice intervention for trans women is well understood, and services are increasing. However, intervention that targets transgender men and nonbinary people, as well as TGD people of color, remains less well developed with limited research. These aspects of clinical practice are discussed in the upcoming sections.

TRANSMASCULINE VOICE TRAINING

In the early 1940s, cisgender women who underwent androgen therapy for various endocrine disorders reported vocal changes.[30] Some complained of hoarseness, while others developed a distinctly masculine character; all voices fatigued quickly. Some of these changes were temporary and some permanent; the dosage and length of hormonal treatment varied between cases. These cases represent the first hormonal therapies available to cisgender women, a practice still denied to transgender men at the time.

TGD individuals have long existed, though, even before the advent of medical transitions. Murray Hall lived his life as a successful man, married twice, and became active in New York politics. After his death in 1901, the coroner revealed Hall's female anatomy, and newspapers latched onto the story and scrambled to explain Hall's "true sex." His story circulated widely across the nation. When the press interviewed his acquaintances and associates, none doubted his status as a man. Some described his voice as nasal and boyish, while others characterized it as deep.[31] Was Hall's voice the result of his own practice, or was it natural? Neither formal voice training nor medical transition was available at the time; these services would not become available until the latter half of the twentieth century and beyond to people like Hall.

By the 1960s, trans men who were able to access an affirming doctor used testosterone to masculinize their bodies as well as their voices.[32] Many found relief from their voice dysphoria by using testosterone, but others remained dissatisfied. Unlike feminizing hormonal therapy, testosterone acts directly on the vocal folds to deepen the voice. Generally, a year of testosterone therapy will lower an individual's vocal range to that of an average cisgender male speaker.[33] However, testosterone does not always lower pitch to normative cisgender male ranges and does not impact other aspects of communication that encode gender, such as intonational patterns or vocabulary.[34]

More recently, researchers addressed the specific concerns around voice and communication services for transgender men. Christie Block, a New York–based speech pathologist, described her experience providing voice workshops at the Philadelphia Trans* Health Conference in 2012 and 2013. The turnout for her workshop on transmasculine voice was twice that of her transfeminine voice lecture.[35] She and other clinicians discussed the need for additional intervention for those who complain of a young-sounding voice or who find that when they speak expressively, their pitch elevates too high.[36] The literature now also attends to vocal health. For example, some trans men smoke cigarettes to develop a husky, masculine voice, increasing the risk of voice disorders,[37] as well as other tobacco-related illnesses.

Since the early 2010s, resources for behavioral modification of voice and communication for trans men now include pitch and resonance training exercises like those used in transfeminine voice modification. Therapists target posture and breathing to provide more vocal support, which can be negatively affected by behaviors used to reduce chest dysphoria, such as slouching or wearing compressive clothing.[38] Trans men can adopt these behavioral methods with or without hormonal therapy. Phonosurgery is also an option for trans men via a procedure known as thyroplasty type III. This surgery reduces the length of the vocal folds and their tension, resulting in a lower pitch. While there is little available data on its efficacy for transmasculine speakers, it is an option for those who cannot undergo hormonal therapy or who are not satisfied with their pitch after testosterone treatment or behavioral alteration.[39]

NONBINARY VOICE

The goals for modifying nonbinary voices are as varied as nonbinary identities. A nonbinary person may wish to change their voice to (1) a single, consistent register or (2) a wide range in voice that aligns with a nonbinary identity or meets the flexible needs of various situations. Currently, voice treatment protocols fail to support multiple speech patterns, clinging to early beliefs about the importance of a single speech pattern. Speech-language pathologists are now researching and debating how best to serve the individualized needs of nonbinary clients who wish to develop multiple registers, a conversation that fundamentally challenges the field of gender-affirming voice modification.[40] Transgender women are also challenging traditional voice training, maintaining that current practices reinforce stereotypical gender norms and pressure them to obtain a "perfect female voice" rather than exploring ways to find the voice that best suits them.[41] Shifting away from earlier binary protocols better serves all trans clients.

In 2018, Azul and colleagues proposed a framework for working with transmasculine clients, suggesting that treatment should assist individuals to modify their gender presentation as well as change their gender attribution, as perceived by listeners.[42] In this framework, speech-language pathologists guided treatment according to the individual's experience and wishes rather than by protocols, which might or might not align with a client's identity. This framework has potential relevance for all gender-diverse people by focusing on client-centered care, specific to the experience and goals of the TGD individual.

GENDER-AFFIRMING VOICE TRAINING AND INTERSECTIONALITY

In describing the history of professional services, we must pay attention to the stories that are *not* told, often due to issues of access. Research on TGD voice often includes only white participants or fails to detail information about the ethnic and racial composition of participants. TGD people of color experience additional, structural barriers to housing, employment, and healthcare access, all of which limit their ability to access voice intervention.[43]

A 2017 survey of trans people of color found that lack of access to gender-affirming voice and communication services stemmed in part from the lack of knowledge, or misinformation about, these services.[44] A separate survey by Sawyer and colleagues revealed that forty-seven percent of trans respondents could not describe services provided by speech-language pathologists, and only three percent expressed interest in seeking voice and communication training. Even in this survey, seventy-eight percent of respondents listed their race as Caucasian; perspectives from people of color are largely missing in this field.[45]

A 2019 demographic analysis of American Speech-Language Hearing Association members revealed that ninety-two percent of speech-language pathologists identified as white, a statistic that all but guarantees that TGD people of color will find their specific needs ignored in the field.[46] The experience of gender is influenced by factors including race and ethnicity, religion, sexuality, and social class.[47] Gender is culturally complex, and in the United States, societal concepts of masculinity and femininity are based on white, Western standards.[48] When examining intonational patterns, for example, ethnolinguistic identity is generally not reported in research as it relates to trans voice, despite the presence of dialectal influences on intonation. This places clinicians and TGD people in a position where they are left to assume what these patterns sound like. For speech-language pathologists, a majority of whom are white, it is likely they will imagine an intonational pattern based on a monolithic "standard" American English, which is often considered to lack specific regional or ethnic characteristics. Without looking critically at these aspects of language, speech-language pathologists may erase their client's own individual linguistic identity by perpetuating this standard pattern.

Borrowing from the field of psychology, Sand Chang and Anneliese Singh noted that when working with trans people of color, white psychologists could not assume what a client meant when they said, "I am a man" or "I am a woman."[49] Similarly, a white speech-language pathologist cannot assume what a client means when they say, "I want my voice to be more feminine" or "I want my voice to be more masculine." Our view as speech-language pathologists now includes an understanding of voice as an individual experience that falls on a spectrum and that therapy must be tailored to the client's needs and desires. This tenet informs cultural competence and humility about gender and race.

ACCESS TO VOICE SERVICES FOR TRANS YOUTH

TGD youth are affected by red tape like TGD adults. They may need to navigate school, an environment that is often not sensitive to the specific needs of TGD students. Little research or services exist around gender-affirming voice intervention for children and adolescents. However, studies document the hardship these children face when they are prevented access to puberty blockers due to misinformed doctors, obstructive insurance, unsupportive parents, or paternalistic legislation that seeks to discriminate against and criminalize TGD lives. Among other effects, puberty blockers prevent testosterone from acting on the larynx in trans girls, preventing their voices from deepening and the Adam's apple from growing. Denying access to care for trans teens leads to dire social and personal consequences, not only around their interactions with peers but also in voice-related activities, such as singing and acting.

Some adolescents may not access puberty blockers before testosterone impacts their voice. Such was the case for J. C., a sixteen-year-old trans girl who sought voice feminization therapy, described in an article on TGD youth by Meredith Russell and Mere Abrams.[50] Alarmed by her conservative living environment, she worried about bullying and harassment from her peers and withdrew from her involvement in theater. She improved self-perception about her voice during therapy and developed a marked change in objective pitch measures. Currently, the dearth of published research on voice intervention for trans youth and lack of described techniques specific to adolescents limit care. Speech-language pathologists must adapt established interventions designed for adults to meet the needs of young clients.

THEATRICAL AND MUSICAL VOICE TRAINING

TGD individuals are also now requesting voice training for singing and performance, bringing new questions and discussion to the field.[51] Anita Kozan, a speech-language pathologist and singing teacher from Minneapolis, Minnesota, wrote the chapter on singing in the seminal 2006 *Voice and Communication Therapy for the Transgender/Transsexual Individual: Comprehensive Clinical Guide*, a new subject for the professional literature—and an important one to singers in the trans community.[52] In 2018, Liz Jackson Hearns and Brian Kremer, two vocal instructors with backgrounds in music, published the first book to address transgender singers: *The Singing Teacher's Guide to Transgender Voice*.[53]

Singing coaches who cling to the notion of male and female vocal roles do more harm than good when working with TGD singers. Eli Conley, a transgender singer and voice teacher, offered his perspective on working with TGD singers.[54] He stressed the importance of reducing dysphoria for TGD singers by referring to their vocal range with the terms, bass, baritone, tenor, alto, or soprano. Research and pedagogy in musicology for trans singers draws heavily on the field of speech-language pathology, and the reverse is also true. Speech therapists use musical notes as targets during voice training and borrow descriptors from musicology as well. Feminine speech is described as "light" and "bright," and speakers are trained to use their "head voice" rather than their deeper, darker "chest voice"—all direct analogues to descriptions of and training for soprano voices. Associating these vocal characteristics with these adjectives as opposed to "masculine" or "feminine" allows for more freedom in vocal expression.

One of the first transgender clients to take part in the Saint Rose program in 2007 was Jaye McBride, a stand-up comedian who has performed around the country and is now located in New York City. She came to us as a referral from a local mental health counselor. In voice training, McBride focused on increasing pitch and inflection, as well as the production of a clearer tone. We employed vocal warm up and conversation to facilitate changes in her voice during sessions and practice at home. McBride collaborated with us as we developed the program, regularly providing feedback and suggestions during our first few months.

As we began to write this chapter, we asked McBride to provide a few words about voice and communication training. In an email from November 20, 2020, McBride said the following:

> It's amazing how often people take their voice for granted. This is something I should've realized when I was in high school, and my dad had laryngeal cancer but I never really grasped this until after I transitioned. Going through life I constantly hoped and prayed that someone didn't hear my voice and immediately recognize it as a male voice both for convenience and even safety. Every year in this country, trans women are murdered just because of who they are, so it's not hyperbole to say that passing can be a matter of life and death. You can have the most feminine body on the planet, but if you sound like Isaac Hayes, it means being clocked as "male" and thereby viewed by many as a freak, a pervert, an abomination. Voice training managed to get me from Isaac Hayes to Bea Arthur (after a couple of cigars) and eventually to Jaye McBride.[55]

A SESSION OF GENDER-AFFIRMING VOICE AND COMMUNICATION TRAINING

The following is a brief description of our intervention at the College of Saint Rose, a program initiated just after the publication of Adler, Hirsch, and Mordaunt's *A Comprehensive Clinical Guide* (2006). The Saint Rose program in Albany, New York, serves predominantly trans women, although in the last few years, trans men, TGD youth, and people who identify as nonbinary have also contacted us for voice training. Gender-affirming voice and communication intervention takes place on Monday evenings during fall, spring, and summer semesters. Sessions take place over a two-hour period and include two supervising clinicians and six to eight graduate students who serve as communication partners and coaches. This program provides a unique opportunity to explore aspects of voice and communication in both group and individual contexts; it has five distinct parts:

1. Mindfulness: Each session starts with a mindfulness activity. Mindfulness brings the group together and allows everyone to be in the moment and focus on relaxation and breathing, both of which contribute to voice production.

2. Vocal warm-up: This part of the session helps each participant develop an individualized process for warming up the voice like a singer would and gain confidence exploring the pitch, resonance, and inflection that is consistent with the client's gender identity. We use modified approaches, based on those developed for voice disorders, to fit the client's needs. Most intervention programs in the United States include vocal warm-up.

3. Individual work on voice and communication: Clients practice aspects of voice and communication that are important to them. It may include additional practice with warm-up and/or conversational activities for practicing aspects of voice and communication that reflect the participants' priorities. The implemented activities vary but are typical of all voice and communication intervention. Our experience suggests resonance and inflection are two common aspects clients focus on for individual work.

4. Group time: The structure of the program and inclusion of graduate students allow for individual and group activities. In a group context, we explore a variety of topics and incorporate peer support into our intervention. We focus on voice health, the use of nonverbal communication, script reading, and vocal projection during group time.

5. Gratitude: We conclude sessions with a shared expression of gratitude, inviting members of the group to use their voices together one final time to end on a positive note.

SURGERY FOR VOICE FEMINIZATION

In the late 1970s, as the growing literature addressed behavioral voice and communication intervention for TGD people, surgeons began to develop pitch-elevating surgery. Among the procedures described in the professional literature, two predominant forms of vocal fold surgery emerged, both specifically designed to increase pitch: cricothyroid approximation and anterior glottal web formation. Cricothyroid approximation increases the tension of the vocal folds by manipulating the cricothyroid muscle, leaving the vocal folds in a state of stretched contraction, which leads to an increase in pitch. Anterior glottal web formation creates a webbing in the front of the vocal folds that decreases the vibrating length of the vocal folds, leading to an increase in vocal pitch. While these surgeries are effective in increasing pitch, other areas of voice and communication are not impacted, like prosody, voice quality, and resonance, which can reduce patient satisfaction postsurgery.

Studies established that pitch-elevating surgery increased the fundamental frequency (the acoustic correlate of pitch) to levels consistent with cisgender female speakers.[56] One systematic review demonstrated that cricothyroid approximation and anterior glottal web formation increased pitch better than behavioral voice and communication intervention alone. Voice quality was negatively impacted in some studies, particularly by surgeries that facilitated anterior glottal web formation. Most patients who underwent pitch-raising surgery reported satisfaction, but there was no research on long-term results, and none of the studies used a control group or random assignment of participants. Thirteen of the twenty studies in the systematic review mentioned some form of behavioral voice intervention before and/or after surgery, but the therapy was not well described.[57]

In 2016, Hyung-Tae Kim, a prominent South Korean surgeon, described a form of anterior webbing called vocal fold shortening and retrodisplacement of the anterior commissure. The study detailed more than three hundred surgical procedures and demonstrated a significant increase in fundamental frequency, improved voice satisfaction, and improved other vocal measures after both surgery and behavioral voice and communication training. Kim noted postsurgical voice disorders, but they did not persist beyond two or three months, improving with healing time and vocal training. He assessed patients preoperatively, seven days postsurgery, and again at two months, six months, and one year. Kim concluded that surgery alone did not adequately feminize the voice and that best results required a combination of careful presurgical assessment, effective surgery, careful postsurgical care, and vocal training.[58] Given the recent research, the combination of pitch-elevating surgery and gender-affirming voice and communication intervention is promising and likely to become a more common treatment option for some trans women.

CONCLUSION

Although trans voices speak throughout US history, professional services dedicated to gender-affirming vocal modification only began to take shape in the 1970s. Initially, the clinical population was limited to adult trans women, but it has now grown to include adolescents, nonbinary people, and trans men. Ultimately, clinical research and service delivery models must attend more closely to these and other emerging client groups along the gender continuum, particularly TGD people who are not white. Listening to these voices forces the field to explore different ways of envisioning and implementing TGD voice and communication services. While the number of gender-affirming services and procedures expand, issues of access remain, and the field requires significant work to address problems around the intersections of age, race, ethnicity, and education. TGD people and the professionals who serve them must continue to offer insight on how best to improve voice and communication services.

NOTES

1. Richard Kenneth Adler, personal conversation with John Pickering, November 3, 2020.
2. Jennifer Oates, personal conversation with John Pickering, October 25, 2020.
3. Kalra, "Voice Therapy with a Transsexual."
4. Bralley et al. "Evaluation of Vocal Pitch in Male Transsexuals."
5. Oates and Dacakis. "Speech Pathology Considerations."
6. Sandy Hirsch, personal conversation with John Pickering, March 29, 2021.
7. Mordaunt, "Group Therapy for Transgender/Transsexual Clients."
8. Sandy Hirsch, personal conversation with John Pickering, March 29, 2021.
9. Dacakis, "Long-term Maintenance of Fundamental Frequency," 553–55.
10. Mount and Salmon, "Changing the Vocal Characteristics of a Postoperative Transsexual Patient," 236–37.
11. Oates and Dacakis, "Voice Change in Transsexuals."
12. Oates and Dacakis, "Inclusion of Transgender Voice and Communication."
13. Gelfer, "Voice Treatment for the Male-to-Female Transgendered Client," 203.
14. Friedenberg, "Working with Male-to-Female Transgendered Clients."
15. Laing, *Speaking as a Woman.*
16. Esocoff, "Melanie Speaks."
17. Esocoff, "Melanie Speaks."
18. Transsexual Voice for the Tone Deaf.

19. Reddit, r/transvoice, "TransVoice."
20. Adler, Hirsch, and Mordaunt, *Voice and Communication*."
21. Dacakis et al., "Transsexual Voice Questionnaire for Male-to-Female Transsexuals."
22. Hancock, "An ICF Perspective."
23. Adler and Pickering, "Supporting the Modification of Voice."
24. American Speech-Language-Hearing Association, "Reimbursement of Voice Therapy Services for Gender Affirmation Services."
25. American Speech-Language-Hearing Association, "Issues in Ethics."
26. Sawyer, Perry, and Dobbins-Scaramelli, "A Survey of the Awareness," 156.
27. Hancock and Haskin, "SLP' Knowledge and Attitudes."
28. Hancock and Haskin, "SLP Knowledge and Attitudes," 209–15.
29. Massenburg et al., "Educational Exposure to Transgender Patient Care."
30. Goldman and Salmon, "LXXXIX the Effect of Androgen Therapy."
31. Skidmore, *True Sex*, 46.
32. Benjamin, "Clinical Aspects of Transsexualism in the Male and Female."
33. Nygren et al., "Effects on Voice Fundamental Frequency."
34. Azul, Arnold, and Neuschaefer-Rube "Do Transmasculine Speakers Present," 30–35.
35. Christie Block, personal conversation with Terren Lansdaal, March 14, 2021.
36. Block, personal conversation with Terren Lansdaal, March 14, 2021; Block, "Making a Case," 34, 36.
37. Azul et al., "Transmasculine People's Voice Function," 261.e12.
38. Azul et al., "Transmasculine People's Voice Function."
39. Bultynck et al.,"Thyroplasty type III."
40. Davies, Papp, and Antoni, "Voice and Communication Change," 121.
41. Ahmed, "Bridging Social Critique and Design," 3.
42. Azul, Arnold, and Neushaefer-Rube, "Do Transmasculine Speakers Present," 37.
43. Grant et al., "Injustice at Every Turn," 6.
44. Downs, "Access to Voice and Communication Services," 49–50.
45. Sawyer, Perry, and Dobbins-Scaramelli, "A Survey of the Awareness of Speech Services," 150–51.
46. Alder, "A Demographic Snapshot of SLPs," 32.
47. Beauchamp and D'Harlingue. "Beyond Additions and Exceptions"; Chang and Singh. "Affirming Psychological Practice," 140.
48. Warner and Shields. "The Intersections of Sexuality, Gender, and Race."
49. Chang and Singh, "Affirming Psychological Practice," 140.
50. Russell and Abrams, "Transgender and Nonbinary Adolescents," 1298–305.
51. Cayari, "Demystifying Trans*+ Voice Education."
52. Kozan, "The Singing Voice."
53. Hearns, Jackson, and Kremer, *The Singing Teacher's Guide*.

54. Conley, "Creating Gender Liberatory Singing Spaces."
55. Personal communication with Jaye McBride, November 20, 2020.
56. Van Damme et al., "The Effectiveness of Pitch-Raising Surgery."
57. Nolan et al., "The Role of Voice Therapy."
58. Kim, "A New Conceptual Approach for Voice Feminization."

WORKS CITED

Adler, Richard Kenneth. "A Demographic Snapshot of SLPs." *ASHA Leader* 24, no. 7 (2019): 32. https://doi.org/10.1044/leader.AAG.24072019.32.

Adler, Richard K., Sandy Hirsch, and Michelle Mordaunt. *Voice and Communication Therapy for the Transgender/Transsexual Individual: A Comprehensive Clinical Guide.* San Diego, CA: Plural Publishing, 2006.

Adler, Richard Kenneth, and Jack Pickering. "Supporting the Modification of Voice and Resonance with Speakers Who Are Transgender." Presentation at American Speech-Language Hearing Association Annual Convention, Denver, CO, November 2015.

Ahmed, Alex A. "Bridging Social Critique and Design: Building a Health Informatics Tool for Transgender Voice." In *Extended Abstracts of the 2019 CHI Conference on Human Factors in Computing Systems*, 1–4. New York: Association for Computing Machinery, 2019.

American Speech-Language-Hearing Association. "Issues in Ethics: Cultural and Linguistic Competence." 2017. Accessed October 3, 2023. https://www.asha.org/Practice/ethics/Cultural-and-Linguistic-Competence/.

American Speech-Language-Hearing Association. "Payment of Gender-Affirming Voice Therapy: Considerations for Speech-Language Pathologists." 1997–2024. Accessed August 6, 2024. https://www.asha.org/practice/reimbursement/reimbursement-of-voice-therapy-for-gender-affirmation-services/.

Azul, David, Aron Arnold, and Christiane Neuschaefer-Rube. "Do Transmasculine Speakers Present with Gender-Related Voice Problems? Insights from a Participant-Centered Mixed-Methods Study." *Journal of Speech, Language, and Hearing Research* 61, no. 1 (2018): 25–39.

Azul, David, Ulrika Nygren, Maria Södersten, and Christiane Neuschaefer-Rube. "Transmasculine People's Voice Function: A Review of the Currently Available Evidence." *Journal of Voice* 31, no. 2 (2017): 261.e9–23.

Beauchamp, Toby, and Benjamin D'Harlingue. "Beyond Additions and Exceptions: The Category of Transgender and new Pedagogical Approaches for Women's Studies." *Feminist Formations* 24, no. 2 (2012): 25–51.

Benjamin, Harry. "Clinical Aspects of Transsexualism in the Male and Female." *American Journal of Psychotherapy* 18, no. 3 (1964): 458–69.

Block, Christie. "Making a Case for Transmasculine Voice and Communication Training." *Perspectives of the ASHA Special Interest Groups* 2, no. 3 (2017): 33–41.

Bralley, Ralph C., Glen L. Bull, Cheryl Harris Gore, and Milton T. Edgerton. "Evaluation of Vocal Pitch in Male Transsexuals." *Journal of Communication Disorders* 11, no. 5 (1978): 443–49.

Bultynck, Charlotte, Marjan Cosyns, Guy T'Sjoen, John Van Borsel, and Katrien Bonte. "Thyroplasty Type III to Lower the Vocal Pitch in Trans Men." *Otolaryngology-Head and Neck Surgery* 164, no. 1 (2020): 157–59.

Cayari, Christopher. "Demystifying Trans*+ Voice Education: The Transgender Singing Voice Conference." *International Journal of Music Education* 37, no. 1 (2018): 118–31.

Chang, Sand C., and Anneliese A. Singh. "Affirming Psychological Practice with Transgender and Gender Nonconforming People of Color." *Psychology of Sexual Orientation and Gender Diversity* 3, no. 2 (2016): 140–47.

Conley, Eli. "Creating Gender Liberatory Singing Spaces: A Transgender Voice Teacher's Recommendations for Working with Transgender Singers." *Eli Conley* (blog), October 9, 2017. Accessed March 14, 2021. https://www.eliconley.com/blog/creating-gender-liberatory-singing-spaces-a-transgender-voice-teachers-recommendations-for-working-with-transgender-singers.

Dacakis, Georgia. "Long-Term Maintenance of Fundamental Frequency Increases in Male-to-Female Transsexuals." *Journal of Voice* 14, no. 4 (2000): 549–56.

Dacakis, Georgia, Shelagh Davies, Jennifer M. Oates, Jacinta M. Douglas, and Judith R. Johnston. "Transsexual Voice Questionnaire for Male-to-Female Transsexuals." *PsycTESTS Dataset* (2013). https://doi.org/10.1037/t28993-000.

Davies, Shelagh, Viktória G. Papp, and Christella Antoni. "Voice and Communication Change for Gender Nonconforming Individuals: Giving Voice to the Person Inside." *International Journal of Transgenderism* 16, no. 3 (2015): 117–59.

Downs, Sierra C. "Access to Voice and Communication Services for Transgender and Gender Non-Conforming People of Color." Master's thesis, George Washington University, 2017.

Esocoff, Sarah. "Melanie Speaks." Interview with Swan Real, Melanie Anne, Sarah Escoff, et al. Sounds Gay podcast. 99% Invisible, Episode 550. August 22, 2023. Accessed August 19, 2024. https://99percentinvisible.org/episode/melanie-speaks/. A transcript is available at https://99percentinvisible.org/episode/melanie-speaks/transcript/.

Friedenberg, Carol Becklund. "Working with Male-to-Female Transgendered Clients: Clinical Considerations." *Contemporary Issues in Communication Science and Disorders* 29 (2002): 43–58.

Gelfer, Marylou Pausewang. "Voice Treatment for the Male-to-Female Transgendered Client." *American Journal of Speech-Language Pathology* 8, no. 3 (1999): 201–08.

Goldman, Joseph L., and Udall J. Salmon. "LXXXIX the Effect of Androgen Therapy on the Voice and Vocal Cords of Adult Women." *Annals of Otology, Rhinology & Laryngology* 51, no. 4 (1942): 961–68.

Grant, Jaime M., Lisa Mottet, Justin Edward Tanis, Jack Harrison, Jody Herman, and Mara Keisling. "Injustice at Every Turn: A Report of the National Transgender Discrimination Survey." Advocates for Trans Equality, 2011. Accessed August 6, 2024. https://transequality.org/sites/default/files/docs/resources/NTDS_Report.pdf.

Hancock, Adrienne. "An ICF Perspective on Voice-Related Quality of Life of American Transgender Women." *Journal of Voice* 31, no. 1 (2017): 115e.1–e.8.

Hancock, Adrienne, and Gregory Haskin. "SLP' Knowledge and Attitudes Regarding Lesbian, Gay, Bisexual, Transgender, and Queer (LGBTQ) Populations." *American Journal of Speech-Language Pathology* 24, no. 2 (2015): 206–21.

Hearns, Liz Jackson, and Brian Kremer. *The Singing Teacher's Guide to Transgender Voices*. San Diego, CA: Plural Publishing, 2018.

Kalra, Meryle A. "Voice Therapy with a Transsexual." In *Progress in Sexology*, edited by Robert Gemme and Connie Christine Wheeler, 77–84. Boston, MA: Springer, 1977.

Kim, Hyung Tae. "A New Conceptual Approach for Voice Feminization: 12 Years of Experience." *Laryngoscope* 127, no. 5 (2017): 1102–08.

Kozan, Anita "The Singing Voice." In *Voice and Communication Therapy for the Transgender/Transsexual Individual: A Comprehensive Clinical Guide*, 2nd ed., 413–58. San Diego, CA: Plural Publishing, 2012.

Laing, Alison. *Speaking as a Woman*. King of Prussia, PA: Creative Design Services, 1987. Digital Transgender Archives. Accessed August 24, 2023. https://www.digitaltransgenderarchive.net/files/9880vq965.

Massenburg, Benjamin B., Shane D. Morrison, Vania Rashidi, et al. "Educational Exposure to Transgender Patient Care in Otolaryngology Training." *Journal of craniofacial surgery* 29, no. 5 (2018): 1252–57.

Mordaunt, Michelle. "Group Therapy for Transgender/Transsexual Clients." In Adler, Richard A., Sandy Hirsch, and Jack Pickering (Eds.), *Voice and Communication Therapy for the Transgender/Transsexual Individual: A Comprehensive Clinical Guide*, 2nd ed., 393–412. San Diego, CA: Plural Publishing, 2012.

Mount, Kay H., and Shirley J. Salmon. "Changing the Vocal Characteristics of a Post-operative Transsexual Patient: A Longitudinal Study." *Journal of Communication Disorders* 21, no. 3 (1988): 229–38.

Nolan, Ian T., Shane D. Morrison, Omotayo Arowojolu, et al. "The Role of Voice Therapy and Phonosurgery in Transgender Vocal Feminization." *Journal of Craniofacial Surgery* 30, no. 5 (2019): 1368–75.

Nygren, Ulrika, Agneta Nordenskjöld, Stefan Arver, and Maria Södersten. "Effects on Voice Fundamental Frequency and Satisfaction with Voice in Trans Men during Testosterone Treatment—A Longitudinal Study." *Journal of Voice* 30, no. 6 (2016): 766.e23–34.

Oates, Jennifer, and Georgia Dacakis. "Inclusion of Transgender Voice and Communication Training in a University Clinic." *Perspectives of the ASHA Special Interest Groups* 2, no. 10 (2017): 109–15.

———. "Speech Pathology Considerations in the Management of Transsexualism–A Review." *British Journal of Disorders of Communication* 18, no. 3 (1983): 139–51.

———. "Voice Change in Transsexuals." *Venereology* 10, no. 3 (1997): 178–87.

Reddit, r/transvoice. "TransVoice: Share, Constructively Criticize, and Have Fun!" https://www.reddit.com/r/transvoice.

Russell, Meredith R., and Mere Abrams. "Transgender and Nonbinary Adolescents: The Role of Voice and Communication Therapy." *Perspectives of the ASHA Special Interest Groups* 4, no. 6 (2019): 1298–305.

Sawyer, Jean, Jamie L. Perry, and Ashley Dobbins-Scaramelli. "A Survey of the Awareness of Speech Services among Transgender and Transsexual Individuals and SLP." *International Journal of Transgenderism* 15, no. 3–4 (2014): 146–63.

Sekoni, Daneen, and Neela Swanson. "Coverage and Coding for transgender Voice Treatment: Insurance Coverage for Transgender Voice Treatment Varies by State and Payer. Here's What SLPs Should Know." *ASHA Leader* 24, no. 2 (2019): 38–39.

Skidmore, Emily. *True Sex: The Lives of Trans Men at the Turn of The Twentieth Century*. New York: New York University Press, 2019, e-book.

"Transsexual Voice for the Tone Deaf." Wayback Machine, March 28, 2000. [No longer available on the internet.]

Van Damme, Silke, Marjan Cosyns, Sofie Deman, Zoë Van den Eede, and John Van Borsel. "The Effectiveness of Pitch-Raising Surgery in Male-to-female Transsexuals: A Systematic Review." *Journal of Voice* 31, no. 2 (2017): 244.e1–e5.

Warner, Leah R., and Stephanie A. Shields. "The Intersections of Sexuality, Gender, and Race: Identity Research at the Crossroads." *Sex Roles* 68, no. 11 (2013): 803–10.

19.1. PROFILE: MUSINGS FROM A TRANS SPEECH AND LANGUAGE PATHOLOGIST

Terren Lansdaal

On cold Seattle days in 2012, I paid my bus fare and hoped for a window seat for my forty-five-minute commute to high school. Exiting the bus, I thanked the bus driver politely; as I struggled to figure out my identity, I began to pitch these *thank-yous* into a lower range as best I could. I had no knowledge of voice modification but was acutely aware that my voice caused me grief. As I settled into my identity and trained as a speech-language pathologist specifically to assist transgender clients, my grief lessened somewhat, but it has not disappeared.

When I applied to graduate school, I requested a meeting with one of my undergraduate professors to ask for a letter of recommendation. I explained my intention to center my training and career on transgender voice therapy, and she frowned. I knew what she was going to ask me—after all, she was a sociolinguist. How would I reconcile my work as a speech-language pathologist with the knowledge that voice does not define someone's gender? Would my work hurt rather than help by imposing binary definitions about masculine and feminine presentation?

I knew she would ask because I had been asking myself this same question. But I knew all too well how upset I felt when I was misgendered—both when I had not disclosed my identity and when I *had*—because of my voice. At school, we might discuss sociolinguistic theory, but the cashier at the gas station listened to my voice and said ma'am, no matter how masculine or androgynous I might appear. While I have not experienced violence due to my voice, that is not the case for many other trans people.

My personal experience in this field has often been painful. As a graduate student, I purposefully disclosed my trans identity and offered myself as a resource to those who wished to learn more about the trans experience and voice training for trans clients. Only a handful of my peers spoke to me about my experience or remembered my pronouns. This experience during training left me with a sense of despair and resignation about the amount of work left to do but also a steely resolve to move this work forward. I also take comfort in the fact that I am far from the only transgender person in this field. The recent growth in research about the trans voice experience gives me hope that improvements in access to voice modification will continue to advance, along with other aspects of trans-related care.

20

HAIR TROUBLES
A History of Hair Removal and Replacement

Dallas Denny and Yuki Arai

The presence of body and facial hair can cause intense dysphoria for transgender and gender-diverse (TGD) people—hair growth inconsistent with body image and gender identity can serve as a constant and visible reminder of an individual's assigned sex at birth and gender incongruence.[1] The loss or absence of body, scalp, and facial hair can similarly result in dysphoria for transgender men, who may rely on the presence of hair for their sense of self and public gender affirmation. This chapter traces the evolution of treatment methods for depilation, epilation, and hair replacement, with a focus on the specific needs of TGD people.

REMOVING HAIR

Long before the first explorers and immigrants from Europe and Asia and enslaved people from Africa arrived in North America, Indigenous peoples across the continent were removing facial and body hair by shaving, plucking, and singeing.[2] European colonists, astonished by the smooth skin of the native peoples, discussed for more than two centuries whether Indigenous Americans were less hairy than other human races and debated whether it was a sign of racial superiority or racial inferiority.[3] Indigenous peoples sometimes had the opposite reaction: "You cannot woo them to wear it on their chins, where it no sooner grows but it is stubbed up by the roots, for they count it as an unuseful, cumbersome, and opprobrious excrement, insomuch as they call him an Englishman's bastard that hath but the appearance of a beard."[4]

Colonists brought with them methods of depilation and epilation not generally mentioned in discussion of precolonial Indigenous Americans: waxing, threading, abrasion with stones and other objects, and the use of caustic chemicals. Some of these techniques had been in use for thousands of years.[5] Caustic chemicals could be life-threatening. In her book *Plucked: A History of Hair Removal*, Rebecca Herzig devotes a harrowing chapter to epilation by potions and describes the transition from homemade remedies to commercial products. She reproduces a recipe from 1540 that calls for caustic burnt lime and poisonous arsenic: "Take new burnt Lime foure ounces, of Arseneck an ounce, steepe both these in a pint of water the space of two days, and then boyle it in a pint to a half. And to prove whether it be perfect, dippe a feather therein, and if the plume of the feather depart off easily, then it is strong enough."[6]

Things only got worse with patent concoctions. Firstly, they were produced in great quantities,[7] reaching far more people, generally women; second, the contents were often disguised to protect trade secrets;[8] and third, new toxic chemicals were introduced, including thallium compounds, which "produced a systemic toxicity that resulted in hair loss as well as nerve damage and death."[9] Effects of these potions could include scarring, blindness, loss of flesh, and sometimes death. They remained in heavy use and relatively unregulated until well into the twentieth century.[10] Fortunately, today's depilatory creams no longer contain such toxic compounds; they can, however, still cause irritation of the skin.[11]

In 1895, Wilhelm Röntgen discovered X-ray radiation, a method almost immediately proposed as a method of discouraging beard growth.[12] Scientists quickly realized and publicized the danger of X-ray radiation.[13] Nonetheless, X-rays were soon put into use for removal of hair.[14]

In an age in which women were increasingly concerned about facial and body hair[15] and in which other methods of depilation were inconvenient, time-consuming, and painful, many felt that getting rid of unwanted growth by sitting for a few minutes in front of a box that emitted invisible "healing" light was a godsend.

Despite growing knowledge of the damage X-rays caused, physicians continued for some time to administer radiation with enthusiasm. "The X-ray method, including the Tricho System, bypassed the inescapable physicality of all other hair-removal technologies," writes Herzig.[16] Before long, several companies were advertising X-ray treatments with names like Vir-O-Gen[17] and Abbott-Martin Method and were selling or licensing X-ray machines; treatments were administered in salons by lay or lightly trained practitioners. The physician Albert C. Geyser's Tricho Company ran as many as seventy-five X-ray clinics in the United States and defended its practices vigorously.[18]

While X-rays effectively removed hair from the areas treated, the medium- and long-range consequences were devasting. Still, patients aware of the dangers continued to demand X-ray hair removal treatments. Ulceration and scarring occurred in many patients, and, eventually, cancer in various forms. "In 1947, an article in the *Journal of the American Medical Association* described in gruesome detail dozens of cases of cancer resulting from depilatory applications of X-rays."[19]

The horrors resulting from radiation exposure after the United States detonated atomic bombs over the Japanese cities Hiroshima and Nagasaki in 1945 also highlighted the dangers of radiation, yet X-ray treatment for hair removal persisted in North America as an underground activity until the late 1940s.[20] Eventually, though, under pressure from patients and their peers, physicians abandoned the practice, but the damage was already done. The long-term effects were horrific and resulted in many premature deaths. "In 1970, a team of researchers found that more than thirty-five percent of all radiation-induced cancer in women could be traced to X-ray hair removal."[21]

Electrolysis involves the removal of hair via the application of electricity through needle-like probes. Its widespread use predated the application of radiation by twenty years. Electrolysis to remove hair began after the 1875 publication of St. Louis ophthalmologist Charles Michel's journal article in which he reported his success in removing ingrown eyelash hairs and speculated about using electrolysis to remove hair on other parts of the body.[22] Soon after, clinicians adopted this suggestion. In an era in which few American cities were electrified and most private homes were without power, electrolysis still came into widespread use.[23]

Before the 1920s, electrology was limited to the galvanic method, which destroys the hair follicle by creating sodium hydroxide (lye), which subsequently dissolves the root. Technicians apply direct current via thin, rounded probes from a battery (historically) or a rectifier, which converts alternating current to direct current.[24] Often, multiple probes are inserted into different hair channels before current is applied. Each administration requires up to thirty seconds.[25] Thermolysis, which uses alternating current, destroys the hair root by heating it. Again, the technician inserts a probe into each hair follicle. Current is applied for only a fraction of a second. Precise placement of the probe is essential because the heated area is small. Thermolysis became available in the 1920s.[26] The blend method—developed in 1948—combines galvanic and thermolytic techniques to remove hair.[27]

To date, electrolysis is the only method of hair removal the US Food and Drug Administration (FDA) allows to be claimed as permanent.[28] And all three types, when applied properly, permanently remove hair. Notably, electrolysis is effective on every part of the body, for every type and color of hair, and for all skin colors; however, tightly curled hair, which is common among people of color, requires extra precision when placing the probe.

Laser is an acronym for light amplification by stimulated emission of radiation. Engineer and physicist Theodore H. Maiman constructed the first such device in 1960 at Hughes Research Laboratories.[29] No one had an idea how it might prove useful; skeptics called it a solution in search of a problem.[30] Sixty years later, lasers come in many types and have thousands of uses in medicine, the exploration of space, and industry; they can be found in almost every US business and residence. In the mid-1990s, the FDA approved the use of the alexandrite laser for hair removal, and this method became commercially available in the United States, where it has subsequently flourished.

Laser hair removal has the advantage, as did X-rays, of removing hair quickly. It is relatively painless, and large areas can be treated in a single session. It is most effective on nonvellus[31] (large) hairs and when there is considerable contrast in skin and hair color, that is, in individuals with light-colored skin and dark hair, which puts people of color and Caucasians with blonde or gray hair at a considerable disadvantage.[32] The laser works by applying light at designated frequencies, causing chromophores—melanin-bearing areas on and under the skin—to heat; this technique damages or destroys hair follicles.[33] The FDA considers laser treatment a form of permanent hair reduction but not permanent removal.[34] A near cousin of laser hair removal, intense pulsed light therapy, is the application of noncoherent light via a laser-like device; one of its applications is reduction of hair.

Laser is not without its problems. When poorly applied, it can cause burns; these are most likely in patients with tanned and dark skin colors and when using lasers with shorter wavelengths. Burns are usually not serious, but they can lead to infection and scarring. Other problems include eye injuries caused by poorly fitting eye protection and skin that becomes darker or lighter after treatment.[35] In a 2006 review, S. P. R. Lim and Sean Lanigan note an abundance of false commercial claims that laser hair removal is without side effects regardless of skin type, but they go on to conclude that when applied by well-trained technicians, in-office laser treatment has a low number of permanent side effects.[36] Other reviewers have reached similar conclusions.[37]

As with electrolysis, the skill of the operator for laser hair removal is of paramount importance. Unfortunately, there are no federal requirements or guidelines for laser hair removal. Licensing and certification vary across states. Most states require oversight by a doctor, nurse, or physician's assistant, but in some cases, the operator need not have a license or formal training. In a 2021 article, *Bloomberg News* called New York, which does regulate electrolysis, the "wild west" when it came to laser hair removal and noted the state was attempting to introduce legislation requiring licensing and education.[38]

TRANSGENDER PEOPLE AND HAIR REMOVAL

Without a doubt, many transgender people, and especially TGD women, availed themselves of early methods of hair removal. Ancient human history is replete with gender-transcendent origin myths, discoveries of cross-gender burials, and hermaphroditic figures. Anthropologist Timothy Taylor documents these phenomena, discusses the rich pharmacopeias of Paleolithic peoples, and speculates that plants with feminizing properties were known and used by many early tribal societies.[39]

Removal of body and facial hair often increases the comfort levels of transfeminine people and is considered medically necessary for the treatment of gender dysphoria.[40] Rachel Butler and colleagues found that transfeminine and transmasculine respondents to the Trans Health Survey reported lower social anxiety after gender-affirming hair removal than respondents who had not received hair removal treatment; $n = 715$ participants.[41] In a study of 281 transfeminine adults, Bradford, Rider, and Spencer (2019) reported ninety percent of transfeminine people were interested in hair removal and forty-one percent had received treatment. They discovered subjects "who had received hair removal services reported lower symptom ratings for depression and anxiety and greater positive affect than those who had not received hair removal services," concluding that hair removal is an important part of treatment for gender dysphoria.[42]

Unfortunately, despite its demonstrated importance to transgender people, most insurance companies reject coverage for hair removal on the grounds of lack of medical necessity.[43] This stance is inconsistent with medical determinations that hair removal is indeed medically necessary.[44] Thoreson and colleagues examined 123 private insurance policies and fifty-one statewide Medicaid policies available on the Affordable Care Act marketplace. They found only eight (or 4.6 percent of the examined policies) covered hair removal for transgender people: "The remaining 166 policies (95.4 percent) broadly excluded or did not mention gender-affirming care; prohibited coverage of hair removal or did not mention it; or permitted coverage of hair removal only preoperatively before genital surgery."[45]

ELECTROLYSIS IN TGD POPULATIONS

Richard Green and John Money recognized the need for epilation in their 1969 edited text *Transsexualism and Sex Reassignment,* which included a chapter on electrolysis by Morton Finifter. Save for occasional mentions, though, hair removal for TGD people seems to have otherwise gone more or less unaddressed in the various professional journals until 1990—at least I (Dallas Denny) found no instances, save Finifter, to include in my comprehensive 1994 bibliography of gender variance.[46] Nevertheless, electrolysis was the standard treatment for those transgender women who wanted it and could afford it—and the fervent wish of many of those who couldn't afford it. Literature produced by the nascent transgender community frequently discussed electrolysis:

> The expense of a full course of electrolysis cannot be ignored. Rarely can it cost less than a thousand dollars before the last has been executed of the thousands of hairs that make up the average beard. Before spending any money for these treatments, it is usually wise to consult with other people who have undergone treatment by him [sic]. Some are expert technicians, with modern and sanitary equipment, but others may be incompetent charlatans of the worst sort. A lack of expertise, combined with obsolete or inadequate equipment can result in acne-like infection and permanent scarring of the surrounding skin. Perfect results can give us cheeks like a young girl.[47]

Electrolysis is expensive, time-consuming, and uncomfortable, although anesthetic products can reduce pain. But, as acknowledged by the FDA, it is effective.[48] Because of these problems, many transgender women never complete—or even start—treatment. Many are discouraged by the long process. It can take hundreds of hours of treatment to clear a face of hair. Some transgender women known to me (Denny) have assumed they were making progress when, in fact, they were not. Their ineffective electrologists removed their hair but failed to kill the roots. When these women could no longer afford treatment or stopped treatment for other reasons, the hair soon grew back.[49]

Regulation of electrology varies by state, with some, for instance, Georgia, requiring no training and providing no license. This is a recipe for producing incompetent clinicians and charlatans and grievously disappointed clients. Some states, for instance, New York, require training, but do not issue licenses; others, for example, New Jersey, require both training and licenses. The American Electrology Association, the leading professional organization in the United States, provides a Certified Professional Electrologist credential that ensures a level of excellence.[50] Some states, for instance, New Jersey, require electrologists to include classes to gain or maintain their licenses.[51] Certainly, chances of effective treatment will be greater in states with regulation.

Good electrology requires an effective electrolysis device, high-quality probes, and a trained, competent operator who is skilled at properly setting the equipment and precisely placing the probe in the hair follicles.[52] There are many factors to consider: Which type of electrolysis will be used? What type(s) of hair does the client have? What are the proper settings for the machine? Is it better to use one hand or both hands when removing hair via electrolysis? These, and basic knowledge of hair growth cycles, are the sorts of skills that are addressed by expert-provided trainings.

Tenderness and swelling are common immediate effects of electrolysis and occur even with skilled practitioners. These are temporary and will resolve after a couple of days. In the hands of an untrained or incompetent practitioner, however, serious scarring, keloid scars, pitting, blisters, and burns can lead to skin discoloration and permanent disfigurement.[53]

How long does it take to clear the face of a transgender woman? Data are, unfortunately, sparse. In her study of a trans support group in the Midwest, anthropologist Anne Bolin includes a table showing total dollars spent on electrolysis to date by nine of her research subjects.[54] The range was $30 to $6,000, and the mean was $1,309 per subject. We should note that most or all of Bolin's subjects were probably still being treated. An average of two hundred hours, or more, may be required to remove a heavy beard.

Denny and Ahoova Mischael (1998) presented data on four adult transsexual women who were retroactively selected as representative of a pool of more than twenty transsexual women who had seen Mischael for treatment. Treatment was by thermolysis. Mean hours to completion for the four subjects was 67.3 hours; the mean for time elapsed between first and last treatments was 19.25 months.[55] More recently, electrologist Yuki Arai tracked treatment hours for three transfeminine subjects. Her results demonstrated variability in duration of treatment in these and other subjects.

Transgender people have influenced the practice of electrology in several ways. First, in the late 1980s, an electrolysis clinic in Texas began to perform marathon hair-removal sessions, with two or more practitioners working on a single client (usually anesthetized topically or by oral pain relievers or anti-anxiety drugs) for many hours in a single day or across several days. This practice enabled clearing of the entire face at each visit, dramatically reducing the time needed to complete treatment.[56]

Electrolysis requires several days of hair growth so the operator can grasp the shaft with tweezers,[57] and an hour-long treatment leaves the face puffy for a day or two. Having visible facial hair is inconvenient and embarrassing for women who work every day, especially when it happens weekly. Taking a day or two off two or three times over the course of a year or so is less of a burden, so it's not surprising transgender women across the United States were soon booking intensive sessions that, over the course of several days, cleared their faces. In response to demand, other clinics now offer this intensive service.[58]

Electrolysis can and has been performed on almost any area of the body. For transgender women, the two primary sites are the face and, in preparation for gender-confirming surgery, the external male genitalia. "Hair within the neovagina serves as a nidus for infection and encrustation of debris."[59] Moreover, it can clog the vagina and render vaginal intercourse painful or impossible. Because tissue previously on the outside of the body is now on the inside and out of easy reach, effective hair removal is difficult or impossible to achieve.[60]

An advisory issued by the Atlanta-based American Educational Gender Information Service in January 1995 awakened surgeons and electrologists—as well as transgender women—to the need for permanent hair removal from the perineal area prior to vaginoplasty: "We recommend that surgeons doing male-to-female SRS [this is the acronym for sex reassignment surgery, the term then in use for what is today called gender-affirmation surgery] become aware that hair-bearing vagina is extremely embarrassing for their transsexual patients, and to provide them with materials educating them about the problem and indicating where they should consider having electrolysis to avoid hair-bearing vagina. We recommend that electrologists be aware that transsexual women who are seeking SRS have legitimate reasons for seeking electrolysis in the perineal area."

Before the release of the American Educational Gender Information Service advisory bulletin,[61] electrologists were generally skeptical about requests for genital clearing preoperatively,[62] and some surgeons were oblivious to the need for this procedure.[63] Some surgeons, for example Toby Meltzer, Eugene Schrang, Pierre Brassard, and Michel Seghers, advised transfeminine patients to undergo genital clearing via electrolysis prior to their vaginoplasties,[64] but in general, most electrologists, transgender women, and surgeons were unaware or minimally aware of the need. The bulletin, which was distributed to electrologists, surgeons, mental health professionals, and trans people around the world, had an immediate and lasting effect. Electrolysis or laser hair removal before transfeminine bottom surgery is now an integral part of the presurgical process.

Finally, the increased popularity of phalloplasty, propelled by new developments like radial forearm free flap phalloplasty,[65] raised awareness that transmasculine people also needed to denude donor sites of hair.[66] As William Zhang and colleagues note: "Hair within a neourethra will obstruct urine outflow, promote urine retention within the urethra, and often become encrusted with stone and sebaceous debris—all of which increase the risk of urinary infections and post-void dribbling of urine."[67]

REGROWTH IN TRANSMASCULINE POPULATIONS

Under the continuing influence of testosterone, inactive hair follicles can and do activate.[68] The resulting new hair growth, sometimes in areas that have been effectively cleared, can induce dysphoria and pose medical dangers when the new growth is inside vaginas or urethras. Even when the new growth is external, it can be profoundly disturbing in both trans men and trans women, deeply undermining treatment goals. André A. Wilson, a health policy consultant and a member of World Professional Association of Transgender Health, notes the frequency of problems with post-phalloplasty hair growth in transmasculine people. Wilson has been raising this issue with clinicians and community members alike, calling for studies, awareness, and training. André provided us with the following comment:

I have an increasing number of reports from individuals that have undergone phalloplasty in recent years (as recently as a year ago and as long ago as fifteen years) who report negative consequences from hair growth inside their urethra and/or, more rarely, inside the penis shaft itself. Most of these individuals had had twelve to eighteen months of electrolysis or, in some cases, laser followed by electrolysis. Many of them are extremely dysphoric, experience deep shame, and are in despair.[69]

The transmasculine population is often already challenged by dysphoria when seeking intimate medical services. Those with internal shaft hair report having painful lumpy masses that often regrow, requiring repeated surgical removal. Those with internal urethral hair describe ongoing urinary pain, infections and blockages, requiring repeated medical visits. Many are now being told they will need essentially lifelong invasive internal laser interventions and/or penile surgeries to repeatedly remove the hairs. Some have been advised that due to scarring from repeated interventions their "best option" is to remove the neo-urethra and live with a hypospadias condition. Some transmasculine people also experience dissatisfaction and dysphoria related to external hair growth especially on the shaft and, to a lesser degree, the scrotum. Inasmuch as most cisgender male penis shafts are hairless, this hair growth is experienced as an indelible mark of difference, which, combined with the ongoing need for hair removal, may be a source of persistent gender dysphoria.

Many report difficulty finding competent and reimbursable service providers for the initial hair removal in preparation for surgery—but this is nothing compared to the difficulty obtaining internal hair removal services locally or even regionally. One individual traveled more than 2,500 miles for specialist care for urethral hair after an exhaustive search in a localized, multistate area.

Others report a deep sense of shame associated with these complications and rarely discuss it. Thus, these fraught outcomes are often not apparent to community members seeking information prior to surgery. Are the referring clinicians or the surgeons aware? Anecdotally, some individuals report being told they did not need hair removal at all from their donor site.

Reports from other transmasculine people seeking surgery suggest that some surgeons still require no hair removal at all, or as little as three to six months, while others want up to eighteen months of permanent hair removal.

The percentage of people who experience complications and/or compromised treatment goals from postsurgical hair growth is hard to say without research. Some individuals with varying presurgical removal treatments report having had zero complications from urethral hair growth. Is this individual variation? Variation in testosterone levels? A difference in technique? Or, more pessimistically, has not enough time has passed for the regrowth to occur?

LASER AND INTENSE PULSED LIGHT IN TGD POPULATIONS

In the mid-1990s, a far faster, less painful, and less expensive treatment became available—laser hair removal. Transgender people quickly availed themselves of this technology. While laser treatment does not destroy the hair follicle, it results in thinner and finer hair; effects can last for years. Some trans women start with laser treatment; then, when laser has reached its limit of effectiveness, they switch to electrolysis; far fewer sessions of electrolysis are required.[70] Because laser hair removal has the advantage of covering large areas in a single treatment, this can minimize both cost and the duration of time in treatment and completely and permanently clear the face or other body part.

In 2016, William Zhang and colleagues reviewed the literature of hair removal via laser for genital surgery. They noted lower patient satisfaction for both transmasculine and transfeminine patients with hair-bearing penile grafts and hair inside the vagina. They cited a systematic review of thirty controlled trials that concluded laser hair removal is more effective than electrolysis.[71] They noted: "Electrolysis may be cheaper per session, but many hours may be required to treat each area of hair; in contrast, laser hair removal will treat the entire area for hair removal during each session with faster procedure times, low occurrence of side effects, and fewer needed sessions."[72] This seems to apply for intense pulsed light as well. Schroeter et al.[73] reported ninety percent permanent hair reduction in twenty-five transgender subjects treated with intense pulsed light. We caution, however, that areas treated by laser hair removal and intense pulsed light are not considered by the FDA to be permanently cleared of hair.

Over the years, laser treatment has grown increasingly more effective. More types of lasers are in use: ruby, alexandrite, diode, neodymium-yttrium and aluminum garnet—and of course, non-laser intense pulsed light. Treatment of light-colored hair and hair on dark skin is now an option, but it requires more skill from the operator than light skin and dark hair. Laser has largely replaced electrolysis for hair removal in transgender people.[74] Unfortunately, electrolysis and laser treatment continue to be unaffordable for many.

Like data on electrolysis, reports on the effectiveness of laser and intense pulsed light treatment have historically been rare. Unfortunately, even when existing follicles are rendered permanently incapable of producing hairs, dormant hair follicles can become active, producing regrowth. This resurgence of hair is most common under the influence of testosterone.

Without a doubt, hair removal techniques will continue to improve, with new and innovative solutions being invented and developed. Rigorous collection of data will help in determining the efficacy of existing and emerging technologies for removing hair. Hopefully, more insurers will come to understand the medical need for permanent hair removal on the face, forearms, and genital areas. Surgeons and hair removal specialists who are aware of the problems their TGD clients face should make a point of educating their peers and clients about the importance of hair removal, especially in genital areas and donor sites. And certainly, the issue of regrowth of hair in genital areas and the medical problems this causes for transmasculine TGD people require immediate attention.

REPLACING HAIR

Baldness is a considerable source of grief and anxiety for many cisgender and transgender men. This distress is amplified for cisgender and transgender women with thinning or vanishing hair, as women in American society are generally expected to have a full head of hair. Hair loss for transgender women may worsen stigmatization and psychological problems. Many cis and trans people attempt to reverse hair loss with minoxidil and finasteride and various hair potions; many wear wigs, toupees, or other hairpieces; and some seek hair transplants and other surgical procedures.

EARLY DEVELOPMENTS (ANTIQUITY–1800S)

Throughout history, balding men and women have resorted to every sort of potion, lotion, ointment, or other concoction and all sorts of devices in their attempts to grow hair. Methods have been many and varied, often odious, and sometimes poisonous or dangerous.[75] None were effective: "Ireland, 1000 AD: One Celtic remedy for baldness instructed patients to stuff mice into a clay jar, seal it, bury it beside a fire, and take everything out after a year."[76] In the absence of effective methods of growing hair, for ceremonial purposes, and sometimes to enhance or transform hairstyles, men and women have, since antiquity, worn hairpieces.[77] They were all the rage in the court of King Louis XIV (1639–1715) in seventeenth century France and in England during the reign of King Charles II (1630–1685)[78] but were common as early as 2700 BCE in Egypt and other early civilizations.[79] Upper-class American colonists, styling themselves after Europeans, wore them as well, but by the time of the American Revolution, wigs among the affluent had been largely replaced by powdered hair.[80] Wigs and other hairpieces continue to be popular today. Improvements like hair extensions and lace underlayment for wigs offer realistic and nearly undetectable options.[81]

For Indigenous Americans, hair is and has been of spiritual and cultural importance.[82] Men and women of some tribes grew their hair long, and those in other tribes wore their hair short. Some plucked or shaved their heads in part and in whole for utilitarian or ceremonial purposes or in keeping within tradition. Hair of men and women was commonly decorated with copper, bone, feathers, and other parts of animals, and headdresses and hats were common. Paintings and drawings by frontier artists like George Catlin (1796–1872)[83] and James Otto Lewis (1977–1858)[84] profusely illustrate this wonderful variability of Indigenous hairstyles.[85]

Androgenic alopecia (male and female pattern baldness) was relatively rare among Indigenous North Americans, but they were not exempt from hair loss caused by aging, friction, trichotillomania, alopecia areata, hormonal imbalances, metabolic disorders, infestation by parasites, infection, psoriasis, hypothyroidism, vitamin deficiencies, disease, and toxins—all of which can cause hair loss.[86] European immigrants were subject to the same factors and were additionally burdened with a higher rate of hair loss due to androgenic alopecia.[87]

IMPORTANT DEVELOPMENTS (1900S–PRESENT)

The first hair transplant surgery was performed in Wurzburg, Germany, in 1822 by then student and soon to be physician Johann Dieffenbach (1792–1847), who used goose quills as trepines (punches) to transplant hair, feathers, and skin in mammals and birds.[88] In 1939, Japanese dermatologist Shoji Okura (1886–1962) used this punch graft technique to successfully transplant hair to various areas of the human body.[89] The first use of grafts for androgenic alopecia occurred in 1952, when US dermatologist Norman Orentreich (1922–2019) successfully used punch grafts with a patient with male pattern baldness. At first, his peers refused to believe his data: "Dr. Orentreich's first article on hair transplantation was submitted to *The Archives of Dermatology*. The reviewers said that the reported results were 'not possible,' and the article was rejected. Ultimately, it was published by the New York Academy of Sciences in 1959."[90] Orentreich trained the first generation of hair graft practitioners,[91] and there have been many innovations in hair transplantation since.

Orentreich realized hairs retained their characteristics after transplantation, which led to his theory of donor dominance: "The fascinating observation from this work was that when hair follicles were transplanted, the hair grafts maintained their characteristics. These characteristics included: length, texture, curl, colour, and most importantly longevity. Excitingly it was determined that any grafts that were harvested from the so called 'safe zone' (where hair was not susceptible to blading or thinning due to androgenetic alopecia) remained healthy after implantation."[92] Early hair grafts were four millimeters in diameter and resulted in a "pluggy" appearance to the transplanted area.[93]

Over the years, a variety of modifications and new techniques have evolved, allowing for more even coverage and natural-looking hairlines. Today, follicular unit transplants are "by an overwhelming majority, the most common procedure used to correct pattern baldness."[94] It should be noted, however, that many patients simply do not have enough hair to provide sufficient donor sites, and that textures and other characteristics of transplanted hairs sometimes change over time. Lack of skill and aesthetic sensibilities of those doing the transplants can result in scarring at donor and recipient sites, irregular or unnatural-looking hairlines, and bald or scarred donor sites.[95] As with any surgery, there is risk of infection, necrosis, and other complications. Little research has been done on the longevity of transplanted hairs.[96]

Regulations for hair transplant surgeries are unfortunately rudimentary in many countries and states, and in some cases, nonexistent. In New Jersey, for instance, any physician can perform transplants.[97] Most sources suggest the procedure should be limited to dermatologists and plastic surgeons because they alone possess the requisite skills;[98] however, this is not regulated. In 2008, a group of surgeons in India developed minimum guidelines for hair transplantation; these were last updated in 2021.[99] They note "There is no uniform opinion as to which specialties can perform [hair transplants]. Even medical councils have not categorically resolved this issue, and different associations have different criteria for membership."[100]

Hair transplantation is a team procedure.[101] Portions of the procedure are often performed by technicians and not by dermatologists or plastic surgeons or even physicians. Indeed, a physician might not even be present while the procedure is being performed. It is, in most locations, simply not regulated. "Be also aware of 'turn-key' hair practices, where essentially a doctor purchases a hair transplant device and hires (usually unlicensed) technicians to then perform the procedure. This is a growing problem particularly in the United States, where patients think their plastic surgeon or dermatologist will be doing the procedure, only to have the experience of most if not all of the procedure performed by these technicians."[102]

Some other surgical hair procedures include pedicle flap, free-form flap, linear or line grafts, scalp expansion and reduction (today called alopecia reduction), and hair lift. In 1982, R. A. Elliott considered the lateral hair flap "a valuable addition to the armamentarium of the trained surgeon who manages the problem of male pattern baldness."[103] In 1992, plastic surgeons Toby Mayer and Richard Fleming authored a chapter in their textbook *Aesthetic and Reconstructive Surgery of the Scalp* in which they discussed the advantages of their Mayer/Fleming flap with and without scalp reduction surgeries over hair transplants. Today, however, some plastic surgeons consider the hair flap and reduction surgeries outdated.[104] Sandeep Sattur, in a review, concluded they "have a very limited or practically no role in the restoration of patients of pattern hair loss because of the invasive nature of these procedures and the concern that surgical outcomes are not commensurate with the perceived added morbidity. Simply put they do not have a very good risk-benefit ratio."[105] Flap and scalp reduction procedures nonetheless have their proponents, and results are immediate and often impressive. The skill of the surgeon is of primary importance with flaps and hair reduction surgeries,[106] and certainly it must be a surgeon, and hopefully an experienced and qualified plastic surgeon, who performs the procedure.[107]

After more than two millennia of potions, tonics, creams, and elixirs that could only claim to regrow hair, two effective prescription medications are now available. The FDA approved minoxidil (marketed as Rogaine) and finasteride (Proscar, Propecia) in 1988[108] and 1992, respectively.[109] Minoxidil is a topical vasodilator, and finasteride (in oral form) blocks the action of the enzyme 5-alpha reductase, inhibiting the conversion of testosterone to dihydrotestosterone, a hormone that may injure the hair follicle.[110] Marketing for many potions, lotions, and other chemicals still persists, but in a final ruling, the FDA stated that "any over-the-counter hair grower or hair loss prevention drug product for external use is not generally recognized as safe and effective and is misbranded."[111]

HAIR REPLACEMENT IN TRANSGENDER POPULATIONS

Human sex hormones exert considerable influence on hair follicles and the hair cycle. Their interplay in doing so is complex.[112] High levels of estrogen typically result in fuller, thicker hair, and with menopause, many cisgender women experience thinning hair and may develop bald spots. This effect is often reversed with hormone replacement therapy.[113]

Androgenic alopecia and unwanted body hair can exacerbate gender dysphoria in TGD women.[114] Fortunately, on feminizing hormone therapy, body hair diminishes. Sometimes, male pattern baldness is arrested, and rarely, one may see regrowth. In a 2016 single case study, Mary Stevenson and colleagues provided photographic evidence of this.[115] Over a period of six months, their subject reported regrowth and thickening of existing hair. Unfortunately, these hormones often fail to restore hair on their heads to previous levels. As a result, many transfeminine people wear wigs or hairpieces, occasionally or even every day. Those who can afford it may seek hair replacement surgery, but in many cases, there simply is not enough money to pay for surgical procedures that are not covered by medical insurance. Insurance companies typically consider hair replacement procedures to be cosmetic treatment and refuse coverage.

Facial hair is an important masculine secondary sex characteristic and an element of sexual selection in humans.[116] Under the continuing influence of androgens and growth hormones, males develop thick terminal facial hairs and increased body hair. The amount and type and the age at which it develops is highly variable among individuals and ethnic groups.[117] In transmasculine people, hair loss can be simultaneously a marker of manhood and at the same time distressing—after all, who wants to lose their scalp hair? Some TGD men, like some cisgender men, resign themselves to baldness. In an attempt to stop or delay hair loss, some may take minoxidil or finasteride. Others may seek surgical hair replacement or wear hats or toupees.

Similarly, lack of facial and body hair can induce feelings of gender dysphoria in TGD men, especially when hair is slow to develop after initiation of testosterone therapy. The age with which hair develops and the density of growth are highly individualized in both cisgender and TGD men and dependent on genetics. The age at which a full beard can be grown can range from the teen years into the thirties: "Anyone who sees today's high schoolers sporting beards will be surprised—or incredulous—to read in Homer's *Iliad* that

Achilles, the greatest warrior among the Greeks at Troy, was still beardless. Yet Plato accepted it as a well-known and unsurprising tradition."[118]

Hair transplantation techniques have been shown to be effective for cisgender men who have lost facial hair because of dermatological problems or burns.[119] Facial hair transplants can provide immediate gratification to transmasculine people who lack facial hair—and both transmasculine and transfeminine people seek hair transplants. In an article about hair transplantation for transgender patients, Anthony Bared and Jeffrey Epstein note an increase in transgender patients seeking "hairline lowering, beard transplantation, and eyebrow transplantation."[120] They note the importance of proper aesthetics in achieving natural-looking hairlines and beard designs:

> Goals in beard design are often established by the patient. Many patients typically present with a specific understanding of how they want their facial hair to appear. The design and density of the beard may be limited by the quality of the donor hair. Transplantation of full beards requires large amount of grafts, and patients are always made aware of the possibility of undergoing secondary procedures after approximately 1 year if further density is desired. . . . Depending on the exact design and density, graft counts can range from 250 to 300 grafts to each sideburn, 400 to 800 grafts to the mustache and goatee, and 300 to 500 grafts per cheek.[121]

Limitations of space preclude further discussion here, but see a 2021 review by Catherine Motosko and Antonella Tosti for a summary of the literature of hair replacement for TGD people.[122]

CONCLUSION

In the future, new technologies will increase the hair removal and replacement options for TGD people and the effectiveness of existing treatments. Hopefully, there will one day be state-level regulations for hair removal techniques and increased knowledge among care providers of the needs to inform their TGD clients about available options. Today, TGD people have resources available to help them make determinations early in life about the directions their lives will take and can delay, prevent, or induce the development of secondary sex characteristics, including the presence or absence of facial and/or body hair, thus reducing the need for hair removal and replacement technologies.

NOTES

1. Finifter, "Facial Hair," 1969; Denny and Mischael, "Electrolysis in Transsexual Women," 335–36.
2. US Food and Drug Administration, "Laser Facts." Depilation refers to the removal of hair at the surface of the skin. Shaving, used by billions of people, is the most common method and no doubt the oldest. Mechanical and electrical razors slice the hair at skin level, and it quickly grows back. Other methods of depilation include threading and the use of abrasives and depilatories. Epilation removes hair below the skin's surface. Methods include plucking, waxing, electrolysis, and photothermolysis via laser or intense pulsed light. Plucking and waxing can be done at home. Both techniques remove hair temporarily, but it grows back after some weeks. Electrolysis, when used by a competent operator, can result in permanent hair loss. Laser and intense pulsed light, when competently applied, can remove hair for months or years, with regrowth being finer and lighter in color.
3. Herzig, *Plucked*, 19–33.
4. Woods, *New England's Prospect*, 1634.
5. Fernandez et al., "From Flint Razors to Lasers."
6. Herzig, *Plucked*, 38, quoting from Rösslin and Raynalde, *The Byrth of Mankynde*, 1526. We retained the original spelling.
7. Herzig, *Plucked*, 40–47.
8. Herzig, *Plucked*, 40–41.
9. Herzig, *Plucked*, 40.
10. Herzig, *Plucked*, 47–49.
11. Fernandez et al., "From Flint Razors to Lasers."
12. Markandeya, "When Deadly X-Rays Were Used."
13. See Wikipedia, "X-ray"; see also Ford, "The Burning Question," 1–5.
14. Herzig, *Plucked*, devotes her chapter 4 to X-ray hair removal, 75–97.
15. Herzig, *Plucked*, 75–76.
16. Markandeya, "When Deadly X-Rays Were Used," quoting Herzig, *Plucked*, 732.
17. Bennett, "X-rays and Hair Removal"; Herzig, *Plucked*, 91.
18. Markandneya, "When Deadly X-Rays Were Used"; Bennett, "X-rays and Hair Removal." Bennett notes, "Geyser himself was well aware of the hazards of X-rays—the fingers of his left hand were so badly disfigured by exposure during his experiments that he had been urged to have them amputated."

19. Herzig, *Removing Roots,* 724, citing Cipollaro and Einhorn, "Use of X-Rays for Treatment of Hypertrichosis" and Martin et al., "Radiation-Induced Skin Cancer of the Head and Neck."

20. Cleveland, "The Removal of Superfluous Hair by X-ray," 35. "Financial transactions were on a C.O.D. basis and no receipts were given."

21. Herzig, *Removing Roots*, 724. The studies she cites are Martin, Strong, and Spiro, "Radiation-Induced Skin Cancer," 1970, and Rosen and Walfish, "Sequelae of Radiation Facial Epilation," 1989.

22. Herzig, *Plucked*, 868, 880.

23. Herzig, *Plucked*, 871–72.

24. Wikipedia, "Electrology," see emancipatedelectrolysis; see also, Hinkel, *Electrolysis*, for an exhaustive discussion of electrolysis in its various forms.

25. Wikipedia, "Electrology," see emancipatedelectrolysis .

26. Wikipedia, "Electrology," see emancipatedelectrolysis .

27. Wikipedia, "Electrology."

28. American Electrology Association, see FAQs about permanent hair removal; Fletcher and Cobb, "How to Remove Hair Permanently."

29. Maiman, "Stimulated Optical Radiation in Ruby."

30. Wikipedia, "Laser," quoting Townes, "The First Laser."

31. Vellus hairs are short, fine, and light-colored hairs that serve to protect the skin. See Vellinus and Cobb, "Vellus Hair."

32. Black, Indigenous, and people of color have been disadvantaged and disparaged in regard to their facial and body hair since the arrival of the first European immigrants on these shores. Herzig, *Plucked*, devotes several chapters of her book to this.

33. Wikipedia, "Laser Hair Removal."

34. US Food and Drug Administration, "Laser Facts."

35. Derma Network, "Potential Risks and Complications"; Lanigan, "Incidence of Side Effects"; Lim and Lanigan, "A Review of the Adverse Effects."

36. Lim and Lanigan, "A Review of the Adverse Effects."

37. Gan and Graber, "Laser Hair Removal." These authors also examined in-home devices and note the need for further studies.

38. Stanton, "New York Tries to Regulate."

39. Taylor, *The Prehistory of Sex*, 7, 18, 67–68, 213.

40. cf. Marks et al., "Excess Hair, Hair Removal Methods."

41. Butler et al., "Social Anxiety Among Transgender."

42. Bradford et al., "Hair Removal and Psychological Well-Being," 5; see also, Butler et al., "Social Anxiety Among Transgender."

43. Bradford et al., "Hair Removal and Psychological Well-Being," citing Ginsberg et al., "A Potential Role for the Dermatologist." Insurance companies may be more likely to cover genital hair removal than facial hair removal.

44. Marks et al., "Excess Hair, Hair Removal Methods."

45. Thoreson et al., "Health Insurance Coverage, 6." Downing, Yee, and Dy, "Hair Removal for Patients Undergoing Feminizing Surgeries," reported the success of 167 of 1372 (12.2 percent) transgender Medicaid beneficiaries in having at least one claim paid by Medicaid in Oregon.

46. Denny, *Gender Dysphoria*; Hage and Bouman, "Surgical Depilation"; Finifter, "Facial Hair."

47. *Turnabout*. Electrolysis is mentioned frequently throughout the issue.

48. Does electrolysis really work? Speaking from personal experience (Denny), my brown-black facial hair was removed entirely by electrolysis. I attribute this success not only to the effectiveness to electrology but to the skill of my electrologists. I was left with only the thin, blonde, almost invisible vellus hairs, which occur naturally on all humans and are a subtle sign of femininity that is erased by shaving and waxing. After ten years, I developed four or five annoying age-related "granny" hairs, which I continue to pluck—but more than thirty years after my last electrolysis session, I am otherwise entirely without facial hair.

49. Of course, there is no requirement for transgender women to remove their facial hair, but for many, it is an unsettling reminder of their biology. It has to be devastating to realize that after spending hundreds of hours and thousands of dollars over a period of years, you have essentially, because of operator error, made no progress. Similarly, lack of facial hair, especially after months or years on testosterone, frustrates and demoralizes many transgender men.

50. Visit the American Electrology Association's website for a state-by-state breakdown of licensure requirements (and lack thereof). https://professionals.electrology.com/be-an-electrologist/electrology-licensing-requirements.html.

51. Electrologists Association of New Jersey, "Licensing Requirements." For the actual New Jersey licensure requirements, see https://www.electrolysisnj.com/pdf/electrolysislaw.pdf.

52. Zhang et al., "Laser Hair Removal."

53. University of Michigan Health, "Electrolysis for Removing Hair." See Trip Advisor website to view an unfortunate result in Ontario or Google "bad electrolysis," accessed December 31, 2022. https://www.tripadvisor.com/LocationPhotoDirectLink-g154996-d7171213-i360157109-Body_Soul_Spa-Mississauga_Ontario.html.

54. Bolin, *In Search of Eve*, 159.

55. Denny and Mischael, "Electrolysis in Transsexual Women," 339.

56. Electrology 3000, "The International Leader in Transgender Hair Removal."

57. Denny and Mischael, "Electrolysis in Transsexual Women," 336–37.

58. cf. 2 Pass Clinic's website.

59. Zhang et al., "Laser Hair Removal," 371.

60. MTFsurgery.net, "A Patient's Guide."

61. Denny and Mischael, "Electrolysis in Transsexual Women," 349.

62. At a 1991 joint meeting of the Georgia Electrologist's Association and Georgia Clinical Electrologists, several practitioners discussed the problem of sketchy men calling to request treatment of their genital areas. See Denny and Schaefer, "Panel Discussion of Transsexualism."

63. I (Denny) was the founder and executive director of AEGIS. I became aware of the issue in late 1994, when I received a call on the help line from a distressed transgender woman who told me her neovagina was choked with hair, making sexual intercourse painful and sometimes impossible, and who asked if anything could be done to clear the area. I had been unaware of the problem and didn't have an answer for her, but I confirmed the issue by talking with other postoperative trans women. The American Educational Gender Information Service soon released and distributed a medical advisory to make gender surgeons and electrologists aware of the problem. It was surprisingly effective.

64. James, "Transgender Hair Removal before Bottom Surgery."

65. The technique debuted in 1984.

66. Kim et al., "The Anatomy of Forearm Free." See Crane Center's website for images of areas that need to be cleared: https://cranects.com/phalloplasty-hair-removal-templates/.

67. Zhang et al., "Laser Hair Removal," 381.

68. André A. Wilson is co-author of this section.

69. André Wilson, personal communication with Dallas Denny, April 30, 2022. My thanks to André Wilson for their prompt response to my query.

70. See Brannon, "The Structure and Growth Cycle," and Huang, "What Happens during the Anagen Phase," for lay discussions of hair growth cycles. Human hairs have a life cycle that differs among individuals and different parts of the body. Hairs grow, age, and are shed, and new hairs grow from the same follicles. Electrolysis and laser are most effective when treating hairs that are in the anagen, or initial stage of growth, so waxing or laser treatment prior to electrolysis can provide a jump start.

71. Zhang et al., "Laser Hair Removal," citing Haedersdal and Gøtzsche, "Laser and Photoepilation," and Haedersdal and Wulf, "Evidence-Based Review of Hair Removal."

72. Zhang et al., "Laser Hair Removal," 382.

73. Schroeter, et al., "Ninety Percent Permanent Hair Reduction in Transsexual Patients."

74. Zhang et al., "Laser Hair Removal."

75. Advanced Hair Clinic, "History of Hair Loss & Timeline"; Hedgecock, "A Short History of Weird Cures for Baldness."

76. Hedgecock, "A Short History of Weird Cures for Baldness."

77. Waxman, "From Medieval Hookers to Lady Gaga." And not only on the head. Merkins, or pubic wigs, have been in use since the 1400s. Originally, they covered areas that had been shaved to control infestations of lice. Today, they are used by actors when doing scenes in the nude.

78. Courts and Tribunals Judiciary, "History of Court Dress."
79. Cox, "History of Wigs."
80. American Battlefield Trust, "The Rise and Fall of the Powdered Wig."
81. McElroy, *Magic Hair*.
82. Stensgar, "The Significance of Hair"; Stergiou, "In Native American Culture."
83. Horan, *North American Indian Portraits*.
84. Hassrick, *The George Catlin Book*; Reese, *James Otto Lewis*.
85. Horan, *North American Indian Portraits*. Both artists began painting portraits of Indigenous people in the 1820s. Many tribes had been decimated by war, alcohol, and smallpox, but traditional dress and hair styles survived, in some instances incorporating Western fabrics and other materials. Most of their portraits are of men. This approach was at the insistence of males in most tribes; Catlin points out that the men insisted they be painted, and not "unimportant" women.
86. Miguel, "5 Reasons Natives Have Lustrous Locks."
87. American Academy of Dermatology Association, "Hair Loss."
88. Simons, "Johann Friedrich Dieffenbach"; Unger, "The History of Hair Transplantation."
89. Okuda, "Clinical and Experimental Studies;" Shigeki and Itami, "Dr Shoji Okuda"; Unger, "The History of Hair Transplantation."
90. Unger, "The History of Hair Transplantation," 191.
91. Unger, "The History of Hair Transplantation."
92. Sure Hair International, "Norman Orentreich."
93. Mayer and Fleming, *Aesthetic and Reconstructive Surgery*.
94. Sattur, "A Review of Surgical Methods"; see Bernstein, Rassman, and Limmer, "Follicular Unit Plain Speak," for descriptions of the various and innovative hair transplant techniques.
95. Kerure and Patwardhan, "Complications in Hair Transplantation."
96. Kumaresan and Subburathinam, "Longevity of Hair Follicles."
97. Casetext, "N. J. Admin. Code."
98. cf. Cleveland Clinic, "Hair Transplant"; Jeffrey Epstein, "Who's Qualified?"
99. Venkat Center, "Important Hair Transplant Guidelines"; Mysore et al., 2021.
100. Mysore et al., "Hair Transplant Practice Guidelines."
101. Venkat Center, "Important Hair Transplant Guidelines."
102. Jeffrey Epstein, "Who's Qualified?"
103. Elliott, "The Lateral Scalp Flap."
104. Vogel et al., "Hair Restoration Surgery."
105. Sattur, "A Review of Surgical Methods."
106. Sattur, "A Review of Surgical Methods."
107. Meyer, personal communication, January 27, 2022. The first author queried Meyer about his current position. He notes that hair flap and scalp reduction surgeries

are difficult but continues to believe them important options. "The flap is, by far, the superior technique because it gives the patients immediate results, no hair texture change, and the most density. Hair flaps will never be as dense, the hair texture changes, and you have to wait for your hair to grow." Dr. Meyer was clear that the procedure requires a skilled and experienced operator.

108. Panagotacos, "Hair Loss Treatment History."
109. Wikipedia, "Finasteride."
110. Wikipedia "Monixidil." Interestingly, finasteride as a remedy for balding came about after physician P. Roy Vagelos (1929–), a research chief at the pharmaceutical company Merck, discovered a 1974 presentation on male pseudohermaphroditism by endocrinologist Julianne Imperato-McGinley and her coworkers, who had worked with affected populations in the Dominican Republic. See Wikipedia, "Finasteride," and Imperato-McGinley et al., "Steroid 5α-Reductase Deficiency in Man."
111. Hair grower and hair loss prevention drug products for over-the-counter human use.
112. Desai, Almeida, and Miteva, "Understanding Hormonal Therapies"; Grymowicz et al., 2020.
113. Grymowicz et al., "Hormonal Effects on Hair Follicles."
114. Stevenson, Wixon, and Safer, "Scalp Hair Regrowth."
115. Stevenson, Wixon, and Safer, "Scalp Hair Regrowth."
116. Darwin, *The Descent of Man*, 383.
117. Dixson and Vasey, "Beards Augment Perceptions."
118. Moller, "The Accelerated Development of Youth, 748.
119. cf. Yaseen, Ahmed, and Ahmed, "Beard Reconstruction."
120. Bared and Epstein, "Hair Transplantation Techniques," 232.
121. Bared and Epstein, "Hair Transplantation Techniques," 228.
122. Motosko and Tosti, "Dermatologic Care of Hair."

WORKS CITED

2 Pass Clinic. "Facial Electrolysis Marathon Session for Trans Women." Accessed November 13, 2022. https://2pass.clinic/en/hair-removal/procedures/facial-hair-clearing.
Advanced Hair Clinic. "History of Hair Loss & Timeline: A Continuing Search to Find the Perfect Hair Loss Remedy." Accessed January 12, 2022. https://www.advancedhair.com.au/information/history-hair-loss/.
American Academy of Dermatology Association. "Hair Loss: Who Gets and Causes." Accessed January 11, 2022. https://www.aad.org/public/diseases/hair-loss/causes/18-causes.

American Battlefield Trust. "The Rise and Fall of the Powdered Wig." Accessed January 12, 2022. https://www.battlefields.org/learn/head-tilting-history/rise-and-fall-powdered-wig.

American Electrology Association. "Electrology Licensure by State." Accessed December 30, 2021. https://professionals.electrology.com/be-an-electrologist/electrology-licensing-requirements.html.

American Electrology Association. "What is Electrolysis?" Accessed August 5, 2024. https://www.electrology.com/faqs-about-permanent-hair-removal/.

Bared, Anthony, and Jeffrey S. Epstein. "Hair Transplantation Techniques for the Transgender Patient." *Facial and Plastic Surgery Clinics of North America* 27, no. 2 (2019): 227–32.

Belgravia Center. "Native Americans and Hair Loss." Accessed January 10, 2022. https://www.belgraviacentre.com/blog/native-americans-and-hair-loss/.

Bernstein, Robert M., William R. Rassman, and Bobby Limmer. "Follicular Unit Plain Speak." *International Society of Hair Restoration Surgery* 17, no. 6 (2007): 201–3. https://doi.org/10.33589/17.6.0201.

Bennett, James. "X-rays and Hair Removal," Cosmetics and Skin, 2019. Accessed December 22, 2021. https://www.cosmeticsandskin.com/cdc/xray.php.

Bolin, Anne. *In Search of Eve: Transsexual Rites of Passage.* Hadley, MA: Bergin & Garvey, 1998.

Bradford, Nova J., G. Nic Rider, and Katherine Spencer. "Hair Removal and Psychological Well-Being in Transfeminine Adults: Associations with Gender Dysphoria and Gender Euphoria." *Journal of Dermatological Treatment* 32, no. 6 (2007): 635–42. https://doi.org/10.1080/09546634.2019.1687823.

Brannon, Heather L. "The Structure and Growth Cycle of Hair Follicles." verywellhealth, 2021. Accessed December 30, 2021. https://www.verywellhealth.com/hair-follicle-1068786.

Butler, Rachel M., Arielle Horenstein, Matt Gitlin, et al. "Social Anxiety among Transgender and Gender Nonconforming Individuals: The Role of Gender-Affirming Medical Interventions." *Journal of Abnormal Psychology* 128, no. 1 (2019): 25–31. https://doi.org/10.1037/abn0000399.

Casetext. "N. J. Admin. Code #13:35-6.21. Current through *Register* 54, no. 13: 2024." Accessed September 6, 2022. https://casetext.com/regulation/new-jersey-administrative-code/title-13-law-and-public-safety/chapter-35-board-of-medical-examiners/subchapter-6-general-rules-of-practice/section-1335-621-hair-replacement-techniques.

Cipollaro, A.C., and M.B. Einhorn, "Use of X-Rays for Treatment of Hypertrichosis is Dangerous. *Journal of the American Medical Association* no. 135 (October 1947): 350.

Cleveland, D. E. H. "The Removal of Superfluous Hair by X-ray. *Canadian Medical Association Journal* 59, no. 4 (1931): 374–77. PMID: 20318346.

Cleveland Clinic. "Hair Transplant." Accessed September 6, 2022. https://my.cleveland clinic.org/health/treatments/21519-hair-transplant.
Courts and Tribunals Judiciary. "History of Court Dress." Accessed January 12, 2022. https://www.judiciary.uk/about-the-judiciary/the-justice-system/history/.
Cox, Caroline. "History of Wigs." Love to Know. Accessed January 12, 2022. https://fashion-history.lovetoknow.com/fashion-history-eras/history-wigs.
Darwin, Charles. *The Descent of Man, and Selection in Relation to Sex.* London: John Murray, 1871.
Desai, Karishma, Bianca Almeida, and Mariya Miteva. "Understanding Hormonal Therapies: Overview for the Dermatologist Focused on Hair." *Dermatology* 237, no. 5 (2021): 786–91. https://doi.org/10.1159/000512888.
Denny, Dallas. *Gender Dysphoria: A Guide to Research.* New York: Garland Publishing, 1994.
Denny, Dallas, and Margeaux Schaefer. "Panel Discussion of Transsexualism." Georgia Electrologist's Association and Georgia Clinical Electrologists Joint Meeting, Atlanta, GA, November 2, 1991.
Denny, Dallas, and Ahoova Mischael. "Electrolysis in Transsexual Women: A Retrospective Look at Frequency of Treatment in Four Cases." In *Current Concepts in Transgender Identity*, edited by Dallas Denny, 335–52. London, UK: Routledge, 1998. Accessed September 6, 2022. http://dallasdenny.com/Writing/2013/05/12/electrolysis-in-transsexual-women-a-retrospective-look-at-frequency-of-treatment-in-four-cases-1997/.
Derma Network. "Potential Risks and Complications of Laser Hair Removal." Accessed May 3, 2022. https://www.dermanetwork.org/article/cosmetic-enhancements/potential-risks-and-complications-of-laser-hair-removal#.
Dixson, Barnaby J., and Paul L. Vasey. "Beards Augment Perceptions of Men's Age, Social Status, and Aggressiveness, but Not Attractiveness." *Behavioral Ecology* 23, no. 3 (2012): 481–90. https://doi.org/10.1093/beheco/arr214.
Downing, Janelle M., Kimberly Yee, and Geolani Dy. "Hair Removal for Patients Undergoing Feminizing Surgeries in Oregon's Medicaid Program." *JAMA Dermatology* 157, no. 3 (2021): 346–48. https://doi.org/10.1001/jamadermatol.2020.5419.
Electrology 3000. "The International Leader in Transgender Hair Removal." Accessed August 5, 2024. https://electrology3000.
Electrologists Association of New Jersey. "Licensing Requirements." Accessed December 31, 2021. https://www.electrolysisnj.com/licensing_requirements.html.
Elliott, Ray A. "The Lateral Scalp Flap for Anterior Hairline Reconstruction." *Clinics in Plastic Surgery* 9, no. 2 (1982): 241–53. https://doi.org/10.1016/s0094-1298(20)30351-5.
Emancipated Electrolysis. "Frequently Asked Questions." Accessed April 27, 2015. http://www.emancipatedelectrolysis.com/electrolysis/frequently-asked-questions/.
Fernandez, Alexandra A., Katlein França, Anna H. Chacon, and Keyvan Nouri. "From Flint Razors to Lasers: A Timeline of Hair Removal Methods." *Journal of Cosmetic Dermatology* 12, no. 2 (2013): 153–62. https://doi.org/10.1111/jocd.12021.

Finifter, Morton B. "Facial Hair: Permanent Epilation with Respect to the Male Transsexual." In *Transsexualism and Sex Reassignment*, edited by Richard Green and John Money, 309–12. Baltimore, MD: Johns Hopkins University Press, 1969.

Fletcher, Jenna, and Cynthia Cobb. "How to Remove Hair Permanently from the Face, Legs, and Body." *Medical News Today*, June 1, 2020. Accessed October 15, 2022. https://www.medicalnewstoday.com/articles/how-to-remove-hair-permanently.

Ford, Benjamin James. "The Burning Question: Early U.S. Radiology and X-ray Burns, 1896–1904." Master's thesis, Salem State University, April 2016. Accessed August 5, 2024. https://www.academia.edu/24445208/The_Burning_Question_Early_U_S_Radiology_and_X_Ray_Burns_1896_1904.

Gan, Stephanie D., and Emmy M. Graber. "Laser Hair Removal: A Review." *Dermatologic Surgery* 39, no. 6 (2013): 823–38. https://doi.org/10.1111/dsu.12116.

Ginsberg, Brian A., Marcus Calderon, Nicole M. Seminara, and Doris Day. "A Potential Role for the Dermatologist in the Physical Transformation of Transgender People: A Survey of Attitudes and Practices within the Transgender Community." *Journal of the American Academy of Dermatology* 74, no. 2 (2016): 303–08. https://doi.org/10.1016/j.jaad.2015.10.013.

Green, Richard, and John Money, eds. *Transsexualism and Sex Reassignment*. Baltimore, MD: Johns Hopkins University Press, 1969.

Grymowicz, Monika, Ewa Rudnicka, Agnieszka Podfigurna, et al. "Hormonal Effects on Hair Follicles." *International Journal of Molecular Sciences* 21, no. 15 (2020): 5342. https://doi.org/10.3390/ijms21155342.

Haedersdal, Merete, and Peter C. Gøtzsche. "Laser and Photoepilation for Unwanted Hair Growth." *Cochrane Database of Systematic Reviews*, 2006. https://doi.org/10.1002/14651858.cd004684.pub2.

Haedersdal, Merete, and Hans C. Wulf. "Evidence-Based Review of Hair Removal Using Lasers and Light Sources." *Journal of the European Academy of Dermatology and Venereology* 20, no. 1 (2006): 9–20. https://doi.org/10.1111/j.1468-3083.2005.01327.x.

Hage, J. Joris, and Freerk G. Bouman. "Surgical Depilation for the Treatment of Pseudofolliculitis or Local Hirsutism of the Face: Experience in the First 40 Patients." *Plastic and Reconstructive Surgery* 88, no. 3 (1991): 446–51. https://doi.org/10.1097/00006534-199109000-00011.

"Hair Grower and Hair Loss Prevention Drug Products for Over-the-Counter Human Use." *Federal Register* 54, no. 12 (1989): 21 CFR Part 310, 28772-28777.

Hassrick, Royal B. *The George Catlin Book of American Indians*. New York: Watson-Guptill Publications, 1977.

Hedgecock, Sarah. "A Short History of Weird Cures for Baldness." *Forbes Magazine*, April 16, 2016. Accessed August 5, 2024. https://www.forbes.com/sites/sarahhedgecock/2016/04/16/a-short-history-of-weird-cures-for-baldness/.

Herzig, Rebecca M. "Removing Roots: 'North American Hiroshima Maidens' and the X Ray." *Technology and Culture* 40, no. 4 (1999): 723–45. https://doi.org/10.1353/tech.1999.0175.

———. "Subjected to the Current: Batteries, Bodies, and the Early History of Electrification in the United States." *Journal of Social History* 41, no. 4 (2008): 867–85. https://doi.org/10.1353/jsh.0.0013.

———. *Plucked: A History of Hair Removal.* New York: New York University Press, 2016.

Hinkel, Arthur Ralph. *Electrolysis, Thermolysis, and the Blend: The Principles and Practice of Permanent Hair Removal.* A. R. Hinkel, 1968.

Horan, James D. *North American Indian Portraits.* New York: Crown Publishers, 1975.

Hu, Hui-min, Shou-bing Zhang, Xiao-hua Lei, et al. "Estrogen Leads to Reversible Hair Cycle Retardation through Inducing Premature Catagen and Maintaining Telogen." *PLoS ONE* 7, no. 7 (2012). https://doi.org/10.1371/journal.pone.0040124.

Huang, Susan J. "What Happens during the Anagen Phase of Hair Growth." verywellhealth, April 16, 2020. Accessed December 30, 2021. https://www.verywellhealth.com/what-is-the-anagen-phase-of-hair-growth-1069411.

Imperato-McGinley, Julianne, Luis Guerrero, Teofilo Gautier, and Ralph E. Peterson. "Steroid 5α-Reductase Deficiency in Man: An Inherited Form of Male Pseudohermaphroditism." *Science* 186, no. 4170 (1974): 1213–15. https://doi.org/10.1126/science.186.4170.1213.

Inui, Shigeki, and Satoshi Itami. "Dr Shoji Okuda (1886–1962): The Great Pioneer of Punch Graft Hair Transplantation." *Journal of Dermatology* 36, no. 10 (2009): 561–62. https://doi.org/10.1111/j.1346-8138.2009.00704.x.

James, Andrea. "How Long Will Electrolysis Take?" Transgender Map, December 14, 2019. Accessed June 9, 2022. https://www.transgendermap.com/medical/hair-removal/electrolysis/how-long-will-electrolysis-take/.

James, Andrea. "Transgender Hair Removal before Bottom Surgery." Transgender Map, November 5, 2019. Accessed December 3, 2022. https://www.transgendermap.com/medical/hair-removal/bottom-surgery/.

Jeffrey Epstein, MD, FACS. "Who's Qualified to Perform a Hair Transplant Procedure." August 5, 2024. https://www.drjeffreyepstein.com/whos-qualified-to-perform-a-hair-transplant-procedure/.

Kayiran, Oguz, and Ercan Cihandide. "Evolution of Hair Transplantation." *Plastic and Aesthetic Research* 5, no. 3 (2018): 9. https://doi.org/10.20517/2347-9264.2017.86.

Kerure, Amit S., and Narendra Patwardhan. "Complications in Hair Transplantation." *Journal of Cutaneous and Aesthetic Surgery* 11, no. 4 (2018): 182–89. Accessed August 5, 2024. https://www.researchgate.net/publication/330787593_Complications_in_Hair_Transplantation.

Kim, S., M. Dennis, J. Holland, M. Terrell, M. Loukas, and J. Schober. "The Anatomy of Forearm Free Flap Phalloplasty for Transgender Surgery." *Clinical Anatomy* 31, no. 2 (2017): 145–51. https://doi.org/10.1002/ca.23014.

Kumaresan, Mithuvel, and Deepa M. Subburathinam. "Longevity of Hair Follicles after Follicular Unit Transplant Surgery." *Journal of Cutaneous and Aesthetic Surgery* 13, no. 4 (2020): 292–97. Accessed August 5, 2024. https://pubmed.ncbi.nlm.nih.gov/33911409/.

Lanigan, Sean W. "Incidence of Side Effects after Laser Hair Removal." *Journal of the American Academy of Dermatology* 49, no. 5 (2003): 882–86. https://doi.org/10.1016/s0190-9622(03)02106-6.

Lim, S. P. R., and Sean W. Lanigan. "A Review of the Adverse Effects of Laser Hair Removal." *Lasers in Medical Science* 21, no. 3 (2006): 121–25. https://doi.org/10.1007/s10103-006-0377-y.

Maiman, Theodore H. "Stimulated Optical Radiation in Ruby." *Nature* 187, no. 4736 (1960): 493–94. https://doi.org/10.1038/187493a0.

Markandeya, Virat. "When Deadly X-Rays Were Used for Hair Removal." Ozy, November 25, 2019.

Marks, Dustin H., Dina Hagigeorges, Athena J. Manatis-Lornell, Erica Dommasch, and Maryanne M. Senna. "Excess Hair, Hair Removal Methods, and Barriers to Care in Gender Minority Patients: A Survey Study." *Journal of Cosmetic Dermatology* 19, no. 6 (2019): 1494–98. https://doi.org/10.1111/jocd.13164.

Martin, Hayes, Elliot Strong, and Ronald H. Spiro. "Radiation-Induced Skin Cancer of the Head and Neck." *Cancer* 25, no. 1 (1970): 61–71. https://doi.org/10.1002/1097-0142(197001)25:1<61::aid-cncr2820250110>3.0.co;2-w.

Mayer, Toby, and Richard Fleming. *Aesthetic and Reconstructive Surgery of the Scalp.* St. Louis, MO: Mosby Year Book, 1992.

McElroy, Dana Kathleen. *Magic Hair: My Experiences with Lace Wigs.* Scotts Valley, CA: CreateSpace Independent Publishing Platform, 2010.

Miguel, Marie. "5 Reasons Natives Have Lustrous Locks: Ancient, Indigenous Hair Remedies." *Indian Country Today News*, March 29, 2017. Accessed August 5, 2024. https://ictnews.org/archive/5-reasons-natives-have-lustrous-locks-ancient-indigenous-hair-remedies.

Moller, Herbert. "The Accelerated Development of Youth: Beard Growth as a Biological Marker." *Comparative Studies in Society and History* 29, no. 4 (1987): 748–62. https://doi.org/10.1017/s0010417500014869.

Motosko, Catherine C., and Antonella Tosti. "Dermatologic Care of Hair in Transgender Patients: A Systematic Review of Literature." *Dermatology and Therapy* 11, no. 5 (2021): 1457–68. https://doi.org/10.1007/s13555-021-00574-0.

MTFsurgery.net. "A Patient's Guide to Pre-operative Hair Removal for Vaginoplasty." Accessed August 5, 2024. https://www.mtfsurgery.net/vaginoplasty-hair-removal-guide.htm.

Mysore, V., M. Kumaresan, A. Garg, et al. Singh. "Hair Transplant Practice Guidelines." *Journal of Cutaneous and Aesthetic Surgery* 14, no. 3 (2021): 265–84. Accessed August 5, 2024. https://www.ncbi.nlm.nih.gov/pmc/articles/PMC8611706/.

Okuda, Shoji. "Clinical and Experimental Studies on Transplanting of Living Hair." *Japanese Journal of Dermatology* 46 (1939); 537–87.

Orentreich, Norman. Autografts in Alopecias and other Selected Dermatological Conditions. *Annals of the New York Academy of Sciences* 83, no. 3 (1959): 463–79. https://doi.org/ 10.1111/j.1749-6632.1960.tb40920.x.

Panagotacos, Peter. "Chapter 5: Hair Loss Treatment History." Hairdoc. Accessed January 12, 2022. https://www.hairdoc.com/contents/chapter-5-hair-loss-treatment-history.

Ratushny, Vlad. "The Evolution of Hair Transplantation: A Brief History from Hair Plugs to Strip Excision and Fue." MassDerm Hair Transplant Institute, July 1, 2019. Accessed January 11, 2022. https://mahairtransplant.com/the-evolution-of-hair-transplantation-a-brief-history-from-hair-plugs-to-strip-excision-and-fue/.

Reese, William S. *James Otto Lewis and his Aboriginal Port Folio*. New Haven, CT: Overland Press, 2008.

Rosen, I. B., and P. G. Walfish. "Sequelae of Radiation Facial Epilation (North American Hiroshima Maiden Syndrome)." *Surgery* 106, no. 6 (1989): 946–50. PMID: 2588120.

Rösslin, Eucharius, and Thomas Raynalde. *The Byrth of Mankynde*. London: Thomas Ray, 1526. Accessed June 16, 2022. https://www.loc.gov/resource/rbctos.2017 english01732/?st=gallery.

Sattur, Sandeep S. "A Review of Surgical Methods (Excluding Hair Transplantation) and Their Role in Hair Loss Management Today." *Journal of Cutaneous and Aesthetic Surgery* 4, no. 2 (2011): 89–97. https://doi.org/10.4103/0974-2077.85020.

Schroeter, Careen Angela, Jan Stephen Groenewegen, Thorsten Reineke, and Hendrik Arend Neumann. "Ninety Percent Permanent Hair Reduction in Transsexual Patients." *Annals of Plastic Surgery* 51, no. 3 (2003): 243–48. https://doi.org/10.1097/01.sap.0000063759.59038.7e.

Simons, Robert L. "Johann Friedrich Dieffenbach." *Archives of Plastic Surgery* 5 (2003): 276–77.

Stanton, Elizabeth. "New York Tries to Regulate the Wild West of Laser Hair Removal." *Bloomberg News*, March 11, 2021. Accessed May 3, 2022. https://www.bloomberg.com/news/articles/2021-03-11/new-york-finally-tries-to-fix-its-laser-hair-removal-licensing-problem.

Stensgar, Barbie. "The Significance of Hair in Native American Culture." Sister Sky, January 4, 2019. Accessed January 10, 2022. https://sistersky.com/blogs/sister-sky/the-significance-of-hair-in-native-american-culture.

Stergiou, Alexandra. "In Native American Culture, Hair Meets Soul Meets Body." Vox Creative Next, May 3, 2017. Accessed January 12, 2022. https://www.vox.com/ad/15453466/chelsey-luger.

Stevenson, Mary O., Naomi Wixon, and Joshua D. Safer. "Scalp Hair Regrowth in Hormone-Treated Transgender Woman." *Transgender Health* 1, no. 1 (2016): 202–04. https://doi.org/10.1089/trgh.2016.0022.

Sure Hair International. "Norman Orentreich (1922–2019)—The Father of Hair Transplantation." Accessed January 13, 2022. https://web.archive.org/web/20211024180416/https://surehair.com/sure-hair-blog/hair-transplantation/norman-orentreich-1922-2019/.

Taylor, Timothy. *The Prehistory of Sex: Four Million Years of Human Sexual Culture.* New York: Bantam Books, 1996.

Thoreson, Nick, Dustin H. Marks, J. Klint Peebles, Dana S. King, and Erica Dommasch. "Health Insurance Coverage of Permanent Hair Removal in Transgender and Gender-Minority Patients." *JAMA Dermatology* 156, no. 5 (2020): 561–65. https://doi.org/10.1001/jamadermatol.2020.0480.

Townes, Charles H. "The First Laser." In *A Century of Nature: Twenty-One Discoveries that Changed Science and the World*, edited by Laura Garwin and Tim Lincoln, 107–12. Chicago: University of Chicago Press, 2003.

Turnabout: A Magazine of Transvestism, no. 10. Abbé de Choisy Press, ca 1968.

Unger, Walter P. "The History of Hair Transplantation." *International Society of Hair Restoration Surgery* 10, no. 4 (2000): 97–108. https://doi.org/10.33589/10.4.97.

US Food and Drug Administration. "Laser Facts." Accessed June 11, 2022. https://www.fda.gov/radiation-emitting-products/resources-you-radiation-emitting-products.

University of Michigan Health. "Electrolysis for Removing Hair." Accessed December 31, 2021. https://www.uofmhealth.org/health-library/ty7422.

Vellinus, Zahn, and Cynthia Cobb. "Vellus Hair: Function and Growth." *Medical News Today*, updated July 14, 2023. Accessed October 15, 2022. https://www.medicalnewstoday.com/articles/319881.

Venkat Center for Skin & Plastic Surgery. "Important Hair Transplant Guidelines: Standard Patient Care: Venkat Center for Hair Skin & Plastic Surgery." Accessed September 6, 2022. https://www.venkatcenter.com/hair-transplant-guidelines/.

Vogel, James E., Francisco Jimenez, John Cole, et al. "Hair Restoration Surgery: The State of the Art." *Aesthetic Surgery Journal* 33, no. 1 (2013): 128–51. https://doi.org/10.1177/1090820x12468314.

Waxman, Jamye. "From Medieval Hookers to Lady Gaga: A Brief History of the Merkin." *LA Weekly*, June 29, 2011. Accessed January 12, 2022. https://www.laweekly.com/from-medieval-hookers-to-lady-gaga-a-brief-history-of-the-merkin/.

Wikipedia. "Electrology." Accessed December 28, 2021. https://en.wikipedia.org/wiki/Electrology.

Wikipedia "Finasteride." Accessed February 26, 2022. https://en.wikipedia.org/wiki/Finasteride.

Wikipedia. "Laser Hair Removal." Accessed December 28, 2021. https://en.wikipedia.org/wiki/Laser_hair_removal.

Wikipedia "Laser." Accessed December 28, 2021. https://en.wikipedia.org/wiki/Laser.

Wikipedia. "Minoxidil." Accessed February 26, 2022. https://en.wikipedia.org/wiki/Minoxidil.

Wikipedia. "X-ray: Hazards Discovered" Accessed December 22, 2021. https://en.wikipedia.org/wiki/X-rays.

Woods, William. *New England's Prospect.* London: Tho. Cotes, 1634. Accessed December 21, 2021. https://www.gutenberg.org/files/47082/47082-0.txt.

Yaseen, Ummer, Shabir Ahmed, and Muzaffar Ahmed. "Beard Reconstruction." *International Journal of Trichology* 13, no. 6 (2021): 4–8. https://doi.org/10.4103/ijt.ijt_40_19.

Zhang, William R., Giorgia L. Garrett, Sarah T. Arron, and Maurice M. Garcia. "Laser Hair Removal for Genital Gender Affirming Surgery." *Translational Andrology and Urology* 5, no. 3 (2016): 381–87. https://doi.org/10.21037/tau.2016.03.27.

Section V

OUR FUTURE

The trouble with compiling a history book such as this is that, eventually, you need to stop writing—even as history continues to unfold. We've been working on this volume for eight years, during which the field of TGD healthcare continued to evolve, and opposing factions of our society made their opinions on TGD Americans known via guidelines, policies, legislation, and sensationalized pieces in the popular press. Neither our field nor our political environment appear poised to slow down anytime soon.

Thus, we face a dilemma. When do we lay down our pens and leave the future to fill someone else's history book? Our answer: the very last minute.

The previous twenty chapters were completed and submitted to SUNY Press in December 2022. However, we chose to update this next and final chapter in December 2023 to capture the feelings of turmoil and uncertainty brought on by the events of the past year.

In chapter 21, the youngest member of our editorial team, Kyan Lynch, contemplates the future of the field of TGD healthcare and his hopes for this compelling and continually evolving medical field.

21

THE FUTURE OF TRANSGENDER MEDICINE

Kyan Lynch

I write this final chapter at 5:38 p.m. on November 5, 2023. This means that you, dear reader, possess more knowledge about the future of transgender medicine than I have because you are living it. For that reason alone, I could declare this task a fool's errand and quit before I begin. In fact, this moment's sociopolitical landscape is so volatile that any predictions about transgender medicine are bound to haunt me.

So, why not quit while I'm ahead?

Three reasons.

First, this chapter is my responsibility, both literally and metaphorically. I am the youngest editor and one of the youngest contributors to this book. My esteemed fellow editors, along with the pioneers named throughout this volume, have cemented their legacies by getting us this far. While my colleagues still have much to contribute, it is my generation that must take up the mantle now. They lit the torch; we must carry it forward.

Second, there is a freedom in knowing that I am doomed to fail. You know more than I do and can fact check as you read. So, why not take some big swings and hope for the best?

Third, while specific predictions about the fate of this or that bill or the timeline of this or that medical breakthrough would be ill-advised, there are some general ideas about which I am confident. Looking to the future is not that different from looking to the past. The great prognosticators throughout history—Orwell, Verne, Bradbury, Wells, to name a few—achieved uncanny success by simply letting what has been indicate what will be.

For these reasons, I persevere. In this conclusion to our history of transgender medicine in the United States, I will explore five themes present throughout the book that I believe will resonate with you, whenever you exist in the future. I will provide evidence for selecting each theme for this future-forward chapter, discuss the likely implications for the future, and where reasonable, infuse my hopes for our tomorrows.

THEME 1: TRANSGENDER PEOPLE WILL CONTINUE TO DRIVE TRANSGENDER CARE

Medical professionals did not invent the concept of gender expansiveness. Transgender people have always existed. In chapter 2, "The Rise of Sexology in Europe," Clayton J. Whisnant described how transgender people woke the Western medical community to the possibility of gender diversity—certainly not the other way around. Early European sexologists struggled to differentiate sexual desire and gender identity, only beginning to disentangle the concepts in the 1920s.

Despite this fundamental misconception, medical professionals became societally appointed arbiters of gender and the recognized experts on gender variance. This, too, was a façade. Chapter 7, "Trans Circles of Knowledge and Intimacy," lays bear the truth: "[T]rans individuals themselves accelerated the learning curve for medical experts."[1] Through detailed written correspondence, photographic documentation, network building, and a willingness to expose themselves (in body and mind) for the greater good, trans individuals built the stage on which Harry Benjamin, Alfred Kinsey, and other revered cisgender scientists would eventually stand.

Indeed, much of this book catalogues the extraordinary efforts of transgender and gender-diverse (TGD) individuals to move medicine forward *from the outside*. During conversations with Dallas Denny and Jamison Green, I learned that the idea that an out transgender individual could play a role *from within* the medical system was fantastical for much of their careers. As late as 1995, Denny wrote the following about the publication of her reference book, *Gender Dysphoria: A Guide to Research*: "[This is] the first time that one of *us*, out of the closet, is the acknowledged expert, the first time one of us has braced the professionals in their own territory" (emphasis in original).[2] Regarding his advocacy work to improve transgender health while relegated to the margins, Green told me, "I just wanted people to have enough knowledge to make informed decisions about their lives and bodies."[3]

Fortunately, times have changed. According to the American Association of Medical Colleges' Matriculating Student Questionnaire, the number of out TGD students entering medical school more than tripled between 2016 and 2022, increasing year over year, though overall reported numbers remain low (209 in 2022).[4] Trans-led and trans-operated health centers and service providers, such as Transhealth Northampton in Massachusetts and Trans Lifeline, now dot the landscape, along with trans-owned healthcare consulting firms. In addition, programs now build and strengthen TGD healthcare professional pathways to increase the number of TGD individuals within the healthcare workforce[5] and improve access to care.

We lack reliable data on the number of healthcare professionals identifying as TGD and these data will likely lag behind the actual rise in numbers. However, that TGD individuals are squarely within the medical mainstream is undeniable. Many of the most highly regarded experts in transgender medicine now openly identify as trans—and a number of them contributed to this volume.

The road for TGD healthcare providers remains filled with obstacles. Studies examining the experiences of TGD students, physicians, and healthcare professionals are relatively few, but they all reveal increased rates of discrimination and mistreatment compared to cisgender peers.[6] Despite these headwinds, I remain convinced that the number of TGD individuals in the healthcare workforce will continue to rise, and that we, as a community, will continue to be a primary driver of medical advancements in the field. I'm inspired by my predecessors who catalyzed so much change to healthcare by applying pressure *from outside* the medical system. I can't wait to see what my successors will accomplish *from within*.

THEME 2: TRANSGENDER PEOPLE WILL BECOME LESS RELIANT ON MEDICAL PROFESSIONALS

Even as TGD professionals join the healthcare workforce and push the boundaries of transgender medical care, the extent to which the medical establishment can claim ownership of the TGD lived experience will continue to diminish. At first glance, this claim may seem counterintuitive. The increasingly advanced and available hormone therapies and procedures would seem to continually reinforce a dependent (or at least codependent) relationship between transgender people and medical professionals. On closer inspection, though, the true arc of this story bends away from medicine as prerequisite for authentic gender expression and toward medical intervention as a (optional) means to that end. The difference may seem subtle, but it is significant, as it dethrones the medical provider from the role of de facto judge of socially accepted gender expression.

Consider the following progression in identity documentation. In the early twentieth century, the legendary German psychiatrist Magnus Hirschfeld provided his patients with "transvestite passes," certified identification documents attesting to an individual's trans status, to protect them from the threat of arrest by police.[7] In 1950s Los Angeles, trans people "craved medical protection" from harassment by the authorities and, lacking formalized Hirschfeld-esque documentation, "quickly recognized that genital surgery could offer some security."[8] As time went on, however, the medical profession's power to either provide or withhold such protection began to slip. In 1987, New York State Commissioner of Motor Vehicles Patricia B. Adduci relaxed the requirements for gender marker change on identity documents; whereas New York State had previously required proof of surgery, the new guidance required only proof of medical, psychiatric, or psychological evaluation, and a medical determination that "one gender predominates over the other."[9] On March 11, 2022, Secretary of State Anthony Blinken announced the medical profession would be sidelined entirely; the State Department no longer requires people to submit any medical documentation for gender marker change on United States passports and has introduced an *X* gender marker option.[10]

This timeline of events echoes a parallel evolution in our conceptual understanding of the doctor-patient relationship. In the time of Hirschfeld, the Western medical profession relished its newfound role as expert.[11] Whereas their predecessors employed ineffective, if not dangerous, treatments based on faulty assumptions,[12] early to mid-twentieth-century physicians embraced their newfound empiric knowledge,[13] seeing themselves as the knowledgeable engineer tasked with mastering a complex machine.[14] This paternalistic schema relegated patients to the role of passive recipient rather than respected partner.[15] As the twentieth century unfolded, the doctor-patient relationship evolved from one of activity-passivity to mutual participation.[16] Psychoanalytical and psychosocial theories began to influence medical practices by stressing the need to center the patient and consider the patient's broader psychosocial context.[17] More recently, the emergence of shared decision making as an established best practice continues to emphasize the value of mutual respect in the patient-clinician relationship.[18]

Given this history, it is no surprise that the arc of gender-affirming care has, too, bent from paternalism toward respect for patient autonomy. The World Professional Association of Transgender Health *Standards of Care* (*SOC*) version eight continues to advocate for the role of mental health professionals in diagnosis and decision making. However, this still represents a philosophical departure from earlier SOC versions that required a person to perform their gender in specific ways to acquire the necessary approval from mental health professionals to access hormonal therapy.[19] The informed consent model, developed within community health centers and endorsed by the World Professional Association of Transgender Health *SOC* versions seven and eight, takes further steps toward eliminating paternalism from transgender medical care, requiring only that a patient attest to understanding the risks and benefits of treatment prior to initiating care.[20] Though not an ethical panacea,[21] the informed consent model interrupts the historical power imbalance between a clinician and gender-diverse patient; the patient's judgment is no longer superseded by that of the prescribing clinician.[22]

Taken together, these three historical progressions point toward a future in which TGD people are empowered to define their genders on their own terms and determine the treatment best suited to meeting their goals, even—or perhaps especially—when that involves no medical intervention. As demonstrated in various ways throughout this book, medical intervention has historically served two intertwined purposes: first, helping a person feel in greater alignment within their own body, and second, providing a measure of safety from transphobic and cisnormative societal elements. As our collective understanding of gender continues to evolve, the rigidity of the binary will continue to relax. Freed from these normative constraints, TGD individuals will no longer be forced to rely on the medical system to succeed in an unappeasably gendered world, thereby significantly reducing clinicians' roles in TGD lives.

THEME 3: WE WILL CONTINUE TO BLUR THE BOUNDARIES OF GENDER

On the subject of gender expansion, all signs in the United States point to a future in which gender is ever more complex and infinitely more flexible than it is now. At this point, I wish to state for the record that I am no gender theorist, nor am I qualified to interpret the work of the past and present giants in that field. But I am living in America in 2023, and I can read the writing on the wall.

According to a May 2022 survey from Pew Research Center, 5.1 percent of American adults younger than thirty years of age identify as trans or nonbinary, with more respondents identifying as nonbinary (3 percent) than as a trans man or woman.[23] The number of respondents identifying as nonbinary is 2.3 times higher for this younger age group than for those aged thirty to forty-nine, and thirty times higher than those older than fifty years.[24] An analysis by the Williams Institute of Data collected by the Centers for Disease Control and Prevention yielded similar results, estimating that teenagers and adults under age twenty-five account for 43 percent of the US transgender population, despite comprising only 19 percent of the overall population.[25] Of the 1.3 million adults who identify as transgender, more than a quarter reported being gender nonconforming.[26] Finally, an October 2018 survey of high school students in an urban Northeastern school district revealed that nine percent of students identified as having a gender identity incongruent with their sex assigned at birth, five times higher than previous estimates.[27] Roughly a third of these students identified as nonbinary.[28] The future will be far less binary than our world today.

One of the most recognizable markers of gender diversity is the use of nonbinary singular pronouns. Here, too, we see signs of expansion. In a study of more than 1.2 million college applications submitted for the 2022–2023 school year, noted researcher Genny Beemyn found that 37,000 students (3 percent) elected to use pronouns other than "she" or "he."[29] "They" was the most used nonbinary pronoun (97 percent), though it was only one of seventy-eight different pronoun sets submitted, alongside 130 different genders.[30]

These data tell a story, but not necessarily the one people claim. These data demonstrate that more people, and particularly young people, are *identifying* as nonbinary or gender nonconforming and *using* nonbinary pronouns and gender descriptors. These data do not demonstrate that *more* people, particularly young people, *are* nonbinary or gender expansive. A core assertion of this book is that TGD people are not new but rather newly entering the mainstream. Therefore, we can read these studies as simply reporting the expected results of more than a century's worth of progress to reveal the truth of gender, thereby creating space for more authentic expression of gender.

In chapter 14, Carolyn Wolf-Gould and Joshua Safer describe a particular peculiarity of the human race: not that we entertain nonbinary notions of gender but that we have so long fought against them! The animal kingdom is replete with examples of gender diversity and, as we see in chapters 1 and 5, so is human history (when viewed honestly and using a non-Western lens). Life beyond the binary has not been absent from American life but rather forcefully suppressed, mostly through mainstream cultural practices. However, while painful to admit, some of that suppression also came from within the TGD community. As Gillian Frank and Lauren Gutterman argue: "[T]he messier realities of trans peoples' lives, including queer desires or gender queer identities, needed to be smoothed out for them to be accepted by physicians and a wider public."[31]

Despite this suppression, and thanks to countless, and in too many cases nameless activists and advocates, the kids appear to be all right. As a society, we have marched from the most rigidly enforced binary gender norms into a state in which third genders are recognized on birth certificates and *X*'s mark the nonbinary spot on passports. Today's nonbinary and nonconforming teens will become not only adults but also parents, teachers, leaders, scientists, artists, and healthcare professionals. They will challenge and change the established rules of gender, and we will all be the better for it.

THEME 4: BACKLASH WILL ALWAYS PERSIST

Reader, you would be forgiven for thinking that I am too optimistic. Throughout the life of this project, I have imagined my existence in far less friendly pasts, and I cannot help but feel gratitude for my present and future. Still, I remain aware of the dangers of the present moment. I cannot recall a day in recent memory in which I did not learn of a new attempt to roll society back to a more repressive time. As of this writing, 586 anti-trans bills have been proposed, 85 having been passed, and 376 currently pending, across forty-nine states in 2023 alone.[35] These bills target a wide array of daily activities, from youth sports to public restroom use to health care provision.[32] On September 21, 2023, Representative Marjorie Taylor Greene brought the anti-trans agenda to Washington, DC, by introducing HR 5636, the "Protect Children's Innocence Act," to the House of Representatives.[33] This proposed amendment to title 18 of U.S.C. chapter 110 would, among other things, make it a class C felony to provide gender-affirming care to minors.[34] This publicity-stunt-turned-bill is building on the momentum of previous anti-trans actions purporting to "protect children," such as the directive Texas Governor Greg Abbott gave to the Texas Department of Family and Protective Services to investigate any reported instances of children receiving gender-affirming care.[35]

To claim that I see a near or even middle-term future in which these attacks cease would be both baseless and a lie. The truth is that these efforts are having their desired impact. Panic about gender ideology is spreading like wildfire. A representative commentary posted in the Gender section of the website for the Heritage Foundation, a long-standing Republican think tank, on July 7, 2021, situates gender identity alongside several other GOP bogeymen, including critical race theory, wokeness, "cancel culture," and "identity politics."[36] Positioned beneath the image of two adorable pairs of baby shoes—one blue, one pink (of course)—the author does not mince words: "This latest iteration of the sexual revolution is profoundly destructive to children and threatens the rights of parents."[37] Fortunately, the author provides parents with an escape hatch: "For parents to succeed in protecting children from 'woke' gender ideology, they will need to do political battle."[38] And, just like that, a parent's love and concern for their child is neatly reimagined as a recruitment tool for the cause.

I cannot and will not say that these attacks are ineffectual, nor will I say that I am optimistic that we will fend them off with any ease or haste. I can say with certainty that these attacks are neither unexpected nor new in the history of LGBTQ+ rights expansion. This book follows two parallel paths: from past to present, from margins to the mainstream. Overall, the arc has bent toward increased access to care, societal recognition, and respect for TGD people, but this path has been filled with setbacks. Every progressive movement has encountered backlash, and the movement for trans rights is no exception. Isaac Newton's third law of physics dictates that, for every action, there is an equal and opposite reaction. Considering the privileges I enjoy today in comparison to my transcestors' lives of a century ago, I assert that when it comes to the struggle for human rights, Newton was only half right. For every step forward, there will always be pushback—but it will never be enough to halt progress altogether.

THEME 5: YOU CANNOT LONG DETER PEOPLE FROM BEING WHO THEY ARE

I don't need their permission to exist; I exist in spite of them.

—Miss Major Griffin-Gracy

We may stumble, we may experience setbacks, we may be beaten, we may succumb to infighting, we may be sued, we may be criminalized, we may be ridiculed, we may be ignored—but we will never cease to exist. If you take nothing else away from this book, please internalize this message: TGD people are and have always been here. We are your siblings, your teachers, your parents, your friends. Though we may never know why, we have been put on this earth with the unmistakable self-knowledge that we have a different kind of living to do. Some of us can hide it, and some of us have been forced to deny it. But in my experience, fighting it is like fighting the urge to lift one's face toward the sun. Whether relegated to the margins or firmly in the mainstream, TGD people will always find a way, just like Pauli and Miss Major, Carla and Otto, Marsha and Sylvia, Carlett and Avon, Osh-Tisch and We'wha, Joseph and Lou, Dallas and Jamison. We are, all of us, across time and space, tethered as if by invisible string to our shared inheritance: a life authentically lived.

NOTES

1. See chapter 7 in this volume.
2. Denny, "Writing Ourselves."
3. Jamison Green, personal communication with author, August 17, 2022.
4. The total numbers reported in this, and similar studies, must be taken with a grain of salt. As long as disclosing a TGD identity risks placing one's safety and career in jeopardy, the prevalence of TGD individuals in any community will be artificially reduced. American Association of Medical Colleges, "Matriculating Student Questionnaire."
5. Sorcher, "Transgender and Nonbinary-Identified Health Care Professionals."
6. Westafer et al., "Experiences of Transgender and Gender Expansive Physicians," 5; Heiderscheit et al., "Experiences of LGBTQ+ Residents," 27; Dimant et al., "Experiences of Transgender and Gender," 212.
7. Timm, "I Am So Grateful to All You Men of Medicine," 85.
8. Bakker et al., *Others of My Kind*, 111.
9. New York State Department of Motor Vehicles, "Change in Required Documentation."
10. US Department of State, "X Gender Marker Available."
11. Mantri, "Holistic Medicine," 178.
12. Lagay, "The Legacy of Humoral Medicine," 206–08; Wynia, "The Short History and Tenuous Future of Medical Professionalism," 567.

13. Starr, "Professionalization and Public Health," S28; Spree, "The Impact of the Professionalization of Physicians," 29–30.
14. Cushing, "History of the Doctor–Patient Relationship," 7.
15. Hellin, "The Physician–Patient Relationship," 450.
16. Kaba and Sooriakumaran, "The Evolution of the Doctor-Patient Relationship," 60–61.
17. Mead and Bower, "Patient-Centredness," 1089.
18. Lee and Emanuel, "Shared Decision Making," 6.
19. Selvaggi et al., "The 2011 WPATH Standards of Care," 4.
20. Schulz, "The Informed Consent Model of Transgender Care," 83–85.
21. Gerritse et al., "Decision-Making Approaches in Transgender Healthcare," 695.
22. Spanos et al., "The Informed Consent Model of Care," 207.
23. Brown, "About 5% of Young Adults in the U.S. Say Their Gender Is Different."
24. Brown, "About 5% Of Young Adults in The U.S. Say Their Gender Is Different."
25. Herman, Flores, and O'Neill, "How Many Adults and Youth Identify as Transgender."
26. Herman, Flores, and O'Neill, "How Many Adults and Youth Identify as Transgender."
27. Kidd et al., "Prevalence of Gender-Diverse Youth," 1–2.
28. Kidd et al., "Prevalence of Gender-Diverse Youth," 1–2.
29. Beemyn, "College Students are Increasingly Identifying.'"
30. Beemyn, "College Students are Increasingly Identifying.'"
31. Frank and Gutterman, "Canary."
32. Track Trans Legislation, "2023 Anti-Trans Bills."
33. Protect Children's Innocence Act, H.R. 5636, 118th Cong. (2023)
34. Ring, "Marjorie Taylor Greene Attempts to Make Gender Care for Youth a Crime."
35. Klibenoff and Oxner, "Texas' Child Welfare Agency."
36. Kao, "Woke Gender."
37. Kao, "Woke Gender."
38. Kao, "Woke Gender."

WORKS CITED

American Association of Medical Colleges. "Matriculating Student Questionnaire: 2021 All Schools Summary Report." 2021. Accessed October 20, 2023. https://www.aamc.org/data-reports/students-residents/report/matriculating-student-questionnaire-msq.

Bakker, Alex, Rainer Herrn, Michael Thomas Taylor, and Annette F. Timm. *Others of My Kind: Transatlantic Transgender Histories*. Canada: University of Calgary Press, 2020.

Beemyn, Genny. "College Students Are Increasingly Identifying Beyond 'She' And 'He.'" *The Conversation*, 2022. Accessed October 20, 2023. https://theconversation.com/college-students-are-increasingly-identifying-beyond-she-and-he-187338.

Brown, Anna. "About 5% Of Young Adults in the U.S. Say Their Gender Is Different from Their Sex Assigned at Birth." *Pew Research Center*, 2022. Accessed October 20, 2023. https://www.pewresearch.org/fact-tank/2022/06/07/about-5-of-young-adults-in-the-u-s-say-their-gender-is-different-from-their-sex-assigned-at-birth/.

Cushing, Annie. "History of the Doctor–Patient Relationship." In *Clinical Communication in Medicine*, edited by Jo Brown, Lorraine M. Noble, Alexia Papageorgiou, and Jane Kidd, chapter 3. Wiley Online Library, 2015. Access September 15, 2024. https://onlinelibrary.wiley.com/doi/10.1002/9781118728130.ch3.

Denny, Dallas. "Writing Ourselves." *Dallas Denny: Body of Work*. 1995. Accessed September 9, 2023. http://dallasdenny.com/Writing/2011/10/05/writing-ourselves/.

Dimant, Oscar E., Tiffany E. Cook, Richard E. Greene, and Asa E. Radix. "Experiences of Transgender and Gender Nonbinary Medical Students and Physicians." *Transgender Health* 4, no. 1 (2019): 209–16.

Drucker, Zackary. "Trans Icon Miss Major: 'We've Got to Reclaim Who the Fuck We Are.'" Vice.com, 2018. Accessed August 1, 2023. https://www.vice.com/en/article/j5z58d/miss-major-griffin-gracy-transgender-survival-guide.

Frank, G., and Gutterman, L. "Canary: The Story of a Transsexual." Hosted and created by Gillian Frank and Lauren Gutterman. Sexing History, 2020, Podcast Season 2, Episode 4. Accessed September 15, 2024. https://www.sexinghistory.com/episode-24.

Gerritse, Karl, Laura A. Hartman, Marijke A. Bremmer, Baudewijntje P.C. Kreukels, and Bert C. Molewijk. "Decision-Making Approaches in Transgender Healthcare: Conceptual Analysis and Ethical Implications." *Medicine, Health Care and Philosophy* 24, 4 (2021): 687–99.

Heiderscheit, Evan A., Cary Jo R. Schlick, Ryan J. Ellis, et al. "Experiences of LGBTQ+ Residents in US General Surgery Training Programs." *JAMA surgery* 157, no. 1 (2022): 23–32.

Hellin, T. "The Physician–Patient Relationship: Recent Developments and Changes." *Haemophilia* 8, no. 3 (2002): 450–54.

Herman, Jody, Andrew Flores, and Kathryn O'Neill. "How Many Adults and Youth Identify as Transgender in the United States?" UCLA School Of Law Williams Institute, 2022. Accessed October 15, 2023. https://williamsinstitute.law.ucla.edu/publications/trans-adults-united-states/.

Kaba, Riyaz, and Prasanna Sooriakumaran. "The Evolution of the doctor-Patient Relationship." *International Journal of Surgery* 5, no. 1 (2007): 57–65.

Kao, Emilie. "Woke Gender." Heritage Foundation, 2021. Accessed October 20, 2023. https://www.heritage.org/gender/commentary/woke-gender.

Kidd, Kacie M., Gina M. Sequeira, Claudia Douglas, et al. "Prevalence of Gender-Diverse Youth in an Urban School District." *Pediatrics* 147, no. 6 (2021): 1–2.

Klibenoff, Eleanor, and Reese Oxner. "Texas' Child Welfare Agency Ordered to Investigate Trans Kids' Families Has Been in Crisis for Years." *Texas Tribune*, March 11, 2022. Accessed October 20, 2023. https://www.texastribune.org/2022/03/11/texas-dfps-trans-teens/.

Lagay, Faith. "The Legacy of Humoral Medicine." *AMA Journal of Ethics* 4, no. 7 (2002): 206–08.

Mantri, Sneha. "Holistic Medicine and the Western Medical Tradition." *AMA Journal of Ethics* 10, no. 3 (2008): 177–80.

Mead, Nicola, and Peter Bower. "Patient-Centredness: A Conceptual Framework and Review of the Empirical Literature." *Social Science & Medicine* 51, no. 7 (2000): 1087–10.

New York State Department of Motor Vehicles. Change in Required Documentation for Proof of Sex Change, Patricia B. Adduci, "C" 15. Albany, NY: Office of the Commissioner, 1987. Accessed September 15, 2024. https://perma.cc/F7UK-2RUV.

Oshima Lee, E., and E. J. Emanuel. "Shared Decision Making to Improve Care and Reduce Costs." *New England Journal of Medicine* 368, no. 1 (2013): 6–8.

Ring, Trudy. "Marjorie Taylor Greene Attempts to Make Gender Care for Youth a Crime." *The Advocate*, 2022. Accessed November 1, 2023. https://www.advocate.com/breaking-news/2022/8/19/marjorie-taylor-greene-attempts-make-gender-care-youth-crime.

Schulz, Sarah L. "The Informed Consent Model of Transgender Care: An Alternative to the Diagnosis of Gender Dysphoria." *Journal of humanistic psychology* 58, no. 1 (2018): 84.

Selvaggi, Gennaro, Cecilia Dhejne, Mikael Landen, and Anna Elander. "The 2011 WPATH Standards of Care and Penile Reconstruction in Female-to-Male Transsexual Individuals." *Advances in Urology* 2012, no. 581712 (2012): 4. https://doi.org/10.1155/2012/581712.

Sorcher, Rachel. "Transgender and Nonbinary-Identified Health Care Professionals Are Changing the Exclusionary Health Care System." BU School of Public Health, 2022. Accessed October 20, 2023. https://www.bu.edu/sph/news/articles/2022/transgender-and-nonbinary-identified-health-care-professionals-are-changing-the-exclusionary-health-care-system/.

Spanos, Cassandra, Julian A. Grace, Shalem Y. Leemaqz, et al. "The Informed Consent Model of Care for Accessing Gender-Affirming Hormone Therapy Is Associated with High Patient Satisfaction." *Journal of Sexual Medicine* 18, no. 1 (2021): 201–08.

Spree, Reinhard. "The Impact of the Professionalization of Physicians on Social Change in Germany During the Late 19th and Early 20th Centuries." *Historical Social Research/Historische Sozialforschung* (1980): 29–30.

Starr, P. "Professionalization and Public Health: Historical Legacies, Continuing Dilemmas." *Journal of Public Health Management and Practice* 15, no. 6 (2009): S28.

Track Trans Legislation, "2022 Anti-Trans Bills." *Tracktranslegislation.com*, 2022. Accessed September 9, 2023. https://www.tracktranslegislation.com/.

US Department of State. "X Gender Marker Available on U.S. Passports Starting April 11." Anthony J. Blinken, Office of the Spokesperson, 2022.

Westafer, Lauren M., Caroline E. Freiermuth, Michelle D. Lall, Sarah J. Muder, Eleanor L. Ragone, and Angela F. Jarman. "Experiences of Transgender and Gender Expansive Physicians." *JAMA Network Open* 5, no. 6 (2022): e2219791.

Wynia, Matthew K. "The Short History and Tenuous Future of Medical Professionalism: The Erosion of Medicine's Social Contract." *Perspectives in Biology and Medicine* 51, no. 4 (2008): 567.

CONTRIBUTORS

Noah Adams, MSW. University of Toronto, Ontario Institute for Studies in Education. Transgender Professional Association for Transgender Health.

Yuki Arai, LE, CPE. New York Electrolysis Office Member of WPATH, American Electrology Association, and New York Electrolysis Association.

Hansel Arroyo, MD. Assistant Professor of Psychiatry in the Icahn School of Medicine at Mount Sinai.

Amy Block, MD. Resident, Department of Psychiatry, Dartmouth-Hitchcock Medical Center.

Alexander Boscia, MS, MD. Graduate Medical Fellow, Maternal-Fetal Medicine, Department of Obstetrics, Gynecology, and Reproductive Science, University of Pittsburgh Medical Center, Magee-Womens Hospital.

George R. Brown, MD, DFAPA. Professor and Associate Chairman of Psychiatry, East Tennessee State University, Quillen College of Medicine. James H. Quillen Veterans Affairs (VA) Medical Center.

Dani Castro, MA MFT. Founding Board Member, Center of Excellence in Transgender Health, University of California San Francisco. Cofounder, Transgender Advocates for Justice and Accountability.

Ms. Bob Davis, MFA. Founder and Director, Louise Lawrence Transgender Archive. GLBT Historical Society, former secretary and board member. City College of San Francisco music faculty, interim Dean of Liberal Arts (retired).

Dallas Denny, BS, MA, Licensed Psychological Examiner (Tennessee, retired). Gender Education & Advocacy, Inc.

Contributors

Aaron Devor, PhD, FSSSS, FSTLHE. Founder and inaugural chair in Transgender Studies. Founder and subject matter expert, Transgender Archives. Founder and host, Moving Trans History Forward Conferences. Professor, Sociology Department, University of Victoria, Canada.

David A. Diamond, MD. Department of Pediatric Urology, University of Rochester School of Medicine and Dentistry.

Diane Ehrensaft, PhD. Developmental and Clinical Psychologist. Director of Mental Health, University of California San Francisco Benioff Children's Hospital Child and Adolescent Gender Center. Professor of Pediatrics, University of California San Francisco.

Cecile A. Ferrando, MD, MPH. Clinical Medical Director, Urogynecology and Reconstructive Pelvic Surgery, Professor of Obstetrics, Gynecology, and Reproductive Services, University of California, San Diego Health.

Jules Gill-Peterson, PhD. Associate Professor, Department of History, Johns Hopkins University. General co-editor, TSQ: Transgender Studies Quarterly.

Zil Goldstein, FNP-BC. Callen-Lorde Community Health Center. City University of New York School of Public Health and Health Policy.

Jamison Green, PhD, MFA. Past President World Professional Association for Transgender Health (WPATH) (2014–2016). Gender Education & Advocacy, Inc.

Katherine Blumoff Greenberg, MD. Associate Professor of Pediatrics, Obstetrics/Gynecology, and University Health. University of Rochester School of Medicine and Dentistry.

Tj Gundling, PhD. Professor and Program Coordinator, Anthropology, Department of Community and Social Justice Studies, William Paterson University of New Jersey.

Alexander B. Harris, MPH, CPH. Clinical Research Manager, Callen-Lorde Community Health Center.

Ashliana Hawelu, President, Kulia Na Mamo.

Tresne Hernandez, MD. University of California, San Francisco, Family & Community Medicine Residency Program at San Francisco General Hospital.

Kenneth Hubbell, MD. Resident, Department of Internal Medicine, University of California San Francisco Medical Center.

Trudie Jackson, MS. American Indian Two Spirit Transgender Elder/Scholar residing in Phoenix, Arizona, originally from the Navajo Nation.

Yongha Kim, MD. Resident, General Adult Psychiatry, Zucker Hillside Hospital, Northwell Health.

Terren Lansdaal, MS, CCC-SLP. Member, American Speech-Language-Hearing Association.

Jennifer Lee, PhD, MPH. Founder and lead organizer, House Lives Matter.

Bambi Lobdell, PhD. Adjunct Professor, State University of New York at Oneonta.

Kyan Lynch, MD, MA. Assistant Professor, University of Rochester School of Medicine and Dentistry.

Serena Nanda, PhD. Professor Emeritus, John Jay College, City University of New York.

Ruth Pearce, MD. Lecturer in Community Development, School of Education, University of Glasgow. Senior Fellow, Center for Applied Transgender Studies.

Jack Pickering, PhD, CCC-SLP. Professor of Practice in Speech Language Pathology. Russell Sage College.

Asa Radix, MD, PhD, MPH. Executive Vice President of Research and Education, Callen-Lorde Community Health Center, and Associate Professor, Columbia University Mailman School of Public Health.

Joshua D. Safer, MD, FACP, FACE. Executive Director, Center for Transgender Medicine and Surgery, Mount Sinai Health System. Professor of Medicine, Icahn School of Medicine at Mount Sinai.

Amrita Sarkar, Advisor, Transgender Wellbeing and Advocacy, India HIV/AIDS Alliance. Member of World Professional Association for Transgender Health, Transgender Professional Association for Transgender Health, Secretary and founding member of International Reference Group of Trans Women and HIV.

Jillian Shipherd, PhD. LGBTQ+ Health Program, Veteran's Health Administration, Washington, DC. National Center for Post Traumatic Stress Disorder, VA Boston Healthcare System, Boston, MA. Department of Psychiatry, Boston University Chobanian & Avedisian School of Medicine, Boston, MA.

Sharon Stuart (a.k.a. Thomas Heitz), JD. Retired Librarian, National Baseball Hall of Fame. Lifetime member of Tri-ESS. Founding Director International Conference on Transgender Law and Employment Policy. Editor and coordinator for development of the International Bill of Gender Rights (1995). Lifetime member of NAACP.

Annette F. Timm, PhD. Professor, Department of History, University of Calgary.

Jaimie F. Veale, PhD. Trans Health Research Lab, School of Psychology, University of Waikato, Aotearoa New Zealand.

Amanda Wang, MD. Resident, Weill Cornell Medical Center, Department of Internal Medicine.

Clayton J. Whisnant, PhD. Chapman Professor of History and the Humanities, Wofford College.

Teri Wilhelm, BA, AS. Albany Damien Center. Trans Health Advocates of New York. Working in coalition:

- Lorena Borjas Transgender Wellness and Equity Fund
- Gender Recognition Act
- Gender Expression Non-Discrimination Act

Carolyn Wolf-Gould, MD. Founder, Gender Wellness Center—Bassett Healthcare Network.

Christopher Wolf-Gould, MD. Gender Wellness Center—Bassett Healthcare Network.

INDEX

Abdur-Rahman, Aliyyah I., 32
Abraham, Felix, 586
ACA. *See* Affordable Care Act
Ackerley, J. R., 56
acquired immunodeficiency disease (AIDS), 150, 299. *See also* HIV/AIDS epidemic
   HBC relation to, 317
activism, 17
   of Denny, 313
   of Green, J., 431–432, 718–719
   healthcare, 8
   of Hirschfeld, 70
   in HIV/AIDS epidemic, 300–301
   for human rights, 20
   of Johnson, M., 417–418
   of Murray, P., 302–303, 304, 305–306
   of Rivera, 421–422
   for sex work, 418–419
   of Two Spirit people, 148, 149
ACTUP. *See* AIDS Coalition to Unleash Power
Adams, Noah, 545, 731
   on ethics, 544
   on Hoff, 571
Adler, Richard, 661, 664, 675
   Voice and Communication Therapy for the Transgender/Transsexual Client of, 667, 674
   WPATH relation to, 667–668
administrative separation from military, cross-dressing and, 538n10
adzáán (primary gender), 131

affirmative mental healthcare models, 553
Affirming Sexual Orientation and Gender Identity Act (2015), 637
Affordable Care Act (ACA), 458, 461, 562–563
   discrimination relation to, 409, 562, 565n48
   gender identity relation to, 668
   insurance coverage relation to, 690
Africa, homosexual relationships, 33
"age of anxiety," 202
"Agnes" (pseudonym), 266–267
AIDS. *See* acquired immunodeficiency disease
AIDS Coalition to Unleash Power (ACTUP), 301
   HIV/AIDS epidemic relation to, 313
   Johnson, M., and, 418
Albany Trust of London, 347, 437–438
alcohol abuse, transgender veterans relation to, 528–529
Alexander, Gerianne, 484
Alford, Blake, 320n60
Allen, Luke Roy, 464
Allen, Robert, 168, 180–182
allies, cisgender people as, 6
Allison, Rebecca, 454, 462
Almaas, Elsa, 453
Altman, Lawrence K., 299
American Association of Medical Colleges, 719
American Association of Sex Educators, Counselors and Therapists, 228, 341

735

American College of Pediatricians, 410
American culture, 1
　Judeo-Christian doctrine relation to, 2
American Educational Gender
　　Information Service, 308, 311, 425,
　　705n63
　Denny relation to, 231, 350, 426, 705
　vaginoplasty relation to, 692–693
American Electrology Association, 691
American Foundation for AIDS Research,
　　253
American Journal of Psychiatry, 520
American Psychiatric Association, 273,
　　462
　transgender medical research relation
　　to, 520
American Scholar (magazine), 377–378
American Speech-Language Hearing
　　Association, 662, 668, 669, 672
American Weekly (magazine), 177
Americans with Disabilities Act (1990),
　　261, 458
amicus briefs, 450, 456, 463
Anderson, Maxwell, 309
androgen insensitivity syndrome, 485
androgen therapy, 556, 557–558
　gender-affirming voice training and,
　　660–661, 670
androgenic alopecia, 697–698. *See also*
　　baldness
　hormones relation to, 700
androgens, 484, 489
　CAH relation to, 485
androgyny, 48
　of bissu, 21
　Hinduism relation to, 18
　in Mexican culture, 25
Angelo, Gen, 174
Angelo, Joseph, 588
animal kingdom, gender diversity in,
　　474–475, 723

Anne (Queen), 99
anterior glottal web formation, 677
anti-trans legislation, 513, 723–724
　in Arkansas, 410, 650, 655
Antoninus, Marcus Aurelius, 584–585
apotemnophilia, 606n74
appendectomy, 227
Arai, Yuki, 692, 731
　on body hair, 685
Archives of Sexual Behavior (journal),
　　268, 451, 636
　Green, R., relation to, 385n14
Argot, Madeline, 571
Argus Pressclipping Bureau, 94
Arkansas, 410, 655
　GAM relation to, 650
Armendarez, Evangelina Trujillo, 333
Armstrong, William L., 458
Arrow Electronics, 333
Arroyo, Hansel, 167, 731
　on psychology, 255
Article 1557, of ACA, 409
As Nature Made Him (Colapinto), 482
Ashley, April, 15, 113, 125–126
Ashton, Aileen, *332*, 333
Asscheman, Henk, 527
Association for the Advancement of
　　Psychotherapy, 186
Atherton, Gerthud, 506
attribution theory, 509
autism spectrum disorder, 261, 276n75,
　　486, 489
autocastration, 210, 215–216, 235n48
　transgender inmates relation to, 534–
　　535
autoeroticism, 53
autogynephilia, 265
Avenue Theatre, 223–224
aversion therapy
　for cross-dressing, 263–264
　Rekers and, 269–270

Azul, Arnold, 672

badé, 134. See also Two Spirit people
Bahuchara Mata, 19
Bailey, J. Michael, 265
Bailey, Marlon, 316
Bak, Robert, 263
bakla, 31
baldness, 696, 707n110
  follicular unit transplants for, 698
Bangladesh, 20
  third gender status in, 33
Banks, Jim, 579, 580n15
bans
  on conversion therapy, 275n59
  on gender-affirming treatment, 655–656
  in military, 10, 549–550
  on sports participation, 410
  TERF relation to, 405–406
Barbarito, William, 185
Barbin, Herculine, 68–69, 84n16
Bared, Anthony, 701
Barlow, Irene, 305
Barnum & Bailey Circus and Shows, 225, 237n82
Battle of the Rosebud, 134
Bauer, Heike, 79
Bauman, Walter, 465
Bay Cities Dog and Cat Hospital, 226
Beachy, Robert, 73
Beaumont, Charles Eon de, 121n69
Becoming a Visible Man (Green, J.), 370, 430, 431
bed nucleus of the stria terminalis (BSTc), 491
Beecroft, Carol, 249
Beemyn, Genny, 245, 722
Begochiddy, 133. See also Diné people
Beh, Hazel Glenn, 483

Belt, Elmer, 363, 623
  gender-affirming surgery relation to, 553, 624–625
Benestad, Esben Esther Pirelli, 453
Benjamin, Harry, 8–9, 14–15, 67, 167, 185–187, 190
  Belt relation to, 624
  Biber relation to, 592
  Erickson relation to, 332, 344–345
  Erskine relation to, 69, 209, 210–214, 216–218, 220–223, 233n4, 235n46, 235n53
  etiology and, 479–480
  funding relation to, 537–538
  on gender roles, 474
  Hirschfeld relation to, 65–68, 74–75, *75*, 83n3, 83n6, 184, 188–189, 235n44
  Hoff relation to, 571
  hormone therapy relation to, 251n1, 519, 556
  hormones relation to, 66, 82
  identification and, 449
  Ihlenfeld relation to, 263
  at International Symposium on Gender Identity, 348–349
  intimate histories relation to, 232
  Jorgensen, C., relation to, 170, 183–184, 187, 193n50, 194n74, 195n76, 197n99, 363, 588
  Kinsey relation to, 65–68, 76–77, 80–81, 85n39, 96, 185, 195n84
  Lawrence, L., relation to, 243
  Money relation to, 436
  Pauly relation to, 271
  Prince relation to, 249–251
  Schaefer relation to, 272
  Self relation to, 124
  Sex Orientation Scale of, 196n92
  Spengler relation to, 93, 95, 195n82
  Steinach relation to, 184, 506

Benjamin, Harry *(continued)*
  transgender medical research of, 518–519, 520–521
  Transsexualism and Sex Reassignment relation to, 366–367
berdache, 130. *See also* Two Spirit people
Berlin, Germany
  Department for Pederasty in, 73
  sexual subcultures in, 65, 71–72, 74
  University of, 43
Berlin Institute for Sexual Science, 8–9
Berlins (Hirschfeld), 84n25
Bettelheim, Bruno, 276n75
Beyer, Dana, 512
bias
  eugenics and, 382–383
  at HBIGDA, 430
  racial, 601–602
  of researchers, 380
  in SOC, 445
Biber, Stanley, 591–593, 607n90
Bibliotheca Historica, 585
Biden, Joe, 409
  Levine, R., relation to, 577, 579
Biden administration, 550
bigender euphoria, 251
bigendered, 250, 251n4
Billings, Dwight, 381
Binghamton Insane Asylum, 288
biocultural diversity, 191n15
biofeedback, 665
biological essentialism, 510, 511–512
biological sex, gender compared to, 182, 190n2, 194n68
birth control pill, 82, 228
bisexuality, 252–253
  Freud relation to, 258
  universal, 92
Bisexuality (Firestein), 452

bisexuals, 58n48
  Kinsey on, 78–79
  psychic hermaphrodites as, 48
bissu, 21–22
Bitter Water, 128
Black Lives Matter movement, 409
black market hormones, 145
Black on Both Sides (Snorton), 205
Black TGD people, 205–206. *See also* people of color
blackmail, 73
Blackstone, Elliot, 400
Blanchard, Ray, 252
  autogynephilia and, 265
Blinken, Anthony, 720
Bloch, Iwan, 51
Block, Amy, 731
  on Belt, 623
Block, Christie, 671
Bloomberg News, 689
Blüher, Hans, 46
Blumenstein, Rosalyne, 453
Bockting, Walter, 252–253, 441, 453, 461–462
  Committee on Lesbian, Gay, Bisexual, and Transgender Health Issues and Research Gaps and Opportunities and, 462
  International Journal of Transgender Health relation to, 465
body hair
  gender incongruence and, 685
  of people of color, 703n32
body modification practices, 17. *See also* gender-affirming surgery
Boerhaave, Hermann, 41
Bogoraz, Nikoalai A., 597
Boisvert, Jeanne "Nanou," 112
Bolin, Anne, 271, 691
  on gender clinics, 375–376

In Search of Eve of, 381, 387n52, 404
Bondy, Phillip, 591
Bonne, Francis, 126
Book of Mormon, 153n2
born-in-the-wrong-body narrative, 197n105
  Jorgensen, C., and, 194n59
"Born This Way," 510–511
born-this-way argument, 512–513
  for human rights, 510–511
Born This Way Foundation, 510–511
Boscia, Alexander, 15, 105, 123, 125
Boston Children's Hospital, GeMS at, 640, 649–652, 653–654
Boston Globe, 288
Boston Medical Center, 651
Boston Phoenix Report, 343
Boswell, Holly, 407
Botzer, Marsha, 441–442, 461
Bouman, F. G., 599
Bowers, Marci, 441, 554, 594, 607n95
  Biber relation to, 593
  WPATH relation to, 465
Bowman, Karl, 245, 247n5
Boysen, Guy, 510
Bradford, Judith, 462
Bradford, Nova J., 689
Bradley, Susan, 635
brain development, 261
Bralley, Ralph, 662
Brassard, Pierre, 594
  on electrolysis, 693
Brazil, 25–27
  Candomblé in, 27–28
Breckenridge, Bunny, 219
Brevard, Aleshia, 624–625
Brewster, Lee, 401
Britain, 51
British colonial period, 19–20

Brown, Carlett, 167
Brown, George R., 330, 456, 550, 731
  on transgender medical research, 517
Brown, John Ronald, 590–591
  apotemnophilia and, 606n74
Brown, Kay, 389n82
Brown v. Board of Education, 304
Brownstein, Michael, 252
Bry, Theodor de, 138
Bryant, Karl, 635
BSTc. *See* bed nucleus of the stria terminalis
Buddhism, 21, 297
  homoeroticism relation to, 24
Bugis, 21–22
Bullough, Bonnie, 228
Bullough, Vern, 346
Bund für Menschenrechte (League for Human Rights), 73
buprenorphine therapy, 510
Bureau of Indian Affairs, 134, 141
Burkholder, Nancy, 406
Burns, Christine, 461
Burou, Georges, 15, 112, 116, 363
  Ashley and, 125
  Dufresnoy and, 126
  penile inversion vaginoplasty and, 588
  Richards, R., relation to, 263
  vaginoplasty and, 15, 105–106, 113, 114–115
Butler, Judith, 146
  on gender identity, 260
Butler, Rachel, 689
Byne, William, 508
Byrd, Jodi, 146, 147

Caen, Herb, 212, 223–224, 233n17
CAH. *See* congenital adrenal hyperplasia
calabai, 22
Calderone, Mary S., 228

California Board of Medical Quality
    Assurance, 590–591
California Department of Insurance, 460
California State University, Long Beach
    (CSULB), 228
California State University, Northridge, 228
Callen-Lorde Community Health Center,
    560
Callo, 585
CAMH. *See* Gender Identity Clinic for
    Children at the Centre for Addiction
    and Mental Health
Campbell, Marie Ciel. *See* Erskine, Carla
    (pseudonym)
*The Canadian Professional Association
    for Transgender Health's Ethical
    Guidelines*, 546
cancer
    hormone therapy relation to, 527–528
    X-rays relation to, 687
candidate gene, 488
Candomblé, 27–28
capitation, 535, 540n40
carcinoma, 598
cardiometabolic impacts, of hormone
    therapy, 654–655
caregiver lists, 379
Carnival, cross-dressing during, 27
Carpenter, Edward, 52
    Ackerley relation to, 56
Casa Valentina, 246
Casablanca, Morocco, 112–113
"Case of Sexual Perversion," 288
Case Western Reserve University, 374
Casper, Johann Ludwig, 42–43, 46, 57
    Westphal relation to, 45
The Cass Review, 389n88
castration, 32, 108, 584
    auto, 210, 215–216, 235n48, 534–535
    chemical, 174

demasculinization and, 117
Freud relation to, 256
homosexuality relation to, 193n43
of Jorgensen, C., 118
Castro, Dani, 731
    on ethics, 544
Catholic Church, 296
    cisgender people relation to, 26
    patriarchy relation to, 25
Catlin, George, 697, 706n85
Cauldwell, David O., 167–168, 205,
    292–294
censorship, of transgender medical
    research, 520
Center for Craniofacial Anomalies,
    601
Center for Medicare and Medicaid
    Services (CMS), 458, 461
    gender identity relation to, 477
Center for Special Problems, 251–252,
    400
Center for Substance Abuse Treatment,
    576
Center of Excellence for Transgender
    Health, 165
    Green, J., relation to, 432
    Keatley and, 576
Center or Sex Research, 228
Centers for Disease Control and
    Prevention, 164, 722
Chacaby, Ma-Nee, 147–148
Chang, Sand, 673
Charing Cross Hospital, 436
Charles II, 697
Chase, Cheryl, 483
chemical castration, 174
Cherchez la Femme (revue), 126
Cherokee Nation Health services, 151
chest binding, 654
Chiland, Colette, 632

Child and Adolescent Gender Center, at University of California, San Francisco, 643
Child Welfare League, 141
children. *See also* TGD youth
　gender-affirming treatment for, 723–724
　gender dysphoria and, 637–638
　gender identity of, 257, 631–632
　intervention model relation to, 631–632
Chiricahua Apache, 135
chorionic gonadotropin, 116
Christian right, 86n48
Christianity, 138
　patriarchy and, 408
　TERF relation to, 405–406
"Christine Jorgensen Reveals," 178
Christopher Street, 417
Chrysalis Quarterly, 372, 426
　Case Western Reserve University and, 374
Church of Jesus Christ of the Latter-day Saints, 128, 296
cisgender people
　as allies, 6
　Catholic Church relation to, 26
cisnormative culture, 3
civil rights, 202
　gender-affirming treatment and, 397
　legal system relation to, 449–450
　Murray, P., relation to, 302–303, 304, 305
　for people of color, 329
Clark, Joanna, 229–230, 349
Clarke Institute of Psychiatry, 275n59
Cleveland, Grover, 135
clinicians, 12n2
　language of, 11
Clinique du Parc, 112

cloacal exstrophy, 483
A Clockwork Orange (film), 264
Close, Roberta, 27
Closing the Gap (Jackson and Vernon), 131, 145, 150
CMS. *See* Center for Medicare and Medicaid Services
Coates, Susan, 632–633
Coccinelle, 15, 113, 126
Cochise, 135
Cohen-Kettenis, Peggy, 462, 650, 653
Cola, Lola, 309, 320n60
Colapinto, John, 482
Cold War, 169, 242
Coleman, Eli, 252
　HBIGDA relation to, 456
　at Program in Human Sexuality, 384n5
　SOC relation to, 461, 464
Colesworthy, Rebecca, 4
College of Medicine in Syracuse, New York, Department of Obstetrics and Gynecology at, 342
College of Saint Rose, 664, 674–676
Collins, Susan, 578
colonialism, 19–20, 31
　in academia, 141–142
　Dutch, 21
　marginalization by, 6
　sexual otherness and, 32
　sexuality relation to, 33
　subcultures relation to, 14
　trauma relation to, 147
colonization, 130
　institutional, 140–141
　researchers relation to, 141–142
　transphobia and, 151
　Two Spirit people relation to, 15, 138–139
colporrhaphy, 109

Columbia University, 66, 303
Combs, Dave, 418
Committee on Lesbian, Gay, Bisexual, and Transgender Health Issues and Research Gaps and Opportunities, 462
communism, 169, 387–398
community health centers, hormone therapy at, 559–561
comorbid, 314
A Comprehensive Clinical Guide (Adler, Hirsch, and Mordaunt), 667–668, 675–676
Compton's Cafeteria riots, 338, 398–400
Condon, Bill, 221
Confessions of a Gender Defender (Ettner), 272
confidentiality, 538n10
"Congenital Absence of the Penis," 109
congenital adrenal hyperplasia (CAH), 261, 485
conjugated estrogen, 558
Conley, Eli, 674
consumer, 439
  Patton as, 229
consumer lobbies, for gender-affirming treatment, 444
contractile tissue, for phalloplasty, 598
contrary sexual feeling, 46
Contrary Sexual Feeling (Westphal), 43–45
Conundrum (Morris), 113, 126
conversion therapy, 196n92, 257, 264
  bans on, 275n59
Cook-Lynn, Elizabeth, 142
Cooke, Suzan, 338
Coolidge, Frederick, 487
Cooper, A. J., 264
Copernicus, Nicolaus, 382
Coquille Tribe, 149

Corporate Equality Index, 431, 457, 460
Count Cajus, 43
County, Jane, 571
A Course in Miracles, 333, 335
courtship rituals, 53
COVID-19 pandemic, 563
  Levine, R., relation to, 578
Cowell, Roberta, 15, 168, 179–180
  Dillon and, 111, 123–124
  Erskine relation to, 235n47
  Gillies relation to, 588
  Jorgensen, C., relation to, 181–182
Cox, Laverne, 205, 207n24, 410–411
craniofacial surgery, 600
  racial bias and, 601–602
cremasteric reflex, 598
Crenshaw, Aleshia, 213, 237n67
  Benjamin relation to, 222
Crenshaw, Kimberlé, 133, 402
Crick, Francis, 475, 486
cricothyroid approximation, 677
crimes against nature, 76
criminalization
  of cross-dressing, 400, 457, 555–556
  of gender-affirming treatment, 537
  of homosexuality, 51
  misinformation relation to, 465
Critische Pfeile (Ulrichs), 45
Cromwell, Jason, 454
cross-dressing, 54, 220
  administrative separation and, 538n10
  aversion therapy for, 263–264
  berdache and, 130
  during Carnival, 27
  criminalization of, 400, 457, 555–556
  EEF relation to, 338
  homosexuality relation to, 95
  Hyde, E., relation to, 99–100
  Prince relation to, 244–246, 247
  prostitution relation to, 234n31

in San Francisco, 214–215
secondary transsexual relation to, 369
Spengler and, 94
support groups for, 229
cross-living men, 100–101
Crow Agency, 134
Crownsville State Hospital for the Negro Insane, 303
Crozier, Ivan, 53
Cryle, Peter, 78
CSULB. *See* California State University, Long Beach
Cullors, Patrisse, 409
cultural acceptance, prevalence relation to, 478
cultural labor, 316
cultural mainstream, marginalized communities in, 17
Cummings, Katherine, 244
Current Concepts in Transgender Identity (Denny), 370, 426
Current Opinion in Endocrinology, Diabetes, and Obesity (journal), 525

D. F. (pseudonym), 226–227
D., Angela, 218, *218*, 219, 235n48
Dacakis, Georgia, 662, 663, 664
    Transsexual Voice Questionnaire of, 667
The Daddies (painting), 148, *149*
Dahl-Iversen, Erling, 258
Dahteste, 135–136
Daily Democrat, 622
Dain, Steve, 252
    Green, J., relation to, 429
    metoidioplasty and, 599
Dakota Access Pipeline, 149
Dallas Museum of Art, 100
damage-centered research, 145
dando santo (giving saint), 28

The Danish Girl (film), 628
Danish Society for Endocrinology, 116
"Dark Testament," 306
Das 3. Geschlecht (periodical), 96
Daughters of Bilitis, 401
Davis, Alvin, 179
Davis, Bob, Ms., 731
    on Lawrence, L., 241
Davis, Kate, 308, 309, 320n60
Davydov technique, 596
Dawkins, Richard, 488
dead names, 7–8, 12n9
Dear Abby, 343
Declaration of Independence, 449
decolonization, 129, 146–147, 148, 150–151
    in HBC, 317
decriminalization, of homosexuality, 70
degeneration, theory of, 47
Deishere, Robert W., 338
demasculinization, castration and, 117
denied care, medicalization relation to, 168
Denny, Dallas, 1, 167, 244, 255
    activism of, 313
    American Educational Gender Information Service relation to, 231, 350, 426
    on body hair, 685
    Brown, J., relation to, 591
    on Eads, 308
    gender-affirming treatment relation to, 314–315, 425
    on gender clinics, 361
    Gender Dysphoria of, 385n25, 426, 718
    Green, J., relation to, 430
    HBIGDA relation to, 452
    on Jorgensen, C., 171
    on Levine, R., 577

Denny, Dallas *(continued)*
  on medicalization, 299
  prejudice and, 12n5
  on psychology, 255
  on silicone, 310
  at Transgender Lives Conference, 4
Department for Pederasty (*Päderastenabteilung*), 73
Department of Defense (DOD), 330, 549
  VHA relation to, 550
Department of Obstetrics and Gynecology, College of Medicine in Syracuse, New York, 342
depilation, 686
  by shaving, 702n2
"The Desire for Change of Sex as Shown by Personal Letters from 465 Men and Women," 118
Deutungsmacht (interpretive authority), 68
Devenir Femme (organization), 126
Devor, Aaron, 270, 461
  on Erickson, 331
Devor, Holly, 453
Dewhurst, C. J., 347, 437–438
Diagnostic and Statistical Manual of Mental Disorders (DSM), 193n40, 262
  gender identity disorder in, 309, 453, 462, 476
  homosexuality and, 300, 301, 318
  transsexualism in, 301, 522–523
Diamond, David A., 649
Diamond, Milton, 474, 482–483
diathermy, 506
Dickinson, Edward, 68
Dieffenbach, Johann, 697
diethylstilbestrol, 315
Digital Transgender Archive, 237n77

dihydrotestosterone, 484
  5-alpha-reductase deficiency relation to, 485
Dillon, Michael, 87n67
  Cowell and, 111, 123–124
  Gillies relation to, 15, 110–111, 363, 597
  testosterone relation to, 556
dimorphic structural sex differences, gender identity relation to, 490–491
Diné Marriage Act (2005), 148
Diné Origin Myth, 133
Diné people, 128–129, 131
Dio, Cassius, 604n6
Directive 53, 296
Directive 1341 (2) VHA, 550
discrimination, 719
  ACA relation to, 409, 562, 565n48
  gender clinics relation to, 371
  health insurance relation to, 457, 460
  in military tribunals, 533–534
  of QPOC, 315
  in San Francisco, 430, 451–452
  sex work relation to, 309
  stigma and, 508
  of travesti, 27
  VHA and, 330
  VHA relation to, 330
  workplace, 10
disinformation, 389n88
disorderly behavior, 255
Diva of Polynesia (pageant), 164
Division of Professional Misconduct, of New York State County Medical Society, 520
DNA, 486
  epigenetics and, 490
Dobbs decision, 450
Dobler, Jens, 72, 73
DOD. *See* Department of Defense

Dolan, Anette, 624
donor dominance, 698
Don't Ask Don't Tell, 627
Doorbar, Ruth Rae, 345
   Green, R., relation to, 364
Douglas, Angela, 380–381, 389n82
Dresden Municipal Women's Clinic, 587
Driskill, Qwo-Li, 130–131, 146–147, 155n69
Drucker, Donna, 78, 87n56
DSM. See *Diagnostic and Statistical Manual of Mental Disorders*
Dufresnoy, Jacques-Charles, 126
Dunwoody, Ann Elizabeth, 580n15
Dusseau, George, 124
Dutch colonialism, 21
Dutch protocol
   GAM compared to, 639
   GeMS relation to, 650, 653–654
Dyke (quarterly), 389n82

Eads, Robert, 308–309, 320n60
East Coast Homophile Organization, 401
East Tennessee State University Institutional Review Board, 524
Eder, Franz, 69–70
Edgerton, Milton, 364
   at HBIGDA, 589
Edwards-Leeper, Laura, 649, 650
EEF. See Erickson Educational Foundation
EEF Newsletter, 339, *340*, 341, 343, 344
Ehrensaft, Diane, 630, 732
   See Gender Affirmative Model (GAM)
   psychoanalytic critique, 631–633
Ehrhardt, Anke, 334
Eichel, Edward W., 86n48
Ekins, Richard, 189, 453
   on Benjamin, 221

Elagabalus, 584–585
   pronouns relation to, 604n6
Elbe, Lili, 15, 84n14, 91, 182
   Cowell compared to, 180
   gender-affirming surgery of, 92, 93, 586–587
Eldorado, 74
electrolysis, 687–688, 689, 690–691
   for facial hair, 704n48
   gender-affirming surgery and, 692–693
   laser hair removal relation to, 695, 705n70
Elgin, Clair, 224
eligibility requirements
   for gender clinics, 362, 367–368, 374–375, 404, 407
   SOC relation to, 444–445
Elkins, Gay, 242
Elliot, Beth, 404–405
Elliott, R. A., 699
Ellis, Albert, 77
Ellis, Havelock, 51–54, 56
   on Eonism, 55
   Murray, P., relation to, 304
embryonic development, Urnings relation to, 45–46
Emory University
   gender-affirming voice training at, 661–662
   gender clinics at, 386n33
The Empire Strikes Back (Stone), 406–407
empiricism, in Western medical practices, 307
Employers Alliance v. EEOC, 565n48
endocrine biology, 49–50
Endocrine Society Guidelines, 462, 557
   GeMS relation to, 653–654
endocrinology, 81, 448
   Hamburger and, 116
   Steinach relation to, 506

Enlightenment, 43
entertainment industry
  kathoey in, 24
  waria in, 22–23
environmental forces, 486
  gender identity relation to, 480–481
d'Eon, Le Chevalière, 15, 54–55, 62–64, *63*, 64nn1–3
Eonism, 54–55, 117, 121n69, 183
Eonism (Ellis), 54
Epic, 461
epidemics, 140
epigenetics, 490
epilation, 686, 690
epilator, 219
Episcopal Church, 305
Epstein, Jeffrey, 701
erasure
  dead names and, 8
  Indian Student Placement Program and, 153n2
  of intersex individuals, 69
  people of color and, 416n52
  of Two Spirit people, 146–147
Erickson, Reed, 9, 329, 331, *332*, 334
  Benjamin relation to, 332, 344–345
  EEF Newsletter and, 339
  EEF pamphlet series and, 341
  Gilbert, J. A., relation to, 620
  HBIGDA relation to, 439
  ketamine relation to, 333
  ONE Inc. relation to, 335
  public opinion relation to, 336
Erickson Educational Foundation (EEF), 189, 229, 295, 329, 337, 350–351
  cross-dressing relation to, 338
  funding relation to, 377, 437, 438
  Guidelines for Transsexuals of, 446–447
  HBIGDA relation to, 344–345

Janus Information Facility relation to, 349
Johns Hopkins Gender Clinic relation to, 345, 364
ONE Inc. relation to, 334–335
public education relation to, 339, 341, *342*, 342–344, 401
public opinion relation to, 331, 336
research grants of, 345–347
Walker relation to, 238n90, 346
erotic desire, 220–221
  sexual revolution relation to, 435
Erskine, Carla (pseudonym), 78, 167, *218*, 233n17
  Benjamin relation to, 69, 209, 210–214, 216–218, 220–223, 233n4, 235n46, 235n53
  Cowell relation to, 235n47
  intimate histories of, 232
  Laub relation to, 224–225, 234nn25–26
  MacLane relation to, 219–220, 235n52
  in Mexico City, 214–215
estradiol, 174
  ethinyl, 558
  Steinach relation to, 506
estrogen
  "Agnes" and, 266
  Benjamin relation to, 66
  cancer relation to, 527
  conjugated, 558
  Denny relation to, 425
  diethylstilbestrol, 315
  at gender clinics, 556
  Progynon, 95
  Reimer relation to, 481
  VHA relation to, 529, *531*, 532
ethical dilemmas, 5
ethical review boards, 547n6
ethics, 86n45
  of American Speech-Language-Hearing Association, 669

in transgender medical research, 544–547
ethics committee, of HBIGDA, 453
ethinyl estradiol, 558
ethnic cleansing, 138, 140
ethnocultural hierarchies, 141
ethnography, rescue, 188
ethnolinguistic identity, 672–673
etiology
  of gender diversity, 9, 329, 509, 519, 537
  gender identity relation to, 483, 508, 510–511, 512
  stigma relation to, 510
  of transsexualism, 479–480
Ettner, Randi, 272
Étude medico-légale sur les attentats aux moeurs (Tardieu), 42
eugenics, 117, 621
  bias and, 382–383
eunuchs, 19–20
Euro-American culture, Judeo-Christian doctrine relation to, 16
Eurocentric beauty standards, 310
Europe
  gender diversity in, 17
  sexology in, 8
The European Professional Association for Transgender Health's Research Policy, 546
Evangelical churches, 296
evidence-based medicine, 307
evolving language, 5

Facial Feminization Surgery (Ousterhout), 601–602
facial hair
  electrolysis for, 704n48
  hair transplant surgery for, 701
  testosterone relation to, 700, 704n49

Fairleigh Dickinson University, 342
fakaleiti, 29
Family Research Council, 269
Fang, R. H., 595–596
Fantasia Fair, 5, 7–8, 12n4
Farewell the Trumpets (Morris), 126
FDA. *See* Food and Drug Administration
Feinberg, Leslie, 408
Feinbloom, Deborah H., 343, 403–404
female liminal roles, 29
femininity, 32
  colonization relation to, 130
  gender clinics relation to, 371
  sexual intermediaries relation to, 48–49
  sexual inversion relation to, 52
  Urnings relation to, 45
  Western standards relation to, 672–673
feminist anthropology, 17
feminist movement, 399. *See also* trans exclusionary radical feminist
feminist standpoint theory, 260
Femme/Butch roles, 384n4
Fenway Health, 560–561
  GeMS relation to, 651
Fernández, Rosa, 489
Ferrando, Cecile A., 15, 105, 123, 125
fetishism, 53
  Eonism relation to, 55
Fierstein, Harvey, 246
finasteride, 699, 707n110
Finifter, Morton, 690
Firestein, Beth, 452
The First Man-Made Man (Kennedy), 111
First Miami Gender Identity Symposium, 342
Fisher, Jack, 590

Fisk, Norman, 252
    Fraser relation to, 442
    Laub relation to, 594
    sex reassignment relation to, 372
fistulae, 597
Fithian, Marilyn, 228
Fitzgerald, Pauline, 303
5-alpha-reductase deficiency, 182, 485
Fleming, Richard, 699
F2M Fraternity, 442–443
Fogh-Anderson, Paul, 348
Folded Arms people, 128
follicular unit transplants, 698
Folx Health, 563
Food and Drug Administration (FDA), 312, 688, 699
    electrolysis relation to, 690–691
Foreman, Madeleine, 489
forensic manuals, 42–43
Fort, Joel, 400
Fort Dix Separation Center, 173
Foucault, Michel, 55, 70
    feminist standpoint theory relation to, 260
    on intersex individuals, 68–69
Fradkin, Howard, 228
Francis (Pope), 296
Frank, Gillian, 69, 723
Frankel, Joseph, 66
Fraser, Lin, 272, 462
    Brown, J., relation to, 591
    Global Education Initiative and, 464
    Green, R., relation to, 436
    HBIGDA relation to, 442
"free love," 228
French Order of Medicine, 112
French Revolution, 64
Freud, Sigmund, 52, 70, 631
    bisexuality relation to, 258
    psychoanalytic drive theory of, 256–257
    Steinach relation to, 506
Freudian psychoanalysis, 46
Freund, Joseph, 561
Frey, Jordan, 600
Friedan, Betty, 305
Friedenberg, Carol, 661–662, 663, 665–666
Frye, Phyllis, 468n44
FTM International, 429–430
FTM Newsletter, 253, 271, 429
Fu Yang, 489
Full Personality Expression, 246, 247
funding
    EEF relation to, 377, 437, 438
    for Johns Hopkins Gender Clinic, 365
    for transgender medical research, 535, 537–538
Furtrell, J. William, 595

Galton, Francis, 486
galvanic method, 687–688
GAM. *See* gender affirmative model
Game Face (documentary), 628
Garfinkel, Harold, 266
Garofalo, Robert, 462
Garza, Alicia, 409
gatekeeping model, of gender-affirming treatment, 426
The Gateway (newsletter), 376
Gay Activists Alliance, 421–422
"gay gene," 488
Gay Liberation Front, 418
    Rivera relation to, 421–422
gay men, 386. *See also* homosexuals
    masculinity and, 24–25
Gay Men's Health Crisis, 301
Gay Pride March, 418

Gay Pride Rally, 422
gay-related immunodeficiency (GRID), 299
Gebhard, Paul, 76
Gelfer, Marylou, 665–666
gender, 404
  biological sex compared to, 182, 190n2, 194n68
  Cold War relation to, 242
  HBC relation to, 316
  racialized, 205
  sex assignment relation to, 258–259
  sexuality relation to, 16–17, 69
  transsexualism and, 373
  Western standards relation to, 672–673
gender affirmative model (GAM), 638–640, 643
  at GeMS, 650
  social transition relation to, 641–642
gender-affirming surgery, 81, 105, 354n87, 362, 583–584. *See also* craniofacial surgery; phalloplasty; vaginoplasty
  Belt relation to, 553, 624–625
  Benjamin relation to, 519
  Bowers relation to, 593
  of Callo, 585
  Cauldwell relation to, 293
  of Dillon, 87n67
  of Elbe, 92, 93, 586–587
  electrolysis and, 692–693
  of Erskine, 69, 209–210, 212
  at GeMS, 650–651
  gender identity relation to, 404
  hair removal relation to, 694–695, 705n63
  Hart and, 596
  health insurance and, 165, 589, 628

  hormone therapy relation to, 116
  hysterectomy as, 620
  income tax relation to, 463
  at Institute for Sexual Science, 585
  at Johns Hopkins Gender Clinic, 361, 374, 388n56, 556
  of Jorgensen, C., 258, 585
  Laub relation to, 593
  Lawrence, A., and, 607n95
  mayhem statutes relation to, 195n85, 624
  Medicare/Medicaid for, 458
  mental health issues relation to, 536–537
  for nonbinary gender identity, 603
  patient satisfaction with, 600
  of Patton, 227
  Paul relation to, 579
  for pitch elevation, 676–677
  psychiatric observation and, 118
  religion relation to, 295–297
  of Roberts, 205
  Steinach relation to, 504
  TERF relation to, 405
  at Transgender Surgical and Medical Center in, 595
  transsexualism and, 189
  VHA relation to, 550
gender-affirming treatment, 264, 550–551
  ACA relation to, 565n48
  bans on, 655–656
  for children, 723–724
  civil rights and, 397
  consumer lobbies for, 444
  Denny relation to, 314–315, 425
  eligibility requirements for, 444–445
  gatekeeping model of, 426
  for gender dysphoria, 519–520

gender-affirming treatment *(continued)*
  at Golisano Children's Hospital, 655–656
  Green, R., relation to, 267
  hair removal as, 689–690
  health insurance for, 310, 410–411, 446, 603
  of Jorgensen, C., 174–175, 176, 262, 556
  in military, 522–523
  mistreatment in, 376–377
  Murray, P., relation to, 306
  patient autonomy in, 720
  for people of color, 203
  research mandate and, 544–545
  silicone relation to, 313
  stigma and, 509
  telehealth for, 562–563
  for TGD youth, 278n122, 406, 553, 631, 650
  transgender inmates relation to, 534–535, 537
  transgender medical research relation to, 533
  for Two Spirit people, 145, 150–151
  Vanderbilt University relation to, 389n87
  VHA relation to, 524–525
gender-affirming voice training, 554, 663–664, 678, 684
  androgen therapy and, 660–661, 670
  biofeedback and, 665
  at College of Saint Rose, 675–676
  at Emory University, 661–662
  for nonbinary gender identity, 671–672
  for people of color, 672–673
  SOC relation to, 660, 666, 668
  for TGD youth, 673–674
  WPATH relation to, 667–668

gender-based behavior, 484
gender binary, 16–17, 384n4, 721
  gender clinics relation to, 361–362, 368, 371, 380, 382, 387n44
  Murray, P., relation to, 319n18
  religion relation to, 296
  in Western philosophy, 31
  in Wild West culture, 101
gender clinics, 10–11, 364, 370, 381, 400. *See also* Johns Hopkins Gender Clinic
  eligibility requirements for, 362, 367–368, 374–375, 404, 407
  at Emory University, 386n33
  funding for, 365
  GeMS, 640, 649–651
  gender binary relation to, 361–362, 368, 371, 380, 382, 387n44
  at Golisano Children's Hospital, 655–656
  hormone therapy at, 556
  intersectionality at, 377
  McHugh relation to, 271, 362
  Papillon Gender Wellness Center, 627–628
  pathologization at, 403
  power dynamics at, 375–376, 381
  PPFA, 228, 561–562
  researchers at, 370–371
  sex reassignment at, 362, 372
  snow-blindedness at, 383
  SOC relation to, 559
  speech-language pathologists in, 669
  stigma at, 372–373
  TGD youth at, 630
  The Transsexual Phenomenon relation to, 366, 373–374
  at UCLA, 267, 268
  at University of Texas Medical Branch, 346, 349, 436

Index   751

at Vanderbilt University, 386n35
VHA, 524–525, 526
"Gender Confirmation Surgery," 603
gender diversity, 12n1, 15, 17
   in animal kingdom, 474–475, 723
   etiology of, 9, 329, 509, 519, 537
   homosexuality relation to, 478, 480
   Indigenous North Americans and, 15, 139
   in Navajo Nation, 132t
   in Polynesia, 28–29
   prevalence of, 476–478, 492n11
   sexual practice relation to, 25–26
gender dysphoria, 10, 105, 193n40, 264–265
   Americans with Disabilities Act relation to, 261
   androgenic alopecia relation to, 700
   children and, 637–638
   in DSM, 462
   EEF relation to, 334
   GAM and, 642–643
   gender-affirming treatment for, 519–520
   gender identity disorder compared to, 652n1
   hair removal relation to, 689, 694
   health insurance relation to, 262
   hormone therapy for, 506
   hormones relation to, 489
   justice system relation to, 534
   media relation to, 170
   mental health issues relation to, 536–537
   in military, 523
   mood disorders relation to, 532
   of Murray, P., 304
   personality disorders relation to, 524
   silicone relation to, 313
   Stuart relation to, 251
   transvestic fetishism relation to, 539n26
   trauma relation to, 632–633
   veterans with, 526
Gender Dysphoria Association, 189
Gender Dysphoria Clinic, at Queen Victoria Hospital, 662
Gender Dysphoria (Denny), 385n25, 426, 718
Gender Education Initiative, 446
gender euphoria, 642–643
gender expansion, 721–722
gender expression, 720
   gender identity compared to, 632
gender fluidity, 48
gender identity, 329, 474, 550. *See also* nonbinary gender identity
   ACA relation to, 668
   CAH relation to, 485
   of children, 257, 631–632
   CMS relation to, 477
   environmental forces relation to, 480–481
   etiology relation to, 483, 508, 510–511, 512
   GAM relation to, 641
   gender-affirming surgery relation to, 404
   gender expression compared to, 631
   gender transposition relation to, 259
   genetics relation to, 486
   hormones relation to, 475, 485
   Indigenous Hawaiian people and, 161
   International Conference on, 229
   International Symposium on, 347–348
   intersex individuals and, 172, 482
   neuroanatomical relation to, 490–491
   pathologization and, 492n11
   performativity of, 260
   polymorphisms and, 488

gender identity *(continued)*
  psychotherapy relation to, 189
  in radical behavioral model, 260
  religion relation to, 296–297
  reparative therapy and, 634–635
  sexual orientation relation to, 478–479
  sexuality relation to, 188, 402
  of TGD youth, 451, 630, 636, 650, 654
  twin studies and, 486–488
  VHA relation to, 550
Gender Identity Clinic, 257, 625
  at National University Hospital, 595
Gender Identity Clinic for Children at the Centre for Addiction and Mental Health (CAMH), 635, 637
gender identity disorder, 309, 453, 462, 476
  gender dysphoria compared to, 652n1
Gender Identity Project, of LGBT Community Center, 443
Gender Identity Research Clinic, at UCLA, 556
gender incongruence, 10, 259, 262, 478
  body hair and, 685
  in *International Classification of Diseases*, 463
  twin studies and, 486–488
gender inversion, 48
Gender (Kessler and McKee), 343, 404
Gender Loving Care (Ettner), 272
Gender Management Services Clinic (GeMS), 640, 649, 652, 653–654
  gender-affirming surgery at, 650–651
gender nonconformity, 14
  sexual inversion relation to, 55
gender programs, 228–229
gender roles, 2, 399, 474
  CAH relation to, 485
  hijra, 18–20

penetration relation to, 26
performativity of, 190n5
Reimer relation to, 481
sexuality relation to, 46
Two Spirit people relation to, 130
Gender Surgical Center of Excellence, of GeMS, 651
gender transposition, 259
gender tropes, 83
Gender Wellness Center, 4, 410
gendercide, 138, 408
General Theological Seminary, 305
Genesis 6, 16
genetic determinism, 488
genetics, 487–489
  gender identity relation to, 486
  of sexuality, 49
genital mutilation, 108, 111
genocide, 138
George Washington University, 664
Georgia Clinical Electrologists, 705n62
Georgia Electrologist's Association, 705n62
Georgia State Medical Examiner's Office, 313
Germany. *See also* Berlin, Germany
  homosexual rights movement in, 46
  sexual inversion in, 51
Geronimo, 135
Geshlecht und Character (Weininger), 48–49
Geyser, Albert C., 687, 702n18
Gilbert, J. Allen, 620, 621
Gilbert, Joshua, 596, 598–599
Gill-Peterson, Jules, 732
  on Lawrence, L., 241
Gillies, Harold, 105, 123
  Cowell relation to, 588
  craniofacial surgery and, 600
  Dillon relation to, 15, 110–111, 363, 597

hypospadias and, 108–109
McIndoe relation to, 587
phalloplasty and, 109–110, 119
tubed pedicle and, 106–107
vaginoplasty and, 108, 115
Ginsberg, Ruth Bader, 304
Give Voice, 664
giving saint (*dando santo*), 28
glandular manipulation, 504–505
Glenn, Fred Kennedy, 313
Glide Memorial United Methodist Church, 399
GLMA: Health Professionals Advancing LGBTQ+ Equality, 462
Global Education Initiative, 464, 465
Global Education Institute, 350
Global Training Institute, 465
globalism, leiti relation to, 30
GnRH analogs, 409–410
for TGD youth, 637
Goddard, Henry H., 382–383
Goffman, Irving, 373
Gohrbandt, Erwing, 586, 587
Golden Gate Girls/Guys support group, 376
Goldschmidt, Richard, 178, 183
Goldstein, Benjamin, 510
Goldstein, Zil, 732
on hormone therapy, 555
Golisano Children's Hospital, at University of Rochester Medical Center, 655–656
gonadotropin-releasing hormone analogs, 653
Goodwin, Chelsea, 422
Goodwin, Willard, 625
Gooren, Louis, 462, 527
Gorman, Michael, 480
Gottlieb, Gerda, 91, 92
Gould, Stephen Jay, 382–383

Gradual Civilization Act (1857), 139
Gradual Enfranchisement Act (1869), 139
Graduate Student Initiative, of WPATH, 464
Graduate Student Union (GSU), 460
Grandma (film), 207n24
Grant, Rosemary, 649
Great Britain, mayhem statutes in, 123
Great Father, 148
Great Society, 399
Greece, gender diversity in, 17
"Greek Love," 52
Green, George, 101, 167
on Sullivan, 251
Green, Jamison, 1, 4, 65, 251, 255, 428
activism of, 431–432, 629, 718–719
on Erskine, 209
on gender-affirming surgery, 583–584
on gender binary, 384n4
on Hirschfeld, 14–15
on psychology, 255
on sexual revolution, 435
Sullivan relation to, 271, 429
WPATH relation to, 430–431, 547n8
Green, Richard, 364, 690
Benjamin relation to, 519
EEF relation to, 345
HBIGDA relation to, 267, 436, 439, 452, 456
Money relation to, 267, 268, 269, 277n98, 363, 436
multidisciplinary model and, 385n14
Sissy Boy Syndrome and the Development of Homosexuality of, 385n14, 633–634
twin studies of, 487
Greenberg, Katherine Blumoff, 653
Greene, Marjorie Taylor, 723
Gregory, Vernon, 224

GRID. *See* gay-related immunodeficiency
Griese, Karl, *72*
Griesinger, Wilhelm, 43
Griffin-Gracy, Miss Major, 724
Grosskurth, Phyllis, 52
GSU. *See* Graduate Student Union
"Guidance and Ethical Considerations for Undertaking Transgender Health Research and Institutional Review Boards Adjudicating this Research," 544
Guidelines for Transsexuals, 446–447
Gundling, Tj, 167, 169
Gutterman, Lauren, 69, 723
Guze, Henry, 345
    Green, R., relation to, 363–364
gynandromorphism, 194n74

Haefele-Thomas, Ardel, 83n3
Hage, J. Joris, 595, 600
    phalloplasty relation to, 596
hair removal, 701, 702n2. *See also* epilation
    electrolysis for, 687–693, 695, 705n70
    gender-affirming surgery relation to, 694–695, 705n63
    health insurance relation to, 690, 703n43
    of Indigenous North Americans, 685–686
    laser, 688–689, 695, 702n2, 705n70
    phalloplasty relation to, 693–695
    testosterone relation to, 696
    vaginoplasty relation to, 692–693
    X-rays for, 686–687
hair replacement, 700
hair transplant surgery, 697–699, 706n107
    for facial hair, 701
hairpieces, 696–697, 700

Hale, C. Jacob, 176–177
Hall, Murray, 670
Hall, Thomas, 98–99
Halperin, David, 45
Hamburger, Christian, 15, 105
    Jorgensen, C., relation to, 106, 116–117, 174, 178, 192n31, 193n50, 193n54
    on patient regret, 117–118
    Roberts relation to, 204
Hampson, Joan, 260, 384n3
Hampson, John, 260, 384n3
Hancock, Adrienne, 667
Hannover, 45
Hanson, Verlyn, 607n90
Harappa, 18
harm reduction, 560
Harrington, Mark, 313
Harris, Alexander B., 555
Harris, Alvin, 235n48
Harris, Jason, 602
Harry Benjamin Foundation, 189
    Hoff relation to, 571
Harry Benjamin International Gender Dysphoria Association (HBIGDA), 230, 252, 347, 455
    Edgerton at, 589
    EEF relation to, 344–345
    ethics committee of, 453
    Fraser relation to, 442
    Green, J., relation to, 430
    Green, R., relation to, 267, 436, 439, 452, 456
    Kirk relation to, 441, 454, 595
    Laub and, 237n77
    Rachlin relation to, 443, 451
    SOC of, 350, 377, 451–453, 467n21, 522
    Walker relation to, 438–439, 557
    WPATH relation to, 440, 456

Hart, Alan, 117, 554, 620–622
  gender-affirming surgery and, 596
Hartin, Deborah, 342
Hartsuiker, Frederik, 219
  Benjamin relation to, 588
Harvard Law School, 303
hastiin, 131. *See also* Two-Spirit people
Hastings, Jen, 561
Hawaii, 161
Hawaiian language, 162
Hawelu, Ashliana, 15, 161–165, *165*
Hayes, Elinor, 224
Hayworth, Christina, 422
HBC. *See* House and Ballroom Community
HBIGDA. *See* Harry Benjamin International Gender Dysphoria Association
Health Care Financing Administration (HCFA), 458
health disparities, 528–529
  in justice system, 534
  people of color and, 205–206, 415n22, 528
Health Information Portability and Accountability Act, 86n45
health insurance
  capitation and, 540n40
  craniofacial surgery relation to, 602
  discrimination relation to, 457, 460
  gender-affirming surgery and, 165, 589, 628
  for gender-affirming treatment, 310, 410–411, 446, 603
  gender dysphoria relation to, 262
  hair removal relation to, 690, 703n43
  hair replacement relation to, 700
  for hormones, 458
  in San Francisco, 459–460
  SOC relation to, 557

speech-language pathologists relation to, 668
Health Resources and Services Administration, 462
healthcare. *See specific topics*
healthcare activism, 8
Hearns, Liz Jackson, 674
Hearst Corporation, 177
Heaven's Command (Morris), 126
Helms, Jesse, 458
Hembree, Wylie, 4
  Endocrine Society Guidelines and, 462
Henningsson, Susanne, 489
Henry, George, 96
Herbert, Brandy, 341
heredity, 487–488
Heritage Foundation, 724
The Hermaphrodite (White-Sun and Dorsey), 133–134
hermaphroditic model, 190n16
hermaphroditism, 182
  homoeroticism relation to, 24
  intersex individuals compared to, 178
  pseudo, 216–217, 304, 585
  psychic, 48, 268, 363
  psychological, 45–46, 49, 54, 183
Hernandez, Tresne, 653
Herrn, Rainer, 210
Herzig, Rebecca, 686–687
heteronormativity, 169
heterosexual social order, 69
Heylens, Gunter, 487
HHS. *See* US Department of Health and Human Services
hijra, 18–20, 584
  waria compared to, 23
Hillary, Edmund, 126
Hinduism, 18, 21
  sexual renunciation in, 19
Hines, Melissa, 484

Hinman, Frank, Jr., 212, 220, 235n46
Hippocrates, 106
Hippocratic Oath, 172, 538n10
Hirsch, Sandy, 664
   Voice and Communication Therapy for the Transgender/Transsexual Client of, 667, 674
Hirschfeld, Magnus, 8–9, 14–15, 53, 56, 258, 720
   Benjamin relation to, 65–66, 74–75, *75*, 83n3, 83n6, 184, 188–189, 235n44
   Berlins of, 84n25
   Elbe relation to, 92
   Griese and, *72*
   Hitler relation to, 587
   homosexuality of, 79
   hormone therapy and, 586
   identification and, 449
   Institut für Sexualwissenschaft of, 363
   Kinsey relation to, 75, 79, 83n11, 87n56
   Psycho-Biological Questionnaire of, 70–71
   on sexual intermediaries, 78
   sexual subcultures and, 71–72, 74
   Die Transvestiten of, 54, 71, 79, 96, 479
   Die Zeitschrift für Sexualwissenschaft of, 50
Hirschfeld Scrapbook, 83n11
historical trauma, 138, 143
Hitler, Adolf, 587
HIV, 163–164, 253, 300
   intravention and, 316
   Sullivan relation to, 429
HIV/AIDS epidemic, 401, 576
   activism in, 300–301
   ACTUP relation to, 313
   Mazzoni Center relation to, 560
   public health and, 402–403
   Tom Waddell Health Center relation to, 559
   transgender veterans relation to, 528–529
HIV (Kirk), 441
Hoff, Jeanne, 554, 571, 572, *572*
Hoffman, Friedrich, 41
Holt, Lester, 627
"Homicidal Transsexuals," 387n55
homoeroticism, 24
homologous structures, 584
homophile movement, 398
homophobia, 130, 139
homosexual relationships, 23
   penetration relation to, 26
   in Polynesia, 33
   psychological disorders relation to, 32
   in Thailand, 24–25
homosexual rights movement, in Germany, 46
homosexuality, 52–53, 252–253
   berdache and, 130
   castration relation to, 193n43
   criminalization of, 51
   cross-dressing relation to, 95
   decriminalization of, 70
   DSM and, 300, 301, 318
   epigenetics relation to, 490
   gender diversity relation to, 478, 480
   of Hirschfeld, 79
   Hitler relation to, 587
   hormones relation to, 49–50
   in Iran, 297
   Krafft-Ebing on, 84n21
   mahu relation to, 162
   McCarthyism relation to, 398
   pathologization of, 299–300
   psychotherapy relation to, 186
   Rekers relation to, 269

Steinach relation to, 504
stigma and, 226
in Tonga, 30
Urnings relation to, 290n29
homosexuals, 259
human rights of, 94
Hooker, Evelyn, 334
Hoopes, John, 364
Biber relation to, 592
Hore, B. D., 487
Hormone Department of Statens Seruminstitut, 116
hormone therapy, 50, 105, 184, 189, 557–558. *See also* gender-affirming treatment
Benjamin relation to, 251n1, 519, 556
cancer relation to, 527–528
cardiometabolic impacts of, 654–655
at Case Western Reserve University, 374
at community health centers, 559–561
of Dillon, 87n67
of Erickson, 332
gender-affirming surgery relation to, 116
gender-affirming voice training and, 670
at gender clinics, 556
for gender dysphoria, 506
of Hart, 622
IHS relation to, 150
inmate medical care providers relation to, 535–536
of Jorgensen, C., 116–117, 588
military relation to, 522, 550
at PPFA, 561
of Richter, 586
in SOC, 444, 555, 595
telehealth for, 562–563
testicular atrophy relation to, 111

for TGD youth, 409–410, 638, 640, 653
at VHA gender clinic, 524
VHA relation to, 529, 531, *531*, 532
hormones, 162–163, 448, 457. *See also* estrogen; testosterone
androgenic alopecia relation to, 700
Benjamin relation to, 66, 82
black market, 145
Denny relation to, 425
gender dysphoria relation to, 489
gender identity relation to, 475, 485
health insurance for, 458
homosexuality relation to, 49–50
Jorgensen, C., and, 174
Kinsey on, 81–82
Kirk relation to, 594–595
mass production of, 258
nonbinary gender identity and, 409, 558
organotherapy and, 190n4
for people of color, 322n95
psychiatric disorders relation to, 485–486
sex-typical childhood behaviors relation to, 261
sexual differentiation relation to, 484–485
sexual intermediaries relation to, 49
travesti and, 26
waria and, 23
Hose and Heels Club, 245
Hot Peaches, 417
Hotel Sir Francis Drake, 211
House and Ballroom Community (HBC), 315
intravention in, 316–317
house ballroom culture, 168
House Committee on Un-American Activities, 169

House of Labeija, 315
Hoyer, Niels, 91, 92–93, 586–587
Hsieh, Sam, 654
Hubbell, Kenneth, 425
Hughes, H. Stuart, 54
Hughes Research Laboratories, 688
human genome, 486
human rights, 10
 activism for, 20
 born-this-way argument for, 510–511
 of homosexuals, 94
Human Rights Campaign Foundation, 431, 460, 655
Human Rights Commission, of San Francisco, 430, 459
Hunter College, 303
Hurst, Michel, 246
Hyde, C., 487
Hyde, Edward, 99–100
hypospadias, 108–109
 Erskine and, 214, 234n26
hysterectomy, 227, 554
 as gender-affirming surgery, 620

I am a Woman Now (documentary), 113
I Am Not This Body (film), 336, 341, 342–343
ICTLET. See International Conference on Transgender Law and Employment Policy
identification, 448–449
 transvestite pass, *74*, 85n33, 220, 720
Ihlenfeld, Charles, 263
IHS. See Indian Health Services
I'm Something Else (documentary), 343
Imperato-McGinley, Julianne, 707n110
Implementing Comprehensive HIV and STI Programmes with Transgender People, 547n7

In Search of Eve (Bolin), 381, 387n52, 404
INAH3. See interstitial nucleus of the anterior hypothalamus 3
income tax, 463
India
 hijra in, 18–20, 23, 584
 third gender status in, 33
Indian Act (1876), 139
Indian Adoption Project, 141
Indian Affairs, 140
Indian boarding schools, 128–129, 140–141
Indian Health Services (IHS), 143, 150–151
Indian Student Placement Program, 128, 153n2
Indiana University, 67
Indigenous Hawaiian people, 161
Indigenous North Americans, 8, 697, 706n85. See also Two Spirit people
 gender diversity and, 15, 139
 hair removal of, 685–686
 joyas of, 99
 knowledge formulation of, 129
 nonbinary gender identity and, 130
 pronouns relation to, 134
 sacred spaces of, 140
 same-sex marriage relation to, 148, 149
 transphobia and, 150–151
 trauma of, 128–129, 138, 143
Indigenous Ways of Knowing program, 150
individualized-care model, 261
Indonesia
 sex/gender pluralism in, 21
 waria in, 23
Information for the Female-to-Male Crossdresser and Transsexual, 238n90, 252

informed consent model, 560–561, 721
Ingersoll Gender Center, 441
inmate medical care providers, hormone therapy relation to, 535–536
Innovative Response Globally for Transgender Women and HIV, 576
Inoubli, Adrien, 490
Inouye, Daniel, 164
Institut für Sexualwissenschaft, 363
Institute for Sexual Science, 70, 71–72, 74–75, 586
  gender-affirming surgery at, 585
  Hitler relation to, 587
  Katter at, 85n33
Institute for the Study of Human Resources, 335
Institute of Medicine, 462
institutional colonization, 140–141
institutional review boards, 546, 547n6
institutionalized racism, 6
intense pulsed light therapy, 688, 695–696, 702n2
inter-Indigenous, 133
International Classification of Diseases, 261–262, 463
International Classification of Functioning, 667
International Conference on Gender Identity, 229
International Conference on Transgender Law and Employment Policy (ICTLEP), 458–459, 468n44
International Council of Two Spirit Societies, 149–150
International Foundation for Gender Education, 379
  Denny relation to, 425
  Green, J., relation to, 431
  Kirk relation to, 440–441

International Gender Dysphoria Symposium, 350
  language at, 387n53
International Journal of Sexology, 217
International Journal of Transgender Health, 464–465
International Journal of Transgenderism, 461, 464
International Psychoanalytic Congress, 267
International Society for Sex Research, 51
International Symposium on Gender Identity, 347–349
International Two Spirit Gathering, 130
Interplast, 224
interpretive authority (*Deutungsmacht*), 68
intersectional identities, 5–6, 129
intersectionality, 133, 402
  at gender clinics, 377
intersex individuals, 17, 68, 84n14, 171, 176
  "Agnes" as, 266
  Allen, R., as, 181
  Cowell as, 124
  erasure of, 69
  gender identity and, 172, 482
  hermaphroditism compared to, 178
  hypospadias and, 214
  Judaism relation to, 297
  sex attitude and, 108
intersex model, 190n16
Intersex Society of North America, 483
intersocial realm, 259
interstitial nucleus of the anterior hypothalamus 3 (INAH3), 491
intervention model, 631–632
intimate histories, 231–232
intravention, 316–317

invert, 290n29
Investigation into Discrimination Against Transgendered People, 430
Iran, 297
Irvine, Janice, 79
isolation, 257
Israel, Gianna, 272–273
Isserman, Maurice, 435

J. H. (pseudonym), 227
Jackson, Trudie, 128
  on gender diversity, 15
  social mores and, 3
Jacoby, Adam, 596
Jahrbuch für sexuelle Zwischenstufen (journal), 84n22
Jahromi, Alireza, 603
Jane Crow, 302
Janssen, Aron, 486
Janus Information Facility, 229–230
  EEF relation to, 349
  Information for the Female-to-Male Crossdresser and Transsexual at, 252
  Walker relation to, 238n90, 346
Jayaram, Bangalore, 595
J2CP, 349
Jehovah's Witnesses, 296
Jenner, Caitlyn, 197n101
Jet (magazine), 204
Jiang-Ning Zhou, 491
Jivaka, Lobzang, 124
John/Joan case, 355n110
Johns Hopkins Gender Clinic, 204, 258, 381, 588
  EEF relation to, 345, 364
  funding for, 365
  gender-affirming surgery at, 361, 374, 388n56, 556
  Green, R., relation to, 267
  McHugh relation to, 377–379, 589–590
  Walker at, 346
Johns Hopkins University, 9
Johnson, Lyndon B., 399
Johnson, Marsha P., 330, 401–402, 417, 419
  Rivera relation to, 418, 419n10, 421
Jones, Howard Jr., 364
Jones, Mary, 102
Jorgensen, Christine (nee George), 9, 80, 167, 172–173, *175*
  Benjamin relation to, 170, 183–184, 187, 193n50, 194n74, 195n76, 197n99, 363, 588
  born-in-the-wrong-body narrative and, 194n59
  castration of, 118
  Cowell relation to, 181–182
  Elbe relation to, 92
  Erskine relation to, 209–210, 212, 216
  gender-affirming surgery of, 258, 585
  gender-affirming treatment of, 174–175, 176, 262, 556
  Hamburger relation to, 106, 116–117, 174, 178, 192n31, 193n50, 193n54
  media relation to, 171, 176–177, 187–188, 192nn37–38, 202–203
  pronouns relation to, 191n20
  public consciousness and, 193n44
  Roberts relation to, 204
  social mores and, 3
  "The Story of My Life" and, 177–179
  Stuart relation to, 250
  vaginoplasty and, 185, 588
Jorgensen, Florence, 172
Journal of the American Medical Association, 183, 258, 262, 687
joyas, 99, 138, 408. *See also* Two-Spirit people

Judaism, 297
Judeo-Christian doctrine
   American culture relation to, 2
   Euro-American culture relation to, 16
justice system, health disparities in, 534

Kaiser Permanente, 477
Kalra, Meryle, 662
Kane, Ariadne, 229
Kanner, Leo, 276n75
Kaplan, Isaac, 598
Karasic, Dan, 273
   American Psychiatric Association relation to, 462
karyotype, 489–490
Kates, Gary, 64n1
kathoey, 24–25, 31
Katter, Eva, 85n33
Kay-des-tizhi, 133
Ke Kulana He Mahu (documentary), 164
Ke Ola Mamo, 163
Keatley, JoAnne, 554, 574–576
   Green, J., relation to, 431
   social mores and, 3
Kelly, Maureen, 562
Kenna, J. C., 487
Kennedy, Pagan, 111
Kenyon, Dorothy, 304
Kertbeny, Karl Maria, 43
Kessler, Suzanne, 271, 343–344, 368
   on gender clinics, 381
   Gender of, 404
   on medical model, 377
   University of Victoria Transgender Archives and, 341
ketamine, 333
Khomeini, Ayatollah, 297
"Kill the Indian, Save the Man," 138
Kim, Hyung-Tae, 677
Kim, Yongha, 627

Kinsey, Alfred, 9, 14–15, 56, 83n12, 85n37
   Benjamin relation to, 65–68, 76–77, 80–81, 85n39, 96, 185, 195n84
   on bisexuals, 78–79
   Christian right relation to, 86n48
   Erskine relation to, 210, 211, 212, 221
   Hirschfeld relation to, 75, 79, 83n11, 87n56
   on hormones, 81–82
   intimate histories relation to, 232
   lavender scare relation to, 192n23
   Lawrence, L., relation to, 243
   orgasm relation to, 221, 236n64
   Pomeroy relation to, 252
   Psycho-Biological Questionnaire and, 71
   sexual revolution relation to, 435
Kinsey Institute for Research in Sex, Gender, and Reproduction, 346
   Hoff relation to, 572
Kirk, Sheila, 440
   HBIGDA relation to, 441, 454, 595
   hormones relation to, 594–595
   SOC relation to, 453
Klah, Hastiin, 136, 137, *137*
knowledge formulation
   of Indigenous North Americans, 129
   personal networks and, 80
Knudson, Gail, 464
   WPATH relation to, 465
Koch, H. C., Jr., 588
Kononen, Mark, 313
Die konträre Geschlechtsgefühl (Ellis, H., and Symonds), 52
Kopp, Heinrich, 73, 74
Kosasa Foundation, 164
Koyama, Emi, 408
Kozan, Anita, 674

Kraepelin, Emil, 51
Krafft-Ebing, Richard von, 47–48, 52, 83n3
  decriminalization relation to, 70
  on homosexuality, 84n21
Kremer, Brian, 674
Kreutz, Werner, 92
Kubrick, Stanley, 264
Kulia Na Mamo, 164–165
Kupperman, Herbert, 345
  Green, R., relation to, 364

Labadie Collection, at University of Michigan, 388n71
Labeija, Crystal, 315
labiaplasty, 176
Lacan, Jacques, 260
Ladies and Gentlemen collection, 417
Lady Gaga, 510–511
Laing, Alison, 666
Lamanites, 128, 153n2
Langley Porter Hospital, 241–243, 245
language
  of clinicians, 11
  evolving, 5
  at International Gender Dysphoria Symposium, 387n53
  mistreatment and, 387n54
  pathologization and, 6–7, 492n11
  public health relation to, 299
  in SOC, 467n22
  in trans-affirming medical publications, 12n1
Lanigan, Sean, 689
Lansdaal, Terren, 554, 660, 683
laparotomy, 109
Larson, Anna, 91
laser hair removal, 688–689, 702n2
  electrolysis relation to, 695, 705n70
lateral hair flap, 699

LaTrobe University, 665
Laub, Donald R., 224–225, 234nn25–26, 598
  Dain relation to, 252
  Fisk relation to, 594
  Fraser relation to, 442
  gender-affirming surgery relation to, 593
  HBIGDA and, 237n77
  intimate histories relation to, 232
  metoidioplasty relation to, 599
  Patton relation to, 227–228, 229
  on penile inversion vaginoplasty, 605n40
  sex reassignment relation to, 372
Lavender Los Angeles, 220
Lavender Scare, 173, 192n23, 398
Lawrence, Anne, 265
  gender-affirming surgery and, 607n95
  SOC relation to, 453
Lawrence, Louise, 77, 168, 233n3, 241–242, *243*, 385n25
  Benjamin relation to, 243
  Cummings relation to, 244
  Erskine relation to, 209, 216, 218, *218*, 219
  intimate histories of, 232
  Prince relation to, 245
League for Human Rights (*Bund für Menschenrechte*), 73
Lee, Jennifer, 168
  on HBC, 315
  on medicalization, 299
legal protections, 522
legal reform, 68, 70
legal rights, 450
legal system, 449–450
Legg, Dorr, 335
leiti, 29–31
Leng, Kirsten, 47

lesbian, 288. *See also* homosexuals
Leser, Hedwig Gruen, 67
Lev, Arlene Istar, 273
Leve, Gerald, 227
Levine, Edward M., 259
Levine, Rachel Leland, 554, 577–579
Levy-Lenz, Ludwig, 586, 587
Lewis, James Otto, 697
Lewis and Clark College, 150
Leydig cells, 505
LGBT Community Center, Gender Identity Project of, 443
LGBTQ+ Health Fellowships, 551
LGBTQ+ Veteran Care Coordinators, 550
liberation movement, 3
Lichtenstern, Robert, 504
Lieninger, Jennifer, 654
Lilly, John, 333, 335
Lim, S. P. R., 689
Lincoln, Pamela, 341
living-in-your-own-skin model, 635–637, 639, 643
   GAM compared to, 641, 642
Lobdell, Bambi, 286
Lobdell, Joseph, 168, 286–288, *289*, 289n5
logical positivism, 307
Long, Iris, 313
"Long-Term Follow-up of Transsexual Persons Undergoing Sex Reassignment Surgery," 536–537
Lorenz, Konrad, 265
Lothstein, Leslie, 257, 270, 387n54
Louis XIV, 697
Louis XVI, 15, 62, 63
Louise Lawrence Transgender Archive, 233n3
Lovaas, Ivar, 269–270
Love Joy Palace, 333
Lozen, 135–136

Lynch, Kyan, 1, 168, 717
   on medicalization, 299
   at SPECTRUM conference, 4
Lynch, Michael, 300, 302
   Johnson, M., relation to, 418

Mackenzie, Roy, 349
MacLane, Dixie, 219–220, 235nn52–53
magnetic resonance imaging (MRI), 475
mahu, 161–165. *See also* Indigenous Hawaiian people
Maiman, Theodore H., 688
The Male Hormone (De Kruif), 173
male pseudohermaphroditism, 585
Male with Female Outlook (Gillies), 111
Man into Woman (Hoyer), 91, 586
The Man-Monster, 102, *102*
Man & Woman, Boy & Girl (Money and Ehrhardt), 346
Manchester Metropolitan University, 431
Mandel, Francie, 649
Manders, Ernest, 595
Manifest Destiny, 138
"Many People, Many Passports," 224
Marcuse, Max, 50, 51, 587
marginalization
   of Black TGD people, 205–206
   by colonialism, 6
marginalized communities, 155n77
   in cultural mainstream, 17
Marriage Equality Act (2011), 149
Marshall, Thurgood, 304
Martin, Clyde, 76
Martin, Mary, 226
Martinez, Fred, 152
Martinez, Lilly, 511
Maryland Blue Cross, 589
masculinity
   colonization relation to, 130
   gay men and, 24–25

masculinity *(continued)*
  gender clinics relation to, 371
  homophile movement relation to, 398
  sexual intermediaries relation to, 48–49
  in Tonga, 29
  Urnings relation to, 45
  Western standards relation to, 672–673
masochism, 53
mass production, of hormones, 258
mastectomy, 603
masturbation, 41, 43
Mate-Kole, Charles, 381
Maternity of Mustapha Hospital, 112
Mattachine Society of New York, 217, 401
Matte, Nicholas, 461
Matzner, Andrew, 164
Mayer, Toby, 699, 706n107
mayhem statutes, 123, 185, 589
  gender-affirming surgery relation to, 195n85, 624
  orchiectomy and, 588
Mazzoni Center, 560–561
McBride, Jaye, 674–675
McCarthyism, 387–398
McGinn, Christine, 554, 627–628
McHugh, Paul, 262, 329, 380
  gender clinics relation to, 271, 362
  Johns Hopkins Gender Clinic relation to, 377–379, 589–590
  Labadie Collection relation to, 388n71
  Meyer, J., relation to, 288n72, 378–379
McIlvenna, Ted, 334
McIndoe, Archibald, 587–588
McKee, Embree, 314, 343–344
  on gender clinics, 381
McKenna, Wendy, 271, 368
  Gender of, 404
  on medical model, 377

McLeod, Charlotte, 194n58
Meaningful Use Incentive Program, 477
media
  gender dysphoria relation to, 170
  at International Symposium, Gender Identity, 347–348
  Johns Hopkins Gender Clinic relation to, 378–379
  Jorgensen, C., relation to, 171, 176–177, 187–188, 192nn37–38, 202–203
Medical, Legal & Workplace Issues for the Transsexual (Rothblatt and Kirk), 441
medical model, of transsexualism, 366, 367–368, 377, 381, 382
Medical Society for Sexual Science and Eugenics, 51
Medical Standards and Guidelines, 561–562
medicalization, 299, 454
  denied care relation to, 168
  HBC relation to, 317
  of homosexuality, 300–301
  mental illness relation to, 449
  Murray, P., relation to, 306–307
  of sexuality, 70
  SOC relation to, 318
Medicare/Medicaid
  for gender-affirming surgery, 458
  for gender-affirming treatment, 603
  hair removal relation to, 690
Meerscheidt-Hüllessem, Leopold von, 73
Melanesia, 32–33
"Melanie Speaks," 666
Meltzer, Toby, 594
  on electrolysis, 693
membership dues, 467n17
  for HBIGDA, 440
  for WPATH, 465
Ménard, Yvon, 594

menopause, 700
mental disorders, 314, 463
mental health issues
   sex reassignment relation to, 536–537
   of transgender veterans, 528
   of Two Spirit people, 145
mental illness, 264, 272, 382
   gender clinics relation to, 361
   gender diversity relation to, 476
   medicalization relation to, 449
   organic diseases compared to, 306–307
   SOC relation to, 453
   stigma and, 387n51
   of transgender inmates, 534
   transsexualism relation to, 366, 383, 404, 519
Merck, 707n110
merkins, 705n77
Mescalero Apache, 135–136
metoidioplasty, 584, 599–600
   nonbinary gender identity and, 603
   patient satisfaction with, 600
   in surgery journals, 451
Metro, 636
Mexican culture, androgyny in, 25
Mexico City, 77
   Erskine in, 214–215
Meyer, Jon, 271, 589–590
   gender clinics relation to, 362
   McHugh relation to, 288n72, 378–379
Meyer, Walter, 462
Meyer-Bahlburg, Heino F.L., 349
Meyerowitz, Joanne, 65, 87n67, 170, 267
   on Green, R., 269
Miami New Times, 270
Michel, Charles, 687
Michigan Womyn's Music Festival (Michfest), 406, 408

microsurgical techniques, for phalloplasty, 596–597, 598–599
Middleton, Lisa, 458–459
Migeon, Claude, 364
Mihailovic, Miodrag, 259
Milbank Estate, 335
military, 522–523
   bans in, 10, 549–550
   Don't Ask Don't Tell in, 627
military tribunals, 533–534
Millard, Ralph, 110
   vaginoplasty and, 115
Milliken, Donald, 387n55
Minnesota Department of Health, 253
Minnesota Multiphasic Personality Inventory test, 446
minority stress, 6
minoxidil, 699
Miranda, Deborah, 408
Mischael, Ahoova, 692
misinformation, 389n88, 465
The Mismeasure of Man (Gould), 382–383
misogyny, 306, 449
Miss Chief Eagle Testickle, 148
Miss Galaxy beauty contest, 30
mistreatment
   in gender-affirming treatment, 376–377
   language and, 387n54
modernism, leiti relation to, 30
Mohenjadaro, 18
Moll, Albert, 51
Money, John, 216, 258, 384n3, 690
   Ashton relation to, 333
   EEF relation to, 334, 345, 346
   gender identity relation to, 260, 480–481
   Green, R., relation to, 267, 268, 269, 277n98, 363, 436
   John/Joan case relation to, 355n110

Money, John *(continued)*
   McHugh relation to, 378
   Real Life Test relation to, 446–447
   Reimer relation to, 267, 481–483
   sexology relation to, 435–436
   in Society for the Scientific Study of Sex, 437
   speaking engagements of, 344
   stigma and, 372–373
Monkman, Kent, 148
Monstrey, Stan, 456, 595
   WPATH relation to, 602
Montgomery, Bernard, 126
Montgomery Medical and Psychiatric Institute, 425
mood disorders, gender dysphoria relation to, 532
Moore, Rusty Mae, 422
moral insanity, 44
moral purity groups, sexuality relation to, 46–47
morality, sexuality relation to, 41–42
Mordaunt, Michelle, 664
   Voice and Communication Therapy for the Transgender/Transsexual Client of, 667, 674
Morehouse School of Medicine, National Advisory Council at the Center of Excellence in Sexual Health at, 627
Morestin, Hippolyte, 106
   Gillies relation to, 597
Morris, Jan, 15, 113, 115, 126
The Most Excellent Order of the British Empire, 126
mother-blame theory, 265–266
mother-child dyad, 257
Motosko, Catherine, 701
Mount, Kay, 664–665
Mountain Home Transgender Veteran Research Protocol, 526, 532

Movement Advancement Project, 275n59
MRI. *See* magnetic resonance imaging
Mughal invasion, 19
multidisciplinary model, of transsexualism, 385n14
Murkowski, Lisa, 578
Murphy, Kirk Andrew, 267, 269–270
Murray, Julia, 422
Murray, Pauli, 12n8, 302–303, 305
   Ellis, H., relation to, 304
   medicalization relation to, 306–307
   pronouns relation to, 319n18
Museum of Navajo Ceremonial Art, 137
Muslims, 297
   bissu relation to, 22
   waria relation to, 23
My Name is Pauli Murray (documentary), 304

nádleehí, 131, 146. *See also* Two-Spirit people
   in Diné Origin Myth, 133
   Klah as, 136
Nanda, Serena, 14, 16
NASA. *See* National Aeronautics and Space Administration
National Academies Press, 462
National Advisory Council at the Center of Excellence in Sexual Health, at Morehouse School of Medicine, 627
National Aeronautics and Space Administration (NASA), 627
National Association of People with AIDS, 301
National Center for Advancing Translational Sciences, 532–533
National Center for Health Care Technology, 405
National Center for Transgender Equality, 532

National Council on Family Relations, 342
National Institute on Drug Abuse, 575
National Institutes of Health, 456
  TGD youth relation to, 654
  translational research of, 532–533
National Native American AIDS Prevention Center, 164
National Organization for Women, 305
National Sex Forum, 252
National Socialist Party, 587
National Transsexual Counseling Unit, 338
National University Hospital, Gender Identity Clinic at, 595
Native Hawaiian Health Care Act (1988), 163
Navajo Nation, 128
  Diné Marriage Act of, 148
  gender diversity in, 132t
  nádleehí relation to, 131
Navajo Studies Conference, 149
Nemoto, Tooru, 575
neocolonialism, 33
neologisms, 187
  transsexualism as, 190n3
nervous system, 47–48
neurons, 491
New England Journal of Medicine, 483
"New Homosexual Disorder Worries Health Officials," 299
New York City Gay Rights Bill, 422
New York Daily News, 176
New York Medical Journal, 95
New York Post, 179
New York State County Medical Society, Division of Professional Misconduct of, 520
New York State Historical Society, 100
New York Times, 101, 288, 628
  The Transsexual Empire and, 405

Newsweek, 179, 343
Newton, Delisa, 167, 205
Ngun, Tuck, 489
Nickle Galleries, 210
nonbinary gender identity, 100, 197n105, 408, 723
  gender-affirming surgery for, 603
  gender-affirming voice training for, 671–672
  Hitler relation to, 587
  hormones and, 409, 558
  Indigenous North Americans and, 130
  pronouns and, 722
nonprocreative sexual activities, 8, 13, 41–42
nonverbal vocalizations, 665
Norgay, Tenzing, 126
Norris, Denise, 354n85
nosology, 476
nullification surgery, 603
Numantius, Numa. *See* Ulrichs, Karl Heinrich
Núñez de Balboa, Vasco, 138

O Au No Keia (Matzner), 164
Oakland Tribune, 224
Oates, Jennifer, 662, 663
Obama, Barack, 409
Obama administration, 526
  DOD relation to, 549
obesity, 510
Obwegeser, Hugo, 600
Odo, Carol, 163
Of Justification by Faith (Calvin), 296
Office of Health Equity, 525
Office of Health Technology, 405
Ogas, Ogi, 378
O'Leary, Jean, 422
Olivia Women's Music Collective, 407
Olson, Kristina, 638

L'Onanisme (Tissot), 41
ONE Inc., 334–335
ONE Institute for Homophile Studies, 335
ONE National Gay & Lesbian Archives, 335
Oosterhuis, Harry, 48, 70
Oprah Winfrey Show, 628
orchiectomy
  of Cowell, 15, 123, 124
  of Elbe, 92, 586–587
  of Erskine, 211
  mayhem statutes and, 588
  of Reimer, 481
  vaginoplasty and, 115
Orentreich, Norman, 697–698
organic diseases, mental illness compared to, 306–307
organotherapy, hormones and, 190n4
orgasm, 221, 236n64
Orientalism (Said), 32
Orticochea, Miguel, 598
Osh-Tish, 134, *136*
otolaryngology, 669–670
Ousterhout, Douglas, 600–602
Out of the Ordinary (Dillon), 111, 124
ovarian cancer, 309
Ovesey, Lionel, 265–266, 368

Päderastenabteilung (Department for Pederasty), 73
Pakistan, 20
  third gender status in, 33
Paleolithic peoples, 689
pamphlet series, of EEF, 339, 341, *342*
Pan-Indianism, 133
Papillon Gender Wellness Center, 627–628
paraffin injections, 311
Pare, Florence, 546

parental practices, 476
Paris Match, 112–113
Parkhurst, Charley, 101
Parks, Rosa, 304
passport application procedures, 449–450
Pastel, Sophia, 313
Pasterski, Vickie, 485
pathologization, 261–262
  at gender clinics, 403
  of homosexuality, 299–300
  Krafft-Ebing and, 48
  language and, 6–7, 492n11
  in transgender medical research, 517
pathologizing beliefs, 9
patient autonomy, in gender-affirming treatment, 720
patient-caregiver relations, 272
patient regret, 117–118
patient satisfaction, 600
patriarchy
  Catholic Church relation to, 25
  Christianity and, 408
Patton, Jude, 167, 225, *230*, 349
  D. F. relation to, 226–227
  Fraser relation to, 442
  Green, R., relation to, 436
  HBIGDA relation to, 439, 441, 454
  Laub relation to, 227–228, 229
  SOC relation to, 453
  WPATH relation to, 440
Paul, Rand, 579
Paul VI (Pope), 593
Pauli Murray Center for History and Social Justice, 319n18
Pauly, Ira B., 227, 265
  Benjamin relation to, 271
  HBIGDA relation to, 452
  Sullivan relation to, 252, 370
Pax Britannica (Morris), 126
Paxton, Ken, 579

Pearce, Ruth, 544, 546
pederasts, 43
pelvic osteopathy, 603
penectomy, 176
penetration
    Candomblé relation to, 28
    gender roles relation to, 26
    sodomy and, 42–43
penile inversion vaginoplasty, 115, 119, 588, 589
    Biber relation to, 592
    Laub on, 605n40
people of color, 167, 421. *See also* Indigenous Hawaiian people; Indigenous North Americans
    body hair of, 703n32
    civil rights for, 329
    electrolysis for, 688
    erasure and, 416n52
    gender-affirming treatment for, 203
    gender-affirming voice training for, 672–673
    at gender clinics, 377
    health disparities and, 205–206, 415n22, 528
    hormones for, 322n95
    research gaps and, 666, 670
    Two Spirit people relation to, 129, 143–144
performativity
    of gender identity, 260
    of gender roles, 190n5
Perina, Barbra Ann, 453–454
Perovic, Sava, 599
Perry, Alan, 320n60
Perry, Marie, 287–288
Person, Ethyl, 265–266, 368–369
personal networks, 80
    HBIGDA, 442
    healthcare, 559, 576, 668

research and, 80, 346, 523, 547n9
TGD community, 95, 164, 241, 271, 317, 442, 464, 718
trans and medical communities, 71, 75, 77, 94, 209–232, 243, 350, 379
personality disorders, assumptions about transgender people, 524
Pew Research Center, 722
phalloplasty, 108, 109–110, 119
    hair removal relation to, 693–695
    patient satisfaction with, 600
    in surgery journals, 451
    techniques for, 596–600
Phelan, Jo, 510
Philadelphia Community Health Alternatives, 560
Philadelphia Trans* Health Conference, 671
Philippines, homosexual relationships in, 23
Phillips, Melanie, "Melanie Speaks," 666
Phoenix, C. H., 484
phonosurgery, 671
Pickering, Jack, 660, 668, 675–676
Piotrowski, Cas, 320n60
pitch elevation, gender-affirming surgery for, 676–677
Pittsburgh, Pennsylvania, Transgender Surgical and Medical Center in, 595
PlanetOut.com, 431
Planned Parenthood Federation of America (PPFA), 228, 561–562
Plucked (Herzig), 686–687
Plume, 563
Polderman, Tinca, 487, 488–489, 512
political will, 450
polygenic threshold model, 488
polymorphisms, 489
    gender identity and, 488
Polynesia, 28–30
    homosexual relationships, 33

Pomeroy, Wardell, 76
  EEF relation to, 345
  Green, R., relation to, 364
  Sullivan relation to, 252
postnatal social programming, 259
Pott, John, 99
Powell, Tia, 511
power dynamics
  at gender clinics, 375–376, 381
  medical institutions, 402
PPFA. See Planned Parenthood Federation of America
Pratt, Richard, 138
pre-natal hormones, 486
prenatal hormonal neurotransmitter levels, 259
Prescod-Weinstein, Chanda, 307
Pretty Eagle (Chief), 134
prevalence, of gender diversity, 476–478, 492n11
Primary Care Protocol for Transgender Care, at University of California, San Francisco, 431
primary gender (*adzáán*), 131
primary transsexual, 368–369
Primrose, Clay, 372–373
Prince, Virginia, 168, 229, *246*, 247n5, 251nn3–4, 385n25
  Benjamin relation to, 249–251
  Cauldwell relation to, 294
  cross-dressing relation to, 244–246, 247
  Denny relation to, 425
  Fraser relation to, 442
  pronouns relation to, 247n1
The Principles and Art of Plastic Surgery (Gillies), 108, 110, 115
privacy, before HIPPA, 86n45
Program in Human Sexuality, at University of Minnesota, 362
  Coleman at, 384n5

Progynon, 95
pronouns, 7
  Elagabalus relation to, 604n6
  Indigenous North Americans relation to, 134
  Jorgensen, C., relation to, 191n20
  Murray, P., relation to, 319n18
  nonbinary gender identity and, 722
  Prince relation to, 247n1
  Reimer relation to, 493n42
  Spengler relation to, 96n2
  Westphal relation to, 57n10
prostitution. See also sex work
  cross-dressing relation to, 234n31
  Department for Pederasty relation to, 73
  silicone relation to, 311
Protect Children's Innocence Act, 723
Protestant religions, 296
pseudo-hermaphrodite, 216–217, 304, 585
pseudotranssexuals, 265
psychiatric disorders, hormones relation to, 485–486
psychiatry, 255–273, 377–378
psychic hermaphrodites, 48, 268, 363
psychic life, sexuality relation to, 56
Psycho-Biological Questionnaire, 70–71
psychoanalysis, 78
psychological hermaphroditism, 45–46, 49, 54, 183
psychology, 255–273
Psychopathia Sexualis (Cauldwell), 47–48, 52, 70, 292–293, 354n85
psychosexual neutrality theory, 260
psychosis, as explanation for gender diversity, 257, 262
psychotherapy, as cure for gender diversity, 186–187, 189
puberty blockers, 409–410, 640, 650
  gender-affirming voice training and, 673

gonadotropin-releasing hormone analogs, 653
  SMR (Tanner stages), relation to, 654
public education, EEF relation to, 339, 341, *342*, 342–344, 401
public health
  HIV/AIDS epidemic and, 402–403
  language relation to, 299
public opinion, EEF relation to, 331, 336
Public Universal Friend, 100

QPOC. *See* queer people of color
Quarter Court, 99
Queen Victoria Hospital, Gender Dysphoria Clinic at, 662
The Queen's Hospital, 107
Queens Liberation Front, 401
Queer Med, 563
queer people of color (QPOC), 315–317. *See also* people of color
queer studies, Two Spirit people relation to, 142, 146–147

Rachlin, Katherine, 442, 451, 463
  WPATH relation to, 443–444
racial bias, craniofacial surgery and, 601–602
racialized gender, 205
racism, 32, 306, 518
  American Indian, 142, 148, 195n85, 686
  Institutionalized, 195–196, 202, 205, 399, 402, 445
  LGBT activism, 401
  Sexology relation to, 56
radical behavioral model, 260
radioimmunoassay, 475, 484
Radix, Asa, 441, 465
  on ethics, 544
  on hormone therapy, 555

Radszuweit, Friedrich, 73
Raskin, Lynn, 341, 342
Ratnam, S. Shan, 595
Raymond, Janice, 262
  CMS relation to, 458
  The Transsexual Empire of, 377, 380–381, 389n81, 405, 406–407
Real Life Test, 445
  Money relation to, 446–447
rectosigmoid vaginoplasty, 594
Reed v. Reed, 304
Rees, Tamara, 194n58
refrigerator mother, 276n75
Regnell, Joan, 664
Reimer, David, 267, 481–483. *See also* John/Joan case
  pronouns relation to, 493n42
Reinisch, June, 346
Reisman, Judith A., 86n48
rejuvenation, 504–505, 506
Rekers, George, 267, 275n59
  aversion therapy and, 269–270
religion
  gender-affirming surgery relation to, 295–297
  Two Spirit people relation to, 131
  Yoruba, 27
religious roles, of bissu, 22
Reminiscences (Benjamin), 74
Renaissance News, 229, 231
reparative therapy, 546, 633–635, 639, 643
rescue ethnography, 188
research gaps, 462, 535–536
  people of color and, 666, 670
research grants, of EEF, 345–347
research mandate, gender-affirming treatment and, 544–545
researchers
  bias of, 380

researchers *(continued)*
  colonization relation to, 141–142
  at gender clinics, 370–371
  Reter, Donna, 378, 589–590
Richards, Barbara Ann, 241
Richards, Renée, 263
Richter, Dora "Dorchen," 586
Rider, Nic, 689
Rivera, Sylvia, 330, 401–402, 420, 423, 430
  Johnson, M., relation to, 418, 419n10, 421
  at Transy House, 422
RKO-Pathe News, 172, 173
Robert Eads, 308–309
  Health Partnership Program, 320n60
Roberts, Monica, x, 3, 6, 167, 203–206, 408
Robinson, Bean, 463
Robinson, Henry, 102
Rocky Mountain News, 592
Rolling Stone, 482
Rome, gender diversity in, 17
Röntgen, Wilhelm, 686
Rooksdown House, 106
Roosevelt, Eleanor, 304
Roscoe, Will, 129
Roselli, Francine, 510
Rosenthal, Stephen, 509
Rothblatt, Martine, 441
Roughgarden, Joan, 475
Ruddick, Edna, 621
Russell, Meredith, 673

S., Judy, 218, *218*, 219
sacred spaces, 140, 149
sadism, 53
Safer, Joshua D., 474
  on nonbinary gender identity, 722–723

SAGE LGBTQ Encyclopedia, 3–4
Said, Edward, 32
Salmon, Shirley, 664–665
Salon d'Automne, 91–92
sambia, 32–33
same-sex desire, 45–46
  gender inversion relation to, 48
same-sex marriage, 409, 449–450
  Indigenous North Americans relation to, 148, 149
  in United Kingdom, 126
San Carlos Reservation, 135
San Francisco, 77, 85n39
  Compton's Cafeteria riots in, 338, 398–400
  cross-dressing in, 214–215
  discrimination in, 430, 451–452
  health insurance in, 459–460
  Human Rights Commission of, 430, 459
  Tom Waddell Health Center in, 559
  University of California, 165, 431, 432, 576, 601, 643
San Francisco Examiner, 215–216
Santana, Sarah, 337
Sarkar, Amrita, 544
Satcher, David, 627
Sattur, Sandeep, 699
Sawyer, Carla, 624
Sawyer, Jean, 669, 672
Schaefer, Leah C., 96, 184, 272
  Fraser relation to, 442
Schechter, Loren, 603
Schering, 95
Schilt, Kristen, 266
Schmid, Andreas, 312
Schrang, Eugene, 594
  on electrolysis, 693
Schroeter, Careen Angela, 695
Schucman, Helen, 335

Schuylkill Metals, 331–332, 333
Science, Johnny, 442–443
The Science of Orgasm (McGinn), 627
Scientific Humanitarian Committee, 65
  Spengler and, 94
Scientific Symposium, 461
Scopes Monkey Trial, 513
Scott, Campbell, 140
Screaming Queens (film), 399–400
scrotoplasty, 599
Sears, Clare, 214
Seattle Counseling Service, 338
Second Interdisciplinary Symposium on Gender Dysphoria Syndrome, 113, 114
secondary transsexual, 368–369
Seghers, Michel, 693
Self (Dillon), 123, 124
Sense8 (series), 431
Sepia (magazine), 205
Serlin, David, 171
Seven Years War, 62
Seventh-Day Adventists, 296
Severa, Aquilia, 604n11
sex assignment, 258–259
sex attitude, 108
sex/gender pluralism, 22
  in Indonesia, 21
Sex Orientation Scale, 196n93
sex reassignment
  at gender clinics, 362, 372
  mental health issues relation to, 536–537
Sex Reassignment Program, at Stanford University, 446
sex steroids, 484
"Sex Transmutation — Can One's Sex Be Changed?," 293
sex-typical childhood behaviors, 261
Sex Without Guilt (Ellis, A.), 77

sex work, 162–163, 575
  activism for, 418–419
  discrimination relation to, 309
  hijra and, 19
  HIV/AIDS epidemic relation to, 402
  kathoey and, 24
  travesti and, 27
  waria, 22
sexo-aesthetic inversion, 54
sexology, 13, 47, 50, 56
  in Europe, 8
  Hitler relation to, 587
  sexual identity relation to, 55–56
  sexual revolution relation to, 435–436
  Ulrichs relation to, 45
Sexology (magazine), 167–168, 205
Sexual Behavior in the Human Female (Kinsey), 67, 76–77, 78, 80, 83n12
  endocrinology in, 81
Sexual Behavior in the Human Male (Kinsey), 67, 75, 76, 80, 83n12
sexual development, 484–485
sexual differentiation, hormones relation to, 484–485
sexual dimorphism, 79–80
sexual identity, 70
  Kinsey relation to, 80–81
  sexology relation to, 55
Sexual Identity Conflict in Children and Adults (Green, R.), 633
"Sexual Identity of 37 Children Raised by Homosexual or Transsexual Parents," 268
sexual intermediaries, 48–49, 78, 94, 479
sexual inversion, 46, 51, 56, 257, 290n29
Sexual Inversion (Ellis, H., and Symonds), 52–53
sexual maturity rating (SMR), 656n6
  puberty blockers relation to, 654

sexual norms, 2
sexual orientation, conflation with gender identity, 478–479
sexual otherness, colonialism and, 32
sexual perversity, interest to sexologists, 47
sexual practices, Travesti, gender diversity relation to, 25–26
Sexual-Probleme (journal), 50
sexual renunciation, in Hinduism, 19
sexual revolution, 435–436
sexual rights movements, 65, 94, 217, 231, 300–301, 304–305, 334, 336, 398–401, 403–406, 409–410
sexual subcultures, 14, 56, 259, 315
  in Berlin, 65, 71–72, 74
  Department for Pederasty relation to, 73
sexuality
  Cold War relation to, 242
  colonialism relation to, 33
  gender identity relation to, 188, 402
  gender relation to, 16–17, 69
  gender roles relation to, 46
  genetics of, 49
  HBC relation to, 316
  medicalization of, 70
  moral purity groups relation to, 46–47
  morality relation to, 41–42
  in Polynesia, 28
  psychic life relation to, 56
  religion relation to, 296
Sexuality Information and Education Council of the United States, 228
Shaiova, Charles H., 259
shaving, depilation by, 702n2
Sherwin, Robert, 364
Shia Islamic philosophy, 21
Shipherd, Jillian, 549
Shoji Okura, 697

Siculus, Diodorus, 585
Sigmundson, Keith, 482
silicone, 310, 312–313, 457
  American Educational Gender Information Services on, *311*
  prostitution relation to, 311
  travesti and, 26
  waria and, 23
silicone embolism syndrome, 312
Simmons-Thorne, Naomi, 319n18
Simon, William, 86n48
Sinclair, Upton, 624
Sing Sing Correctional Facility, 102
Singh, Anneliese, 673
singing, gender-affirming voice training and, 674
The Singing Teacher's Guide to Transgender Voice (Herns and Kremer), 674
Sissy Boy study, 267, 268–269, 277n98
Sissy Boy Syndrome and the Development of Homosexuality (Green, R.), 385n14, 633–634
Sister (journal), 381
Skidmore, Emily, 100–101
  on Jorgensen, C., 171
Skinner, B. F., 260
Slater, George, 287, 289n5
slavery, 32, 99
Slavitz, Harriet, 341
2SLGBTS. *See* Two Spirit people
Smith, Martin, 591–592
Smith, Phoebe, 379, 384n13
SMR. *See* sexual maturity rating
Snorton, C. Riley, 205
snow-blindedness, 382–383
SOC. See *Standards of Care*
Socarides, Charles, 262
  Hoff relation to, 571
Social Problems (journal), 381

social roles, 260
social transition, 117
  GAM relation to, 641–642
  Utrecht University Hospital and, 653
  in watchful waiting model, 638
Society for the Scientific Study of Sex, 228
  Money in, 437
Society for the Second Self (Tri-Ess), 246, 249
  Denny relation to, 425
sodomy
  colonialism relation to, 32
  penetration and, 42–43
Song, Colin, 598
South Sulawesi, 21
Southern Comfort Conference, 308, 309, 320n60
Southern Comfort (film), 308, 309, 320n60
Southern Poverty Law Center, 269
Spack, Norman, 409–410, 640
  Endocrine Society Guidelines and, 462
  GeMS and, 649–650, 653–654
Speaking as a Woman (Laing), 666
speaking engagements, of EEF, 343–344
Spector, Scott, 43
SPECTRUM conference, 4
speech-language pathologists, 660–661, 683–684
  ethnolinguistic identity relation to, 673
  in gender clinics, 669
  health insurance relation to, 668
  singing relation to, 674
Spence, James, 590
Spencer, Katherine, 689
Spengler, Otto, 15, 94, 96
  Benjamin relation to, 93, 95, 195n82
  intimate histories of, 232
  pronouns relation to, 96n2

spermatogenesis, 505
spironolactone, 529, *531*, 532
sports participation, 723
  anti-trans legislation and, 655
  bans on, 410
St. Amand, Colt, 464
Staley, Peter, 313
Standards of Care (SOC), 318, 435, 440, 448, 460, 466, 557, 594
  Americans with Disabilities Act relation to, 261
  bias in, 445
  Coleman relation to, 461, 464
  eligibility requirements relation to, 444–445
  Fraser on, 442
  GAM relation to, 643
  Garofalo relation to, 462
  gender-affirming voice training relation to, 660, 666, 668
  gender clinics relation to, 559
  Gender Education Initiative and, 446
  Green, J., relation to, 430–431
  of HBIGDA, 189, 267, 350, 377, 451–453, 467n21, 522
  health insurance relation to, 557
  hormone therapy in, 444, 555, 595
  informed consent model in, 560, 721
  Kirk relation to, 595
  language in, 467n22
  legal rights and, 450
  mental health and, 721
  Rachlin relation to, 443
  Radix relation to, 465
  surgical care and, 375–376, 594, 695
  transgender inmates and, 535
  voice and communication and, 660, 668
Standing Rock, 149
Stanford Gender Dysphoria Program, 271

Stanford Symposium, 115
Stanford University, Sex Reassignment Program at, 446
Stanford University School of Medicine, 224
STAR. *See* Street Transvestite Action Revolutionaries
STAR House, 418, 421, 422
Stark, Inez, 621
State University of New York at Stony Brook, 342–343
States' Laws on Race and Color (Murray, P.), 304
Statistical Manual of Mental Health Disorders, 5th edition, 165
Steinach, Eugen, 49–50, 81, 329, 478, 587
  Benjamin relation to, 184, 506
  glandular manipulation by, 504–505
Steinachfilm (film), 50
Steiner, Betty, 372
Stephens, Elizabeth, 78
Stevenson, Mary, 700
Stevenson, Matilda Coxe, 135
stigma, 1–6, 508, 518–519, 636, 655
  baldness and, 696
  biological validation and, 509–510
  Black TGD people and, 205–206
  colonization relation to, 139, 142, 152
  discrimination and, 508
  etiology relation to, 510
  gender-affirming treatment and, 373, 509
  at gender clinics, 372–373
  gender diversity and, 475
  healthcare disparities and, 575
  homosexuality and, 24, 30, 226, 259
  kathoey and, 24, 25
  Lili Elbe and, 92
  mental illness and, 261, 387n51, 404
  in military, 522–523
  waria and, 22
Stoller, Robert J., 257
  "Agnes" relation to, 267
  Belt relation to, 624
  Gender Identity Research Clinic relation to, 556
  Green, R., relation to, 268
  intervention model of, 631–632
  Money relation to, 436
  mother-blame theory of, 265–266
  sex reassignment relation to, 372
  Sissy Boy Syndrome and the Development of Homosexuality relation to, 633
  twin studies of, 487
Stone, Allucquére Rosanne "Sandy," 370, 385n25
  The Empire Strikes Back of, 406–407
Stonewall Uprising, 398, 400–401
  Johnson, M., relation to, 417–418
  Rivera relation to, 421
"The Story of My Life" (Jorgensen, C.), 177–179, 193n54
Street Transvestite Action Revolutionaries (STAR), 401, 418, 421
Strewe, Bernhard, 73
Stryker, Susan, 65, 222
  on MacLane, 219
  Screaming Queens of, 399–400
Stuart, Sharon, 168, 250–251
  on Benjamin, 249
Studies in Ethnomethodology, 266
Studies in the Psychology of Sex (Ellis, H.), 53
"Studying Trans," 546
Stürup, George, 258
  at International Symposium on Gender Identity, 348

subcultures, 2, 14, 56, 259
  in Berlin, 65, 71–72, 74
  colonialism relation to, 14
  Department for Pederasty relation to, 73
  HBC, 315–316
Substance Abuse and Mental Health Services Administration, DHH, 149–150, 164, 576
Sudduth, Henry, 226
Sudduth, Lorraine, 226
Suharto (President), 21–22
suicidal behaviors, 526–527
Sullivan, Louis G., 168, 251–253, 370, 386, 429
  Green, J., relation to, 271, 429
  Green, R., relation to, 436
  Information for the Female-to-Male Crossdresser and Transsexual of, 238n90, 252
  social mores and, 3
Sunday Kansas City Star, 250
Sunrise Films, 341
Suplee, Zelda, 334, 336–337, 342
  EEF Newsletter and, 339
  at International Symposium on Gender Identity, 348
  Janus Information Facility relation to, 349
support groups, for cross-dressing, 95, 229, 245–246, 249
Supreme Court, Dobbs decision in, 450
Suquamish Tribe, 149
surgical transition, 117. *See also* gender-affirming surgery
Swaab, Dick, 508–509
Swenson, Erin, 386n33
"swishes," 398
Swope, Robert, 246
Sylvia Rivera Law Project, 422–423

Sylvia Rivera Prize for Best Book in Transgender Studies, 430
Symonds, John Addington, 51–52
Szasz, Thomas, 262
  on *The Transsexual Empire*, 405

TAAF. *See* Tribal Alliance Against Frauds
Tahiti, 31
Talmey, Bernard, 95
Tangpricha, Vin, 462
Tardieu, Ambroise, 42
Tarver, Donald E., II, 272–273
Taylor, Michael Thomas, 210
Taylor, Timothy, 689
Teec Nos Pos, 128
telehealth, 562–563
TERF. *See* trans exclusionary radical feminist
Tessier, Paul, 600, 601
testicular atrophy, hormone therapy relation to, 111
testosterone, 173, 484
  Benjamin relation to, 66
  brain development relation to, 261
  chemical castration and, 174
  facial hair relation to, 700, 704n49
  finasteride relation to, 699
  gender-affirming voice training and, 670
  at gender clinics, 556
  hair removal relation to, 696
  metoidioplasty relation to, 599
  Patton and, 227
  Reimer relation to, 483
  secondary transsexual relation to, 369
  Steinach relation to, 506
  VHA relation to, 529, *531*, 532
Texas T Parties, 523
TGD. *See* transgender and gender-diverse

TGD youth. *See also* gender affirmative model
  at GeMS, 650
  gender-affirming surgery for, 603
  gender-affirming treatment for, 278n122, 406, 553, 631, 650
  gender-affirming voice training for, 673–674
  gender identity of, 451, 630, 636, 650, 654
  GnRH analogs for, 637
  hormone therapy for, 409–410, 638, 640, 653
Thailand, 23, 595–596
  kathoey in, 24–25
thallium compounds, 686
thermolysis, 688, 692
third gender status, 33
Thomas, Wesley, 131, 132, 133, 151
Thompson, Fred, 524, 539n17
Thongpeaw, Prakob, 595
Thoreson, Nick, 690
thyroplasty type III, 671
Ti-Shang Chang, 598
Tiewtranon, Preecha, 595
Time, 410
  Money in, 482
The Times, 126
Times Higher Education, 364
Timm, Annette F., 65, 167
  on Erskine, 209
  on Hirschfeld, 14–15
Tissot, Samuel-Auguste, 41
Title VII workplace protections, 449–450
Tom Waddell Health Center, 273, 559
Tometi, Opal, 409
Tonga, leiti of, 29–31
top surgery, 227, 320n60, 596
Tosti, Antonella, 701
trans-affirming medical publications, language in, 12n1

Trans (documentary), 628
Trans Education and Action Capacity for Health, 576
trans exclusionary radical feminist (TERF), 405–406
Trans Health Survey, 689
trans history. *See specific topics*
Trans Lifeline, 719
trans-representation, 191n16
trans studies. *See* transgender studies
Trans Thrive, 576
The Transexual Menace, 354n85, 453
transgender and gender-diverse (TGD). *See specific topics*
Transgender and HIV (Bockting and Kirk), 441
transgender athletes, 537
Transgender Care (Gianna and Tarver), 273
Transgender Emergence (Lev), 273
Transgender Health & Education Alliance's Peach State Conference, 320n60
transgender inmates, 534–535, 537
Transgender Law and Policy Institute, 431
Transgender Liberation (Feinberg), 408
Transgender Lives Conference, 4
transgender medical research, 518–519, 521
  censorship of, 520
  ethics in, 544–547
  funding for, 535, 537–538
  gender-affirming treatment relation to, 533
  pathologization in, 517
Transgender Professional Association for Transgender Health, 545
Transgender Resource and Neighborhood Space, 576
Transgender Rights Committee, 231

transgender studies, 385n25, 408, 430
Transgender Surgical and Medical Center, 595
transgender veterans
   Directive 1341 (2) relation to, 550
   health disparities and, 528–529
   justice system relation to, 534
   suicidal behaviors of, 526–527
transgenderist, 250
Transgriot (blog), 206
Transhealth Northampton, 719
TransHealthCare.org, 119
transition. *See specific topics*
translational research, of National Institutes of Health, 532–533
transphobia, 139
   Indigenous North Americans and, 150–151
   Two Spirit people and, 151–152
The Transsexual Empire (Raymond), 377, 380–381, 389n81
   The Empire Strikes Back relation to, 406–407
   TERF relation to, 405
The Transsexual Phenomenon (Benjamin), 210–211, 227, 314, 342, 354n85, 480
   gender clinics relation to, 366, 373–374
   hormone therapy in, 556
   transgender medical research and, 518
Transsexual Voice for the Tone Deaf, 666
Transsexual Voice (publication), 379
Transsexual Voice Questionnaire, 667
transsexualism, 189, 190n5, 196n90, 227, 336
   Cauldwell relation to, 292
   in DSM, 301, 522–523
   etiology of, 479–480
   gender and, 373

   karyotype relation to, 490
   medical model of, 366, 367–368, 377, 381, 382
   mental disorders relation to, 314, 463
   mental illness relation to, 366, 383, 404, 519
   multidisciplinary model of, 385n14
   prevalence of, 477
   psychoanalytic drive theory relation to, 256–257
   psychotherapy relation to, 186–187
   transvestism compared to, 185–186, 190n3
Transsexualism and Sex Reassignment (Green, R., and Money), 216, 271, 314, 345, 364
   Benjamin relation to, 366–367
   electrolysis in, 690
   gender clinics relation to, 373–734
   multidisciplinary model and, 385n14
   Real Life Test in, 447
Transsexualism Religious Aspects (pamphlet), 295
TransTrans (exhibition), 210, 222
Transvestia (magazine), 245, 247, 250
transvestic fetishism, 527
   gender dysphoria relation to, 539n26
transvestism, 180, 183
   in DSM, 301
   erotic desire and, 220–221
   Erskine relation to, 210
   Hamburger on, 117
   Jorgensen, C., relation to, 177
   Kinsey on, 76, 78
   Spengler relation to, 94
   Talmey on, 95
   transsexualism compared to, 185–186, 190n3
   Yoruba religion and, 27
transvestite pass (*Transvestitenpass*), 74, 85n33, 220, 720

Die Transvestiten (Hirschfeld), 54, 71, 79, 479
  Spengler relation to, 96
Transvestites and Transsexuals (Feinbloom), 343, 403–404
"Transvestivism," 95
Transy House, 422
TransYouth Family Allies, 431
TransYouth Project, 638
trauma, 11
  colonialism relation to, 147
  gender dysphoria relation to, 632–633
  of Indigenous North Americans, 128–129, 138, 143
travesti, 25–27
Tresckow, Hans von, 73
Tri-Ess. *See* Society for the Second Self
trial period, 446–447. *See also* Real Life Test
Tribal Alliance Against Frauds (TAAF), 155n69
Tribal Equity Toolkit, 150
Tribal Self Governance Act (1994), 140
Tribal Training and Technical Assistance Center, 149–150
Tricho System, 687
Trinidad, Colorado, 591–594, 607n90
Trump, Donald J., 409, 549, 628
tubed pedicle, 107–108
Tuck, Eve, 145
Tuckniss, Morris, 126
TV-TS Tapestry Journal, 379
twin studies, 486–488
A Two Spirit Journey (Chacaby), 147
Two Spirit people, 129, 143, 408
  activism of, 148, 149
  colonization relation to, 15, 138–139
  gender-affirming treatment for, 145, 150–151
  gender roles relation to, 130
  in Indian boarding schools, 141
  queer studies relation to, 142, 146–147
  religion relation to, 131
  sacred spaces relation to, 140
  transphobia and, 151–152

UCLA. *See* University of California, Los Angeles
Ulrichs, Karl Heinrich, 45–46, 48, 73
  on Urnings, 290n29
unisex bathroom, 524
United Kingdom, same sex marriage in, 126
United Mine Workers Clinic, 591
United States Transgender Survey Report on the Experiences of American Indian & Alaskan Native Respondents, 142–144, 144t, 145, 155n77
universal bisexuality, 92
University of Berlin, 43
University of California, Los Angeles (UCLA), 257, 625
  gender clinics at, 267, 268
  Gender Identity Research Clinic at, 556
University of California, San Francisco
  Center for Craniofacial Anomalies at, 601
  Center of Excellence for Transgender Health at, 165, 432, 576
  Child and Adolescent Gender Center at, 643
  Primary Care Protocol for Transgender Care at, 431
University of Ghent, 595
University of Michigan, Labadie Collection at, 388n71
University of Minnesota, 252
  Program in Human Sexuality at, 362, 384n5

University of North Carolina, 303
University of Prague, 49
University of Rochester Medical Center, Golisano Children's Hospital at, 655–656
University of Texas Medical Branch, 346, 349
    Walker at, 436
University of Victoria Transgender Archives, 341
University of Washington, 664
Urban, Thomas, 381
Urban Indians, 133
Urnings, 45–46, 73
    homosexuality relation to, 290n29
US Department of Health and Human Services (HHS), 262, 565n48
    Levine, R., relation to, 577–578
    Substance Abuse and Mental Health Services Administration of, 149–150, 164, 576
US Professional Association for Transgender Health (USPATH), 440
    Rachlin relation to, 444
US Public Health Service Commissioned Corps, 578
USTS. See *United States Transgender Survey Report on the Experiences of American Indian & Alaskan Native Respondents*
Utrecht University Hospital, 653

VA. See Veteran Affairs
Vagelos, P. Roy, 707n110
vaginoplasty, 124
    Ashley and, 125
    at Boston Medical Center, 651
    Burou and, 15, 105–106, 113, 114–115
    Cowell and, 180
    Davydov technique, 596
    Gillies and, 108, 115
    hair removal relation to, 692–693
    Hoff and, 571
    Jorgensen, C., and, 185, 588
    McIndoe relation to, 587–588
    penile inversion, 115, 119, 588, 589, 592, 605n40
    rectosigmoid, 594
    Richter and, 586
    in surgery journals, 451
    in Thailand, 595–596
Valadier, Auguste, 106
    Gillies relation to, 597
Van Kesteren, Paul, 527
Vanderbilt University, 381, 425
    gender-affirming treatment relation to, 389n87
    gender clinics at, 386n35
vasectomy, 505
Veale, Jaimie F., 544
venereal disease, 41
venous thromboembolism, 558
Veritas Meeting Solutions, 465
Vernon, Irene, 131
vestal virgins, 604n11
Veteran Affairs (VA), 525
Veterans Administration Hospitals, 477
Veteran's Health Administration (VHA), 530
    Directive 1341 (2) of, 550
    discrimination and, 330
    gender clinic of, 524–525, 526
    hormone therapy relation to, 529, 531, *531*, 532
    LGBTQ+ Health Fellowships relation to, 551
VHA Office of Health Equity, 526
Victorio, 135
Vietnam War, 399

Vincent, Ben, 546
Vindex (Ulrichs), 290n29
Violante, Monica, 607n90
Vladicka, Theresa, 461
vocal characteristics, 662, *663*, 664–665
Vogel, David, 510
Vogue, 125
Voice and Communication Therapy for the Transgender/Transsexual Client (Adler, Hirsch, and Mordaunt), 667, 674
voyeurism, 231–232
Vries, Annelou C. V. de, 653
Vrije Universiteit Medical Center, 637–638

Walker, Paul, 252, 524
   EEF relation to, 328n90, 346
   Fraser relation to, 272
   HBIGDA relation to, 438–439, 557
   Janus Information Facility relation to, 238n90, 349
   at University of Texas Medical Branch, 436
Wang, Amanda Yijun, 417
Warhol, Andy, 417
waria, 22–23
   kathoey compared to, 24
Warnekros, Kurt, 587
Warren, Barbara, 272
Warren, Earl, 624
Watanyusakul, Suporn, 596
watchful waiting model, 637–639
   GAM compared to, 642
Watson, James, 475, 486
Watson, Steve, 417
Wegener, Einar, 91–93
Weininger, Otto, 48–49
   Ackerley relation to, 56
Wen-Yi Hwang, 598

Wesser, David, 598
West Coast Lesbian Conference, 404–405
Western philosophy, gender binary in, 31
Western standards, race, gender and voice, 672–673
Westphal, Carl, 43–45, 46, 290n29
   pronouns use for Ha, 57n10
Westside Planned Parenthood Clinic, 561
Wetzell, Richard, 68
We'Wha, 134–135, *136*
Wheeler, Christine
   on Benjamin, 184
   Fraser relation to, 442
   Schaefer relation to, 272
Wheeler, Connie, 96
Wheelwright, Mary Cabot, 137
While, Cole, 64
Whisnant, Clayton J., 41, 62, 718
   on d'Eon, 62–64
   on nonprocreative sexual activities, 13
white empiricism, 307
Whitman-Walker, 560
Whitmore, Earl, 215–216
Whittle, Stephen, 408
   Green, J., relation to, 431
   HBIGDA relation to, 454, 455
   WPATH relation to, 441
"Who Stole Native American Studies?," 142
Wicker, Randy, 418
wigs, 697
   merkins, 705n77
Wilchins, Riki Anne, 354n85
Wilcox, Richard, 241
Wild West culture, 101
Wilhelm, Teri, 420
   on Green, J., 428
   on Keatley, 574
Wilkinson, Jemima, 100

Willard Insane Asylum, 288
Williams Institute, 460, 477, 722
Wilson, André, 456–457, 460, 693–694
Wilson, Avon, 167
Wise, P. M., 288
Wolf, Tom, 579
Wolf-Gould, Carolyn, 1, 3–4, 98, 295
  on Cauldwell, 292
  on civil rights, 397
  on Elbe, 91
  on gender-affirming surgery, 583
  on gender identity, 474
  on Hart, 620
  on Jorgensen, 202
  on medicalization, 299
  on Murray, P., 302
  on nonbinary gender identity, 722–723
  on religion, 295
  on Rivera, 420
  on Roberts, 203
  on Spengler, 93
  on Steinach, 504
  on stigma, 508
  on transgender medical research, 517
Wolf-Gould, Christopher, 93
Wolff, Samantha, 508–509
Wollman, Leo, 342
  EEF relation to, 345
  Green, R., relation to, 363–364
  speaking engagements of, 344
Woodson, Carter G., 206
Wordon, Frederic G., 219
World Association for Sexual Health, 437
World Health Organization, 261–262
  International Classification of Functioning of, 667
  WPATH relation to, 456, 463
World League for Sexual Reform, 51
World Professional Association for Transgender Health (WPATH), 197n108, 344, 347. See also *Standards of Care*
  Adler relation to, 667–668
  Benjamin relation to, 519
  ethics and, 545
  Fraser relation to, 442
  "Gender Confirmation Surgery" and, 603
  Graduate Student Initiative of, 464
  Green, J., relation to, 430–431, 547n8
  HBIGDA relation to, 440, 456
  Monstrey relation to, 602
  Rachlin relation to, 443–444
  Veritas Meeting Solutions relation to, 465
  Whittle relation to, 441
  World Health Organization relation to, 456, 463
World Transgender Conference, 165
World's Columbian Exposition, 136
Wounded Arrow, Jamie, 152
WPATH. *See* World Professional Association for Transgender Health

X-rays, 702n18
  for hair removal, 686–687
Xavier, Jessica, 462

Yale University, Pauli Murray and, 304
Yeats, William Butler, 506
Yoruba religion, 27

Die Zeitschrift für Sexualwissenschaft (journal), 50
Zhang, William, 693, 695
Zucker, Kenneth, 269, 275n59
  HBIGDA relation to, 452
  living-in-your-own-skin model and, 635–637